Point-of-Care Ultrasound

Point-of-Care Ultrasound

Second Edition

NILAM J. SONI, MD, MS
Professor of Medicine, Division of General & Hospital Medicine and Division of Pulmonary & Critical Care Medicine, University of Texas Health San Antonio, San Antonio, Texas

ROBERT ARNTFIELD, MD, FRCPC
Associate Professor of Medicine, Division of Emergency Medicine and Division of Critical Care Medicine, Schulich School of Medicine & Dentistry, Western University, London Health Sciences Centre, London, Ontario, Canada

PIERRE KORY, MD, MPA
Associate Professor of Medicine, Division of Allergy, Pulmonary, and Critical Care Medicine, University of Wisconsin School of Medicine and Public Health, Madison, Wisconsin

ELSEVIER

1600 John F. Kennedy Blvd.
Ste 1800
Philadelphia, PA 19103-2899

POINT-OF-CARE ULTRASOUND, SECOND EDITION

ISBN: 978-0-323-54470-2

Notices

Knowledge and best practice in this field are constantly changing. As new research and experience broaden our understanding, changes in research methods, professional practices, or medical treatment may become necessary.

Practitioners and researchers must always rely on their own experience and knowledge in evaluating and using any information, methods, compounds, or experiments described herein. In using such information or methods they should be mindful of their own safety and the safety of others, including parties for whom they have a professional responsibility.

With respect to any drug or pharmaceutical products identified, readers are advised to check the most current information provided (i) on procedures featured or (ii) by the manufacturer of each product to be administered, to verify the recommended dose or formula, the method and duration of administration, and contraindications. It is the responsibility of practitioners, relying on their own experience and knowledge of their patients, to make diagnoses, to determine dosages and the best treatment for each individual patient, and to take all appropriate safety precautions.

To the fullest extent of the law, neither the Publisher nor the authors, contributors, or editors, assume any liability for any injury and/or damage to persons or property as a matter of products liability, negligence or otherwise, or from any use or operation of any methods, products, instructions, or ideas contained in the material herein.

Previous edition copyrighted 2015 by Saunders, an imprint of Elsevier Inc.

Library of Congress Cataloging-in-Publication Control Number: 2019937376

Senior Content Strategist: Sarah Barth
Senior Content Development Manager: Lucia Gunzel
Publishing Services Manager: Shereen Jameel/Catherine Jackson
Project Manager: Nadhiya Sekar/Kristine Feeherty
Design Direction: Bridget Hoette

Printed in India

Last digit is the print number: 9   8   7

Working together
to grow libraries in
developing countries

www.elsevier.com • www.bookaid.org

Mohammed M. Abbasi, MD
Division of Pulmonary and Critical Care
Albert Einstein College of Medicine
Montefiore Medical Center
Bronx, New York

Sara Ahmadi, MD, ECNU
Assistant Professor of Medicine
Division of Endocrinology
Duke University Medical Center
Durham, North Carolina

Stephen Alerhand, MD
Assistant Professor
Department of Emergency Medicine
Rutgers New Jersey Medical School
Newark, New Jersey

Phillip Andrus, MD, FACEP
Assistant Professor of Emergency Medicine
Assistant Director of Emergency Ultrasound
Icahn School of Medicine at Mount Sinai
New York, New York

Shane Arishenkoff, MD, FRCPC
Assistant Clinical Professor
Division of General Internal Medicine
Department of Medicine
University of British Columbia
Vancouver, British Columbia, Canada

Robert Arntfield, MD, FRCPC
Associate Professor of Medicine
Division of Emergency Medicine and Division
  of Critical Care Medicine
Schulich School of Medicine & Dentistry
Western University
London Health Sciences Centre
London, Ontario, Canada

Uché Blackstock, MD
Assistant Professor
Co-Director of Emergency Ultrasound
  Fellowship
Department of Emergency Medicine
New York University School of Medicine
New York University Langone Health
New York, New York

Michel Boivin, MD
Professor of Medicine
Division of Pulmonary, Critical Care, and
  Sleep Medicine
Department of Medicine
University of New Mexico
Albuquerque, New Mexico

Brian M. Buchanan, BSc, MD, FRCPC
Assistant Professor of Critical Care Medicine
Department of Critical Care Medicine
University of Alberta
Edmonton, Alberta, Canada

Jose Cardenas-Garcia, MD
Assistant Professor of Medicine
Director of Interventional Pulmonology
Division of Pulmonary & Critical Care
  Medicine
Department of Medicine
University of Michigan
Ann Arbor, Michigan

Anita Cave, MD, FRCPC
Assistant Professor
Department of Anesthesia and Perioperative
  Medicine
Schulich School of Medicine & Dentistry
Western University
London Health Sciences Centre
London, Ontario, Canada

Alfred B. Cheng, MD
Assistant Professor of Emergency Medicine
Director of the Division of Emergency
  Medicine Ultrasound
Department of Emergency Medicine
Cooper Medical School of Rowan University
Camden, New Jersey

Gregg L. Chesney, MD
Assistant Professor of Emergency Medicine
Department of Emergency Medicine and
  Division of Pulmonary, Critical Care, and
  Sleep Medicine
New York University School of Medicine
New York University Langone Health/
  Brooklyn Medical Center
New York, New York

Alan T. Chiem, MD, MPH
Associate Clinical Professor
Director of Emergency Ultrasound
Department of Emergency Medicine
University of California Los Angeles
Olive View–UCLA Medical Center
Los Angeles, California

Thomas W. Conlon, MD
Assistant Professor of Pediatrics
Department of Anesthesiology and Critical
  Care Medicine
Perelman School of Medicine at the University
  of Pennsylvania
Children's Hospital of Philadelphia
Philadelphia, Pennsylvania

Sara Crager, MD
Assistant Clinical Professor
Division of Critical Care
Departments of Anesthesia and Emergency
  Medicine
University of California Los Angeles
Los Angeles, California

Ria Dancel, MD, FHM, FAAP, FACP
Associate Professor of Medicine and Pediatrics
Director of Medicine Procedure Service
Division of Hospital Medicine
Departments of Medicine and Pediatrics
University of North Carolina
Chapel Hill, North Carolina

Christopher Dayton, MD
Clinical Assistant Professor
Division of Pulmonary & Critical Care
  Medicine
Departments of Medicine and Emergency
  Medicine
University of Texas Health San Antonio
San Antonio, Texas

Eitan Dickman, MD, MMM, FACEP, FAIUM
Executive Vice Chairman and Medical
  Director
Department of Emergency Medicine
Maimonides Medical Center
New York, New York

Maili Drachman, MD
Assistant Professor
Department of Emergency Medicine
University of Arizona Health Sciences
Tucson, Arizona

John Eicken, MD, Ed.M.
Clinical Assistant Professor
Division of Emergency Ultrasound
Department of Emergency Medicine
University of South Carolina School of
  Medicine Greenville
Greenville Health System
Greenville, South Carolina

Lewis A. Eisen, MD
Professor of Medicine
Division of Critical Care Medicine
Albert Einstein College of Medicine
Montefiore Medical Center
New York, New York

James F. Fair III, MD, FASE, FACEP
Assistant Professor of Emergency Medicine
Division of Emergency Medicine
Department of Surgery
University of Utah Health Sciences Center
Salt Lake City, Utah

Daniel Fein, MD
Assistant Professor of Medicine
Division of Pulmonary Medicine
Department of Medicine
Albert Einstein School of Medicine
Montefiore Medical Center
Bronx, New York

Stephanie Fish, MD
Associate Professor of Medicine
Division of Endocrinology
Department of Medicine
Memorial Sloan Kettering Cancer Center
New York, New York

John Christian Fox, MD
Professor of Emergency Medicine
Interim Chair of the Department of
  Emergency Medicine
University of California Irvine
Orange, California

María V. Fraga, MD
Associate Professor of Clinical Pediatrics
Division of Neonatology
Department of Pediatrics
Perelman School of Medicine at the University
  of Pennsylvania
Children's Hospital of Philadelphia
Philadelphia, Pennsylvania

Ricardo Franco-Sadud, MD
Associate Professor of Medicine
Director of Academic Hospital Medicine and
  Point of Care Ultrasound
University of Central Florida College of
  Medicine
Naples Community Hospital
Naples, Florida

Kelly S. Gibson, MD
Assistant Professor
Department of Obstetrics/Gynecology-
  Maternal Fetal Medicine
Case Western Reserve University School of
  Medicine
University Hospitals Cleveland Medical
  Center
Cleveland, Ohio

Laura K. Gonzalez, MD, FAAP
Attending Physician
Division of Emergency Ultrasound
Department of Emergency Medicine
Maimonides Medical Center
New York, New York

Ben Goodgame, MD, RDMS
Attending Physician
Critical Care Medicine
Centennial Medical Center
Nashville, Tennessee

Behzad Hassani, MD, CCFP (EM)
Assistant Professor
Division of Emergency Medicine
Schulich School of Medicine & Dentistry
Western University
London Health Sciences Centre
London, Ontario, Canada

Ahmed F. Hegazy, MB BCh, MPH, FRCPC
Assistant Professor
Division of Critical Care Medicine
Department of Anesthesia and Perioperative
  Medicine
Schulich School of Medicine & Dentistry
Western University
London Health Sciences Centre
London, Ontario, Canada

Patricia C. Henwood, MD
Assistant Professor of Emergency Medicine
Associate Chief of the Division of Emergency
  Ultrasound
Department of Emergency Medicine
Harvard Medical School
Brigham and Women's Hospital
Boston, Massachusetts

Hailey Hobbs, MD, FRCPC
Assistant Professor of Medicine
Department of Critical Care
Queen's University
Kingston, Ontario, Canada

J. Terrill Huggins, MD
Professor of Medicine
Division of Pulmonary, Critical Care, Allergy,
  and Sleep Medicine
Medical University of South Carolina
Charleston, South Carolina

Sahar Janjua, MBBS
Attending Physician
Division of Rheumatology
Department of Medicine
Frisbie Memorial Hospital
Rochester, New Hampshire

Maykol Postigo Jasahui, MD
Assistant Professor of Medicine
Interventional Pulmonary Medicine
Division of Pulmonary/Critical Care
University of Kansas Medical Center
Kansas City, Kansas

Robert Jones, DO, FACEP
Professor of Emergency Medicine
Director of Emergency Ultrasound
Department of Emergency Medicine
Case Western Reserve Medical School
MetroHealth Medical Center
Cleveland, Ohio

David O. Kessler, MD, MSc, RDMS/APCA
Assistant Professor of Pediatrics
Department of Pediatrics
Columbia University College of Physicians
  and Surgeons
New York Presbyterian–Morgan Stanley
  Children's Hospital
New York, New York

Chan Kim, MD
Instructor of Rheumatology
Division of Rheumatology
Boston University School of Medicine
Boston, Massachusetts

Jae H. Kim, MD, PhD
Professor of Clinical Pediatrics
Divisions of Neonatology & Pediatric
  Gastroenterology, Hepatology and Nutrition
University of California San Diego
Children's Hospital of San Diego
La Jolla, California

Eugene Kissin, MD
Associate Professor of Medicine
Program Director of Rheumatology Fellowship
Division of Rheumatology
Boston University School of Medicine
Boston, Massachusetts

Starr Knight, MD
Associate Clinical Professor of Emergency
  Medicine
Co-Director of Emergency Ultrasound
  Fellowship
Department of Emergency Medicine
University of California San Francisco School
  of Medicine
San Francisco, California

Pierre Kory, MD, MPA
Associate Professor of Medicine
Division of Allergy, Pulmonary, and Critical
  Care Medicine
University of Wisconsin School of Medicine
  and Public Health
Madison, Wisconsin

Daniel Lakoff, MD, FACEP
Assistant Professor of Clinical Emergency
  Medicine
Department of Emergency Medicine
Weill Cornell Medical College
New York, New York

Viera Lakticova, MD
Assistant Professor of Medicine
Director of Bronchoscopy and Interventional
  Pulmonology
Division of Pulmonary, Critical Care, and
  Sleep Medicine
Long Island Jewish Medical Center and North
  Shore University Hospital
Donald and Barbara Zucker School of
  Medicine at Hofstra/Northwell
Hempstead, New York

Elizabeth Lalande, MD, FRCP
Department of Emergency Medicine
Centre Hospitalier de l'Université Laval
  (CHUL) de Québec
Université Laval
Quebec City, Quebec, Canada

Justin R. Lappen, MD
Assistant Professor
Department of Reproductive Biology
Case Western Reserve University School of
  Medicine
University Hospitals Cleveland Medical
  Center
Cleveland, Ohio

Vincent I. Lau, MD, FRCPC
Adjunct Professor
Division of Critical Care Medicine
Schulich School of Medicine & Dentistry
Western University
London, Ontario, Canada

Alycia Paige Lee, BS, RDCS, RVT
Liberty University College of Osteopathic
  Medicine
Lynchburg, Virginia

Peter M. Lee, MD
Assistant Professor of Medicine
Director of Interventional Pulmonology &
  Lung Cancer Screening
Division of Pulmonary & Critical Care
Hunter-Holmes McGuire Veterans Affairs
  Medical Center
Virginia Commonwealth University
Richmond, Virginia

W. Robert Leeper, MD, MEd, FRCSC, FACS
Assistant Professor of Surgery
Trauma, and Critical Care Medicine
Division of General Surgery
Department of Surgery
Schulich School of Medicine & Dentistry
Western University
Victoria Hospital
London Health Sciences Centre
London, Ontario, Canada

Shankar LeVine, MD
Department of Emergency Medicine
Alameda Health System
Highland General Hospital
Oakland, California

Ken E. Lyn-Kew, MD
Associate Professor of Medicine
Section Head of Critical Care Medicine
Division of Pulmonary, Critical Care, and
  Sleep Medicine
University of Colorado
National Jewish Health
Denver, Colorado

Irene Ma, MD, PhD, FRCPC, FACP, RDMS, RDCS
Associate Professor of Medicine
Division of General Internal Medicine
Cumming School of Medicine
University of Calgary
Calgary, Alberta, Canada

Haney Mallemat, MD, MS
Associate Professor of Emergency and Internal
  Medicine
Departments of Emergency Medicine and
  Critical Care Medicine
Cooper Medical School at Rowan University
Camden, New Jersey

Daniel Mantuani, MD, MPH
Department of Emergency Medicine
Alameda Health System
Highland General Hospital
Oakland, California

Michael Mayette, MD, FRCPC
Associate Professor of Medicine
Division of Critical Care Medicine
Department of Medicine
Université de Sherbrooke
Sherbrooke, Québec, Canada

Paul Mayo, MD
Professor of Clinical Medicine
Academic Director of Critical Care
Division of Pulmonary, Critical Care, and
  Sleep Medicine
Long Island Jewish Medical Center and North
  Shore University Hospital
Donald and Barbara Zucker School of
  Medicine at Hofstra/Northwell
Hempstead, New York

Paul G. McHardy, MD, FRCPC
Assistant Professor of Anesthesia
Department of Anesthesia
University of Toronto
Sunnybrook Health Sciences Centre
Toronto, Ontario, Canada

Scott Millington, MD, FRCPC
Associate Professor of Medicine
Department of Critical Care Medicine
University of Ottawa and the Ottawa Hospital
Ottawa, Ontario, Canada

Paul K. Mohabir, MD
Clinical Professor of Medicine
Director of Critical Care Medicine Fellowship
Director of Adult Cystic Fibrosis Program
Division of Pulmonary and Critical Care
  Medicine
Stanford University School of Medicine
Stanford, California

Patrick Murphy, MD, MPH, MSc, FRCSC
Division of General Surgery
Department of Surgery
Schulich School of Medicine and Dentistry
Western University
London, Ontario, Canada

Arun Nagdev, MD
Director of Emergency Ultrasound
Alameda Health System
Highland General Hospital
Oakland, California

Mangala Narasimhan, DO, FCCP
Professor of Clinical Medicine
Regional Director of Critical Care Medicine
Northwell Health
Donald and Barbara Zucker School of
  Medicine at Hofstra/Northwell
Hempstead, New York

Bret P. Nelson, MD, FACEP
Professor of Emergency Medicine
Chief of the Division of Emergency
  Ultrasound
Department of Emergency Medicine
Icahn School of Medicine at Mount Sinai
New York, New York

Vicki E. Noble, MD
Professor of Emergency Medicine
Vice Chairman of Academic Affairs
Program Director of Emergency Medicine
Case Western Reserve School of Medicine
University Hospitals Cleveland Medical
  Center
Cleveland, Ohio

Paru Patrawalla, MD
Assistant Professor of Medicine
Program Director of Pulmonary/Critical Care
  Fellowship
Division of Pulmonary, Critical Care, and
  Sleep Medicine
Icahn School of Medicine at Mount Sinai
New York, New York

Daniel R. Peterson, MD, PhD, FRCPC, RDMS
Clinical Assistant Professor
Academic Department of Emergency Medicine
University of Calgary
Foothills Medical Centre
Calgary, Alberta, Canada

Nitin Puri, MD, FCCP
Associate Professor of Medicine
Program Director of Critical Care Medicine
  Fellowship
Interim Division Head of Critical Care
  Medicine
Cooper Medical School of Rowan University
Camden, New Jersey

Xian Qiao, MD
Division of Pulmonary and Critical Care
  Medicine
Virginia Commonwealth University Health
  System
Richmond, Virginia

Aviral Roy, MD
Consultant
Critical Care Medicine and Internal Medicine
Medical Institute of Critical Care
Medica Superspecialty Hospital
Kolkata, India

Lewis Satterwhite, MD, FCCP
Associate Professor of Medicine
Division of Pulmonary, Critical Care, and
  Sleep Medicine
University of Kansas School of Medicine
Kansas City, Kansas

Daniel J. Schnobrich, MD, FACP
Assistant Professor of Medicine
Divisions of General Internal Medicine and
  Hospital Pediatrics
University of Minnesota School of Medicine
Minneapolis, Minnesota

Shideh Shafie, MD
Assistant Professor of Emergency Medicine
Department of Emergency Medicine
Brown University
Providence, Rhode Island

Ariel L. Shiloh, MD
Associate Professor of Medicine and
  Neurology
Division of Critical Care Medicine
Departments of Medicine and Neurology
Albert Einstein College of Medicine
Montefiore Medical Center
Bronx, New York

Craig Sisson, MD, RDMS
Clinical Associate Professor
Chief of the Division of Emergency
  Ultrasound
Department of Emergency Medicine
University of Texas Health San Antonio
San Antonio, Texas

Jessica Solis-McCarthy, MD
Assistant Clinical Professor
Assistant Director of Ultrasound Education
Department of Emergency Medicine
University of Texas Health San Antonio
San Antonio, Texas

Nilam J. Soni, MD, MS
Professor of Medicine
Division of General & Hospital Medicine
  and Division of Pulmonary & Critical Care
  Medicine
University of Texas Health San Antonio
San Antonio, Texas

Kirk T. Spencer, MD, FASE
Professor of Medicine
Section of Cardiology
Department of Medicine
University of Chicago-Pritzker School of
Medicine
Chicago, Illinois

Erik Su, MD
Division of Pediatric Cardiology
Department of Pediatrics
Stanford University School of Medicine
Palo Alto, California

Christopher R. Tainter, MD, RDMS
Clinical Associate Professor
Division of Critical Care
Departments of Anesthesiology and
Emergency Medicine
University of California San Diego School of
Medicine
San Diego, California

Nathan Teismann, MD
Associate Clinical Professor
Department of Emergency Medicine
University of California San Francisco School
of Medicine
San Francisco, California

Felipe Teran, MD, MSCE
Clinical Instructor
Division of Emergency Ultrasound and
Center for Resuscitation Science
Department of Emergency Medicine
University of Pennsylvania
Hospital of the University of Pennsylvania
Philadelphia, Pennsylvania

David M. Tierney, MD, FACP
Program Director of Internal Medicine
Residency
Department of Medical Education
Abbott Northwestern Hospital
Minneapolis, Minnesota

Matthew D. Tyler, MD, RDMS
Division of Critical Care Medicine
Department of Emergency Medicine
Advocate Christ Medical Center
Oak Lawn, Illinois

Marsia Vermeulen, DO, RDMS, RDCS, FACEP
Assistant Professor of Emergency Medicine
Department of Emergency Medicine
New York University School of Medicine
New York University Langone Health/
Bellevue Hospital Center
New York, New York

Stephen D. Walsh, MD, FRCPC
Departments of Critical Care Medicine and
General Internal Medicine
Dalhousie University
Halifax, Nova Scotia, Canada

Gabriel Wardi, MD, MPH
Clinical Assistant Professor
Division of Pulmonary, Critical Care, and
Sleep Medicine
Department of Emergency Medicine
University of California San Diego School of
Medicine
San Diego, California

Michael Y. Woo, MD
Associate Professor
Program Director of Emergency Medicine
Ultrasound Fellowship
Department of Emergency Medicine
University of Ottawa and Ottawa Hospital
Research Institute
Ottawa, Ontario, Canada

Gulrukh Zaidi, MD, FCCP
Assistant Professor of Medicine
Division of Pulmonary, Critical Care and
Sleep Medicine
Long Island Jewish Medical Center and North
Shore University Hospital
Donald and Barbara Zucker School of
Medicine at Hofstra/Northwell
Hempstead, New York

This book is dedicated to all the compassionate and hardworking clinicians who stay at the bedside to provide the best possible care to their patients.

To my colleagues, whose passion for ultrasound invigorates me.

To my patients, whose journeys have taught me more than medicine.

To my family, whose limitless support, sacrifices, and love make it all possible.

NS

With gratitude to my family, my mentors, and my patients.

RA

To my angels, Amy, Ella, Eve, and Violet, along with my dear parents, Leslie and Odile, for their unwavering patience, support, and love.

PK

Point-of-care ultrasound (POCUS) has been shown to make procedures safer, expedite and increase the accuracy of diagnoses, and raise confidence in clinical decision-making. POCUS is one of few new technologies that brings providers closer to patients, putting them right at the bedside, enriching the experience for patients and providers alike.

The first edition of *Point-of-Care Ultrasound* was published in 2014 and established a foundation for sharing knowledge across multiple specialties that utilize varied bedside ultrasound applications. Since its initial publication, the book has been translated into Chinese and Spanish, with thousands of copies distributed worldwide. As more providers have learned *what* POCUS is, they have turned to this book to learn *how* to use POCUS. Given the visual and dynamic nature of ultrasonography, this book provides a rich experience with its online video-based version. Its handbook style, concise chapters, high-yield figures, and practical teaching points are attractive to busy clinicians seeking to improve their knowledge of ultrasound.

In this second edition, we expanded the content in multiple ways. First, we added six new chapters on hemodynamics, transesophageal echocardiography, second and third trimester pregnancy, pediatrics, neonatology, and transcranial ultrasound. Second, we increased the online video content from approximately 300 to over 1000 videos demonstrating normal and pathologic ultrasound findings. Third, we added new clinical cases and review questions at the end of each chapter emphasizing the key learning points of each chapter. Finally, we kept pace with this rapidly evolving field by updating the literature, images, and figures in every chapter.

Covered in detail are the principles and broad applications of POCUS that are most generalizable to health care providers from any discipline or practice setting. We are confident that the diverse interests of health care providers interested in learning POCUS will be met through this second edition of our book.

Nilam J. Soni
Robert Arntfield
Pierre Kory

ACKNOWLEDGMENTS

For contributing ultrasound images:

Atul Jaidka, MD (Lead Contributor)
Department of Medicine
Western University
London Health Sciences Centre
London, Ontario, Canada

Jeremy Boyd, MD
Assistant Professor
Department of Emergency Medicine
Vanderbilt University
Nashville, Tennessee

Arben Brahaj, MD, RMSK
Assistant Clinical Professor
Department of Orthopedics and
  Rehabilitation
Yale School of Medicine
VA Connecticut Healthcare System
West Haven, Connecticut

John P. Corcoran, BM BCh, MRCP
Oxford Centre for Respiratory Medicine
Oxford University Hospitals NHS Trust
Oxford, United Kingdom

Janeve Desy, MD, FRCPC
Assistant Professor
Division of General Internal Medicine
University of Calgary
Calgary, Alberta, Canada

Danny Duque, MD, RDMS, FACEP
Assistant Professor
Department of Emergency Medicine
Elmhurst Hospital Center
New York, New York

Laleh Gharahbaghian, MD
Clinical Associate Professor
Department of Emergency Medicine
Stanford University Medical Center
Stanford, California

Horiana Grosu, MD
Assistant Professor
Department of Pulmonary Medicine
The University of Texas MD Anderson
  Cancer Center
Houston, Texas

Jennifer Huang, DO, FACEP
Assistant Professor
Department of Emergency Medicine
Icahn School of Medicine at Mount Sinai
New York, New York

Christian B. Laursen, MD, PhD
Associate Professor
Institute of Clinical Research
University of Southern Denmark
Odense, Denmark

Alycia Paige Lee, BS, RDCS, RVT
Liberty University College of Osteopathic
  Medicine
Lynchburg, Virginia

Roya Etemad Rezai, MD, FRCPC
Associate Professor
Department of Diagnostic Radiology and
  Nuclear Medicine
Western University
London Health Sciences Centre
London, Ontario, Canada

Rebecca Riggs, MD
Assistant Professor
Department of Pediatric Anesthesiology and
  Critical Care Medicine
Johns Hopkins University
Baltimore, Maryland

Christopher Schott, MD, MS
Assistant Professor
Department of Critical Care Medicine
University of Pittsburgh
Pittsburgh, Pennsylvania

Allen Shefrin, MD, FRCPC
Assistant Professor
Department of Pediatrics
University of Ottawa
Children's Hospital of Eastern Ontario
Ottawa, Ontario, Canada

Jason Stoller, MD
Associate Professor
Division of Neonatology
Perelman School of Medicine at the University
  of Pennsylvania Medical School
Philadelphia, Pennsylvania

Ee Tay, MD, FAAP
Assistant Professor
Department of Emergency Medicine and
 Pediatrics
Icahn School of Medicine at Mount Sinai
New York, New York

Drew Thompson, MD, FRCPC
Associate Professor
Department of Emergency Medicine
Western University
London Health Sciences Centre
London, Ontario, Canada

Brita E. Zaia, MD, FACEP
Director, Emergency Ultrasound
Department of Emergency Medicine
Kaiser San Francisco Medical Center
San Francisco, California

For serving as reviewers:

Jason Filopei, MD
Assistant Professor of Medicine
Division of Pulmonary, Critical Care, and
 Sleep Medicine
Department of Medicine
Icahn School of Medicine at Mount Sinai
New York, New York

Elizabeth K. Haro, MPH
Division of Pulmonary & Critical Care
 Medicine
Department of Medicine
University of Texas Health San Antonio
San Antonio, Texas

Robert Nathanson, MD, FACP
Assistant Professor
Division of General & Hospital Medicine
Department of Medicine
University of Texas Health San Antonio
New York, New York

Kevin Proud, MD, FCCP
Assistant Professor of Medicine
Division of Pulmonary Diseases & Critical
 Care Medicine
Department of Medicine
University of Texas Health San Antonio
San Antonio, Texas

Katie Wiskar, MD, FRCPC
Division of General Internal Medicine
Department of Medicine
University of British Columbia
Vancouver, British Columbia, Canada

For developing original illustrations and photography:

Victoria Heim, CMI
Medical Illustrator
Loganville, Georgia

Jordan Hill, BA
Health and Fitness Consultant
P&G Professional
San Antonio, Texas

Jade Myers
Graphic Designer
Matrix Art Services
York, Pennsylvania

Sam Newman
3D Medical Animator
University of Texas Health San Antonio
San Antonio, Texas

Lester Rosebrock
Photographer
Lester Multimedia
San Antonio, Texas

For serving as a mentor and educator:

Paul H. Mayo, MD
Professor of Clinical Medicine
Academic Director of Critical Care
Division of Pulmonary, Critical Care, and
 Sleep Medicine
Long Island Jewish Medical Center and North
 Shore University Hospital
Donald and Barbara Zucker School of
 Medicine at Hofstra/Northwell
Hempstead, New York

CONTENTS

Fundamental Principles of Ultrasound

CHAPTER 1

Evolution of Point-of-Care Ultrasound

Nilam J. Soni ■ Robert Arntfield ■ Pierre Kory

KEY POINTS

- Point-of-care ultrasound is defined as a goal-directed, bedside ultrasound examination performed by a health care provider to answer a specific diagnostic question or to guide the performance of an invasive procedure.
- Diagnostic ultrasound was first developed and used in medicine during the 1940s, but point-of-care ultrasound has been integrated into diverse areas of clinical practice since the early 1980s.
- Important considerations when using point-of-care ultrasound include provider training and skill level, patient characteristics, and ultrasound equipment features.

Background

Point-of-care ultrasound has revolutionized the practice of medicine, influencing how care is provided in nearly every medical and surgical specialty. For more than a century, clinicians had been limited to primitive bedside tools, such as the reflex hammer (c. 1888) and stethoscope (c. 1816), but with bedside ultrasound, providers are equipped with a tool that allows them to actually see what they can only infer through palpation or auscultation. The technologic miniaturization of ultrasound devices has outpaced integration of these devices into clinical practice. Many specialty professional societies, patient safety organizations, and national health care agencies have recognized the potent benefits of point-of-care ultrasound and have endorsed its routine use in clinical practice. In 2001 the American Medical Association stated, "Ultrasound has diverse applications and is used by a wide range of physicians and disciplines. Ultrasound imaging is within the scope of practice of appropriately trained physicians."[1] Thus it has been well recognized for nearly 2 decades that providers from diverse specialties can be trained in the use of ultrasound relevant to their specialty. This chapter reviews the major milestones in the history of medical ultrasound, with a focus on important considerations for point-of-care ultrasound.

History

Acoustic properties of sound were well described by ancient Greek and Roman civilizations. In the 20th century, the sinking of the *Titanic* followed by the start of World War I served as catalysts for the development of sonar, or sound navigation and ranging, which was the first real-world application of the principles of sound.[2,3]

Although several physicians were simultaneously competing to be the first to use ultrasound in medicine, Karl Theodore Dussik, an Austrian psychiatrist and neurologist, is credited as being the first physician to use ultrasound in medical diagnostics when he attempted to visualize cerebral ventricles and brain tumors using a primitive ultrasound device in 1942 (Fig. 1.1).

During the 1940s and 1950s, many pioneers advanced the field of medical ultrasound. John Julian Wild described various clinical applications of ultrasound, including the difference in appearance of normal and cancerous tissues. Douglass Howry and Joseph Holmes focused on ultrasound equipment technology. They built immersion-tank ultrasound systems, including the "somascope" in 1954 (Fig. 1.2), and they published the first two-dimensional ultrasound images. Ian Donald contributed significant amounts of research to obstetric and gynecologic ultrasonography. Inge Edler and Carl Hellmuth Hertz investigated cardiac ultrasound and established the field of echocardiography in the early 1950s. Shigeo Satomura, a Japanese physicist isolated from the pioneers in the United States and Europe, is credited as being the first physician to use Doppler ultrasound in his studies of cardiac valve motion.[3]

Advancements in ultrasound technology accelerated the field in the 1960s and 1970s. Early ultrasound machines used open-shutter photography to capture screen images. Multiple still images of moving structures were captured, sequentially displayed, and interpreted by imagining the structures in motion. In 1965, Siemens released the Vidoson, the first real-time ultrasound scanner that could display 15 images per second. The Vidoson was quickly incorporated into obstetric care over the next decade and became a standard component of assessing pregnant women. Sector scanning became possible with development of phased-array transducers in the early 1970s, giving rise to echocardiography as an independent field.[3]

Ultrasound technology continued to advance during the 1970s and 1980s with the development of more sophisticated transducers, along with refinements in image quality. Following the early adopters of ultrasound, namely radiology, cardiology, and obstetrics/gynecology, ultrasound began to be used in emergency care, a role that marked the beginning of the era of point-of-care ultrasound.[3] For the first time, life-threatening conditions could be diagnosed rapidly at the bedside with

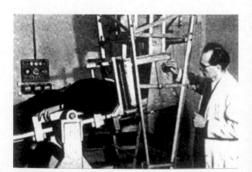

Figure 1.1   Karl Theodore Dussik and the First Medical Ultrasound Device in 1946. (From Frentzel-Beyme B. Vom Echolot zur Farbdopplersonographie. *Der Radiologe.* 2005;45(4):363–370.)

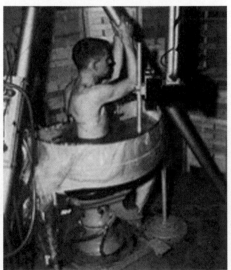

Figure 1.2   Immersion-Tank Ultrasound Machine From the 1950s. (From Hagen-Ansert SL. *Textbook of Diagnostic Sonography.* 7th ed. St Louis: Mosby; 2011.)

portable ultrasound. Frontline physicians, mostly surgeons and emergency medicine physicians, started assessing trauma patients with ultrasound in the 1970s, and the term FAST exam, or Focused Assessment with Sonography in Trauma, was coined in the early 1990s.[4-6] The FAST exam was incorporated into Advanced Trauma Life Support (ATLS) guidelines in the late 1990s.[7,8] From its early description in the 1970s in Europe to its incorporation into ATLS guidelines in the 1990s in the United States, the FAST exam established a precedent for defining point-of-care ultrasound applications and incorporating these applications into routine clinical practice.

Since the 1990s, point-of-care ultrasound has been integrated into nearly every specialty's practice. In addition to defining specific point-of-care ultrasound applications in the 1990s, such as the FAST exam, general medical ultrasound applications, broadly applicable to many specialties, started to emerge. In the 1980s, ultrasound artifacts of the lung—an organ long felt to have little utility in ultrasound diagnostics—began to be described. Correlation of lung ultrasound artifacts with discrete lung pathologies was codified by Daniel Lichtenstein, a French critical care physician. His work gave rise to the field of lung ultrasonography.[9] Even though lung ultrasound was first used by intensivists to evaluate critically ill patients, lung ultrasound is broadly applicable to any patient with pulmonary symptoms, is more accurate than chest x-ray, and can be used by any health care provider with appropriate training.[10]

Another broad application that emerged was the use of ultrasound to guide invasive bedside procedures. Multiple studies since the 1990s have demonstrated reduced mechanical complications and increased procedure success rates when ultrasound is used to guide bedside procedures, in particular the insertion of central venous catheters.[11,12] Current guidelines from multiple professional societies and patient safety organizations recommend that all providers use ultrasound guidance when placing internal jugular central venous catheters.

Ultrasound technology was well advanced by the 2000s, when three-dimensional ultrasound emerged for select diagnostic applications; however, use of two-dimensional ultrasound has remained the standard of care for the majority of indications. The most important change during the 2000s was continued reduction in

the size and price of ultrasound machines. The increased portability and affordability of ultrasound devices led to an exponential increase in the use of ultrasound by providers from different specialties. Subsequently, many professional societies published practice guidelines on use of point-of-care ultrasound, including the American Institute of Ultrasound in Medicine (AIUM), American College of Emergency Physicians (ACEP), American College of Chest Physicians (ACCP), and American Society of Echocardiography (ASE). Furthermore, consensus guidelines between imaging and specialty societies have been established, such as the guidelines on obstetrical ultrasound collaboratively developed by the American College of Radiology (ACR), American College of Obstetricians and Gynecologists (ACOG), AIUM, and Society of Radiologists in Ultrasound (SRU). Another consensus guideline between two societies is the ACEP–ASE statement on focused cardiac ultrasound in the emergent setting.[13,14] Specialty-specific guidelines also emerged, such as the American Association of Clinical Endocrinologists guidelines on thyroid ultrasound that defined a pathway for endocrinologists to earn a certificate of competency in thyroid and neck ultrasound.[15]

Medical educators recognized the importance of teaching basics of ultrasound in the early 2000s and began to explore how to incorporate ultrasound training into curricula for medical students, residents, and fellows. The Accreditation Council for Graduate Medical Education (ACGME) began to mandate certain residencies and fellowships in the United States include basic ultrasound education; for example, pulmonary/critical care fellowships are now required to include training in general critical care ultrasound, ultrasound-guided thoracentesis, and ultrasound-guided central venous catheterization. Many medical schools worldwide have started to expose their students to the principles and practice of ultrasound, most often in conjunction with anatomy and physical examination courses.[16-19] The coming generation of physicians will thus be more adept at point-of-care ultrasound applications and will consider use of ultrasound to be routine in most clinical encounters. Whereas past generations' contributions established the utility of ultrasound as a valuable bedside tool in diagnostics and procedures, the next generation will advance the field by studying how point-of-care ultrasound can be best incorporated into

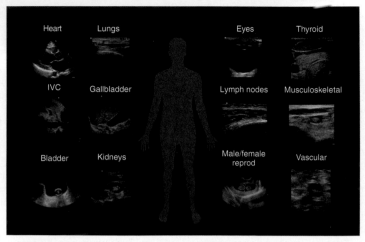

Figure 1.3   Common Diagnostic Applications of Point-of-Care Ultrasound. *IVC,* Inferior vena cava.

patient care algorithms and its effect on health care outcomes, cost-effectiveness, and patient experience.

Key Considerations

Point-of-care ultrasound exams differ from comprehensive ultrasound exams in several aspects. Point-of-care ultrasound is most often used to detect acute, potentially life-threatening conditions, where detection at the bedside expedites patient care. Point-of-care ultrasound exams are dedicated exams of a single or few organs to answer specific clinical questions at the bedside. In contrast, comprehensive ultrasound exams thoroughly evaluate an entire anatomical region related to an organ or organ system. The workflow of ordering, performing, interpreting, and reporting such comprehensive ultrasound exams usually takes hours, whereas acquisition and interpretation of point-of-care ultrasound exams takes minutes, providing real-time clinical information to guide decision-making.[20]

Key considerations to improve the efficiency and quality of point-of-care ultrasound examinations include optimization of provider training, patient factors, and ultrasound equipment features.

CLINICAL APPLICATIONS

A point-of-care ultrasound exam is aimed at answering a specific clinical question through a focused, goal-directed evaluation and can be used to evaluate most organ systems (Fig. 1.3). Generally the goal is to "rule in" or "rule out" a specific condition or answer a "yes/no" question. Clinical applications can be categorized as follows:

- *Procedural guidance:* Ultrasound guidance has been shown to reduce complications and improve success rates of invasive bedside procedures. Procedures commonly performed with ultrasound guidance include vascular access, thoracentesis, paracentesis, lumbar puncture, arthrocentesis, and pericardiocentesis.
- *Diagnostics:* Based on the patient's presenting signs and symptoms, an ultrasound exam can narrow the differential diagnosis and guide treatment, or additional investigations, especially in urgent or emergent situations. Focused ultrasound exams are commonly performed to evaluate the lungs, heart, gallbladder, aorta, kidneys, bladder, gravid uterus, joints, and lower-extremity veins (Fig. 1.3).
- *Monitoring:* Serial ultrasound exams can be performed to monitor a patient's condition or to monitor the effects of a therapeutic intervention without exposing patients to ionizing radiation or intravenous contrast. Common applications include monitoring inferior vena cava distention and collapsibility during fluid resuscitation, monitoring left ventricular contraction in response to inotrope initiation, and monitoring for

resolution or worsening of a pneumothorax or pneumonia on lung ultrasound.

- *Resuscitation:* Use of ultrasound during resuscitation for cardiac arrest is a unique but underutilized application. Bedside ultrasound can direct emergent interventions by rapidly assessing for a pneumothorax, cardiac tamponade, or massive pulmonary embolism. In addition, ultrasound can be used to assess cardiac activity to help guide prognosis in cardiac arrest. Visualization of cardiac standstill or clotting within the heart chambers allows providers to stop futile interventions, whereas visualization of subtle or weak cardiac contractions typically justifies the continuation of resuscitative efforts.

- *Screening:* Screening with ultrasound is potentially advantageous because it is noninvasive and avoids ionizing radiation. Although screening for abdominal aortic aneurysm or asymptomatic left ventricular function using point-of-care ultrasound has been described, more widespread screening applications have been slow to develop due to the challenge of weighing benefits of early detection against the harms of false-positive findings that can lead to unnecessary testing or procedures.[21-23]

PROVIDER TRAINING

The amount of training required to achieve competency in point-of-care ultrasound applications varies by provider skill acquisition and ultrasound exam complexity. Prior experience with ultrasound greatly facilitates learning new applications. The training required to achieve competency in the use point-of-care ultrasound will vary based on the provider's scope of practice; for example, a rheumatologist may be proficient with musculoskeletal ultrasound but less proficient with cardiac or abdominal ultrasound, whereas the opposite may be true for a critical care physician. Protocols from published studies on ultrasound education have differed, but it is generally accepted that training must include hands-on image acquisition and interpretation practice, supplemented by focused didactics. Current studies have provided general guidance on the average number of practice exams needed to acquire the skills to perform specific types of exams; for example, novice users have been able to achieve an "acceptable" skill level in focused cardiac ultrasound after performing 20 to 30 limited cardiac examinations.[24] Although a minimum number of exams will likely continue to be required for certain certifications, future generations will focus on competency-based education, with competency determined by achievement of certain milestones rather than completion of a predetermined number of exams.

PATIENT FACTORS

Body habitus, positioning, and acute illness are important considerations when imaging patients. Similar to plain film radiography, ultrasound waves are attenuated by adipose tissue, and ultrasound has limited penetration in morbidly obese patients. Lower frequencies must be used for deeper penetration, resulting in lower-resolution images. Positioning can limit ultrasound examination; for example, acquisition of apical cardiac ultrasound images is often limited in patients who cannot be placed in a left lateral decubitus position. Similarly, providers often have to adjust their own position to evaluate pleural effusions and perform thoracentesis when patients are unable to sit upright. On the contrary, ascites and pleural effusions improve visualization of deep organs due to propagation of sound waves in fluid.

ULTRASOUND EQUIPMENT

Early adopters of point-of-care ultrasound were often faced with using large, full-platform ultrasound machines, where lack of familiarity with the features and controls presented a barrier to use. Fortunately, a wide variety of portable ultrasound machines designed specifically for point-of-care use with ease-of-use as a priority are now available. These machines range from pocket-sized devices to laptop-style machines. Most recently, a surge of handheld and pocket-sized devices has entered the marketplace and are being purchased by individuals as personal devices. Thus, availability of ultrasound machines, the most commonly reported barrier to use of point-of-care ultrasound, is a problem that may soon be solved.[25,26]

The diminution in size of portable ultrasound machines comes with certain limitations: small screen size, limited transducer selection, few imaging modes, and few adjustable parameters to optimize the image. However, new

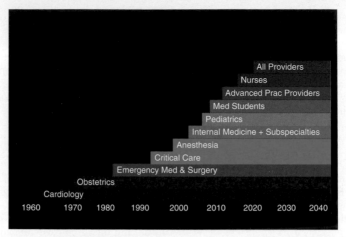

Figure 1.4   Integration of Point-of-Care Ultrasound in Medical Specialties.

pocket-sized devices are being built to overcome these known limitations and can perform the vast majority of common diagnostic applications at the bedside. Transducer availability is an important consideration because certain exams can be performed with multiple transducer types, whereas others can be performed with only a single transducer type; for example, a curvilinear or phased-array transducer can be used to evaluate the abdomen but only a phased-array transducer can be used to evaluate the heart. Providers must be familiar with basic operation of the ultrasound equipment that is available to them, including entering patient information, selecting the appropriate imaging mode, and adjusting the image depth and gain.

Vision

Point-of-care ultrasound use has spread rapidly over the past 20 years. We anticipate that nearly all health care providers, including nurses, advanced practice providers, and physicians, will be using point-of-care ultrasound in their clinical practice over the next 10 years (Fig. 1.4). Health care systems throughout the world are striving to provide high-quality, cost-effective health care, and point-of-care ultrasound can contribute to achieving these goals by reducing procedural complications, expediting care, decreasing costs of ancillary testing, and reducing imaging that utilizes ionizing radiation. Realizing such objectives can further the ultimate goal of improving patient experience and health care outcomes.

CHAPTER 2

Ultrasound Physics and Modes

Michael Mayette ■ Paul K. Mohabir

KEY POINTS

- Ultrasonography utilizes sound waves to visualize internal organs; in comparison, plain radiography and computed tomography utilize ionizing radiation.
- High-frequency transducers produce higher-resolution images but penetrate less deeply compared to low-frequency transducers, which produce lower-resolution images but penetrate deeper.
- The most common imaging mode used in point-of-care ultrasound is B-mode, or two-dimensional mode. M-mode and Doppler ultrasound are also used for specific applications.

Background

Ultrasound has been used for diagnostic purposes in medicine since the late 1940s, but the history of ultrasound physics dates back to ancient Greece. In the sixth century BC, Pythagoras described the unique characteristics of sound waves by studying the harmonics of stringed instruments. By the late eighteenth century, Lazzaro Spallanzani had developed a deeper understanding of sound-wave physics based on his echolocation studies in bats. Pierre and Jacques Curie described the piezoelectric properties of certain materials in 1880, one of the most important milestones in the evolution of the field of ultrasonography.[1] Multiple other milestones, such as the invention of sonar by Fessenden and Langevin after the sinking of the *Titanic* and the development of radar by Watson-Watt, continued to build our understanding of ultrasound physics. Ultrasound entered the field of medicine in the late 1940s with the works of George Ludwig and John Wild in the United States and Karl Theodore Dussik in Europe.[2-4]

Even though advances in technology have improved ultrasound devices and image quality, modern ultrasound machines still rely on the same original physical principles from centuries ago. Understanding ultrasound physics helps providers acquire and interpret images correctly. This chapter reviews fundamental principles of ultrasound physics and imaging modes.

Principles

Sound waves are emitted by piezoelectric material, most often synthetic ceramic material (lead zirconate titanate [PZT]), which is contained in ultrasound transducers. When a rapidly alternating electrical voltage is applied to piezoelectric material, the material experiences corresponding oscillations in mechanical strain. As this material expands and contracts rapidly, vibrations in the adjacent material are produced and sound wave are generated. Mechanical properties of piezoelectric material determine the range of sound wave frequencies that are generated. Sound waves propagate through media by creating compressions and rarefactions of particles (Fig. 2.1). This process of generating mechanical strain from the application of an electrical signal to piezoelectric material is known as the *reverse piezoelectric effect*. The opposite process, or generation of an electrical signal from mechanical strain of piezoelectric material, is known as the *direct piezoelectric effect*. Transducers produce ultrasound waves by the reverse piezoelectric effect, and reflected ultrasound waves, or echoes, are received by the same transducer and converted

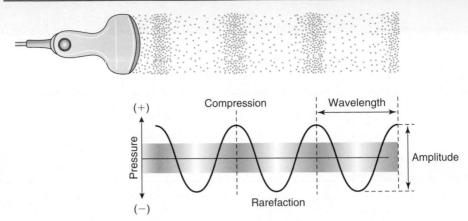

Figure 2.1 Sound Wave Properties. Sound waves are mechanical waves propagated through media by creating compressions and rarefactions, corresponding to high- and low-density regions of particles. Amplitude is the magnitude of the pressure change between the peaks and nadirs and represents the "strength" of the sound wave. Wavelength is the distance between successive compressions or rarefactions and depends on the sound wave frequency and propagation speed in a given tissue.

to an electrical signal by the direct piezoelectric effect. The electrical signal is analyzed by a computer processor, and based on the amplitude of the signal received, a gray-scale image is displayed on the screen. Key parameters of ultrasound waves include frequency, wavelength, velocity, power, and intensity.[5]

FREQUENCY AND WAVELENGTH

The term ultrasound refers to sound waves at a frequency above the normal human audible range (>20 kHz). Frequencies used in medical ultrasonography typically range from 1 to 15 MHz. Frequency (f) is the number of sound wave cycles per second, or hertz (Hz); it is inversely proportional to wavelength (λ) and directly proportional to the propagation speed of sound in a given tissue (c) according to the formula: $f = c/\lambda$. Frequency is determined by properties of the piezoelectric crystals, whereas propagation speed is determined by the density and stiffness of a tissue. The average propagation speed of ultrasound in tissues is 1540 m/s.

Two important considerations in ultrasonography are the penetration depth and the resolution, or sharpness, of the image; the latter is generally measured by the wavelength used. For example, when wavelengths of 1 mm are used, images examined at scales smaller than 1 mm appear blurry. Ultrasound waves with shorter wavelengths have higher frequency and produce higher resolution images but penetrate to shallower depths. Conversely,

ultrasound waves with longer wavelengths have lower frequency and produce lower resolution images but penetrate deeper. The relationship between frequency, resolution, and penetration of a typical biologic material is demonstrated in Fig. 2.2. Maximizing axial resolution while maintaining adequate penetration is a key consideration when choosing an appropriate transducer frequency. Higher frequencies are used in linear-array transducers to visualize superficial structures, most commonly vasculature, soft tissues, and joints. Lower frequencies are used in curvilinear and phased-array transducers to visualize deep structures in the thorax, abdomen, and pelvis.

POWER AND INTENSITY

Average power is the total energy incident on a tissue in a specified time (W). Intensity is the concentration of power per unit area (W/cm²). The intensity of ultrasound waves determines how much heat is generated in tissues. Heat generation is generally insignificant in diagnostic ultrasound imaging as long as the manufacturer's recommended settings are used. However, heat generation becomes important in therapeutic ultrasound applications, such as lithotripsy (see "Safety" below).

Resolution

Image resolution is divided into axial, lateral, elevational, and temporal components (Fig. 2.3).

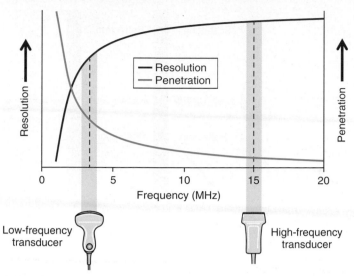

Figure 2.2 Relationship of Frequency, Penetration, and Resolution. High-frequency ultrasound waves produce higher-resolution images but penetrate less deep. Low-frequency ultrasound waves produce lower-resolution images but penetrate deeper.

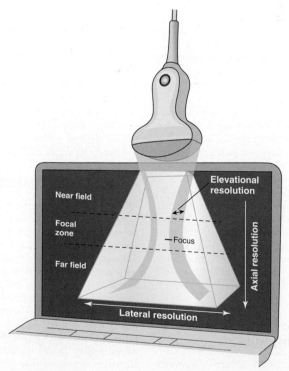

Figure 2.3 Types of Resolution. Axial, lateral, and elevational image resolution in relation to the ultrasound beam and display.

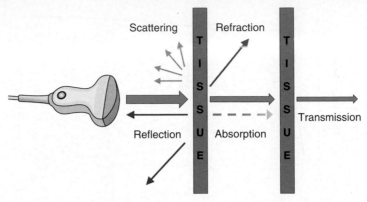

Figure 2.4   Ultrasound-Tissue Interactions. Ultrasound waves are reflected, refracted, scattered, transmitted, and absorbed at tissue interfaces.

Axial resolution is the ability to differentiate two objects along the axis of the ultrasound beam and is the vertical resolution on the screen. Axial resolution depends on transducer frequency. Higher frequencies generate images with better axial resolution, but higher frequencies have shallower penetration. Lateral resolution, or horizontal resolution, is the ability to differentiate two objects perpendicular to the ultrasound beam and is dependent on the width of the beam at a given depth. Lateral resolution can be optimized by placing the target structure in the focal zone of the ultrasound beam. The ultrasound beam has a curved shape, and the focal zone is the narrowest portion of the ultrasound beam with the highest intensity. Lateral resolution decreases as deeper structures are imaged due to divergence and increased scattering of the ultrasound beam. Elevational resolution is a fixed property of the transducer that refers to the ability to resolve objects within the height, or thickness, of the ultrasound beam. The number of individual PZT crystals emitting and receiving ultrasound waves, as well as their sensitivity, affects the overall image resolution. Temporal resolution refers to the clarity, or resolution, of moving structures. (See Chapter 3 for additional details about image resolution.)

Generation of Ultrasound Images

Sound waves are reflected, refracted, scattered, transmitted, and absorbed by tissues due to differences in the tissues' physical properties (Fig. 2.4). Ultrasound images are generated by sound waves reflected back to the transducer. Transducers receive and record the intensity of the returning sound waves. Specifically, mechanical deformation of the transducer's piezoelectric material generates an electrical impulse proportional to the amplitude of these returning sound waves. Electrical impulses cumulatively generate a map of gray scale points seen on the screen as an ultrasound image. Depth of structures along the axis of the ultrasound beam is determined by the time delay for echoes to return to the transducer. The process of emitting and receiving sound waves is repeated serially by the transducer, generating a dynamic image (Fig. 2.5). The reflection and propagation of sound waves through tissues depend on two important parameters: acoustic impedance and attenuation.

ACOUSTIC IMPEDANCE

Propagation speed is the velocity of sound in tissues and varies depending on the physical properties of tissues. Acoustic impedance is the resistance to propagation of sound wave through tissues and is a fixed property of tissues determined by mass density and sound wave speed in specific tissues (Table 2.1). Differences in acoustic impedance determine reflectivity of sound waves at tissue interfaces. Greater differences in acoustic impedance lead to greater reflection of sound waves. For example, sound waves reflect in all directions, or scatter, at air-tissue interfaces due to a large difference in acoustic impedance between air and bodily tissues. Scattering of sound waves at air-tissue

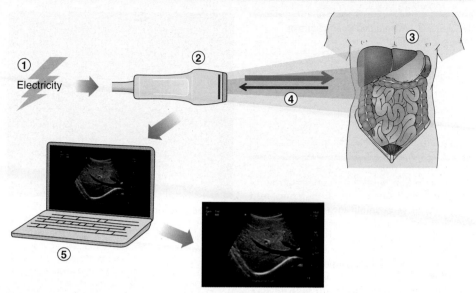

Figure 2.5 Generation of Ultrasound Images. (1) Oscillating voltage is applied to piezoelectric elements. (2) Piezoelectric elements vibrate rapidly, producing sound waves. (3) Ultrasound beam penetrates tissues. (4) Echoes (reflected sound waves) return to transducer. (5) Echoes are converted to electrical signals that are processed into gray scale images.

TABLE 2.1 **Acoustic Impedance of Different Tissues[6–8]**

Tissue or Material	Density (g/cm³)	Speed of Sound (m/s)	Acoustic Impedance (kg/[s m²]) × 10⁶
Air	0.001225	340	0.0004
Fat	0.95	1450	1.38
Blood	1.055	1575	1.66
Liver	1.06	1590	1.69
Bone	1.9	4080	7.75
Metal (e.g., titanium)	4.5	5090	22.9

interfaces explains why a liquid medium, most commonly gel, is needed to seal the interface between the transducer and skin surface, allowing sound waves to enter the body. Ultrasound machines are calibrated to rely on small differences in impedance because only 1% of sound waves are reflected back to the transducer. The majority of sound waves (99%) are scattered, refracted, or absorbed and do not return to the transducer.

ATTENUATION

As sound waves travel through tissues, energy is lost, and this loss of energy is called *attenuation*. Attenuation is due to absorption,

deflection, and divergence of sound waves and is dependent on the attenuation coefficient of tissues, frequency of sound waves, and distance traveled by sound waves.[9] Each type of tissue has an intrinsic attenuation coefficient (Table 2.2). Absorption, the most important cause of attenuation, refers to sound wave energy transferred to tissues as heat. Heat production is an important safety consideration of ultrasonography (see "Safety" below).[10] Absorption is also the most important determinant of depth of ultrasound penetration. High-frequency sound waves are more readily absorbed and therefore penetrate shallower than low-frequency sound waves. Deflection, a second cause of attenuation, refers collectively

TABLE 2.2 **Attenuation Coefficients of Different Materials**

Tissue or Material	Attenuation (dB/cm/MHz)
Water	0.0022
Blood	0.15
Soft tissues	0.75
Air	7.50
Bone	15.00

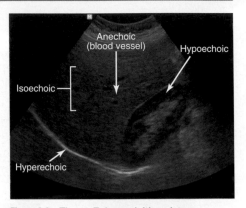

Figure 2.6 Tissue Echogenicities. A two-dimensional ultrasound image of the right upper quadrant demonstrates the isoechoic character of normal liver parenchyma, anechoic blood vessels within the liver, hypoechoic renal cortex compared with the liver parenchyma, and hyperechoic diaphragm.

to the reflection, refraction, and scattering of energy within tissues. Deflection results in a reduction in echo amplitude, especially when the observed interfaces between tissues are not perpendicular to the beam. Divergence refers to loss of ultrasound beam intensity as the beam widens and a fixed amount of acoustic energy is spread over a wider area. Attempts to overcome attenuation can be made by increasing the gain or amplifying the signal in postprocessing. However, increasing gain affects both signal and noise. Adjusting gain manipulates only the computer-generated image and does not improve signal quality.

Modes

Different ultrasound imaging modes permit the evaluation of different characteristics of the same structures. Here we discuss the following imaging modes: two-dimensional (2D) or brightness mode (B-mode); motion mode (M-mode); and Doppler modes (D-mode).

TWO-DIMENSIONAL MODE

The majority of diagnostic ultrasound imaging is performed using two-dimensional (2D) mode, the default mode of most ultrasound machines. This mode is also called *B-mode*, or brightness mode, because the echogenicity, or "brightness," of observed structures depends on the intensity of reflected signals. Structures that transmit all sound waves without reflection are described as being *anechoic* and appear black. Structures containing fluid—such as blood, bile, and urine—generally will appear anechoic. Structures that reflect relatively fewer sound waves than surrounding structures are described as being *hypoechoic*, such as the renal cortex relative to the liver. Structures that reflect sound waves similar to surrounding structures are described as being *isoechoic*.

Both hypoechoic and isoechoic structures appear as shades of gray, commonly seen with solid organs, soft tissues, and muscle. *Hyperechoic* structures reflect most sound waves and appear bright white on ultrasound. Calcified and dense or fibrous structures, such as the diaphragm or pericardium, appear hyperechoic. Some hyperechoic structures, such as bones, create shadows due to the near total reflection of sound waves and often preclude the visualization of underlying structures. Fig. 2.6 illustrates different tissue echogenicities in the right upper quadrant of the abdomen.

M-MODE

M-mode, or motion mode, is an older imaging mode but is still frequently used today to analyze the movement of structures over time.[11] After acquiring a 2D image, an M-mode cursor is applied along a single line within the 2D image. A single-axis beam is emitted along the cursor line and movements of all tissues along that line are plotted over time. The dimensions of cavities or movement of structures can be evaluated. M-mode is often used to measure the size of cardiac chambers or movement of cardiac valves throughout the cardiac cycle (Fig. 2.7). Other frequent point-of-care applications include measurement of respiratory variation of the inferior vena cava and evaluation of the lung-pleura interface in the assessment of pneumothorax.

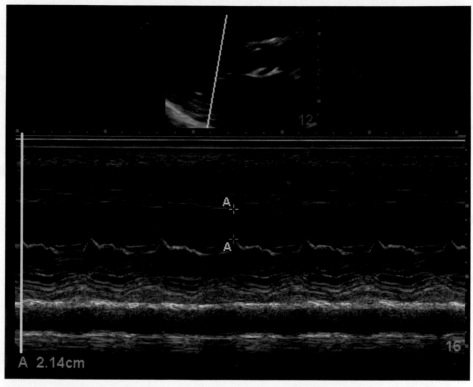

Figure 2.7 M-Mode Ultrasound. The *top panel*, a parasternal long-axis view, shows a two-dimensional image with the M-mode cursor placed on the tip of the anterior mitral valve leaflet. The *bottom panel* shows the motion of the mitral valve toward the septum over time. The separation of the anterior leaflet from the septum during early diastole is measured here and is abnormal at >9 mm (see Chapter 15 for more details).

DOPPLER IMAGING

The Doppler effect is a shift in the frequency of sound waves due to relative motion between the source and observer.[12] In ultrasonography, the primary source of sound waves is the transducer, and the same transducer is the observer for returning echoes. Movement of tissues, most often blood flow, produces a shift in frequency of returning sound waves. Blood flow moving toward the transducer shifts the echoes to a higher frequency, whereas blood flow moving away from the transducer shifts the echoes to a lower frequency (Fig. 2.8). The change in frequency between the emitted and received sound waves is called the *Doppler shift*.[13] Variables that determine the amount of Doppler shift are:

1. Frequency of ultrasound waves
2. Velocity of blood flow
3. Angle of insonation

The Doppler equation is:

Doppler shift = [2 × (ultrasound beam frequency) × (Velocity of blood flow) × (cosine of angle of insonation)]/ propagation of speed of ultrasound in tissues

The angle of insonation, or angle between the ultrasound beam and direction of the measured flow, is critical in the Doppler equation (Fig. 2.9). The Doppler shift can be increased by increasing the frequency of the ultrasound beam, increasing velocity of blood flow, or decreasing the angle of insonation. A correctional factor for the angle of insonation is used in the Doppler equation to better estimate velocities. No Doppler shift can be measured when the ultrasound beam is perpendicular to the direction of blood flow. Ideally the ultrasound beam should be placed parallel to the

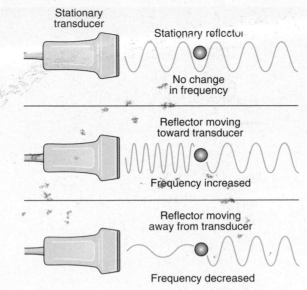

Figure 2.8 Doppler Shift. Movement of the source or reflector of sound waves toward each other causes an increase in sound wave frequency (positive Doppler shift), whereas movement of either the source or reflector apart from one another causes a decrease in sound wave frequency (negative Doppler shift).

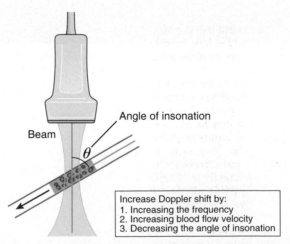

Figure 2.9 Doppler Interrogation. The angle of insonation is the angle measured between the ultrasound beam and direction of flow. The operator can increase the Doppler shift by increasing the sound wave frequency or decreasing the angle of insonation.

direction of blood flow, but a near-parallel intercept angle between 0 and 60 degrees is more often achievable. Angling the ultrasound beam toward the direction of blood flow causes a positive Doppler shift, whereas angling the ultrasound beam away from the direction of blood flow causes a negative Doppler shift (Fig. 2.10).

Spectral Doppler

Doppler effect may be represented graphically using velocity (y-axis) plotted over time (x-axis) in a display called *spectral Doppler*. By convention, the frequency shifts displayed above the baseline represent velocities toward the transducer, and shifts below baseline represent velocities moving away from the transducer.

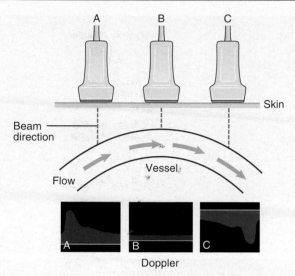

Figure 2.10   Ultrasound Beam Alignment and Doppler Shift. (A) Aligning the ultrasound beam toward the direction of flow causes a positive Doppler shift. (B) No Doppler shift is created when the ultrasound beam is perpendicular to the direction of blood flow. (C) Aligning the ultrasound beam away from the direction of blood flow causes a negative Doppler shift.

Spectral Doppler permits quantitative assessment of velocities and is divided into pulsed-wave and continuous-wave Doppler ultrasound (Fig. 2.11).

Pulsed-wave Doppler refers to the emission of sound waves in pulses that allows measurement of Doppler shift at a precise location. After a pulsed signal is sent into tissues, the transducer must await the returning echo before emitting another pulse. This cycle of emitting a wave into tissues and capturing the returning echo is repeated rapidly at a rate called *pulse repetition frequency* (PRF). Ideally the maximum possible PRF is used; however, the maximum PRF is determined by wave travel time, and wave travel time is limited by tissue depth. Deeper depths require longer wait times for returning echoes, reducing the maximum PRF before ambiguous signaling, or *aliasing*, occurs. When aliasing occurs, the true velocity and vector direction cannot be determined. The maximum Doppler frequency or velocity that can be measured before aliasing occurs is called the *Nyquist limit*. This limit is one half of the PRF because ultrasound waveforms must be sampled at least twice per wavelength to reliably assess velocity and direction (Fig. 2.12).[14] The significance of the Nyquist limit can be exemplified by considering severe aortic

stenosis. The aortic valve is a relatively deep structure, which limits the PRF and makes accurate measurement of the high velocities of severe aortic stenosis difficult. Techniques to avoid aliasing include maximizing the PRF (or velocity scale) to raise the Nyquist limit, shifting the baseline to increase the Nyquist limit in a particular direction, reducing the imaging depth, selecting a lower transducer frequency, or switching to continuous-wave Doppler imaging. In addition to its spatial precision, pulsed-wave Doppler introduces less interference from surrounding structures. Its main disadvantage is susceptibility to aliasing because of the Nyquist limit.

In contrast to spatially precise pulsed-wave Doppler imaging, continuous-wave Doppler measures blood flow velocities along the entire ultrasound beam. This technique relies on two different sets of piezoelectric crystals to continuously emit and receive signals; therefore, there is no PRF or Nyquist limit and aliasing does not occur. Continuous-wave Doppler is most often used to measure high velocities that pulsed-wave Doppler cannot accurately measure, such as severe aortic stenosis. The main limitation of continuous-wave Doppler is the inability to measure velocities at specific depths because Doppler signals are received from all tissues

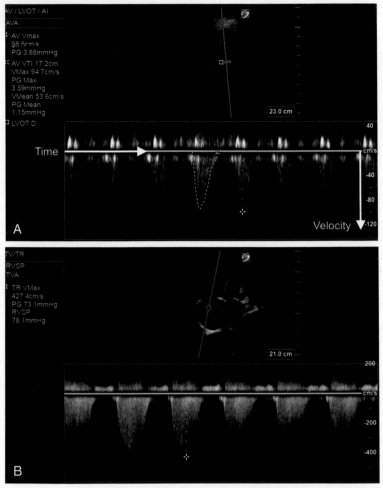

Figure 2.11   Spectral Doppler Ultrasound. (A) Pulsed-wave Doppler ultrasound measuring flow through the left ventricular outflow tract. (B) Continuous-wave Doppler ultrasound measuring regurgitant flow through the tricuspid valve.

along the path of the ultrasound beam. In both pulsed- and continuous-wave Doppler imaging, the accuracy of measurements depends on signal quality, which governs the visual clarity of the spectral peaks and curves used to determine velocities.

Color Flow Doppler

Color flow Doppler images display color-coded maps representing Doppler shifts that are superimposed on 2D ultrasound images (Fig. 2.13 and Video 2.1). Color flow Doppler relies on the same principles as pulsed-wave Doppler but shorter pulses are obtained from multiple small areas to build a color-coded map. When velocities exceed the Nyquist limit, pixels appear as a mosaic color pattern (blue, red, and white) as the direction of flow cannot be reliably ascertained. In color flow Doppler imaging, the color corresponds to the velocity and direction of flow. Conventionally, blue represents blood flow away from the transducer (longer wavelengths) and red represents blood flow toward the transducer (shorter wavelengths). It is important to note that red or blue is not specific for arteries or veins because the color depends on the direction of flow relative to the transducer (Video 2.2). If the ultrasound

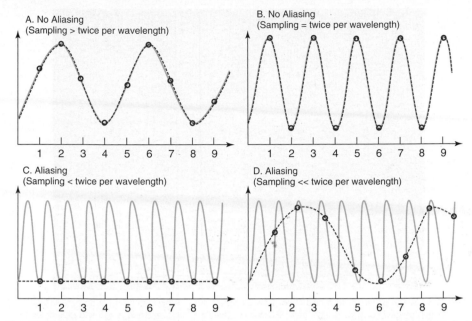

Figure 2.12   Aliasing. (A and B) When sampling *(red circles)* is at least twice per full wavelength *(blue line)*, the signal can be recreated and analyzed reliably *(red dashed line)*. (C and D) When sampling is less than twice per wavelength (above the Nyquist limit), a reliable signal cannot be obtained, leading to aliasing.

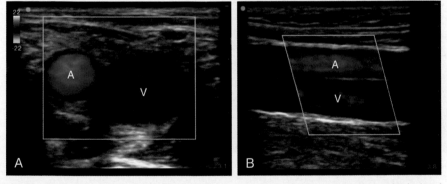

Figure 2.13   Color Flow Doppler Ultrasound. Color flow Doppler displays the direction and velocity of flow. An artery and vein are shown in transverse (A) and longitudinal (B) views. Using the conventional color flow map, blood flow toward the transducer appears red, whereas blood flow away from the transducer appears blue.

beam is perpendicular to the direction of flow, no Doppler shift can be detected, resulting in an ambiguous red and blue color flow pattern (Fig. 2.14 and Video 2.3).

Power Doppler

Power Doppler assesses echo signals similar to color flow Doppler but has unique characteristics.[15] Power Doppler analyzes only the amplitude of returning echoes (Fig. 2.15 and Video 2.4). Thus, power Doppler is superimposed on a 2D ultrasound image and the levels of brightness correlate with the magnitude of flow. Sensitivity for detecting flow is three to five times higher than with conventional color flow Doppler. Two important limitations of power Doppler are (1) no information regarding direction of flow is given, limiting its use in

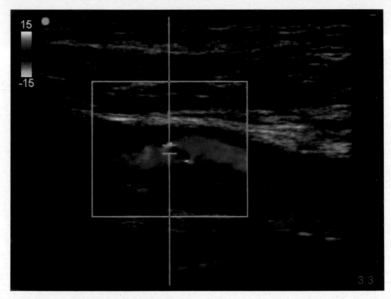

Figure 2.14 Angle of Insonation and Color flow Doppler. If the ultrasound beam is perpendicular to the direction of flow, no Doppler shift can be detected, resulting in an ambiguous red and blue color flow pattern.

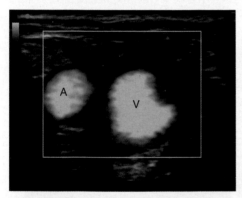

Figure 2.15 Power Doppler Ultrasound.
Power Doppler ultrasound is nondirectional and displays only the magnitude of flow. The common femoral artery (A) and vein (V) are shown in a transverse view. Both the artery and vein appear yellow-orange.

cardiac imaging; and (2) images are more susceptible to artifacts, called *flash artifacts*, caused by surrounding soft tissue motion. Compared to color flow Doppler, two advantages of power Doppler are less angle dependence and no aliasing because the integrated power of the Doppler signal is displayed, rather than the mean frequency shift. Practical uses of power Doppler include tissues with low blood flow

velocities, such as joints or testicles, or when direction of flow is not critical, such as tumor flow studies.[16]

Tissue Doppler imaging. Tissue Doppler imaging (TDI) refers to the use of Doppler ultrasound to measure the movement of muscles, most commonly the myocardium. TDI can be acquired as either pulsed-wave or color flow Doppler to measure patterns of muscle contraction and relaxation. Compared with the high-frequency, low-amplitude signals of blood flow, myocardial tissues generate low-frequency, high-amplitude signals. Tissue Doppler images are most often acquired using pulsed-wave Doppler on a specific segment of myocardium (Fig. 2.16) or color flow mapping of the heart. Tissue Doppler imaging permits a more precise assessment of left or right ventricular systolic and diastolic function by measuring muscle velocities instead of changes in intracavitary size. Longitudinal left ventricular contraction and relaxation can be assessed using pulsed-wave TDI by positioning the Doppler sample gate immediately adjacent to the mitral annulus to measure mitral annular motion.

TDI is limited in its ability to discriminate between active and passive motion. Doppler strain imaging, a newer modality, allows the

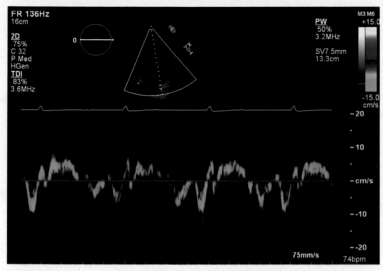

Figure 2.16 Pulsed-Wave Tissue Doppler Imaging. The velocity of the lateral mitral annulus is measured using pulsed-wave tissue Doppler to assess left ventricular diastolic performance and filling pressures.

differentiation of active versus passive motion by assessing the relative change in tissue length. The fractional change in the length of a muscle segment, or deformation, is called *strain* and is expressed as a percentage of change from its baseline length (Fig. 2.17 and Video 2.5).

Safety

Ultrasound imaging is considered to be a very safe imaging modality, but its limitations must be recognized. When applied to tissues, intense ultrasound beams can potentially cause thermal (heat generation) and nonthermal (cavitation) injuries. The intensities generated by current ultrasound systems range from 10 to 430 mW/cm^2, with the highest intensity occurring with pulsed-wave Doppler imaging due to its focused target zone. Current recommendations from the American Institute of Ultrasound in Medicine include exposure to intensities below 1 W/cm^2, which corresponds to a calculated possible elevation of tissue temperature less than 1°C above baseline.[17] The exact elevation of temperature in the human body is difficult to measure. Temperatures rapidly dissipate, especially with high-perfusion organs and blood vessels, but they could theoretically be as high as 4°C with prolonged exposure at the focal point.[18] Because of this theoretical risk, societies advocate the As Low As Reasonably Achievable (ALARA) principle, with minimization of duration of exposure at a single point being the most important modifiable risk factor.[19] These principles are especially important when imaging sensitive tissues, such as fetuses and eyes.

Modern ultrasound machines provide operators with an easy way to estimate potential risk from ultrasound by displaying two measures: mechanical index (MI) and thermal index (TI). TI is subdivided into TIs (soft tissues), TIb (bone), and TIc (cranium). Both MI and TI are calculated ratios. TI is a ratio of total emitted acoustic power to theoretical power required to raise tissue temperature by 1°C and reflects the risk of an ultrasound beam causing thermal injury. Mechanical index is a ratio of the peak negative pressure and reflects the risk of an ultrasound beam causing tissue damage primarily from cavitation. Thermal index is generally recommended to be below 1.0 with lower limits (<0.7) for obstetric ultrasonography. The mechanical index is recommended to be below 0.7 with lower limits (<0.4) for gas-filled structures and for the use of contrast agents.[20,21]

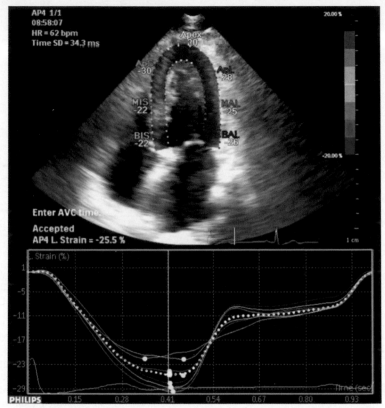

Figure 2.17   **Doppler Strain Imaging.** The *top panel* shows the computer tracking of myocardial deformation of the left ventricle (LV). The *lower panel* shows longitudinal strain over time throughout the cardiac cycle. During systole the strain becomes more negative, and during diastole three discrete phases of strain are seen. The most common clinical utility is the detection of reduced longitudinal strain due to subclinical LV systolic dysfunction, despite normal LV ejection fraction.

CHAPTER 3

Transducers

Alan T. Chiem

KEY POINTS

- The four common types of ultrasound transducers—linear, curvilinear, phased-array, and intracavitary—differ by crystal arrangement, size, and footprint, which determine their suitability in different applications.
- High-frequency transducers produce high-resolution images of superficial structures, whereas low-frequency transducers produce low-resolution images of deep structures.
- Resolution of ultrasound images is divided into four different types: axial, lateral, elevational, and temporal.

Background

The transducer is a fundamental component of ultrasound imaging. Piezoelectric crystals inside the transducer generate fine vibrations with the application of electricity, a phenomenon called the *reverse piezoelectric effect*. The vibrating crystals, also known as *piezoelectric elements*, generate ultrasonic waves that are transmitted to tissues. Reflected sound waves return to the transducer and cause mechanical distortion of the crystals, which is converted to an electrical current via the *direct piezoelectric effect*. The electrical current is processed by the ultrasound machine's computer and rendered into an image. Point-of-care ultrasound users should have a basic understanding of the characteristics and construction of different types of transducers as well as the determinants of image resolution.

Transducer Construction

Ultrasound transducers are designed for the optimal transmission and reception of sound waves (Fig. 3.1). An *electrical shield* lines the transducer case to prevent external electrical interference from distorting sound wave transmission. A thin *acoustic insulator* dampens vibrations from the case to piezoelectric elements and also prevents transmission of

spurious electrical current to the machine's computer processor. At the tip of the transducer, a thin *matching layer* improves efficiency of sound wave transmission from piezoelectric elements to skin and deeper structures. *Backing material* is an essential component of transducers. Backing material is fixed behind the layer of piezoelectric elements to dampen ongoing vibrations of elements. Sound wave energy is absorbed by the backing material when piezoelectric elements send and receive sound waves.[1]

Transducers are sensitive instruments, and the internal components of the transducers, especially the piezoelectric elements, can be damaged easily with minor impact. Providers must be trained to safeguard transducers at all times. Transducers should be hung on the manufacturer's rack or held firmly in hand when in use. Additionally, providers should avoid stepping on or rolling the machine over the transducer cables. The transducer cables should be lifted off the ground to remove any excess slack, especially when pushing the machine.

Resolution

The total resolution of ultrasound images depends on three complementary properties of the transducer: axial, lateral, and elevational

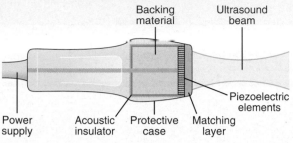

Figure 3.1   **Transducer Construction.** An electrical current causes the piezoelectric elements to vibrate and generate sound waves. The matching layer minimizes reverberations as sound waves travel to the skin. The backing material dampens crystal vibrations to prevent unintended continued sound-wave transmission. An acoustic insulator, electrical shield, and case serve to protect the piezoelectric elements from external electrical and acoustic interference.

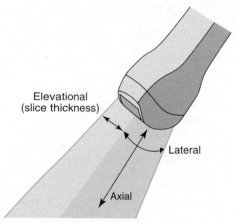

Figure 3.2   **Types of Resolution.** The axial, lateral, and elevational resolution describe the resolution along the length, width, and slice thickness, respectively, of the ultrasound beam.

resolution (Fig. 3.2). *Axial resolution* is the ability to differentiate objects on the same trajectory as the ultrasound beam. Axial resolution is determined by sound wave frequency, with higher frequencies giving better axial resolution (Fig. 3.3A). *Lateral resolution* is the ability to differentiate objects that are perpendicular to the ultrasound beam. Lateral resolution is determined by width of the ultrasound beam, which is influenced by the diameter and frequency of the transducer's piezoelectric crystals. Small-diameter crystals that produce high-frequency pulses generate narrow ultrasound beams and thereby increase lateral resolution.[2] More importantly, the narrowest portion of the ultrasound beam, the focal zone,

has the greatest lateral resolution. Depth of the focal zone can be adjusted to the level of the target structure to maximize lateral resolution (Fig. 3.3B). Ultrasound computer processors adjust sound-wave frequency to maximize axial and lateral resolution when depth settings are changed.

Elevational resolution, referred to as slice-thickness resolution, is the type of resolution least influenced by the diameter of the piezoelectric crystal or sound wave frequency (Fig. 3.4). In point-of-care ultrasound systems, elevational resolution is determined primarily by the thickness of the ultrasound beam and the imaging depth. Sound waves return to the transducer from the various planes that constitute the ultrasound beam, and signals from these various planes are averaged to produce a single two-dimensional image. Elevational resolution is analogous to looking into a swimming pool from above, where shallow and deep objects are blended into one plane. Thus an important principle in ultrasonography is to visualize structures in two planes to account for limitations of elevational resolution.

Temporal resolution refers to the visualization of moving structures, similar to the frame rate or shutter speed of a camera. High temporal resolution indicates a high frame rate and better capture of movement. Both transducer pulse frequency and imaging depth affect temporal resolution. Pulse frequency is the rate at which transducers emit sound waves and is distinct from the frequency range of transducers. A higher pulse frequency and shallower depth increase temporal resolution because reflected sound waves can be received by the transducer in more rapid succession.[3] The limiting factor

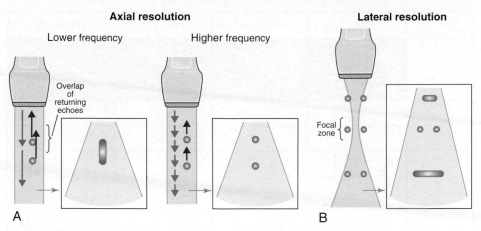

Axial resolution

Lower frequency   Higher frequency

Overlap of returning echoes

Lateral resolution

Focal zone

Figure 3.3   Axial and Lateral Resolution. (A) Axial resolution depends on the frequency of the ultrasound wave. Higher-frequency sound waves have shorter wavelengths, generating images with better axial resolution. (B) Lateral resolution depends on beam width and is highest in the focal zone, the narrowest portion of the ultrasound beam.

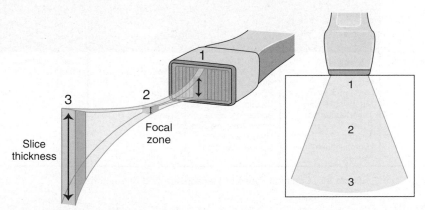

Slice thickness

Focal zone

Figure 3.4   Elevational Resolution. The elevational, or slice thickness, resolution is determined by actual ultrasound beam thickness. Elevational resolution is greatest in the focal zone and least in the far field, where the ultrasound beam diverges.

of temporal resolution with many point-of-care ultrasound machines is computer processing speed.

Transducer Types

Transducers typically contain 60 to 600 piezoelectric elements and are described by the arrangement of their elements as well as by their function and beam shape. There are four common types of transducers: linear, curvilinear, phased-array, and intracavitary (Fig. 3.5).

Linear transducers have elements that are arranged in a flat matrix, producing parallel,

linear ultrasound beams and generating a rectangular image format (Fig. 3.6, Video 3.1). Generally, linear transducers generate high-frequency (5 to 10 MHz), shorter-wavelength sound waves with excellent axial and lateral resolution. Linear transducers also have excellent elevational, or slice thickness, resolution because the shape of the ultrasound beam is relatively flat.[4] However, linear transducers are limited to the visualization of superficial structures in a relatively narrow field of view to maximum depths of 6–9 cm. Linear-array transducers are ideal for evaluating superficial structures, including blood vessels, muscles, nerves, and

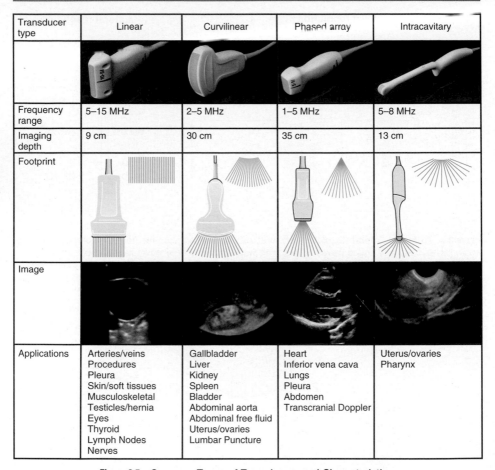

Transducer type	Linear	Curvilinear	Phased array	Intracavitary
Frequency range	5–15 MHz	2–5 MHz	1–5 MHz	5–8 MHz
Imaging depth	9 cm	30 cm	35 cm	13 cm
Footprint				
Image				
Applications	Arteries/veins Procedures Pleura Skin/soft tissues Musculoskeletal Testicles/hernia Eyes Thyroid Lymph Nodes Nerves	Gallbladder Liver Kidney Spleen Bladder Abdominal aorta Abdominal free fluid Uterus/ovaries Lumbar Puncture	Heart Inferior vena cava Lungs Pleura Abdomen Transcranial Doppler	Uterus/ovaries Pharynx

Figure 3.5   Common Types of Transducers and Characteristics.

joints, and for performing ultrasound-guided procedures.

Curvilinear transducers are named for the curvilinear or convex arrangement of crystals. The ultrasound beam is broad and trapezoidal with a wide field of view, but this type of transducer has lower resolution compared with the linear transducers (Video 3.2). Overlap of transmitted ultrasound waves in deep tissues provides consistent lateral resolution. Curvilinear transducers utilize lower frequencies (2 to 5 MHz) with longer wavelengths that penetrate deep structures with relatively less attenuation, particularly for structures 5 to 25 cm deep.[5] Curvilinear transducer beams have a greater slice thickness and lower elevational resolution than linear transducers because a greater number of structures are averaged into a single two-dimensional image on the display.

Curvilinear transducers are ideal for imaging abdominal and pelvic organs—including the liver, spleen, kidneys, and bladder—and for imaging larger musculoskeletal structures such as the hips and spine. Curvilinear transducers are not optimal for imaging the heart or superficial structures because of poor near-field resolution.

Phased-array transducers produce diverging, low-frequency ultrasound beams (1 to 5 MHz) that generate a pie-shaped image format with adjustable focusing and steering (Fig. 3.6, Video 3.3). Differential excitation of piezoelectric elements creates rapid electronic beam sweeping by sequentially pulsing multiple small crystals within the transducer (Fig. 3.7). Steering and focusing of the ultrasound beam allows for a wider field of view than with linear transducers.[6] Phased-array technology allows for more

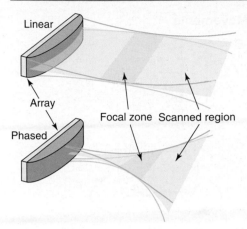

efficient two-dimensional imaging and is ideal for moving structures, such as the heart. The ability to steer ultrasound beams with phasing permits accurate velocity measurements when the vector of movement is not completely parallel with the beam. These unique characteristics make phased-array transducers ideal for cardiac and thoracic imaging.

Intracavitary transducers combine a small, microconvex footprint with a high-frequency range (5 to 8 MHz). The field of view is wider than linear transducers but with similar high image resolution (Video 3.4). Intracavitary transducers are ideal for transvaginal and transrectal imaging, as well as intraoral evaluation for peritonsillar abscess.[7] Similar to linear transducers, they are not ideal for deep structures, such as abdominal organs.

Several other types of transducers are used in point-of-care ultrasound. Microconvex transducers are similar in construction to curvilinear transducers but produce higher-frequency sound waves (5 to 8 MHz) that are limited in penetration to 10 to 15 cm. The small footprint of microconvex transducers is ideal for

Figure 3.6   Ultrasound Beam Contours. Linear-array transducers produce a series of parallel beams that generate a rectangular image format. Phased-array transducers fire sequentially in different directions, producing diverging beams that generates a pie-shaped image format.

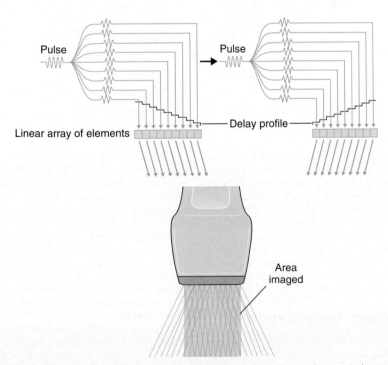

Figure 3.7   Beam Steering. Phased-array transducers electronically steer sound waves to image a wider field of view and improve image resolution over a wider range of depths.

Transducer Movements

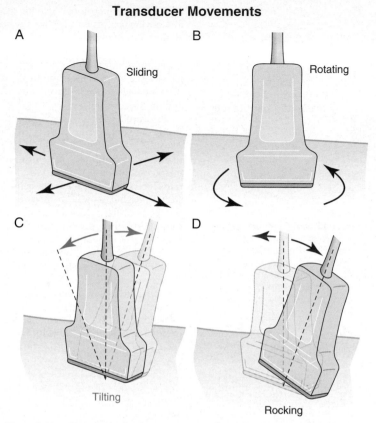

Figure 3.8 **Transducer Manipulation.** (A) Sliding is relocation of the transducer on the skin surface. (B) Rotating refers to twisting the transducer along its central axis. (C) Tilting refers to changing the angle of the imaging plane to obtain serial cross-sectional images. (D) Rocking refers to aiming the ultrasound beam toward or away from the transducer orientation marker to center the image on the screen.

intercostal imaging of the heart and lungs, as well as for pediatric and neonatal applications. Linear transducers are available with a "hockey stick" design for imaging small superficial structures. Ultra-high-frequency linear transducers utilize frequencies as high as 70 MHz and produce very high-resolution images of skin and superficial structures from 1 to 4 cm deep. Transesophageal echocardiography utilizes a unique transducer that is described in a later chapter (see Chapter 20).

TRANSDUCER MANIPULATION

Four principal transducer movements are described in ultrasound imaging. The use of standard definitions is important for training and communication. Standard nomenclature

was defined by the American Institute of Ultrasound in Medicine (AIUM) in 1999. Although other conventions exist, the AIUM nomenclature is the most cited across specialties. The following definitions are used throughout this textbook (Fig. 3.8):

- Sliding: Sliding is relocating the transducer on the skin surface; it is the process of physically moving the point of contact between the transducer and skin. This maneuver helps identify the optimal location to obtain desired views, particularly when imaging in between ribs.
- Rotating: Rotating refers to twisting the transducer on its central axis, like a corkscrew. Rotation is often used to align the ultrasound beam with the long or short axis of a structure.[3,4]

- Tilting: Tilting is also called *fanning* or *sweeping.* The transducer is held in place on the skin and the angle of the imaging plane is changed. Tilting allows visualization of serial cross-sectional images of a structure from a single acoustic window. Tilting is often used to obtain serial cross-sectional images of solid organs, such as the kidney, to appreciate the entire structure of interest from left to right or from cranial to caudal.
- Rocking: Rocking refers to aiming the ultrasound beam either toward or away from the transducer orientation marker while maintaining the point of contact with the skin surface. Rocking is similar to tilting but in a perpendicular plane of motion. This "in-plane" movement pushes one of the transducer corners into the skin surface and allows centering of the image on the screen.

PEARLS AND PITFALLS

- Transducers are sensitive instruments and expensive to replace. The internal components of the transducer head, especially the piezoelectric elements, can break easily with minor impact. Safeguard the transducers by holding them firmly or hanging them on the ultrasound rack.
- Linear transducers are ideal for imaging superficial structures less than 6 cm deep, such as blood vessels, muscles, joints, nerves, and eyes. Ultrasound-guided procedures using real-time needle tracking are most often performed with a linear transducer.
- Low-frequency transducers are optimal for visualizing structures deeper than 5 cm. In general, curvilinear or phased-array transducers are used for abdominal and pelvic imaging. Phased-array transducers are the only transducer type that can be used to properly evaluate the heart.
- Axial resolution is determined primarily by sound-wave frequency, and lateral resolution is determined primarily by beam width. To improve lateral resolution when deep structures are being imaged, adjust the depth or focal zone position to make sure that the target structure is within the focal zone.

CHAPTER 4

Orientation

Sara Crager ■ Paul K. Mohabir

KEY POINTS

- Providers must understand the spatial relationships between the transducer, ultrasound screen, operator, and patient because ultrasound images are two-dimensional views of three-dimensional structures.
- The body is divided into transverse, sagittal, and coronal planes. The sagittal and coronal planes are along the long axis of the body and often referred to as the *longitudinal* plane. The *transverse* plane is along the short axis of the body.
- The transducer orientation marker is generally pointed to the operator's left side when imaging in a *transverse* plane or pointed to the patient's head when imaging in a *longitudinal* plane.
- When real-time ultrasound guidance is being used for invasive procedures, the needle tip is tracked using either a longitudinal (in-plane) or a transverse (out-of-plane) approach.

Introduction

Point-of-care ultrasound allows providers to perform focused exams at the bedside to answer specific clinical questions and guide management.[1] An important advantage of real-time ultrasound scanning is the ability to visualize structures in multiple planes. An understanding of the orientation of three-dimensional structures being displayed in two dimensions on the ultrasound screen is critical to accurate interpretation. This chapter reviews the standard imaging planes and orientation between the transducer, ultrasound screen, operator, and patient.

Transducer Orientation

All transducers have an orientation marker that corresponds to the screen orientation marker. The transducer marker has traditionally been located between the head and body of the transducer, such that it can be easily felt by rubbing one's thumb along the side of the transducer. The transducer orientation marker is also called the notch or index marker.

Modern ultrasound transducers usually have additional divots or plastic ridges to attach needle guides; these should not be confused with the transducer marker (Fig. 4.1). Some modern transducers have a small red or green light rather than a plastic notch.

The transducer should be held gently in the scanning hand, like a pen, with the thumb and index finger. The remaining fingers can be held against the transducer or spread out on the patient's body to anchor the transducer for stability. This grip improves patient comfort by minimizing pressure applied to the skin by the transducer and allows better operator control to make fine adjustments.

Screen Orientation

During the evolution of diagnostic ultrasonography from the 1940s until the 1970s, various conventions emerged for screen orientation by different specialties and countries. Screen orientation can be confusing for providers to understand because of differing conventions. The screen orientation marker is usually a small colored circle or square that can be positioned

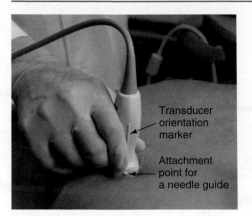

Figure 4.1 **Transducer Marker.** All ultrasound transducers have a marker ("notch") that corresponds with the screen orientation marker. Transducers should be held gently, like a pencil, with the thumb and index finger.

in any of the four corners of the screen (Fig. 4.2, Videos 4.1–4.4). When the screen orientation marker is positioned in the *upper* corners of the screen, superficial structures are viewed at the top of the screen and deep structures at the bottom. The opposite is true when the screen orientation marker is positioned in the *lower* corners of the screen. For example, some providers may choose to invert images generated by transvaginal ultrasound so that structures nearest the transducer are viewed at the bottom of the ultrasound screen.

In North America and Europe, general medical and cardiac ultrasound imaging uses two different conventions for screen orientation. General medical ultrasonography utilizes a convention with the screen orientation marker in the upper *left* corner of the screen. Most specialties performing diagnostic ultrasound imaging, including radiology, follow this convention. In contrast, cardiac ultrasound imaging utilizes a convention with the screen orientation marker in the upper *right*

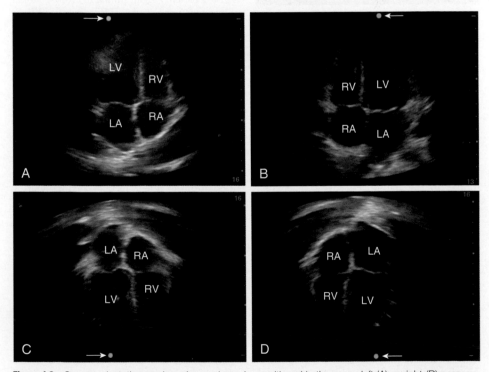

Figure 4.2 Screen orientation markers *(arrows)* can be positioned in the upper left (A) or right (B) corners or the lower left (C) or right (D) corners.

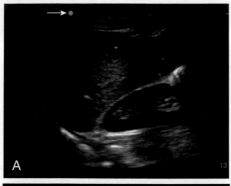

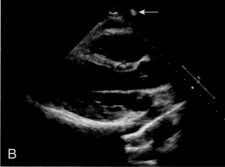

Figure 4.3   Screen Orientation Marker. (A) The general medical ultrasound convention has the screen orientation marker in the upper left corner of the screen *(arrow)*. (B) The cardiac ultrasound convention has the screen orientation marker in the upper right corner of the screen *(arrow)*.

corner (Fig. 4.3). This orientation is utilized by most specialties performing cardiac ultrasound imaging.[2]

The screen orientation marker corresponds to the transducer marker. Therefore, in general medical ultrasonography, when the screen marker is in the *upper left* corner, the transducer marker is pointed to the operator's *left*-hand side to obtain transverse images. To obtain longitudinal images (sagittal or coronal planes), the transducer marker is pointed to the patient's head (see Imaging Planes, later).

Operator Orientation

Traditionally, providers have performed bedside ultrasound exams standing on the patient's right side (left side of the bed), similar to the physical examination, with the ultrasound machine directly in front of them. One hand

holds the transducer on the patient while the other hand operates the ultrasound machine. Providers may stand on the patient's left side (right side of the bed) when scanning the heart, especially to obtain cardiac apical views.[2] The height of the patient's bed can be adjusted, as can the position of the ultrasound machine, to optimize both patient and operator comfort. A systematic approach using the same setup with the transducer held in the same hand can help to develop muscle memory.

Patient Orientation

Although optimal patient positioning varies based on the ultrasound exam being performed, the orientation of the transducer marker remains constant with the convention being used. Using the general medical ultrasound convention, the screen orientation marker is in the upper left corner of the screen. When the operator faces the patient from the foot of the bed and the transducer marker is pointed toward the operator's left, the left side of the screen corresponds to the operator's left and the patient's right, similar to cross-sectional computed tomography (CT) images. When the transducer marker is pointed toward the patient's head, the left side of the screen corresponds to the patient's head and the right side to the patient's feet.

It is important to recognize that provider-to-screen orientation does not change, regardless of patient position, as long as the transducer marker is pointed toward the operator's left in a transverse plane or toward the patient's head in a longitudinal plane. For example, when standing at the head of the bed to place an internal jugular central line, the operator's orientation to the screen is maintained by keeping the transducer marker pointed toward the operator's left, which is the patient's left side in this situation.

Imaging Planes

The body is divided into three primary planes in ultrasonography: sagittal, transverse, and coronal. Oblique imaging planes that are not parallel to these three standard planes may also be utilized, most often in cardiac ultrasound imaging. The sagittal and coronal planes are often referred to as the *long-axis* plane, or longitudinal plane, and the transverse plane is often referred to as the *short-axis* plane (Fig. 4.4).

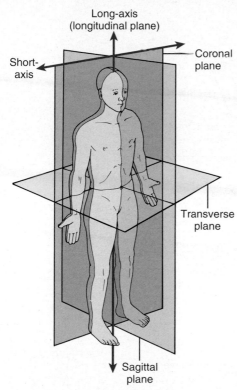

Long-axis
(longitudinal plane)

Coronal
plane

Short-
axis

Transverse
plane

Sagittal
plane

Figure 4.4   Ultrasound Imaging Planes. The sagittal and coronal planes are often referred to as *longitudinal* or *long-axis* planes and the transverse plane is often referred to as the *short-axis* plane.

SAGITTAL PLANE

The sagittal plane is a vertical plane that divides the body into left and right halves. The midsagittal plane is the plane running through the midline of the body, passing through all midline structures such as the bladder. Parasagittal planes are vertical planes parallel to the midline. By standard convention, the transducer marker is directed superiorly toward the patient's head such that superior structures are seen on the left side of the ultrasound screen. The term *sagittal view* refers to an image acquired in either the midsagittal plane or one of the parasagittal planes (Fig. 4.5, Video 4.5).

CORONAL PLANE

The coronal plane, also known as the *frontal plane*, is the plane that divides the body into

ventral and dorsal, or anterior and posterior, halves. By standard convention, the transducer marker is kept pointed toward the patient's head, creating a long axis or longitudinal image with the patient's head toward the left side of the screen and feet toward the right side (Fig. 4.6, Video 4.6).

TRANSVERSE PLANE

The transverse plane, also known as the *short-axis plane*, is the plane that divides the body into superior and inferior parts and is perpendicular to the sagittal and coronal planes. These are the same planes seen in CT scans. By standard convention, the transducer marker points to the operator's left side so that the patient's right-sided structures appear on the left side of the screen (Fig. 4.7, Video 4.7).[4]

Needle Orientation

Many invasive procedures, such as central venous catheter insertion, are performed with real-time ultrasound guidance to decrease the risk of complications. Maintenance of appropriate needle orientation with the transducer and screen allows tracking of the needle tip using a longitudinal (in-plane) or transverse (out-of-plane) approach (Fig. 4.8).[3]

LONGITUDINAL APPROACH (IN-PLANE)

Using a longitudinal approach, the transducer is placed lengthwise over the long axis of the target structure. The transducer marker should be facing the operator. The needle tip is inserted in the center of the short side of the transducer. The needle and syringe trajectory must be aligned with the center of the transducer, which is the long axis of the ultrasound beam. The needle insertion angle relative to the skin depends on the depth of the target structure. Insertion angles are typically 30 to 60 degrees. Shallow insertion angles are used for more superficial structures, such as joints and superficial veins, whereas steep angles are used for deep structures, such as the femoral vein (Video 4.8).

The primary challenge in using a longitudinal or in-plane approach is keeping the needle within the narrow plane of the ultrasound beam. If the needle tip is outside the plane of the ultrasound beam, the shaft of the needle

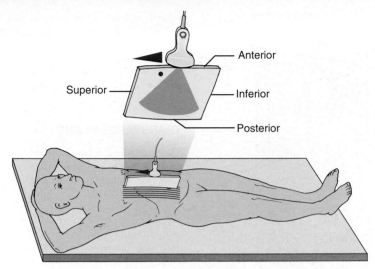

Figure 4.5 Sagittal Plane.

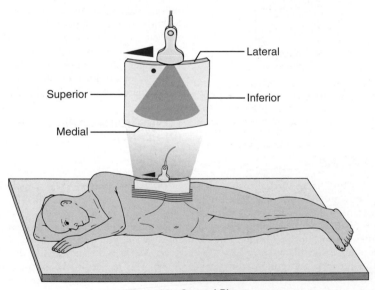

Figure 4.6 Coronal Plane.

may be the only portion visualized, giving a false impression of seeing the needle tip. Steep insertion angles (60 to 90 degrees) place the needle nearly parallel to the ultrasound beam, resulting in poor visualization of the needle tip because fewer echoes are reflected back to the transducer.

TRANSVERSE APPROACH (OUT-OF-PLANE)

A transverse view is obtained by placing the transducer on the short axis of the target structure with the transducer marker pointed to the operator's left. The target structure is

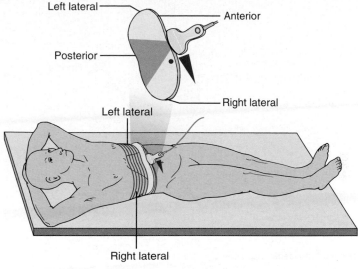

Figure 4.7 Transverse Plane.

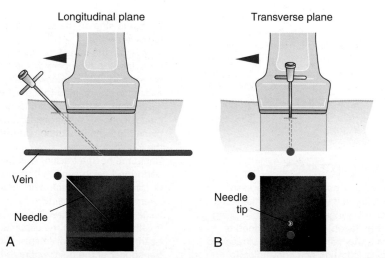

Figure 4.8 (A) Longitudinal (in-plane) and (B) transverse (out-of-plane) approaches to real-time needle insertion.

centered on the screen and the operator's hand is fixed in place. Ideally, the needle is inserted as perpendicular as possible to the ultrasound beam to maximize visualization, but the needle insertion angle depends on depth of the target structure, as described earlier. The needle is inserted in the center of the transducer, and once the needle is under the skin, the needle tip should be identified directly above the target structure as a hyperechoic dot. As the

needle is advanced toward the target structure, the transducer must be tilted to track the tip with the ultrasound beam (Fig. 4.9, Video 4.9).

It is important to ensure correct orientation of the transducer marker, screen marker, and operator when performing real-time ultrasound-guided procedures. When the transducer marker or screen marker is flipped, the needle tip is seen moving in the opposite direction on the screen (i.e., leftward movement of the

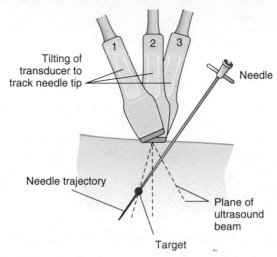

Figure 4.9 Tracking the Needle Tip. When a transverse (out-of-plane) approach is being used, the ultrasound beam is initially aimed toward the operator *(1)*; as the needle is advanced *(2)*, the transducer is tilted to aim the beam away from the operator to track the needle tip *(3)*.

needle tip in the patient is seen as rightward movement on the screen). Another common mistake is to visualize the needle shaft in cross section and think that it is the tip while the actual tip is much deeper. Thus it is critical to maintain the needle tip in the plane of the ultrasound beam for direct visualization.

PEARLS AND PITFALLS

- Even though conventions for screen orientation differ by specialty, the same imaging findings can be identified using any orientation. It is recommended to use a systematic approach to ultrasound imaging following one convention to avoid missing important findings.
- Transducer orientation markers, also called *probe markers* or *notches,* vary in appearance by brand and type of transducer. Plastic attachment points for needle guides are often mistaken for the transducer markers.
- To confirm transducer orientation, touch one end of the transducer and look for movement on the ultrasound screen. The end of the transducer being touched should be aligned with the same side on the screen displaying movement.
- In general, the transducer marker should be pointed to the operator's left side when imaging in a transverse (short-axis) plane or pointed to the patient's head when imaging in coronal or sagittal planes (long-axis). Coronal and sagittal planes together are often referred to as the *longitudinal plane.*
- Real-time needle tracking can be performed using either a longitudinal or transverse approach. With both approaches it is imperative to maintain visualization of the needle tip by keeping it within the plane of the ultrasound beam. Fine tilting movements of the transducer at the point where the needle tip disappears on the screen will confirm the location of the tip.
- It is imperative to establish proper orientation between the transducer and screen in using real-time ultrasound guidance for procedures. If the transducer is mistakenly oriented opposite the screen, the needle will be guided in the opposite direction, increasing the risk of complications until the operator realizes that the transducer must be rotated 180 degrees.

CHAPTER 5

Basic Operation of an Ultrasound Machine

Michel Boivin

KEY POINTS

- The most common imaging modes available on portable ultrasound machines include two-dimensional (2D) or brightness mode (B-mode), motion mode (M-mode), and Doppler mode (color flow and spectral). The vast majority of point-of-care ultrasound applications are performed using 2D mode.
- Depth and gain are the two settings that most often need adjustment to optimize ultrasound images. Acquisition of high-quality ultrasound images is essential for accurate interpretation.
- M-mode, or motion-mode imaging, displays movement of structures over time and is used to assess rapidly moving structures. Color and spectral Doppler display blood flow direction and velocity. Specific machine adjustments are required to optimize Doppler images.

Preparation

Adequate preparation is necessary to acquire the highest quality images while minimizing any discomfort to the patient and provider.

- Ideally, the battery of the ultrasound machine should be fully charged prior to use. When performing real-time ultrasound-guided procedures, it is recommended to keep the machine connected to an electrical outlet in case of battery failure or exhaustion.
- Clean the ultrasound machine, especially the transducers and keyboard, with an approved antiseptic wipe according to local standards. Some antiseptic wipes may contain alcohol or other cleaners that can damage the ultrasound machine's screen, keyboard, and transducers. Consult the manufacturer's operating manual for a list of approved antiseptic wipes.
- An option for patients in contact isolation is the use of disposable clear plastic covers to enclose the entire ultrasound machine.
- Ensure that an adequate supply of gel is available before beginning an ultrasound exam or ultrasound-guided procedure. Sterile gel is required for real-time ultrasound-guided procedures and is often included in sterile transducer cover kits. Gel warmers are commercially available to improve patient comfort.
- Dim the room lighting to ensure optimal viewing of the ultrasound images on the screen.
- For general ultrasound scanning, stand on the patient's right side and position the machine directly in front of you. For cardiac ultrasound scanning, some providers may choose to stand on the patient's left side (see Chapter 4).
- After turning on the power of the ultrasound machine, select the most appropriate transducer for the exam to be performed (see Chapter 3).
- Enter the patient's data (name, medical record number, date of birth) and provider name. Select the type of exam to be performed.
- The patient is generally positioned supine, but position will vary with the type of exam. Cardiac views from the apical or parasternal

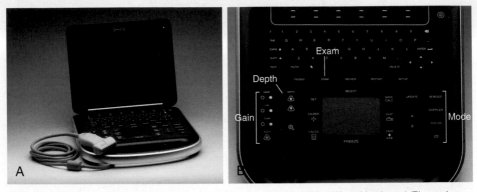

Figure 5.1   Ultrasound Keyboard. A typical portable ultrasound machine (A) and keyboard (B) are shown highlighting the primary controls.

windows are often better acquired with the patient in a left lateral decubitus position. The left and right upper quadrants may be better imaged with the patient in a right or left lateral decubitus position, respectively. Scanning of the posterior chest—including the lungs, pleura, and spine—is best performed with the patient in a seated position. Patient and provider comfort should be optimized prior to starting.

- Keep the patient adequately covered to respect privacy and expose only the body area or areas to be scanned. Body towels are ideal for covering a patient and removing gel postprocedure. Make sure that the room's curtains and door are closed, and consider having a chaperone.
- Sterile transducer sheaths should be used for real-time ultrasound-guided procedures. Sterile gel should be applied to the transducer head, or placed inside the plastic sheath, before covering the transducer with the sterile sheath. The sheathed transducer should be placed on the sterile field pre-procedure.

Image Acquisition

After preparing the ultrasound machine and positioning the patient, the provider must select the most appropriate transducer type, exam preset, and imaging mode to begin acquiring images. Acquisition of high-quality ultrasound images is essential for accurate interpretation. Poor-quality images or imprecise machine settings can lead to missed or incorrect diagnoses. An understanding of the principles of image optimization will allow providers to obtain the highest-quality images. Providers must be familiar with the primary controls on the keyboard of an ultrasound machine (Fig. 5.1).

IMAGING MODES

The most common imaging modes available on portable ultrasound machines include two-dimensional (2D) or brightness mode (B-mode), motion mode (M-mode), and Doppler mode (spectral, color flow). The vast majority of point-of-care ultrasound applications are performed using 2D mode (Fig. 5.2).

Two-Dimensional Mode

Exam presets. Exam presets adjust the ultrasound machine settings—including gain, power, and frame rate—to optimally image different structures. The exam presets will vary depending on the active transducer. Common exam presets include abdominal, cardiac, vascular, obstetrical, musculoskeletal, nerve, and small parts. Only linear transducers have vascular presets, and only phased-array transducers have a cardiac preset. Providers should select the most appropriate exam preset for the organ being scanned and then make fine adjustments manually to optimize the image.

Depth. Depth should be adjusted to position the structure of interest in the center of the screen (Fig. 5.3). Start scanning with a greater depth setting to visualize surrounding structures, especially if an ultrasound-guided procedure is planned; afterward, reduce the depth to center the target structure on the screen. If the depth is too shallow, structures in deep tissues are not visualized and may be missed. If the

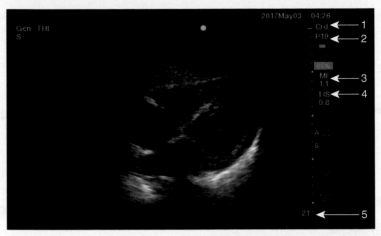

Figure 5.2 Two-Dimensional or B-Mode. A 2D image of a normal subcostal four-chamber view. Note the exam preset (1), transducer type (2), mechanical index (3), thermal index (4), and depth (5).

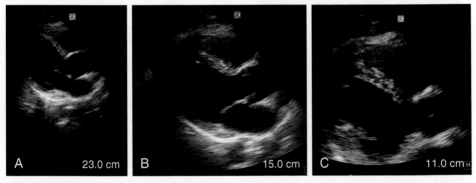

Figure 5.3 Depth. (A) Too deep: the target structure is seen only in the near field. (B) Appropriate depth: target structure is in the center of the screen. (C) Too shallow: the target structure extends beyond the screen and only a portion is visualized. Note the image depth in the lower right hand corner of the screen.

depth is too deep, target structures are seen in the near field but appear small and with lower resolution (Videos 5.1 to 5.3). Additionally, many compact, portable ultrasound devices do not have an adjustable focal zone and the best resolution is obtained with the target structure in the center of the screen.

Gain. Ultrasound waves are attenuated, or weakened, as they travel away from the transducer, reducing the number of returning echoes from deep structures. Thus, the same structure will appear more hyperechoic if it is moved closer to the transducer from the far field to the near field due to less attenuation of sound waves in the near field. Ultrasound

machines compensate for attenuation by automatically increasing gain as depth increases; this is referred to as *time gain compensation.*[1] Most ultrasound machines allow providers to control the amount of time gain compensation by adjusting gain at specific depths using sliders or knobs for near-field and far-field gain adjustments.

Gain adjusts amplification of echoes returning to the receiver. Appropriately adjusted gain is important for accurate image interpretation. When gain is appropriately adjusted, fluid appears black (anechoic), and solid tissues appear along a spectrum from gray to white (hypoechoic, isoechoic, and hyperechoic) as determined by tissue properties (see Chapter

2) (Fig. 5.4). Increasing gain results in brighter images, and decreasing gain results in darker images. The terms *undergained* and *overgained* refer to images that appear too dark or too bright, respectively, due to incorrect gain settings. Undergained images can lead to missed findings because structures appear darker than usual (Fig. 5.5, Videos 5.4 to 5.6).

Zoom. Many ultrasound machines have a zoom feature that allows providers to magnify a structure of interest. Zoom is especially useful in evaluating small structures, such as cardiac valves (Videos 5.7 and 5.8), or when accurate

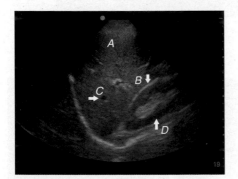

Figure 5.4 Tissue Echogenicity. This normal right-upper-quadrant view demonstrates the isoechoic character of the liver parenchyma *(A)*, hyperechoic fascia between the kidney and liver *(B)*, anechoic blood vessels within the liver *(C)*, and hypoechoic renal cortex relative to the liver parenchyma *(D)*.

measurements are needed, such as the diameter of the common bile duct. Ordinary zoom enlarges the image without changing the resolution, whereas high-resolution zoom increases the resolution of the magnified area.

Focus. The focal zone is the narrowest portion of the ultrasound beam and has the best lateral resolution. Some compact, portable ultrasound devices have the focal zone fixed in the center of the screen, but many ultrasound machines allow the operator to adjust the number and depth of the focal zone or zones. The operator can move the focal zone to the level of the target structure in the near or far field. The primary benefit of increasing the depth of the focal zone is improvement of lateral resolution of deep structures.[1]

Frame rate. When imaging rapidly moving structures such as the heart, the frame rate, or number of frames displayed per second, should be increased on the ultrasound machine. Operators can maximize the frame rate by adjusting two settings: reducing the depth of imaging or narrowing the angle of view (sector angle).[2,3]

M-Mode

M-mode, or motion mode, displays the movement over time of all structures along a single scan line (Fig. 5.6). The main advantage of M-mode is its high sampling rate, which provides good temporal resolution of rapidly moving structures. To use M-mode, center the target structure on the screen in

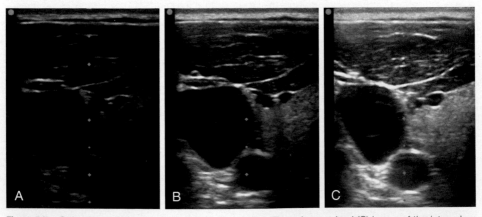

Figure 5.5 Gain. An undergained (A), appropriately gained (B), and overgained (C) image of the internal jugular vein and common carotid artery are shown. Note the poor discrimination between tissues in the undergained image and the artifactual echoes within the internal jugular vein in the overgained image.

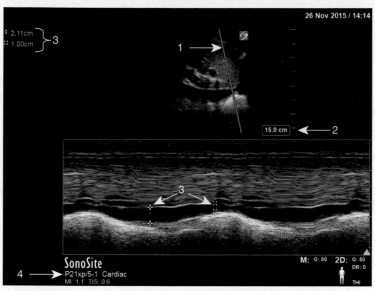

Figure 5.6 **M-Mode.** An M-mode image showing respiratory variation of the inferior vena cava (IVC). Note the M-mode cursor line (1) and depth (2) in the 2D image *(top)*, measurements of IVC collapse (3) in the M-mode image *(bottom)*, and the transducer type and exam preset (4).

2D mode, place the M-mode cursor line over the target structure or structures, and then start M-mode to display the movement of the structures over time. Measurements can be taken by freezing the image. The main utility of M-mode is visualization or measurement of rapidly moving structures, most often the pleura, inferior vena cava, cardiac chambers, and cardiac valves. When measuring distances with M-mode, it is critical to place the cursor line perpendicular to the target structures to obtain accurate measurements.

Doppler Imaging

Color Doppler. Color flow Doppler and power Doppler imaging are used to visualize blood flow. Color flow Doppler is directional and, with conventional settings, blood flow toward the transducer is red and blood flow away from the transducer is blue. The color map on the screen displays the color coding that corresponds to the Doppler shift. Blood flow going toward the transducer has a positive Doppler shift (top of scale) and flow going away from the transducer has a negative Doppler shift (bottom of scale) (Fig. 5.7, Video 5.9). Power Doppler is nondirectional and is more sensitive for low-flow states. Flow velocity is depicted by varying intensities of yellow-orange pulsations

regardless of the direction of flow. Power Doppler is used to assess tissues with low-flow velocities, including the thyroid, synovium of joints, testicles, and urinary jets in the bladder. (Video 5.10).

To utilize color flow or power Doppler, start with a 2D image, center the target structure on the screen, and place the color Doppler box over the target structure. Reduce the size of the color Doppler box to focus on the area of interest. Too large a color Doppler box lowers the frame rate and resolution of the superimposed 2D image.[2,3] The ultrasound beam must be tilted toward or away from the direction of blood flow, ideally with an intercept angle of 0 to 60 degrees. Flow will not be detected if the ultrasound beam is perpendicular to the direction of flow (see also Fig. 2.10). For vascular imaging, the color Doppler box should be steered parallel to blood flow when vessels are being imaged longitudinally.

Gain for color Doppler has to be adjusted, similar to 2D imaging. After activating the color Doppler mode, adjust the gain so that only a few individual color pixels appear on the screen intermittently, with the majority of the color box appearing black. If the gain is set too high, images become cluttered with random color noise, whereas if the gain is set too low,

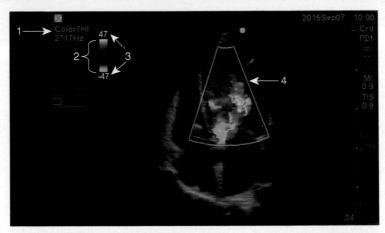

Figure 5.7   Color Flow Doppler Mode. A color flow Doppler image in the apical 5-chamber view showing severe aortic regurgitation. In color flow Doppler mode (1), a color map (2), velocity range or pulse repetition frequency (3), and color box (4) are displayed.

flow will not be detected. Additionally, the velocity scale must be set for low-, medium-, or high-flow velocity.[4] The velocity scale is revealed by the pulse repetition frequency on the color map (Fig. 5.7). When the velocity scale is set too high, low-flow states may not be detected. Conversely, when the velocity scale is set too low for high-flow states, ambiguous signaling, or aliasing, will occur.

Spectral Doppler. Spectral Doppler imaging is particularly useful to measure velocities of blood flow in order to calculate pressure gradients and flow rates. Spectral Doppler signals are presented in graphic format with tracking of velocity or area over time (Fig. 5.8). Spectral Doppler imaging includes pulsed-wave and continuous-wave Doppler. Pulsed-wave Doppler measures velocities in a specific area (sample volume). For vascular imaging, the sample volume gate is centered over the flow of interest and an angle correction line is aligned parallel to the blood flow. For cardiac imaging, the sample volume gate is simply placed over the area of interest without angle correction when the intercept angle is close to 0 degrees. Aliasing, or ambiguous signals, occurs at high velocities above the Nyquist limit, which is the main disadvantage of pulsed-wave Doppler. Techniques to overcome aliasing include increasing the velocity scale, shifting the baseline, using a lower frequency, increasing the angle of insonation (reducing the Doppler shift), reducing the imaging depth, or switching

to continuous-wave Doppler. Continuous-wave Doppler measures velocities over the entire beam. It is not limited by a maximum velocity and sampling occurs along the entire area of interest without any manipulation. Range ambiguity due to measuring velocities in overlapping incident and receiver beams is the main disadvantage of continuous-wave Doppler. See also Chapter 2 for additional details regarding Doppler ultrasound.

Measurements and calculations. Most ultrasound machines have a caliper function to measure distances. Some structures that are commonly measured include the inferior vena cava, left ventricular outflow tract, aorta, bladder, and fluid collections. Most machines have software to calculate measurements into physiologically relevant values, such as bladder volume or cardiac output. Other calculations include measurement of peak velocities or area under the curve of velocity profiles using Doppler mode. Calculations and measurements can be saved and archived with images.

Image storage. Ultrasound machines have internal memory to save still images and video clips. Ultrasound still images and video clips should be archived for the serial monitoring of patients, provider-to-provider communication, and billing requirements (see Chapter 50). Findings from ultrasound exams can be documented in the medical record, either as a separate report or within a standard progress note.

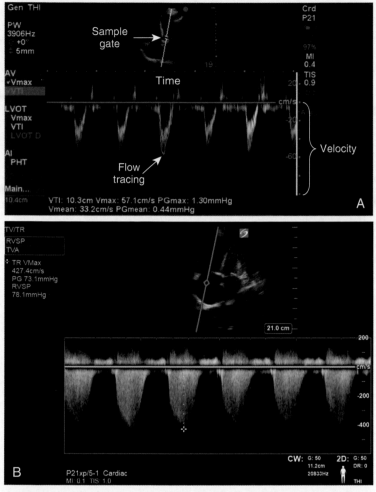

Figure 5.8 Spectral Doppler Mode. Pulsed-wave Doppler (A) is shown measuring the velocity of blood flow through the left ventricular outflow tract. Continuous-wave Doppler (B) is shown measuring the regurgitant jet velocity of severe tricuspid regurgitation.

Postexamination

After completing the ultrasound exam, it is important to place the patient in a safe and comfortable position.

- Clean gel from the patient's skin, raise the bed rails, adjust the bed height, and restore lighting.
- Explain your ultrasound exam findings to the patient. Be cautious to comment only on the structures evaluated and within the scope of the exam performed. Avoid broad, overly simplified statements such as, "Everything looks normal; don't worry about anything."
- End or close the ultrasound exam on the machine so the patient data and images are protected. Ending the exam prevents inadvertently saving another patient's images in the same file. Also, ending the ultrasound exam initiates image archiving in some systems.
- Clean the ultrasound transducer(s) and machine with an approved antiseptic solution or wipe.

• Avoid pushing the ultrasound cart over the transducer cords while transporting the machine to prevent shearing of the cords. Return the ultrasound machine to its storage location.

PEARLS AND PITFALLS

• Gel is the coupling agent that allows ultrasound waves to travel from the transducer to the body. Copious amounts of gel should be used, especially when sliding the transducer over a large skin area. If ultrasonic gel is not available, any liquid-based medium can be used, including water and lubricant gel.

• As depth is increased, gain may have to be adjusted, especially in the far field. Adjust the gain to be appropriately balanced from top to bottom of the screen. Gain slider controls allow fine adjustments at different levels.
• Doppler gain should be set prior to commencing imaging with color flow Doppler. To minimize noise, reduce the Doppler gain until only a few occasional streaks of color appear with the transducer off the patient.
• Be wary of making diagnoses from images with poor gain settings, inappropriate depth, or poor image resolution. Spend enough time to optimize images before interpreting them and making clinical decisions.

CHAPTER 6

Imaging Artifacts

Alfred B. Cheng ■ Alycia Paige Lee ■ Ben Goodgame ■ Nitin Puri

KEY POINTS

- Artifacts are false images or parts of images that do not represent true anatomic structures.
- Artifacts arise when one or more assumptions of sound-wave properties are violated.
- Artifacts disappear when visualized in different planes, whereas true anatomic structures persist when visualized in different planes.

Introduction

Artifacts are false images or parts of images that do not represent true anatomic structures.[1,2] Providers should have a basic understanding of ultrasound artifacts to improve their skills of image acquisition and interpretation at the bedside. Barring equipment malfunction, artifacts originate from erroneous ultrasound signaling due to violation of one or more of the following assumptions:[3-5]

- The speed of sound is constant in all types of human tissue (1540 m/s).
- The ultrasound beam is a single uniform beam of negligible width and thickness.
- Ultrasound waves always travel on a straight path, and reflected ultrasound waves (echoes) return on the same path after reflecting off only one object.
- The attenuation, or decrease in energy, of ultrasound echoes is uniform.
- The amplitude of returning echoes depends on the properties of the reflecting object and the distance to the reflecting object is proportional to the round-trip travel time.
- The time for image processing and reconstruction is negligible.

Artifacts frequently provide insight into tissue makeup and are diagnostic for certain pathologies, such as gallstones and pulmonary edema. Most artifacts can be categorized based on one of four underlying mechanisms:

artifacts of wave propagation, beam characteristics, velocity errors, or attenuation.[6] This chapter reviews some of the most common artifacts encountered in point-of-care ultrasound.

Artifacts of Wave Propagation

REVERBERATION

Sounds waves reflect at tissue interfaces where there is a large difference in the speed of sound between two tissues. This measure of resistance to passage of ultrasound waves through a tissue is called *acoustic impedance*. The amount of sound waves reflected at tissue interfaces is directly proportional to the *difference* in acoustic impedance between two adjacent tissues. If there is no difference in acoustic impedance between two adjacent tissues, no sound waves are reflected. In contrast, if there is a large difference in acoustic impedance, a large proportion of sound waves are reflected.

Reverberation artifact occurs at tissue interfaces with large differences in acoustic impedance, including those with air, metal, and calcium. Reverberation artifact occurs when two or more highly reflective structures are parallel to each other and the ultrasound beam's path is perpendicular to these structures. Ultrasound pulses reflect multiple times between the highly reflective structures. The ultrasound machine displays these reflections as a series of

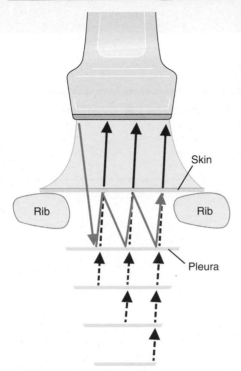

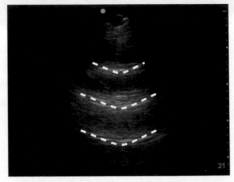

Figure 6.2 Reverberation Artifact. A-lines are an example of reverberation artifact due to repetitive reflections between the pleural surface and skin-transducer interface.

Figure 6.1 Reverberation Artifact. Reverberation artifact results from repetitive reflections between highly reflective surfaces. Reverberation at the pleural surface produces a series of horizontal lines called A-lines.

bright, parallel lines at uniform intervals deep to the reflective structure or structures; these lines dissipate in brightness with depth (Fig. 6.1). The ultrasound machine assigns depth to structures based on the time delay for the echoes to return to the transducer. Echoes that return to the transducer after a single reflection are assigned the actual depth, in contrast to echoes with multiple reflections, which are assigned progressively deeper depths.[6]

A classic example of reverberation artifact, called A-lines, occurs in the lung at the pleural surface (Fig. 6.2; Video 6.1). This specific reverberation artifact is caused by multiple reflections between the highly reflective pleural surface and the skin-transducer interface. A-lines are seen with normal lungs but also with pneumothorax (see Chapter 9 for more details).[7] Reverberation artifacts can be useful in assessing tissue characteristics but they hinder the visualization of deeper structures.

A particular type of reverberation artifact, known as *comet-tail* artifact, is produced when sound waves are reflected between two highly reflective surfaces in very close proximity. The "stacking" of closely spaced reverberations creates an image of bright tapering vertical lines, or comet-tails. After several reflections, the amplitude of returning echoes is decreased, which often appears as tapering of the lines compared with the original echo (Video 6.2).[2] Comet-tail artifacts can be seen in normal and abnormal lungs and are described in more detail in Chapter 9.[8]

Ring-down artifact is similar to comet-tail artifact but is produced by a different mechanism (Fig. 6.3). The source of ring-down artifact is resonant vibrations within a tetrahedron of air bubbles with a central pocket of fluid.[2,9] The ultrasound beam contacts a pocket of trapped fluid, sound waves resonate within the fluid, and a continuous echo is transmitted back to the transducer. The resonant vibrations detected by the ultrasound transducer are displayed as a vertical white band that extends deep to the focus of gas (Video 6.3). Ring-down artifact can be useful in identifying abnormal foci of air in abscesses, vessels (e.g., portal venous gas), or tissue walls (e.g., emphysematous cholecystitis). It is important to recognize that ring-down artifact is caused by air, which is distinct from foreign bodies or calcium, which cause comet-tail artifacts.

A few techniques can minimize the effects of reverberation artifacts. Because reverberations

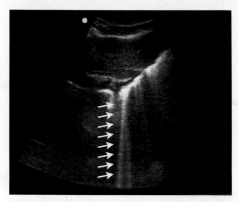

Figure 6.3 Ring-Down Artifact. Ring-down artifact is caused by resonant vibrations in a pocket of fluid surrounded by a tetrahedron of air bubbles, seen here in the hepatic flexure of the colon.

are most pronounced when the ultrasound beam is perpendicular to highly reflective structures, tilting the transducer to change the angle of insonation or imaging plane may lessen reverberations. Similarly, decreasing the distance between the object of interest and ultrasound transducer can reduce reverberation artifact. Tissue harmonic imaging (THI) can reduce artifacts by filtering the fundamental frequencies used and narrowing the width of the ultrasound beam. THI reduces reverberation artifact but improves visualization of comet-tail artifacts.[10] Spatial compounding imaging averages images from multiple planes and reduces visualization of both ring-down and comet-tail artifacts. Therefore, THI should be turned on to enhance visualization of comet-tails, whereas spatial compounding imaging should be turned off to enhance visualization of both comet-tail and ring-down artifacts.[2]

MIRRORING

Mirror-image artifact is created by the reflection of sound waves between a transducer, strong reflector, and target structure, creating a false image behind the reflector. Compared with sound waves reflecting directly to and from a target structure, there is a delay of sound waves reflecting off a strong reflector before returning to the transducer. This delay results in the ultrasound machine displaying a structure identical to the target structure at a deeper depth. The target structure is displayed

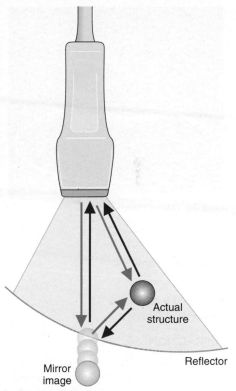

Figure 6.4 Mirror-Image Artifact. The time delay for echoes to reflect off a specular reflector results in the ultrasound machine displaying a mirror image of the actual structure deep to the reflector.

at its actual depth, whereas the mirror image is displayed deep to the strong reflector (Fig. 6.4). The appearance of a mirror image is determined by the shape, sound permeability, and smoothness of the reflector, as well as the angle of insonation of the ultrasound beam.[4] In contrast to reverberation artifacts, which are repetitive reflections of tissue interfaces, mirror-image artifacts are reflections of entire structures or organs.[11] A mirror image can appear deep to any strong reflector, most commonly the diaphragm, pericardium, aorta, bladder, or bowel. Mirror images of the liver or spleen across the diaphragm are normal and should not be confused with a consolidated lower lobe of lung (Fig. 6.5; Videos 6.4 and 6.5). Techniques to reduce mirroring include changing the angle of insonation and decreasing the gain.[2]

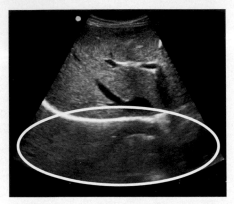

Figure 6.5 Mirror-Image Artifact. A mirror image of the liver is seen above the diaphragm due to the delay in echoes returning to the transducer after reflecting off the diaphragm.

Artifacts Due to Velocity Errors

REFRACTION

Refraction refers to a change in the direction of sound waves at oblique angles as sound waves pass from one tissue to the next. Refraction results from differences in the speed of sound transmission in tissues with differing acoustic properties.[6] The degree of deflection is proportional to the difference in speed of sound of tissues and the angle of incidence of the ultrasound beam. As the differences in speed of sound and angle of incidence increase, the magnitude of refraction increases. Therefore, refraction is most pronounced at fat-soft tissue interfaces, due to differences in speed of sound, and at highly oblique interfaces, such as the lateral aspect of curved structures.[2]

Refraction artifacts include misregistration (displacement of structures), ghosting (duplication of structures), and edge shadowing. *Edge artifact* or *lateral cystic shadowing* is a refractive shadow that occurs at the edges of curved specular reflectors, such as the gallbladder, liver, kidney, bladder, and blood vessels (Fig. 6.6). Specular reflectors are surfaces that reflect sound waves well and send a significant percentage of sound waves back to the ultrasound transducer. At the point where a specular reflector curves, there is a major change in the angle of incidence, and the majority of echoes are refracted rather than reflected, creating

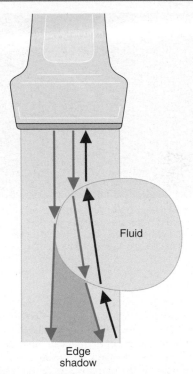

Fluid

Edge shadow

Figure 6.6 Refraction Artifact. Refraction artifact occurs at tissue interfaces that are oblique or curved and have a difference in the speed of sound transmission.

edge artifact, a refractive shadow distal to the curve (Fig. 6.7; Videos 6.6 and 6.7). Edge shadowing can be reduced by changing the angle of insonation and should be differentiated from true shadowing due to stones.[2]

Artifacts Due to Beam Characteristics

LOBE ARTIFACTS

An ultrasound beam is composed of a main lobe and multiple secondary lobes. Side and grating lobes are secondary lobes that project at different angles from the main beam (Fig. 6.8). Side lobes have only 1% of the ultrasound energy of the main beam and typically do not create images.[12] Side-lobe artifacts are created when a strong reflector is in the path of a lobe beam. The machine interprets the reflected sound waves as coming from the main beam and displays the structure on the main beam's

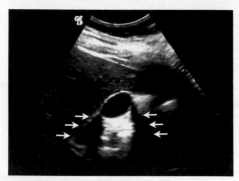

Figure 6.7   Edge Artifact. Edge artifact, a type of refraction artifact, is seen as shadowing along the curved edges of the gallbladder *(arrows).*

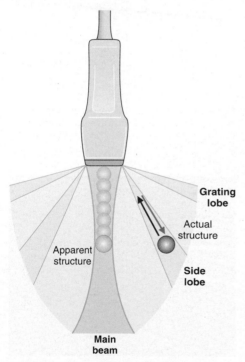

Figure 6.8   Side-Lobe Artifact. Side-lobe artifact is created by reflected sound waves from structures along the path of a side lobe that are displayed as coming from the main ultrasound beam.

path. Side-lobe artifacts are usually seen in the near field of anechoic structures with curved walls—such as the gallbladder, bladder, or heart—or in association with highly reflective interfaces such as air or bone (Video 6.8). If an anechoic or hypoechoic area is not in the near field, lobe artifacts may not be seen.[2] Grating lobes artifacts may be seen when imaging with phased-array transducers.

Multiple techniques can reduce secondary lobe artifacts for more accurate image acquisition. Decreasing gain will reduce low-energy secondary lobes, and using THI can decrease side lobe artifacts. Additionally, secondary lobe artifacts can be reduced by repositioning the patient, changing the angle of insonation, or using a different imaging window. *Apodization,* a common built-in feature of modern portable ultrasound machines, reduces side-lobe artifact by decreasing the pulse amplitude and echo amplification of the outer transducer elements.

Beam-width and *slice-thickness* artifact are two other artifacts attributed to beam characteristics. Beam-width artifact occurs due to limitations of lateral resolution and is most common distal to the focal zone where the ultrasound beam splays to a width greater than the proximal beam. As the beam sweeps from side to side during scanning, structures in the far field appear linear or stretched horizontally (Fig. 6.9). Slice-thickness artifact is due to limitations of elevational resolution. As the ultrasound beam advances distal to the focal zone, the thickness of the beam increases, capturing objects above and below the beam. The ultrasound machine averages the echoes received, and objects may appear linear or fused vertically on the ultrasound display (see Chapter 3 for additional details about image resolution). Techniques to reduce beam-width and slice-thickness artifacts include narrowing the ultrasound beam at the level of the target structure by adjusting the depth of the focal zone(s) or using a standoff pad for superficial structures.[2] THI can reduce these artifacts by narrowing the imaging plane, improving lateral resolution, and reducing the slice thickness.[4,10]

Artifacts Due to Wave Attenuation

ACOUSTIC SHADOWING

Acoustic shadowing is seen distal to highly attenuating structures that either reflect, scatter, or absorb the majority of ultrasound waves (Fig. 6.10). Acoustic shadowing results from violation of the assumption that sound is propagated and attenuated equally throughout the

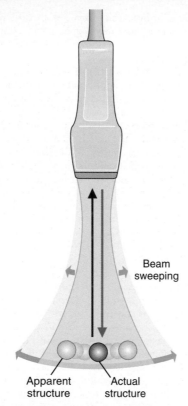

Figure 6.9 Beam-Width Artifact. As the ultra-sound beam widens in the far field, lateral resolution is decreased and structures appear stretched horizontally.

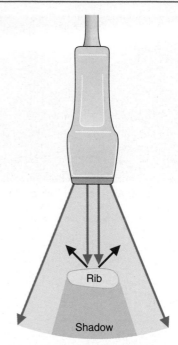

Figure 6.10 Acoustic Shadowing. Acoustic shadowing is seen deep to highly attenuating structures, such as bones, stones, and foreign bodies.

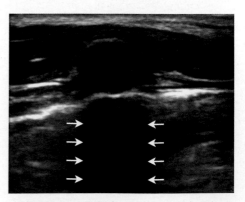

Figure 6.11 Acoustic Shadowing. A rib casting a shadow deep to the pleura.

body. Distal to highly attenuating structures, the amplitude of sound waves is diminished, few echoes return to the transducer, and an area of hypoechogenicity, or *shadowing*, is created (Fig. 6.11; Video 6.9). Acoustic shadowing aids in the diagnosis of gallstones or renal stones (Video 6.10) but hinders the visualization of deep organs. Use of higher frequencies and THI can enhance shadowing. Spatial compounding imaging, excessive beam width, and inappropriate focal zone placement decrease shadowing.[2]

ACOUSTIC ENHANCEMENT

Acoustic enhancement, also called posterior acoustic enhancement, is commonly seen deep to fluid-filled structures. Sound travels through a low-attenuating fluid-filled structure

unimpeded. Therefore, the intensity of the sound waves is preserved as they exit the fluid-filled structure, and high-amplitude echoes are reflected back to the transducer from the tissues deep to the fluid-filled structure. The high-energy echoes returning to the transducer create a bright, hyperechoic appearance of the

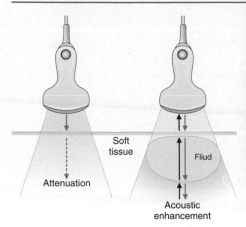

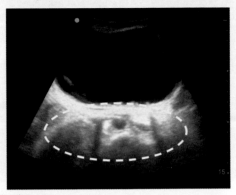

Figure 6.13 Acoustic Enhancement. Acoustic enhancement causes tissues deep to the bladder to appear hyperechoic.

Figure 6.12 Acoustic Enhancement. Fluid-filled structures propagate sound waves unimpeded, causing acoustic enhancement, or hyperechogenicity, of tissues deep to the fluid-filled structure.

deep tissues (Fig. 6.12). Acoustic enhancement is normally seen behind fluid-filled structures, including the bladder (Fig. 6.13; Video 6.11), gallbladder, and large vessels (Video 6.12). Decreasing the far-field gain reduces acoustic enhancement, whereas the use of THI increases acoustic enhancement.[1,2]

PEARLS AND PITFALLS

- Structures should be visualized in at least two planes. If the structure does not persist when visualized in different planes, it is most likely an artifact.
- Reverberation can be diagnostic in the case of A-lines in the lungs. To minimize the presence of reverberation artifact, adjust the transducer's angle of insonation or decrease the distance between the transducer and target structure.
- Tissue harmonic imaging (THI) improves visualization of comet-tail artifacts, whereas spatial compounding imaging reduces visualization of both ring-down and comet-tail artifacts.

- Edge artifact is due to refraction and appears as vertical shadows along the curved surface of structures, such as the gallbladder. By changing the angle of insonation, edge artifact can be differentiated from acoustic shadowing due to stones.
- Beam-width and slice-thickness artifacts are best minimized by adjusting the depth of the focal zone to the level of the target structure.
- Mirroring of the liver or spleen across the diaphragm must be differentiated from lower lobe consolidation by changing the angle of insonation or sliding the transducer cephalad to directly visualize the lower lobe.
- Acoustic shadowing is seen deep to any highly attenuating structure, including stones, bones, foreign bodies, and air. Clean shadows are created by stones and bones, whereas dirty shadows are created by air.
- Acoustic enhancement occurs deep to any fluid-filled structures and can be minimized by reducing the far-field gain to decrease the echogenicity of deep structures.

Lungs and Pleura

CHAPTER 7

Overview

Ken E. Lyn-Kew

KEY POINTS

- Ultrasound waves scatter at an air interface. Normal or partially aerated lungs produce artifacts in discrete patterns that correlate with underlying pathology.
- Thoracic ultrasonography is superior to traditional physical exam or chest radiography and has nearly the same diagnostic accuracy as CT scans in evaluating the causes of acute dyspnea.
- The literature supporting the use of bedside lung ultrasonography (LUS) continues to grow, but the training and credentialing of providers continues to lag behind.

Background

Early descriptions of localizing pleural effusions with ultrasound date back to the 1960s[1]; however, radiologists did not further explore LUS applications owing to a misperception that LUS would be of limited utility due to the highly reflective properties of air. In the 1980s, descriptions of equine LUS emerged in the literature.[2] In the 1990s, innovative research by Daniel Lichtenstein and others demonstrated that ultrasound artifacts created by the pleural line could be correlated with underlying parenchymal and pleural pathologies in critically ill patients.[3-8] These findings included descriptions of lung sliding correlating with an intact parietal and visceral pleural interface and B-lines in pathologic states correlating with interlobular and intralobular septal thickening.[3,5] Building on these findings,

Lichtenstein recognized that consolidated (i.e., airless) lung parenchyma was easily visualized with ultrasound, thus expanding the potential applications of the LUS exam.[9] Further elucidation of these easily recognizable artifacts, combined with the technologic advancement of portable ultrasound machines, has made LUS a common and indispensable application for health care providers.

Indications and Applications

Currently LUS is practiced in nearly all clinical settings, ranging from emergency departments to ambulatory clinics. LUS can facilitate the differential diagnosis of acute respiratory failure by identifying pneumonia, acute pulmonary edema, and pneumothorax; it can also strongly suggest obstructive lung disease or pulmonary embolism using the BLUE (bedside

LUS in emergency) protocol described by Lichtenstein.[10] Trauma services use ultrasound to rapidly diagnose pneumothorax, hemothorax, and lung contusions at the bedside with equal or greater diagnostic accuracy compared with physical exam and chest radiography combined.[11] LUS can also characterize pleural effusions and identify a safe needle-insertion site for drainage, thus reducing the risk of postprocedure complications.[6,12-25]

LUS has been shown to have a diagnostic accuracy that is superior to traditional chest radiography and similar to chest computed tomography (CT) scans. In critically ill patients, LUS has been shown to be a more accurate diagnostic tool than traditional chest radiography for interstitial syndrome (sensitivity 94% vs. 46%), consolidation (sensitivity 100% vs. 38%), pleural effusion (sensitivity 100% vs. 65%),[26] and pneumothorax (sensitivity 88% vs. 52%).[27] Two meta-analyses comparing LUS versus chest CT scans or radiography to diagnose pneumonia reported LUS to have pooled sensitivity and specificity of 85% to 88% and 86% to 93%, respectively.[28,29] In acute care settings, particularly emergency departments and intensive care units, LUS has been shown to expedite diagnosis and reduce the number of imaging studies.[30,31]

LUS can be used to characterize the echogenicity and volume of pleural effusions, thus guiding management.[12-14] Characterization of pleural fluid based on echogenicity and complex features, such as septations, can help to differentiate exudates from transudates. Such characterization of pleural effusions can guide decisions about the timing and method of drainage by thoracentesis, tube thoracostomy, or surgical intervention. Assessment of pleural fluid volume, guidance for thoracentesis, and postprocedure evaluation are all applications of LUS that are supported in the literature, with the added benefit of decreasing complications, radiation exposure, and cost.[16-25] Additionally, LUS can immediately rule out a postprocedure pneumothorax in real time.[32-35]

As the use of pulmonary artery catheters has been shown to be of limited benefit in acute respiratory distress syndrome (ARDS),[36] various papers have looked at differentiating ARDS from acute pulmonary edema by LUS. One study demonstrated that finding areas of interstitial sparing and thickened irregular pleura differentiated ARDS from acute pulmonary edema nearly perfectly.[37] LUS has also

been used to guide lung recruitment during mechanical ventilation.[38] Quantification of extravascular lung water in animal models[39] and patients with congestive heart failure,[40] estimation of pulmonary capillary wedge pressure,[41] as well as response to diuresis and hemodialysis can all be assessed by LUS.[42]

The utilization of LUS extends beyond acute care settings. LUS has been utilized to screen for early interstitial lung disease in patients with systemic sclerosis, thus potentially limiting radiation exposure.[43] LUS can be used in clinics or outpatient procedure centers, as in the intensive care unit (ICU) setting, to guide pleural drainage or the placement of an indwelling catheter in patients with malignant pleural effusions.[44] Postbronchoscopic LUS assessment can evaluate for pneumothorax, thus eliminating the cost, delay, and radiation exposure of chest radiography, which has lower sensitivity than LUS.[32,33]

Limitations

Although LUS is a powerful tool, it has limitations. Inability to acquire high-quality ultrasound images of the lungs is occasionally encountered, as in morbidly obese patients or those with large surgical dressings; the poor resolution of images in these patients limits their interpretation. Similarly, large pneumothoraces interpose air between the chest wall and lung, limiting evaluation of the underlying lung until the pneumothorax is decompressed. In general, the most common barriers to the implementation of point-of-care ultrasound from the perspective of providers include the limited availability of portable ultrasound machines, need for training, and resistance from other specialties using ultrasound.[45-49] Specifically for LUS, an important barrier to implementation into routine clinical practice has been the paucity of trained providers. Although training is increasingly being mandated in graduate medical education, the pool of well-trained faculty to conduct training and apply LUS at the bedside has been limited. Credentialing providers in lung ultrasonography has been a hindrance because there is limited literature on how to demonstrate and maintain competency. Various professional society guidelines describe the equipment, training, and skills needed to perform LUS, offering some guidance in education and credentialing.[50-53] Despite all of the barriers, the field of LUS continues to grow, with more providers using it in their daily practices.[37]

Conclusions

The decreasing size of portable ultrasound machines and evolving software packages have made operation of these machines easier, giving rise to a growing body of literature demonstrating the higher or equivalent sensitivity and specificity of LUS compared with other imaging modalities. By combining clinical and radiographic findings at the bedside, point-of-care LUS serves a powerful diagnostic tool that empowers clinicians to guide management decisions and improve patient care.

CHAPTER 8

Lung and Pleural Ultrasound Technique

Daniel Fein ■ Mohammed M. Abbasi

KEY POINTS

- Low-frequency, phased-array transducers are recommended for complete lung ultrasound (LUS) exams. High-frequency, linear transducers can be used to assess lung sliding, as well as evaluation of pleural pathologies.
- Providers should orient the transducer longitudinally within rib interspaces and ensure that the ultrasound beam is perpendicular to the pleural surface so that reverberation artifacts can be produced. In most clinical circumstances, we advocate for examination of at least three interspaces per hemithorax.
- The interpretation of LUS largely relies on knowledge of the images and artifacts produced at or deep to the pleural line. These findings allow for differentiation of lung pathologies according to their respective air / fluid ratios.

Background

Although often called *lung* sonography, images obtained by ultrasound over the thoracic cage arise largely from the pleural line, making *pleural* sonography a more appropriate descriptor. The reason why pleural-line sonography is diagnostically impactful stems from two insights: (1) In cases of acute respiratory distress or failure, over 90% of attributable pathology will involve the pleural line; and (2) specific pleural-line patterns or "artifacts" correlate with discrete causes of respiratory dysfunction.[1,2]

Unlike chest radiography, whereby an entire view of the thorax is obtained in one image, LUS relies on examination of the pleural surfaces at multiple sites over each hemithorax. The LUS exam points may be considered analogous to traditional physical exam points, but they have a higher sensitivity and specificity than physical examination or chest radiography for multiple diseases states. Multiple clinical studies have shown LUS to have a diagnostic accuracy for acute respiratory pathology nearly equal to that of a computed tomography (CT) scan.[3,4] By first interrogating standard LUS exam points, providers can generate a "mental map" of the distribution of the pleural-line artifacts. The patterns of distribution can then be correlated to specific causes of acute respiratory symptoms (see Chapter 9, Table 9.1). Skilled providers have published multiple reports describing the excellent diagnostic utility of LUS.[5-7] This chapter reviews how to acquire optimal LUS images while avoiding common errors.

Normal Anatomy

The external thorax consists of skin overlying a layer of soft tissue and muscles covering the rib cage. On the inner surface of the ribs lie the parietal pleura. Lubricated by a thin layer of pleural fluid, the visceral pleura slides with respiration against the parietal pleura. The visceral and parietal pleura together are 5 μm thick but are easily visible as a single, hyperechoic, curved line when imaged with ultrasound. Although the two surfaces are indistinguishable on ultrasound, in cases of pneumothorax or pneumonectomy only the parietal pleura will make up the sonographic pleural line.

Deep to the visceral pleura are millions of air-filled alveoli within lobules that are subtended by the interlobular septa. These septa cannot be seen in normal lungs because their width lies below the resolution of ultrasound. The power of LUS to discriminate normal from abnormal lung tissue largely stems from the differentiation between normal and abnormal interlobular septa. When the septa widen from either hydrostatic or permeable fluid infiltration, they then fall within the resolution of ultrasound, allowing the ultrasound waves to propagate into the lung; this results in the imaging artifact called B-lines (see Chapter 9, Fig. 9.8). It should be noted that the fissures that separate the lobes of the lung are made up of the apposition of two pleural surfaces and therefore may normally generate a B-line. Thus, to be considered pathologic, at least three B-lines must be present in a single interspace (see Chapter 9).

Correlation of lung anatomy with position on the chest wall is essential when performing a LUS examination (Fig. 8.1). Anatomically the chest wall is divided into anterior (between the sternum and anterior axillary line), lateral (between the anterior and posterior axillary lines), and posterior (between the posterior axillary line and spine) areas. The upper lobes are seen on the anterior chest wall, the middle lobe (right) and lingula (left) are seen along the anterolateral chest wall, and the lower lobes are seen on the posterolateral chest wall. The costophrenic recesses are generally deepest along the posterolateral chest wall, but the exact intercostal space overlying the costophrenic recesses will vary based on the height of the diaphragm.

Image Acquisition

TRANSDUCER SELECTION

A low-frequency transducer is needed to visualize the deep structures of the thorax. The most common and versatile transducer for LUS imaging is a 3.5- to 5.0-MHz phased-array transducer. Alternatively, some providers may use a curvilinear or microconvex transducer for lung ultrasonography.

A high-frequency linear transducer can also be used but is best limited to evaluate the anterior lung surface for sliding, as in pneumothorax, or to look for pleural irregularities that would distinguish hydrostatic (e.g., cardiogenic pulmonary edema) from inflammatory causes of interstitial syndromes (e.g., acute respiratory distress syndrome [ARDS]).[6] It is also useful for

the evaluation of specific pleural or chest wall pathologies, such as plaques, abscess, tumors, hematoma, or rib fracture.[8] However, the poor penetration of linear transducers of 6 to 9 cm is a major barrier for performing LUS examinations, making it appropriate only for the complete lung evaluation of pediatric patients. The depth limitation becomes especially prohibitive when an examiner aims to identify consolidation, atelectasis, or pleural effusion in an adult.

Pocket ultrasound devices are becoming more accessible to clinicians. It should be recognized that small pocket-sized ultrasound devices, as well as special probes that can connect directly to a smart device, are currently available and may be convenient for performing point-of-care lung ultrasonography. Although most studies have focused on the use of pocket ultrasound devices for echocardiography, there have been studies showing the utility of these devices to diagnose pleural effusions,[9] evaluate for interstitial lung disease,[10] and aid in the diagnosis of dyspnea in a hospitalized patient.[11] Despite these studies, we caution providers that when selecting a pocket device intended for LUS, common limitations of these devices include poor near-field resolution, which limits evaluation of the pleural line; low image resolution quality, which limits the assessment of complex pleural effusions for procedure planning; and reduced imaging depth, which limits the utility of ultrasound in obese patients.

ULTRASOUND SETTINGS

Selecting an appropriate "exam" setting is critical to ensure optimal image resolution. Many new ultrasound machines have an exam preset titled "lung"; however, it is important to note that turning off dynamic filters may improve the visualization of artifacts. The lung exam preset has pre- and postprocessing adjustments, as well as tissue harmonic and compound imaging techniques; these can make the appearance of lung artifacts suboptimal.[12] Therefore our standard approach is to use the "abdominal" exam setting, which is just as effective, if not superior to, the specific lung exam preset. Adjusting the image for minimal gain will help to avoid the common error of acquiring overgained images. Last, in the setting of complex pleural effusions, we have found superior image quality when a "cardiac" exam setting is used because of its improved ability to contrast between areas of fluid, debris, and septations.

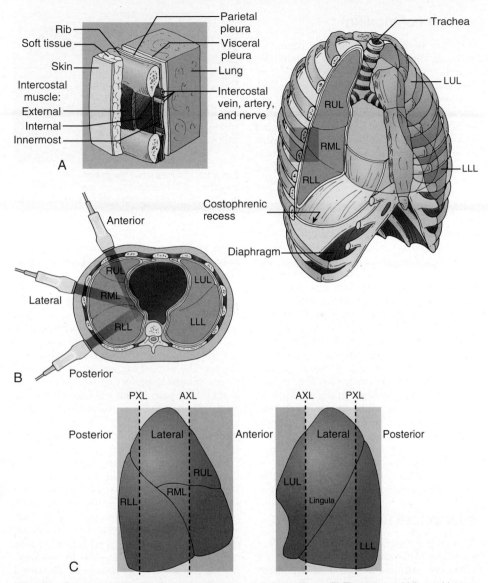

Figure 8.1 Chest Anatomy. (A) Chest wall anatomy of rib interspaces. (B) The upper, middle, and lower lung lobes can be visualized as the transducer is moved on the anterior, lateral, and posterior chest wall. (C) Lateral view of the lung lobes and fissures in relation to the anterior and posterior axillary lines. The upper lobe is primarily anterior, middle lobe/lingula is anterolateral, and the lower lobe is posterolateral. *AXL,* Anterior axillary line; *LLL,* left lower lung; *LUL,* left upper lung; *PXL,* posterior axillary line; *RLL,* right lower lung; *RML,* right middle lung; *RUL,* right upper lung.

Color Doppler is an ultrasound modality often used to determine the direction and velocity of blood or fluid flow within vascular or pleural spaces. Color Doppler has been applied in the evaluation of traumatic pleural communications, intrapulmonary shunting, pneumonia, atelectasis, malignancy, pneumothorax, and lung infarction.[13-15] Despite these potential applications, this modality is not routinely used in point-of-care lung ultrasonography.

PATIENT POSITIONING

LUS may be performed with the patient in essentially any position—supine, semirecumbent, or sitting upright. Owing to the gravity dependence of fluid in the thorax, patient positioning may alter the appearance of the size and character of a pleural effusion. Similarly, interstitial syndromes, with B-line patterns induced by widening of interlobular septa, may be more pronounced in a supine patient. With these exceptions, most patterns of lung pathology are not substantively altered by patient position.

The highest diagnostic yield is often provided by examining the most posterolateral point, or posterolateral alveolar pleural syndrome (PLAPS) point (see below). Given that the majority of consolidations and pleural effusions are found here, the provider must take special care to place the probe at the most posterolateral aspect of the chest wall, just above the level of the diaphragm in a supine patient. This maneuver often requires a gentle lifting or rolling of the patient away from the side being examined, which may be challenging, especially when patients are critically ill, restrained, sedated, or obese. In these instances, it may prove prudent to obtain help to roll the patient to a semidecubitus position or to raise the arms off the bed so that clinically significant findings are not missed. When examining a patient in the recumbent position, certain maneuvers, such as raising the patient's arm to rest over the chest and abdomen or having the patient perform a deep inspiration, may widen the intercostal spaces, thus improving visualization.

TRANSDUCER HANDLING

The transducer should be held like a pen, perpendicular to the patient's chest wall with the transducer orientation marker always pointing toward the head (Fig. 8.2). The screen marker should be set to the upper left side of the screen, a location that is standard when using an "abdominal" or "lung" exam setting but must be switched if using a "cardiac" setting to evaluate a pleural effusion. Thus, when imaging the thorax, the left side of the screen will be cephalad and the right side will be caudad. When visualizing the diaphragm in this orientation, the area to the left of the diaphragm is within the thorax, whereas the area to the right is within the abdomen. If the machine was previously used with a cardiac

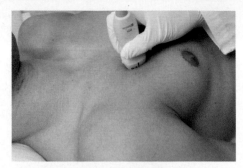

Figure 8.2   Transducer Orientation. The transducer should be held like a pen, oriented with the transducer marker pointed cephalad, and centered over a rib interspace.

exam preset, the screen marker will be on the right side of the screen, with potential for an error in orientation.

NORMAL LUNG PATTERN

It is important to recognize the normal appearance of lungs and pleura before discussing specific techniques to acquire high-quality images. The normal appearance of lungs and pleura must be recognized in intercostal spaces over (1) lung parenchyma and (2) costophrenic recesses (Fig. 8.3). Two characteristics define normal, healthy lungs: (1) "lung sliding," a shimmering or sliding of the visceral pleura against the parietal pleura during respiration (Video 8.1), and (2) A-lines, hyperechoic horizontal lines that are equidistant from the pleural line (Fig. 8.4, Video 8.2). A-lines are reverberation artifacts created by repetitive reflection between the pleural line and transducer. A-lines are best seen when the transducer is positioned perpendicularly to the curved surface of the lung. A-line pattern signifies the absence of other pathologic ultrasound signs, such as pleural effusion, consolidation, and interstitial syndrome. The next chapter (Chapter 9) provides an in-depth discussion of LUS interpretation.

TECHNIQUE

Holding the transducer like a pen, the provider must first center the transducer longitudinally with the transducer orientation marker pointed cephalad over an intercostal space so that rib shadows are seen on either side of the screen. Rib shadows result from failure of ultrasound

Chest Wall

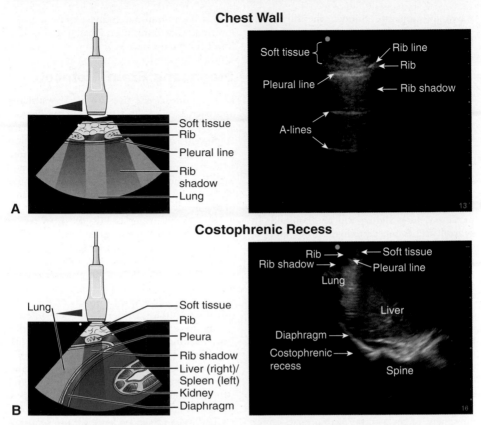

Costophrenic Recess

Figure 8.3   Normal Lung and Pleura. (A) With the screen marker in the upper-left corner, the transducer is centered in between two ribs in a longitudinal plane. The chest wall—with soft tissue, ribs, pleura, and A-lines—is seen. (B) The diaphragm, subdiaphragmatic organs, and inferiormost portion of lung are seen in a costophrenic recess.

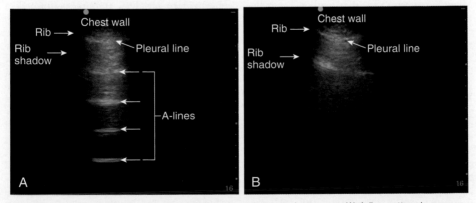

Figure 8.4   A-Lines. These two images are taken from the same interspace. (A) A-line pattern is seen when the transducer is perpendicular to the pleural surface. (B) A nondiagnostic pattern is shown when the transducer is tilted slightly away from the perpendicular plane.

waves to propagate through the rib's bony structure. Rib shadows obscure underlying lung tissue but serve to orient the provider to the image on the screen. The superficial edge of the ribs forms the *rib line*, an approximately 2-cm hyperechoic curvilinear line. The *pleural line* is the first horizontal, curvilinear, hyperechoic line; it is 5 mm deep to the rib line and represents the apposition of the parietal and visceral pleura (see Fig. 8.3).

Lung sliding with repeated A-lines separated by an equal distance are seen in normal lungs. Sliding should not be relied upon as the defining characteristic of the pleural line because, in pathologic conditions such as pneumothorax, lung sliding will be abolished. In general, the A-line pattern must be "brought out" by the provider aligning the transducer perpendicular to the pleural surface; otherwise a nondiagnostic pattern is seen, often referred to as a "non-A, non-B" pattern. (see Fig. 8.4, Video 8.2). If the pleural line, A-line, or other pathologic findings (B-lines, consolidation, or pleural effusion) are not visualized, the provider should gently tilt, rock, or slide the transducer on the chest wall until one of these patterns can be clearly identified.

If lung sliding is subtle or indeterminate using 2D ultrasound then M-mode, or "motion" mode, can be used to evaluate for movement of the visceral pleura. First, center the transducer over an intercostal space and then press the M-mode button. Next, align the M-mode cursor line perpendicular to the pleural line. Press the M-mode button again, or "start," and the motion of the tissues along the cursor line will be displayed over time. The M-mode pattern called the "seashore" sign signifies the presence of normal lung sliding, and the "bar code" or "stratosphere" sign signifies the absence of lung sliding (Fig. 8.5).

Providers should be mindful of the varying depth settings required in examining different points on the thorax and different pathologies. When focusing primarily on the pleural line, a maximum depth of 7.5 to 10 cm should be used to optimize the pleural line's resolution and avoid attenuation of diagnostic artifacts. When evaluating the underlying lung parenchyma, especially the lower lung fields where the majority of consolidations and pleural effusions occur, depths of at least 13 to 16 cm should be used to adequately visualize the diaphragm and thoracic structures. Recall that structures deeper than 6-9 cm cannot be seen

with a linear transducer, and require use of a low-frequency transducer (phased-array, curvilinear, or microconvex).

Diagnostic Exam Protocol

LUS is most effective when a systematic approach is used. Prior investigations demonstrating the clinical utility of LUS have employed a variety of structured examination protocols,[2,16-18] with the number of rib interspaces examined ranging from 3 to 16 over each hemithorax. From these studies, it should be recognized that similar and large amounts of diagnostic information can be acquired from focused exams using as little as three points per hemithorax.[1] Some experts advocate for tailoring the exam protocol depending on the clinical question. For example, in a rapid evaluation of pneumothorax, the provider should focus on imaging one to two interspaces over the most nondependent portion of the anterior lung surface (i.e., the inferior anterior thorax in a supine patient or the superior anterior thorax in a semirecumbent patient). If interstitial syndrome is suspected, interrogation of multiple points over the anterior and lateral chest should be performed. For pleural effusions and consolidations, inclusion of posterolateral areas is essential.[19]

The most robust evidence for use of a thoracic ultrasonography exam protocol in critically ill patients comes from the landmark study, "The Relevance of Lung Ultrasound in the Diagnosis of Acute Respiratory Failure," by Daniel Lichtenstein.[2] This study introduced the BLUE (bedside Lung Ultrasound in emergency) protocol. The authors performed a six-point per hemithorax LUS exam, examining three zones with two interspaces per zone (upper and lower areas in each zone). The three zones encompassed the anterior chest wall, lateral chest wall, and posterolateral chest wall, respectively. Patients with acute respiratory failure were evaluated for the presence and location of A-lines, B-lines, lung sliding, alveolar consolidation, and pleural effusion, as well as both upper and lower extremity deep venous thrombosis. Associating the LUS patterns with the causes of disease, patients were given a diagnosis of pulmonary edema, pulmonary embolism, pneumonia, chronic obstructive pulmonary disease (COPD)/asthma, or pneumothorax (see Chapter 9, Table 9.1). These diagnoses derived from LUS findings alone

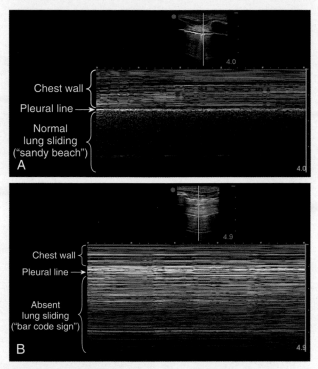

Figure 8.5 Lung Sliding in M-Mode. (A) Normal lung sliding is seen as a seashore pattern (chest wall = ocean waves; normal aerated lung = sandy beach). (B) Absent lung sliding is seen as a bar-code pattern (horizontal lines throughout the image).

proved to be correct in an astonishing 90.5% of examined patients. Lichtenstein later further simplified this exam protocol, advocating for a "three-point" anatomic exam—that is, interrogating only one interspace in the upper lobe, middle lobe/lingula, and lower lobe.[1]

Based on Lichtenstein's work and our own experience, we advocate for a simplified lung exam protocol with three distinct anatomic zones per hemithorax for its accuracy, simplicity and efficiency. An important difference with this three-zone exam is that we avoid limiting interrogation to a specific point on the chest wall or intercostal space but rather focus on imaging the anterior, lateral, and posterior zones, which approximate the upper, middle/lingular, and lower lobes (Fig. 8.6). When interrogating a lung zone, the operator can quickly survey an intercostal space above, below, and next to the presumed center of the lobe or area of pathology and save a single clip of the most abnormal intercostal space of the zone being examined. Certain circumstances—such as prone positioning, presence of surgical

dressings, subcutaneous emphysema, or burn injury—can limit LUS imaging, and the exam protocol may have to be modified.

The most posterior point, also called the "PLAPS" point (posterolateral alveolar pleural syndrome), is generally the highest-yield view, yielding a large number of pleural effusions and alveolar consolidations that would otherwise have been overlooked.[2,7] In a supine patient, it is imperative to image the most posterior point by gripping the transducer in the palm, as one would hold a flashlight, ensuring the transducer face points up from the horizontal plane, "toward the sky." The importance of inserting the transducer between the bed and patient while pointing the transducer face upward cannot be overemphasized. Scanning critically ill, obese, sedated, or restrained patients is often challenging, but failure to insert the transducer between the bed and patient with the probe pointing upward can be a major source of error. An off-axis image of the skin and soft tissue of the axilla can be created if the probe face is not perpendicular

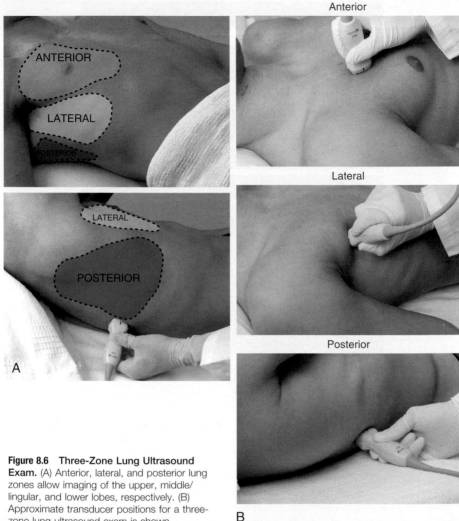

Figure 8.6   Three-Zone Lung Ultrasound Exam. (A) Anterior, lateral, and posterior lung zones allow imaging of the upper, middle/lingular, and lower lobes, respectively. (B) Approximate transducer positions for a three-zone lung ultrasound exam is shown.

to the chest wall and can be mistaken for pneumonia, known as *pseudoconsolidation*. Of equal importance is ensuring that the most posterior view includes definitive identification of the diaphragm. This view allows visualization of pathology in the most dependent portion of the lower lobe next to the diaphragm. The diaphragm is positioned toward the right of the screen (Fig. 8.7).

Interstitial Syndrome Protocols

The presence of bilateral multiple B-lines, also referred to as *interstitial syndrome*, was found

to have a 97% sensitivity and 95% specificity for cardiogenic pulmonary edema in critically ill patients with acute respiratory failure using Lichtenstein's six-point per hemithorax BLUE protocol.[1]

The International Consensus Conference on Lung Ultrasound recommends a four-zone per hemithorax scanning method in the semiquantitative evaluation of interstitial syndrome,[20] recognizing that, solely for diagnosis, a two-zone protocol has also been shown to be sufficient.[6,21] Note that in the protocol using four zones per hemithorax, only the anterior and lateral lung surfaces are examined. The presence of interstitial syndrome is defined as two or more positive interspaces bilaterally, where a positive region is defined as the presence of three or more B-lines between two rib spaces.[6] This was found to have a sensitivity of 85.7% and a specificity of 97.7%, respectively, for alveolar-interstitial syndrome compared with chest radiography.[12]

Sensitivity for identifying interstitial syndrome can be increased by scanning more regions. In scanning 10 zones, Copetti et al. identified that the presence of interstitial syndrome was 100% sensitive for both pulmonary edema and ARDS.[6] More extensive protocols have also been described, including a 12-zone method[22] and a 28-zone method.[18] The 28-zone method has been shown to be highly predictive of volume removal in dialysis patients,[23] and LUS findings have been shown to be superior to physical exam findings.[24] In patients with congestive heart failure, the quantification of B-lines prior to discharge (>15, using the 28-zone method) was found to be associated with a greater than 11 times risk of readmission for heart failure by 6 months.[25]

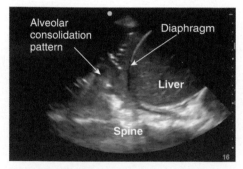

Figure 8.7 Diaphragm. Identification of the diaphragm is an essential step when evaluating the posterior lung zone. A dependent alveolar consolidation is seen in the lower lobe just above the diaphragm.

PEARLS AND PITFALLS

- The screen orientation marker should be set to the upper left of the screen for lung and pleural sonography. This is a common source of error if the machine was previously used with the cardiac exam preset.
- Depth should be appropriately adjusted during a thoracic exam: 7.5 to 10 cm to examine the pleural line and at least 13 to 16 cm to examine the lung parenchyma, particularly along the posterolateral lung surface and diaphragm.
- Upon placing the transducer on the chest, if a nondiagnostic (non-A-line, non-B-line) pattern is seen, the provider should first make sure that the transducer is longitudinally oriented in between two ribs. The pleural line is 5 mm deep to the ribs. Second, tilt the transducer to align the ultrasound beam perpendicular to the pleural surface, so that A-lines can be generated if present.
- Adjust the image to have minimal gain and thus avoid the common error of acquiring overgained images (Fig. 8.8).

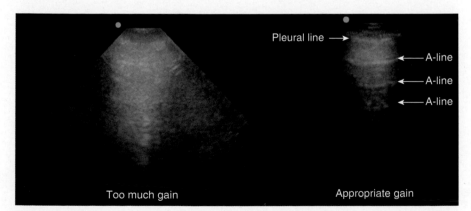

Figure 8.8 Gain Setting. (A) An overgained image makes it difficult to appreciate A-lines and may be mistaken to indicate pulmonary edema. (B) An appropriately gained image taken from the same location reveals the presence of A-lines.

An overgained LUS image may lead to the false appearance of an interstitial disease pattern or debris within a pleural effusion.

- It is imperative to evaluate the most posterior point attainable at the level of the diaphragm. Imaging at this point may sometimes require an additional provider to help lift or roll the patient. Point the transducer face at least partially "to the sky" to ensure an exam of the most posterior dependent lung.

CHAPTER 9

Lung Ultrasound Interpretation

Irene Ma ■ Vicki E. Noble

KEY POINTS

- Normal lung aeration pattern on ultrasound is defined by pleural sliding and A-lines throughout the lungs as well as curtain sign at the lung bases. Although termed "normal aeration", this pattern can be seen in diseases such as asthma, obstructive lung disease, and pulmonary embolism.
- Presence of lung sliding rules out pneumothorax at the point of interrogation, but absence of lung sliding can be due to causes other than pneumothorax.
- In alveolar consolidation patterns, differentiation between atelectasis and pneumonia requires a visual assessment of lung volume loss vs. gain of the consolidated lobe, and inclusion of other clinical data.

Background

A sonographic assessment of discrete points over the chest wall allows providers to gather a global, accurate assessment of underlying lung pathology.[1-3] The interpretation of lung ultrasound patterns requires knowledge and understanding of the unique interactions of ultrasound waves within air-fluid interfaces in both normal and pathologic states. This chapter reviews the characterization of discrete lung ultrasound patterns that allow immediate clinical application in the management and monitoring of patients.

Lungs are predominantly filled with air in the normal state. The lung parenchyma has a fine architecture of pulmonary lobules surrounding respiratory bronchioles. A small amount of serous fluid lubricates the space between the visceral and parietal pleura. Air within the normal lung, directly beneath the visceral pleura, serves as an acoustic barrier to the penetration of ultrasound waves. The normal interlobular and intralobular septa are below the resolution of common ultrasound frequencies, and ultrasound waves cannot propagate in air-filled, "dry" lungs with microns-thick septa. The inability of ultrasound waves to propagate in normal lungs is the key characteristic

defining the utility of lung ultrasound. As soon as the septa are widened or distended with interstitial fluid due to either permeability deficits or elevated hydrostatic pressure, ultrasound waves can propagate into the lung, and the earliest finding of lung fluid accumulation is seen as B-lines. As fluid continues to accumulate in the interstitium, alveoli, and eventually pleura, the pathologic findings progress along a spectrum of air/fluid ratios, from B-lines to alveolar consolidation to pleural effusion (Fig. 9.1).[1]

Image Interpretation

NORMAL LUNG

The normal lung has three sonographic features: A-lines, lung sliding, and the curtain sign at the lung bases.

A-lines appear as horizontal lines deep to the pleural line. They are produced by pleural line reverberations from sound waves trapped between the skin/transducer interface and pleura. The distance between two successive A-lines is the same as the distance between the transducer and the pleural line (Fig. 9.2, Video 9.1). The pleura's dense fibrinous nature makes it highly reflective. There are two reasons why normal aerated lung parenchyma

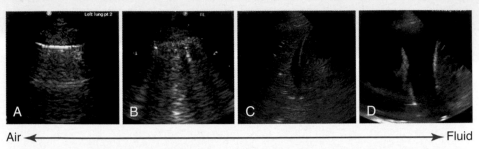

Air ◄──► Fluid

Figure 9.1   Air/Fluid Ratios and Lung Artifacts. (A) A-lines are seen in a "dry" lung, with no fluid-filled or thickened interlobular septa. (B) B-lines appear as fluid begins to widen the interlobular septa. (C) Consolidation pattern is seen when fluid completely fills the alveoli, displacing air. (D) Pleural effusion with consolidation pattern from compressive atelectasis is seen with fluid accumulation in the pleural space.

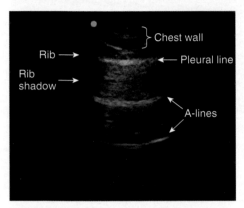

Figure 9.2   A-Lines. A-lines are a type of reverberation artifact that appears as horizontal, hyperechoic lines seen deep to the pleural line, repeating at the same distance as between the transducer and the pleural line.

is not visualized by ultrasound: (1) air beneath the pleural line scatters any sounds waves that penetrate through the pleura and (2) normal subpleural interlobular septa are so thin that they fall below the resolution of ultrasound. Therefore A-lines are horizontal lines beneath the pleura that occur at regular intervals, signify that air is present below the pleural line, and are seen with normal air-filled lung parenchyma.

Lung sliding is a dynamic finding seen in healthy lungs when the visceral and parietal pleural surfaces are apposed and the visceral pleural surface moves freely with respirations (Videos 9.2 and 9.3). This dynamic movement of the pleural line has a shimmering appearance. The movement may be difficult to appreciate where there is less lung movement, such

as at the lung apices, or when the patient is taking shallow breaths. Providers use M-mode to confirm lung sliding, especially when lung sliding is not obvious by two-dimensional ultrasound. M-mode depicts the movement of all tissues along a single scan line over time. The normal respiratory movement of the visceral pleura by M-mode is referred to as the "seashore" sign (Fig. 9.3).[4] The chest wall is less mobile, appearing as a series of horizontal lines, whereas the lung parenchyma is more mobile; it moves back and forth, giving it a grainy appearance by M-mode. The chest wall represents the "calm sea" and the lung parenchyma represents the "rough sand" of the seashore sign. Additionally, normal pleura should be uniformly thin (<0.3 mm) and without irregularities.[5] Zooming into the pleura may help to better characterize pleural irregularities.

Adjacent to the diaphragm, the normally aerated lung base appears as an impenetrable "curtain" that obscures the area where the diaphragm and subdiaphragmatic structures (i.e., liver/spleen) were seen before respiratory descent (Fig. 9.4 and Video 9.4).

A normal lung ultrasound exam shows a thin pleural line with lung sliding and A-lines throughout both hemithoraces and the curtain sign at the lung bases. These findings allow clinicians to conclude that the lung parenchyma is normally aerated or "dry." When these normal findings appear bilaterally in a dyspneic patient, the differential diagnosis is similar to that of a dyspneic patient with a normal chest radiograph: (1) obstructive airway diseases, such as chronic obstructive pulmonary disease (COPD) or asthma; (2) pulmonary embolism; or (3) nonpulmonary causes (neurologic, neuromuscular, or acid/base disorders; or disorders with reduced oxygen-carrying capacity).

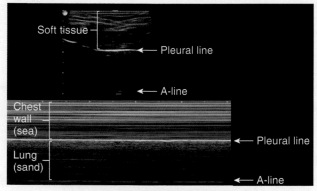

Figure 9.3   Normal Lung in M-Mode ("Seashore Sign"). The horizontal lines above the pleural line represent the "sea" which is the relatively immobile soft tissue of the chest wall. The grainy tissue below the pleural line represents the "sand" which is the relatively mobile aerated lung parenchyma.

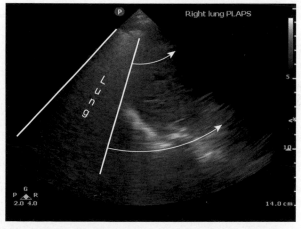

Figure 9.4   Curtain Sign. Air within the descending lung base obscures the area above the descending diaphragm as the lung descends during inspiration.

The main utility of the identification of diffuse normal sonographic findings is to effectively rule out the presence of significant pulmonary edema, pneumonia, and pneumothorax. To further evaluate the undifferentiated dyspneic patient, the ultrasound approach may include a search for deep venous thrombosis (DVT; see Chapter 34), assessment of the inferior vena cava (IVC; see Chapter 17), and evaluation of left ventricular systolic function (see Chapter 15). The presence of a positive DVT scan in patients with acute respiratory failure but normal lung ultrasound may result in a specificity and positive predictive value for pulmonary embolism as high as 99% and 94%, respectively.[1]

PATHOLOGIC LUNG

The diseased lung can generally be characterized by looking at three abnormal findings: absence of lung sliding, B-lines, and consolidation (Table 9.1).

ABSENCE OF LUNG SLIDING

As discussed previously, lung sliding is caused by independent respiratory movements of the visceral pleural surface when directly apposed against the parietal pleura. When lung sliding is absent, it is pathologic, and suggests the possibility of a pneumothorax. Air accumulation in between the visceral and parietal pleura

TABLE 9.1   **Summary of Pathologic Lung Ultrasound Findings**

Condition	Ultrasound Findings
Cardiogenic pulmonary edema	• Diffuse bilateral B-lines • Normal lung sliding • Pleural effusion may be present
Pneumonia	• Early: Focal unilateral B-lines, normal lung sliding • Advanced: Consolidation bounded by B-lines, dynamic air bronchograms, reduced or absent lung sliding • Pleural effusion may be present
COPD or asthma	• Bilateral A-lines with normal lung sliding • Reduced or absent lung sliding without lung point in severe COPD/asthma
Pulmonary embolism	• Bilateral A-lines • Deep venous thrombosis
Pneumothorax	• Absent lung sliding <u>with</u> lung point • Absent anterior B-lines

COPD, Chronic obstructive pulmonary disease.

obscures visualization of the visceral pleura which is displaced away from the parietal pleura by air (Videos 9.5 and 9.6). However, pneumothorax is not the only cause of absent lung sliding, given that pleurodesis (chemical pleurodesis, infectious or inflammatory states, or fibrotic lung diseases), lung volume loss (complete atelectasis, mucous plugging, pneumonectomy), and reduced or absent lung ventilation (apnea, mainstem intubation) also cause a lack of lung sliding (Video 9.7).[6] Thus absence of lung sliding is not specific to pneumothorax, but presence of lung sliding definitively rules out pneumothorax with 100% specificity at the site of interrogation.[7]

When absence of lung sliding is due to causes other than pneumothorax, the absence of lung sliding is "real"—the visceral pleura is truly not moving even though the visceral and parietal pleura are apposed. However, in pneumothorax, the visceral pleura is moving, but this movement cannot be visualized because the air trapped in the pleural space scatters all ultrasound waves, preventing them from propagating deep enough to reflect off the visceral pleura. Thus, only the immobile parietal pleura is seen, resulting in visualization of absent lung sliding. Lack of movement deep to the parietal pleura can be confirmed using M-mode. The static appearance of the M-mode pattern both above and below the pleural line result in a pattern commonly called the "barcode sign" or "stratosphere sign" (Fig. 9.5).[2]

Fortunately, there is a sign that is relatively specific to pneumothorax called the *lung point*. This dynamic sign is caused by an edge of normal aerated lung sliding into view within an interspace where absent lung sliding and A-lines are seen. As the visceral pleura expands and slides into the interspace being examined, pleural air from the pneumothorax is pushed away by normal lung, and the sliding visceral pleura can be seen (Fig. 9.6, Video 9.8). Lung point is defined as a sudden appearance of lung sliding and should not be confused with the inferior edge of the lung sliding into view along the heart border or at the lung bases where the "curtain sign" is seen (Fig. 9.7 and Video 9.9). Lung point is 100% specific for pneumothorax and may be localized by sliding the transducer laterally. An estimation of the size of a pneumothorax can be performed by assessing the distance laterally between the sternum and lung point. Large pneumothoraces will have a more lateral lung point.[4,8,9]

Although only one sign *(lung point)* is specific for pneumothorax, the presence of a number of findings can rule out pneumothorax at the site of ultrasound interrogation, including lung sliding, B-lines (see below), and lung pulse.[7] Lung pulse is observed as rhythmic pleural pulsations due to the transmission of cardiac contractions to the pleura. Lung pulse signifies that the visceral and parietal pleura are apposed (Video 9.10).[10]

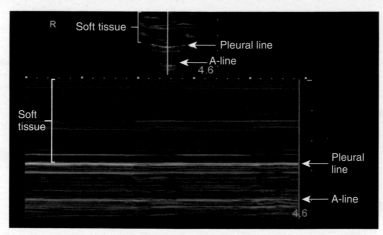

Figure 9.5 **Absent Lung Sliding in M-Mode ("Barcode Sign").** The horizontal lines both above and below the pleural line represent the relatively immobile chest wall and lack of movement just below the parietal pleura, respectively.

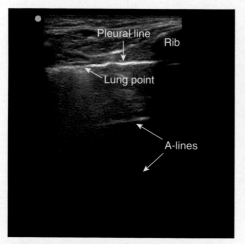

Figure 9.6 **Lung Point.** A lung point is the boundary between aerated lung and air in the pleural space (pneumothorax).

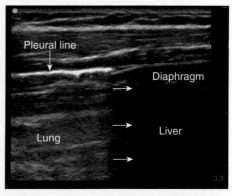

Figure 9.7 **Pseudo-Lung Point.** As the diaphragm and liver descend, the inferior most portion of lung slides into the costophrenic recess, giving the false appearance of a lung point.

Characteristics of the pleura may give clues to the underlying etiology causing a lack of lung sliding. If the pleura is thickened, scarred, and irregular, a more chronic lung process is suggested, whereas a very thin, uniformly smooth pleura suggests an acute process, such as spontaneous pneumothorax. In addition, vertical reverberation artifacts, or comet-tail artifacts, are seen emanating from the pleural line only when the visceral and parietal pleura are apposed. Thus, the lack of lung sliding in the presence of comet-tail artifacts signifies that the pleural surfaces are adhered, most often due to pleurodesis or scarring.

B-LINES

Normal subpleural interlobular septa fall below the resolution of ultrasound. However, interlobular septa can become thickened in a number of diseased states. Thickening of the interlobular septa may be due to fluid accumulation from increased hydrostatic pressure, such as pulmonary edema; increased capillary permeability caused by infectious states, such as pneumonia, acute lung injury,

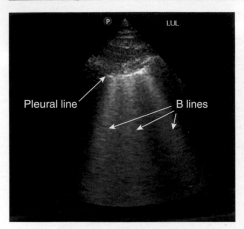

Figure 9.8   B-Lines. B-lines are seen when interlobular septa are thickened due to fluid or scarring. B-lines are also called "lung rockets."

or pulmonary hemorrhage; or from collagen, fibrous tissue, or cellular deposition, such as lymphangitic carcinomatosis, interstitial lung diseases, sarcoidosis, or other inflammatory diseases. In these conditions, the widened interlobular septa propagate ultrasound waves, producing a comet-tail reverberation artifact known as B-lines (Fig. 9.8 and Video 9.11).[7,11] B-lines are often remembered as being similar to Kerley B-lines seen on conventional chest radiographs.[12] Isolated B-lines can been seen in the lung bases due to gravity-dependent fluid widening the septa.[11] Fissures can also produce a single B-line. To be pathologic, three or more B-lines must be present in a single rib interspace.[7]

Mapping the distribution of B-lines can assist in narrowing the differential diagnoses, similar to interpreting bilateral versus unilateral opacities on chest radiographs. Bilateral B-lines are present in conditions such as pulmonary edema, diffuse interstitial pneumonitis/infections, acute respiratory distress syndrome, and interstitial lung disease.[7,13,14] Unilateral or focal B-lines are commonly seen in conditions such as focal pneumonia, atelectasis, lung contusion, pulmonary infarct, or malignancy.[15]

B-lines are commonly confused with other vertically appearing artifacts. B-lines are defined by the following distinctive features, which should be noted during interpretation:
- B-lines are ray-like, hyperechoic, vertical, and discrete.
- B-lines emanate from the pleural line, never above the pleural line.

- B-lines move with lung sliding.
- B-lines extend to the periphery of the far field on the screen.

The artifacts that are sometimes confused with B-lines include E-lines and Z-lines. E-lines are similar in appearance to B-lines except that they do not arise from the pleural line.[6] Seen in subcutaneous emphysema, E-lines are artifacts caused by the presence of air in the subcutaneous tissues. Although Z-lines do arise from the pleural line, they have the following features that allow them to be differentiated from B-lines[2]:
- Z-lines do not extend to the bottom of the screen and usually attenuate after 2 to 4 cm.
- Z-lines are less echogenic than the pleural line.
- Z-lines are not as discrete as B lines and do not move with the pleural line.
- Z-lines have no pathologic significance and are often seen in normal patients.

CONSOLIDATION

When the alveoli are filled with fluid (pneumonia) or are collapsed (atelectasis), the lack of air in the lung parenchyma facilitates propagation of ultrasound waves, allowing visualization of the lung. Lung parenchyma becomes well defined with echogenicity similar to the liver, referred to as *hepatization* (Fig. 9.9 and Video 9.12). Large basilar consolidations by the liver, spleen, and dome of the diaphragm can easily be detected by ultrasound though often remaining occult on portable chest radiographs.[16-19] It is important to understand that "alveolar consolidation pattern" is descriptive and not diagnostic, given its multiple possible etiologies. Additional clinical findings can help differentiate between consolidation due to pneumonia versus compressive or resorptive atelectasis.

Pneumonia

Compared with chest radiographs, lung ultrasound has higher sensitivity for the diagnosis of pneumonia.[20,21] In a systematic review, the pooled sensitivity of lung ultrasound was 93% compared with 54% for chest radiographs for the diagnosis of pneumonia, using chest computed tomography as the gold standard.[21]

Lobar pneumonia results in consolidation, which appears as a tissue-like density of the lung (hepatization) without volume loss (Video 9.13).[22] Consolidation that is not translobar

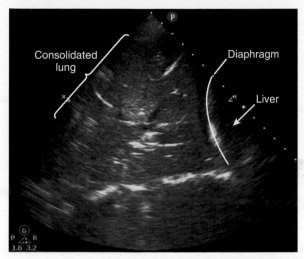

Figure 9.9   Alveolar Consolidation. A consolidation pattern is seen just above the diaphragm (left half of image). Echogenicity of the consolidated lung is similar to that of the liver; this is described as "hepatization" of the lung.

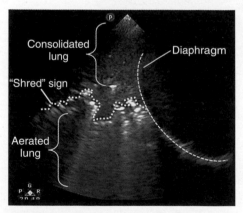

Figure 9.10   "Shred Sign." In the far field, an irregular jagged hyperechoic line traverses the lung at the interface of the aerated lung (far field) and consolidated lung (near field); this is called the "shred sign."

may have the "shred sign," which is seen as a jagged edge within the consolidated lobe. The shred sign appears at the interface between partially aerated alveoli and completely airless or fluid-filled alveoli from pneumonia (Fig. 9.10 and Video 9.14).[22] Two additional features may be seen in pneumonia. First, pleural-line thickening and irregularities can be seen due to inflammation or infection.[7] Second, dynamic air bronchograms may be seen.[23] Dynamic air bronchograms appear as mobile, hyperechoic,

punctiform particles (air bubbles) within the bronchioles that move toward the lung periphery with respirations (Videos 9.15 and 9.16).[2] Although dynamic air bronchograms can be seen in up to 6% of patients with atelectasis, they are far more commonly seen in pneumonia.[2,23] Subpleural consolidation may be present (Fig. 9.11, Video 9.17).

If a pleural effusion is present, the pleural fluid should be characterized. A parapneumonic effusion is suggested by floating debris or air bubbles ("plankton sign"), with multiple tiny echoes swirling within fluid and loculations (Fig. 9.12, Videos 9.18 to 9.20) (see Chapter 10). A well-defined hypoechoic area within a lobe with pneumonia suggests necrosis or abscess (Fig. 9.13 and Video 9.21).

Atelectasis

Basilar resorptive atelectasis is commonly found in patients on ventilators due to hypoinflation of lungs or in patients with proximal bronchial obstruction (Video 9.22). A loss of lung volume and "static" air bronchograms are seen with atelectasis (Video 9.23). Static air bronchograms represent trapped air bubbles within the bronchioles and can be seen in up to 40% of patients with pneumonia. Therefore clinical context must be considered in interpreting these findings. Compressive atelectasis from a pleural effusion leads to volume loss, with lung floating within the effusion, and the

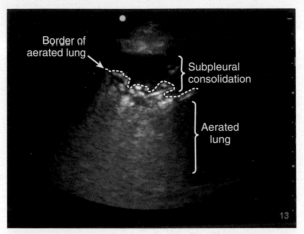

Figure 9.11 Subpleural Consolidation. Alveolar consolidation is shown just beneath the pleural line along the anterior chest wall.

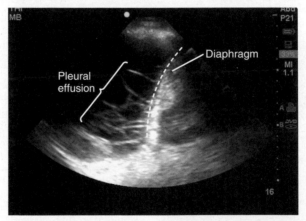

Figure 9.12 Complex Septated Pleural Effusion. An anechoic space above the diaphragm with linear echogenic septations in a patient with an empyema.

lung tip displays sinusoidal movements during respirations (Fig. 9.14, Video 9.24). This movement suggests a simple pleural effusion, as higher-viscosity parapneumonic effusions will result in a loss of sinusoidal movements.

A mirror image of the liver or spleen can be seen above the diaphragm due to a delay in sound waves returning to the transducer after reflecting off the diaphragm (see Chapter 6). A positive curtain sign, negative spine sign, and mirror image of the liver/spleen above the diaphragm are all normal findings that confirm aerated lung is abutting the diaphragm (Video 9.25). However, when a lower lobe pneumonia

or pleural effusion is present, the vertebral bodies are usually visualized extending above the diaphragm (positive spine sign) (Video 9.26) (See Chapter 10).

DIAGNOSTIC APPROACH TO ACUTE DYSPNEA

Most acute dyspnea resulting in respiratory failure is largely caused by one of four processes: (1) COPD/asthma, (2) pneumonia, (3) pulmonary edema, or (4) pulmonary embolism.[1,24,25] Fortunately, the lung ultrasound findings discussed previously allow for a highly

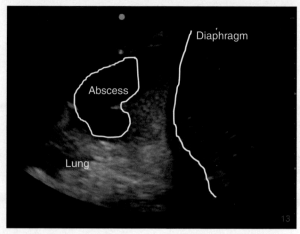

Figure 9.13   Lung Necrosis. An anechoic/hypoechoic area of lung necrosis is seen within an area of alveolar consolidation just above the diaphragm.

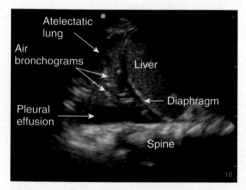

Figure 9.14   Compressive Atelectasis. A pleural effusion is compressing the lower lobe, causing atelectasis with air bronchograms.

accurate (>90%) determination of these underlying conditions in acutely dyspneic patients.[1] Given the high sensitivity of lung ultrasound for the causes of acute respiratory failure and to avoid ordering unnecessary and expensive diagnostic tests, a thoracic ultrasound exam is recommended after obtaining a history and performing a physical exam.[17,18,24] For common conditions such as congestive heart failure, the presence of positive bilateral B-lines in two or more bilateral lung zones is associated with a high positive likelihood ratio (>7) to diagnose acute heart failure.[26] In addition to performing a lung ultrasound exam, providers must be able to associate the various findings described previously with the corresponding

lung pathologies (Fig. 9.15).[27] See Chapter 12 for a case-based illustration of using ultrasound in the evaluation of acute dyspnea.

A summary of lung ultrasound patterns in common conditions is shown in Table 9.2.

PEARLS AND PITFALLS

- Patients with dyspnea but a normal lung ultrasound pattern should be evaluated for COPD/asthma, pulmonary embolism, or nonpulmonary pathologies.
- Presence of lung sliding rules out pneumothorax, but absence of lung sliding can be due to pneumothorax or other causes, such as pleurodesis, lung volume loss, or reduced/absent lung ventilation.
- B-lines are discrete and vertical; they arise from and move with the pleura. B-lines extend to the far field on the screen. For B-lines to be considered pathologic, three or more must appear in a single rib interspace.
- Z-lines should not be confused with B-lines. Although Z-lines are vertical and arise from the pleural line, they do not extend to the far field and are not discrete. Z-lines have no pathologic significance.
- Recall that B-lines can normally be seen in lower lung zones due to gravity-dependent edema and may not be

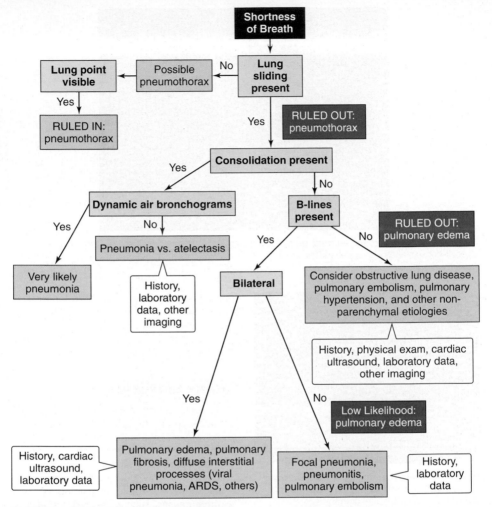

Figure 9.15 Algorithm for Shortness of Breath.

pathologic. Multiple B-lines in the upper lung zones are always pathologic.
- Findings that suggest pneumonia as the cause of consolidation are hepatization, dynamic air bronchograms, the shred sign, loss of sinusoidal movement at the lung tip, preserved or increased lung volume, and an associated

pleural effusion that contains complex features (floating debris or air bubbles, septations).
- Consolidation due to atelectasis is suggested by loss of lung volume, sinusoidal movement of the lung tip with surrounding pleural effusion, and static air bronchograms.

TABLE 9.2 **Summary of Lung Ultrasound Findings**

Lung and pleural exam findings

Condition	Upper Lobe *(Anterior)*	Middle Lobe *(Anterolateral)*	Lower Lobe *(Posterior Basal)*	Comments
Normal			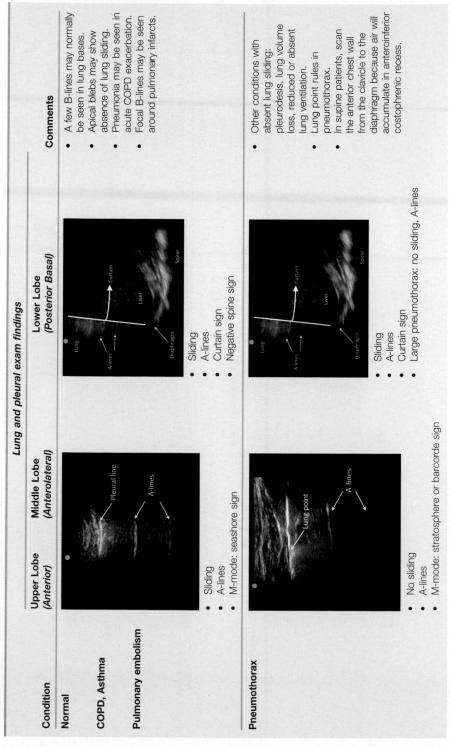	
COPD, Asthma			Spine / Curtain / Liver / A-lines / Lung / Diaphragm	
Pulmonary embolism		Pleural line / A-lines	• Sliding • A-lines • Curtain sign • Negative spine sign	• A few B-lines may normally be seen in lung bases. • Apical blebs may show absence of lung sliding. • Pneumonia may be seen in acute COPD exacerbation. • Focal B-lines may be seen around pulmonary infarcts.
		• Sliding • A-lines • M-mode: seashore sign	Spine / Curtain / Liver / A-lines / Lung / Diaphragm	
Pneumothorax		Lung point / A-lines	• Sliding • A-lines • Curtain sign • Large pneumothorax: no sliding, A-lines	• Other conditions with absent lung sliding: pleurodesis, lung volume loss, reduced or absent lung ventilation. • Lung point rules in pneumothorax. • In supine patients, scan the anterior chest wall from the clavicle to the diaphragm because air will accumulate in anteroinferior costophrenic recess.
		• No sliding • A-lines • M-mode: stratosphere or barcorde sign		

Continued

TABLE 9.2   Summary of Lung Ultrasound Findings—cont'd

Lung and pleural exam findings

Condition	Upper Lobe (Anterior)	Middle Lobe (Anterolateral)	Lower Lobe (Posterior Basal)	Comments
Pulmonary edema				• Nonsevere pulmonary edema may have areas with A-lines. • ARDS shows bilateral patchy B-lines interspersed with A-lines and thickened pleural line.
	• Diffuse bilateral B-lines • Sliding • Thin pleural line		• B-lines • Simple pleural effusion may be present	

Pneumonia

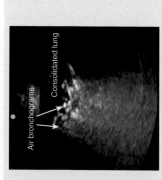

- Early: focal unilateral B-lines, sliding
- Advanced: consolidation, dynamic air bronchograms, shred sign, thickened pleural line, reduced sliding

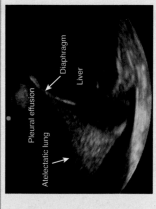

- Early and advanced: same as upper lobe findings
- Complex pleural effusion may be present
- Subpleural consolidation may be present.

Atelectasis

- Reduced/absent lung sliding with pronounced lung pulse (resorptive)
- Consolidation
- Static air-bronchograms
- Focal B-lines

- Pleural effusion (compressive)
- Elevated hemidiaphragm (resorptive)
- Consolidation
- Static air-bronchograms
- Focal B-lines
- Atelectasis is most common in the most dependent portions of the lower lobes.

ARDS, Acute respiratory distress syndrome; *COPD*, chronic obstructive pulmonary disease.

CHAPTER 10

Pleura and Diaphragm

Ria Dancel ◼ Xian Qiao ◼ Peter M. Lee

KEY POINTS

- Ultrasound can rapidly differentiate conditions that cause lower lobe opacification on chest radiographs, including pleural effusions, pneumonia, atelectasis, elevated hemidiaphragm, and masses.
- Ultrasound can detect as little as 20 mL of pleural fluid, with sensitivity reaching 100% for pleural effusions greater than 100 mL.
- Characterization of pleural fluid echogenicity and presence of septations can guide decision-making regarding timing and method of pleural drainage.
- Diaphragmatic function can be assessed by measuring excursion and thickness using two-dimensional or M-mode ultrasound.

Background

Pleural ultrasound is predicated on the sonographic characteristics of ribs and lungs. Ribs cast shadows due to near total reflection of ultrasound waves, preventing visualization of deeper structures. Aerated lungs completely scatter ultrasound waves, generating characteristic artifacts. Most pleural diseases, except for pneumothorax, involve the accumulation of fluid or growth of soft tissue in the pleural space, which are readily visualized with ultrasound. This chapter reviews the use of ultrasound to evaluate pleural pathologies and the diaphragm.

Pleural Effusion

Ultrasound is well suited for the identification and evaluation of pleural effusions. Pleural fluid propagates sound waves, allowing for optimal visualization of the borders around fluid-filled spaces and soft tissues contained within them. Ultrasound is more accurate than chest radiography in detecting pleural effusions and differentiating effusions from atelectasis or pleural thickening.[1,2] Although normal physiologic amounts of pleural fluid (3-5 mL) may be detected,[3] a minimum of 20 mL of pleural fluid is more reliably seen by ultrasound.[4] Sensitivity of ultrasound reaches 100% for pleural effusions greater than 100 mL.[5] In contrast, blunting of the costophrenic recesses and obliteration of the hemidiaphragm on posteroanterior chest radiographs is seen after the accumulation of more than 200 mL and 500 mL of pleural fluid, respectively.[6] Ultrasound is particularly useful in the intensive care unit, given the poor performance of portable chest radiographs to differentiate basilar opacities. Using chest computed tomography (CT) scan as a gold standard, pleural ultrasound was found to have a superior diagnostic accuracy of 93% compared with bedside chest radiography and auscultation (47% and 61%, respectively) for detecting pleural effusions in critically ill patients.[7] A meta-analysis of four studies calculated a pooled sensitivity and specificity of ultrasound for the detection of pleural effusions as 93% and 96%, respectively.[8] In addition, the complexity of pleural effusions and presence of pleural irregularities are better appreciated with ultrasound than with chest CT.[9]

TECHNIQUE

The technique to perform a complete lung and pleural ultrasound examination is described in

Chapter 8. Important technical considerations of pleural ultrasonography are described in the following paragraphs.

Pleural ultrasonography requires a transducer that fits between rib interspaces, typically a phased-array (2–5 MHz) or a microconvex (4–10 MHz) transducer. High-frequency linear transducers (5–15 MHz) provide better resolution of the pleural surface and permit real-time ultrasound-guided pleural procedures but have limited penetration of 6 to 9 cm.

By convention, the screen orientation marker is located in the upper left corner and the transducer is positioned on the chest with the marker pointing cephalad. By maintaining this orientation, the patient's head is always toward the left of the screen.

Ultrasound examination of the pleura in ambulatory patients is usually performed with the patient in an upright position, whereas hospitalized or critically ill patients are usually examined in a supine or semi-recumbent position. Pleural fluid accumulates in the posterolateral costophrenic recesses, the most dependent portions of the thorax in upright patients. The transducer should be extended from the posterior axillary line to the midscapular line posteriorly in supine patients, and the ultrasound beam should be aimed anteriorly to avoid missing a layering pleural effusion or a posterior pleural pathology. Additional providers may be needed to roll or lift the patient, especially if obese. After performing a general scan of deep structures, the depth and gain should be adjusted to focus on a specific segment of lung and pleura.

IMAGE INTERPRETATION

The highly reflective pleura is seen as the first hyperechoic line approximately 0.5 cm deep to the ribs. Near-complete visualization of the pleura can be obtained by sequentially evaluating each interspace by sliding the transducer longitudinally along the anterior, lateral, and posterior chest walls. From the costophrenic recesses, the right diaphragmatic pleura is usually easier to visualize than the left diaphragmatic pleura, especially in the absence of pleural fluid. Three sonographic findings can help rule out a pleural effusion: presence of the curtain sign, presence of mirror-image artifact, and absence of spine sign. Normally aerated lung descends into the scanning field at the level of the diaphragm during inspiration and blocks visualization of deeper structures, which is called the *curtain sign* (Videos 10.1 and 10.2). Additionally, if a mirror-image artifact is seen above the diaphragm, the presence of air (i.e. absence of pathology) above the diaphragm is confirmed. (Video 10.3). Normally the spine is not seen above the level of the diaphragm because air-filled lungs scatter sound waves (Video 10.4). However, the spine can be well seen above the level of the diaphragm when there is fluid above the diaphragm. This is called a positive *spine sign* and is most commonly due to a pleural effusion (Video 10.5); however, it can also be seen with a severe lower lobe pneumonia (Video 10.6).

To diagnose the presence of a pleural effusion, providers should confirm the following three characteristics (Fig. 10.1):

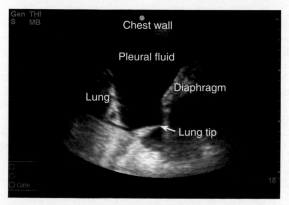

Figure 10.1 Simple Anechoic Pleural Effusion Subtended by Diaphragm, Atelectatic Lung, and Chest Wall.

1. Anatomic boundaries: Identify the diaphragm and subdiaphragmatic organs (liver or spleen), chest wall, and atelectatic lung. An atelectatic lobe of lung will have a tissue-like echogenicity similar to the liver and may have static air bronchograms (Video 10.7).

2. Anechoic space: A relatively anechoic space surrounded by typical anatomic boundaries is most commonly a pleural effusion.

3. Dynamic changes: Characteristic changes of the anechoic space should be identified, including (1) typical movement of the lung in a pleural effusion, also called "lung flapping" or the "jellyfish sign," and (2) diaphragmatic movements (Video 10.8).

Color flow Doppler and M-mode ultrasound can be utilized to determine if pleural fluid is free-flowing. Free-flowing pleural effusions will demonstrate diffuse flow by color Doppler (Video 10.9), and movement of the floating lung toward and away from the chest wall will have an undulating pattern using M-mode, often called the *sinusoid sign*. Dense pleural loculations, pleural thickening, and peripheral lung or pleural masses will show absence of flow (Video 10.10).

Various formulas have been derived to calculate the volume of the pleural fluid.[10-15] The volume of moderate-sized pleural effusion can be estimated using the formula,

Volume of pleural fluid (mL)
= 16 × distance between visceral and parietal pleura (mm)

with the interpleural distance measured between the lung base and mid-diaphragm from a longitudinal view at the midscapular line. Pragmatically, a maximal pleural effusion depth ≥10 cm or effusion spanning more than three intercostal spaces in a sitting patient will likely result in a drained volume greater than 1 L.[13,14] However, a qualitative assessment of pleural effusion volume as small, moderate, or large is sufficient to guide clinical management in most patients.[16,17]

Pleural effusions are qualitatively categorized as simple or complex based on their sonographic appearance. Simple pleural effusions are anechoic and free-flowing. Transudative effusions are almost always simple unless they are chronic. Exudative effusions can be simple or complex.[18,19]

Complex pleural effusions are homogeneously or heterogeneously echogenic and are

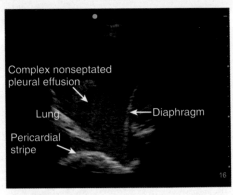

Figure 10.2 Complex Nonseptated Pleural Effusion. Note the echogenic debris homogeneously distributed within the pleural fluid.

subcategorized as either complex nonseptated (Fig. 10.2; Video 10.11) or complex septated (Fig. 10.3; Video 10.12).[18] Complex effusions are almost always exudative.[18,19] Pleural ultrasound is superior to CT scan in visualizing septations within a pleural effusion.[20] Presence of septations or loculations is highly suggestive of an exudative effusion. Although highly echogenic pleural fluid is likely to be exudative, chronic transudates can rarely develop complex features, and therefore, echogenicity is sometimes an imperfect discriminator.[19] Echogenicity can be characterized as being homogeneous or heterogeneous.[18] Heterogeneously echogenic pleural fluid is often seen as swirling debris or air bubbles, called the "plankton sign" (Video 10.13). Homogeneously echogenic pleural fluid usually has high cell counts and may be a hemothorax or empyema.[21] Hemothoraces are initially anechoic but become more echogenic as the blood clots, leading to thrombus formation and septations (Video 10.14). Empyemas usually have a homogeneously echogenic and sometimes speckled appearance (Video 10.15).

Parapneumonic effusions are most commonly exudative.[22] In the first stage, there is an outpouring of exudative fluid, which may be echogenic by ultrasound, into the pleural space. In the second stage, the fibropurulent stage, the pleural fluid is infected and becomes progressively loculated. Loculated pleural effusions are typically in nondependent areas, do not change with body position, and often fail to drain completely with thoracentesis. Chest tube insertion should be considered next as the presence of septations on ultrasound correlate with increased likelihood of needing

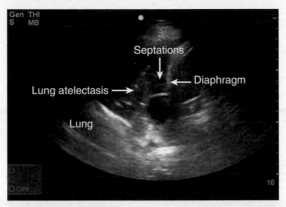

Figure 10.3 Complex Septated Pleural Effusion. Numerous septations are seen between the diaphragm and lower lobe of the lung.

intrapleural fibrinolytic therapy (OR=2.79) or surgical intervention (OR=3.92).[21,23-27] In the third stage, there is fibroblast growth in the pleural fluid from the visceral and parietal pleura, leading to the development of a thick pleural peel.

Ultrasound may help differentiate an empyema from an abscess when the pleural-parenchymal interface is indeterminate by CT. Empyemas tend to cause compressive atelectasis with uniformly thickened parietal pleura. Parenchymal lung abscesses tend to show irregular margins without any uniformity. Detection of color flow Doppler signal along the pericavitary consolidation has been shown to be most characteristic of a lung abscess with high diagnostic accuracy. (Video 10.16).[28]

Solid Pleural Pathology

Normal pleural thickness is 0.2 to 0.3 mm when the visceral and parietal pleura are apposed.[29] Solid pleural lesions may be mistaken for small pleural effusions in up to 20% of patients, and color flow Doppler can be used to differentiate these pathologies with sensitivity of 89% and specificity of 100%.[30] Pleural thickening can be due to various types of pleural injury. Pleural effusions with a parietal pleural thickness greater than 10 mm, diaphragmatic pleural thickness greater than 7 mm, and pleural nodularity are sonographic predictors of malignancy.[20,31] Pleural fibrosis causes diminished or absent respiratory movement of the visceral pleura.[17]

Solid pleural abnormalities may be seen as echogenic structures within the pleural space,

including mesotheliomas, lipomas, and chondromas (Fig. 10.4; Video 10.17). Benign tumors have a distinct capsule and will not invade surrounding tissues. Medical thoracoscopy is preferred for direct visualization to better evaluate a solid pleural mass[32] because chest CT scans have low sensitivity and specificity for characterizing pleural masses.[33,34] Malignant mesotheliomas show hypoechoic thickening of the pleural surface with irregular or indistinct borders and may invade the diaphragm or chest wall. Malignant mesotheliomas can also be nodular in character. Pleural metastases will often be accompanied by a pleural effusion (Fig. 10.5; Video 10.18). Metastatic lesions are frequently multiple with variable echogenicity, and chest wall and diaphragmatic invasion may be evident.[35,36]

Diaphragm

Evaluation of diaphragm function is important in patients who are mechanically ventilated, postoperative, or with neuromuscular diseases. Ultrasound has several advantages over fluoroscopy to assess the diaphragm, including visualization of both supra- and subdiaphragmatic structures, ability to measure excursion, avoidance of geometric and magnification errors of radiography, and avoidance of ionizing radiation. The portability of ultrasound allows for serial imaging at the bedside with high reproducibility, which is particularly relevant in mechanically ventilated patients.[37-39] The two principal sonographic techniques to assess diaphragm function are measurement of diaphragm excursion and thickness.[40,41] To

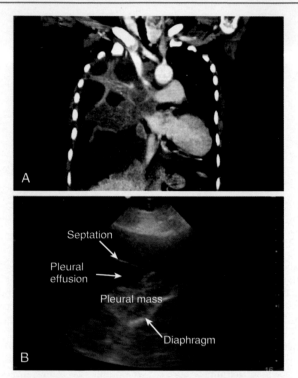

Figure 10.4 Pleural Masses. (A) Chest computed tomography scan demonstrating numerous pleural masses. (B) Irregularly shaped pleural masses are seen within a complex septated pleural effusion.

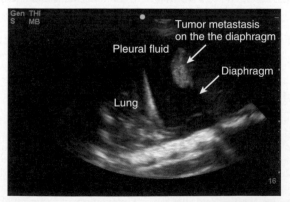

Figure 10.5 Pleural Metastasis. Pleural metastasis appearing as a well-circumscribed hyperechoic mass attached to the diaphragm.

measure excursion, the patient is positioned supine or semirecumbent. A phased-array transducer (3.5–5 MHz) is placed below the costal margin between the midclavicular line and anterior axillary line with the transducer orientation marker pointed cephalad (Fig. 10.6). The right side is most commonly imaged first, as the liver provides a good acoustic window compared with the left, where stomach gas frequently obscures the diaphragm. The ultrasound beam is aimed slightly medially and cranially so the ultrasound beam is directed toward the posterior third of the hemidiaphragm.[40,42] Once the transducer is in position, inspiratory diaphragmatic excursion is measured using M-mode. The M-mode cursor line should be as perpendicular as possible to the middle or posterior diaphragm for accurate measurements (Fig. 10.7; Video 10.19). Normal diaphragmatic excursion in healthy males during quiet breathing, deep breathing, and voluntary sniffing has been reported to be 1.8 ± 0.3, 7.0 ± 0.6, and 2.9 ± 0.6 cm, respectively. For females during quiet breathing, deep breathing, and voluntary sniffing, diaphragmatic excursion measures 1.6 ± 0.3, 5.7 ± 1.0, and 2.6 ± 0.5 cm, respectively.[37] The M-mode tracing can also be used to measure inspiratory time, rate of diaphragm contraction, and duration of the cycle.[41] Diaphragmatic excursion greater than 1.1 cm predicts successful extubation with sensitivity of 84% and specificity of 83%.[43]

It is worth noting that posture may affect diaphragmatic excursion. In the upright position, the posterior and lateral regions of the diaphragm typically have greater range of motion compared with anterior and medial regions. However, in the supine position, dependent regions are shifted cephalad and exhibit less diaphragmatic movement due to shifts in intra-abdominal pressure.[44,45] We recommend a semirecumbent position for optimal imaging.

The second technique to assess diaphragm function is measurement of diaphragm thickness. A higher-frequency linear transducer (6–13 MHz) is placed on the midaxillary line where the diaphragm meets the ribs, known as the zone of apposition (Fig. 10.8). With a high-frequency linear transducer, the diaphragm is typically visualized as a thin hyperechoic stripe with three distinct layers: an isoechoic layer of muscle sandwiched between two hyperechoic layers, the pleura and peritoneum. Diaphragm thickness is measured using either two-dimensional mode or M-mode (Fig. 10.9; Video 10.20). In most normal healthy individuals, thickness at end-expiration can vary between 1.8 and 3 mm.[42] A diaphragmatic thickening fraction is calculated to assess for weakness [(thickness at end-inspiration−thickness at end-expiration)/thickness at end-expiration].[41,42] A thickening fraction of less than 20% suggests diaphragmatic weakness in a variety of disease states, such as critical illness polyneuromyopathy, amyotrophic lateral sclerosis, and muscular dystrophies.[41,46]

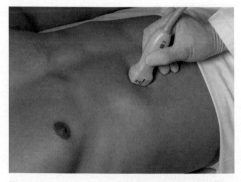

Figure 10.6 **Transducer Position to Measure Diaphragm Excursion.**

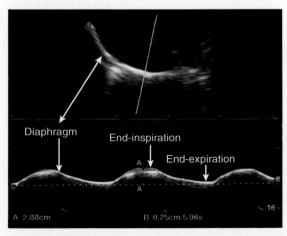

Figure 10.7 **Diaphragmatic Excursion.** Inspiratory diaphragmatic excursion is measured at the posterior third of the diaphragm using M-mode.

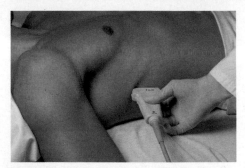

Figure 10.8   Transducer Position to Measure Diaphragm Thickness in the Zone of Apposition.

Pleural processes (effusions, chest wall masses), subdiaphragmatic organs (liver, spleen, and kidneys), and abdominal pathologies (ascites), if present, should be clearly identified. The main limitations to clearly visualize the diaphragm and its neighboring structures are body habitus, rib shadows, bowel gas, and interposition of aerated lung, as well as the angle of the ultrasound beam.[40]

PEARLS AND PITFALLS

- A complete lung and pleural exam includes visualization of three areas: the anterior, lateral, and posterior chest walls. To detect a pleural effusion in supine patients, it is critical to examine the postero-lateral chest wall and aim the ultrasound anteriorly, or "toward the sky."
- Blunting of the costophrenic recesses and obliteration of the hemidiaphragm on a posteroanterior chest radiograph is seen only after accumulation of more than 200 mL and 500 mL of pleural fluid, respectively, but providers can use ultrasound to rapidly rule out pleural effusions greater than 100 mL.
- In obese patients, the pleural line may be difficult to identify deep within the subcutaneous tissue. Therefore providers should first identify a rib and then search for the pleural line 0.5 cm deep to the rib.
- Color flow Doppler can be used to differentiate pleural masses from pleural effusions and determine if pleural fluid is free-flowing to guide decision-making about drainage.
- Pleural effusions are most commonly quantified as small, moderate, or large. An interpleural distance ≥10 cm or effusions involving more than three intercostal spaces correspond with a pleural effusion volume greater than 1 L.
- Although exudative effusions can appear simple or complex, the presence of high levels of echogenicity or septations is most consistent with an exudative effusion.
- Pleural irregularities on ultrasound, such as nodularity or masses, when accompanied by a unilateral pleural effusion, are highly suspicious for metastatic disease. Confirmatory studies, including fluid analysis and/or thoracoscopy, are warranted.
- Diaphragmatic function can be assessed by measuring diaphragmatic excursion or thickness with respirations. Normally the diaphragm thickness increases by more than 20% during respiration.

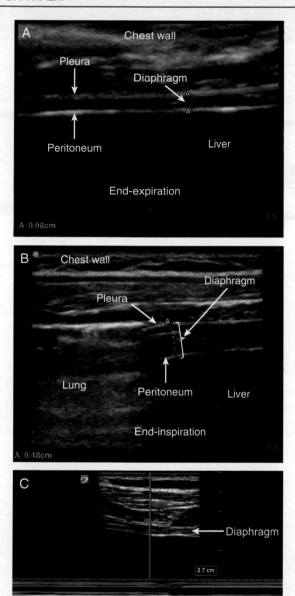

Figure 10.9 Diaphragm Thickness. The three layers in the zone of apposition are the pleura, diaphragm, and peritoneum. (A) Measurement of diaphragm thickness at end-expiration. (B) Measurement of diaphragm thickness at end-inspiration. (C) Measurement of diaphragm thickness using M-mode at end-inspiration and end-expiration.

CHAPTER 11

Lung and Pleural Procedures

Jose Cardenas-Garcia ■ J. Terrill Huggins

KEY POINTS

- Use of ultrasound for preprocedural site marking achieves high safety and success rates as long as patient position is maintained between site marking and procedure performance.
- A minimum pleural effusion depth of 1.5 cm measured by ultrasound is recommended to perform a diagnostic thoracentesis.
- Ultrasound-guided biopsy of peripheral lung masses can achieve higher histologic yields than computed tomography-guided biopsy because ultrasound can readily differentiate solid tissue from fluid.

Background

This chapter reviews key principles in the use of ultrasound to guide lung and pleural procedures. Procedural techniques and details about indications, contraindications, and postprocedure management are described elsewhere.[1-3] Use of ultrasound to guide lung and pleural procedures has advantages compared with computed tomography (CT) or fluoroscopy, including avoidance of radiation exposure, low cost, ease of use, portability, and lack of need for dedicated procedure suites.

Use of ultrasound to guide pleural procedures has several advantages compared with traditional methods, including the following:

1. Evaluation for complications immediately after completion of the procedure, such as pneumothorax (Video 11.1) or hemothorax (Video 11.2) resulting from thoracentesis or pleural biopsies.
2. Monitoring for resolution of pleural effusion or pneumothorax after chest drainage, which can expedite decision making regarding removal of the catheter.[4]
3. Characterization of pleural fluid allows selection of the most appropriate drainage method: thoracentesis for a simple anechoic pleural effusion (Video 11.3); small-bore chest tube for a complex, septated pleural

effusion (Video 11.4); large-bore chest tube for hemothorax (Video 11.5); or tunneled pleural catheter for serial drainage when pleural metastases are observed (Video 11.6).

Two techniques are used for insertion of pleural drainage devices: site marking and real-time needle visualization. Site marking is sufficient in the majority of patients, however, when performing pleural or lung biopsies or when a small pleural fluid collection is present, we recommend using real-time ultrasound guidance either with a free-handed technique or with a needle guide (Fig. 11.1).

Technique

EQUIPMENT

A portable ultrasound machine with both a high-frequency linear transducer and low-frequency phased-array or curvilinear transducer should be available. A high-frequency linear transducer is used to
- Biopsy peripheral lung nodules or pleural masses
- Assess characteristics of the pleural line
- Evaluate for vascular structures with color Doppler at the needle insertion site

A phased-array transducer is suitable for most pleural drainage procedures. The

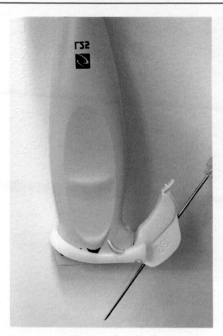

Figure 11.1 Needle Guide. Several disposable needle guidance systems are available that snap onto the transducer and stabilize the needle through a side channel, ensuring real-time visualization of the needle as it is inserted into tissue.

transducer orientation marker is pointed cephalad to obtain longitudinal views during initial scanning of the lungs and pleura and may be turned 90 degrees counterclockwise to obtain transverse views for further evaluation. The screen indicator is placed in the upper left corner of the screen to maintain spatial orientation between the target lesion and surrounding structures. The ultrasound machine is positioned next to the operator with the screen in the operator's direct line of sight.

PATIENT POSITIONING

When marking a site for an ultrasound-guided procedure, it is important to avoid changing the patient's position after the needle insertion site has been selected. If the patient's position changes after site marking, then site selection and marking should be reperformed.

Pleural Effusions

Non-loculated pleural effusions will collect in the posterolateral costophrenic recesses;

thus stable patients should be seated on the edge of the bed with their feet supported and their torso supported by leaning forward onto a raised, portable bedside table with a pillow under the arms for comfort. In critically ill patients with a pleural effusion who cannot maintain a sitting position, they can be placed either in a nearly upright position (head of bead elevated 60–90 degrees) or lateral decubitus position with the ipsilateral arm restrained over the head or chest. Careful attention must be paid to the endotracheal tube and other indwelling devices.

Pneumothorax

The patient is placed in semirecumbent position (head of bed elevated 45 degrees), which will favor the distribution of air to the anterior apical area.

Lung and Pleural Biopsy

Patient positioning for these procedures will depend on the location of the lesion. Prone position is ideal for posterior lesions as it decreases the respiratory movement of the thoracic cage.

SITE SELECTION

Pleural Effusions

Care should be taken in identifying the anatomic boundaries, dynamic findings, and internal elements of a pleural effusion as discussed in Chapter 9. Operators must positively identify the diaphragm to avoid inserting a needle or tube into the subdiaphragmatic organs. The level of the diaphragm varies greatly between patients. In mechanically ventilated patients on low tidal volumes, the diaphragm is often elevated in the thoracic cavity. In patients with an elevated diaphragm or concurrent ascites, first identify the hepatorenal or splenorenal recess in a longitudinal plane and then slide the probe cephalad to find the diaphragm.

Pneumothorax

Post-procedure, the presence of lung sliding, B-lines, lung pulse, or any non-A line pattern will rule out pneumothorax.[5] An A-line pattern with lack of lung sliding strongly suggests pneumothorax, in particular if lung sliding was noted pre-procedure. Thus, operators should look for these signs before and after performing a lung or pleural procedure. Only the presence of a lung point rules in pneumothorax,[6]

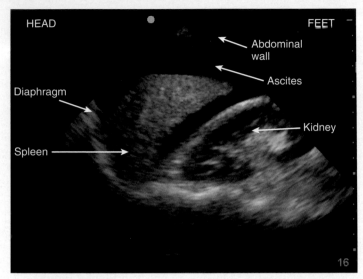

Figure 11.2 Pseudodiaphragm. The curved hyperechoic renal capsule can be mistaken for the diaphragm ("pseudodiaphragm"). When this occurs, the spleen can be mistaken for consolidated lung, as seen in this image. A key difference to differentiate diaphragm and kidney capsule is noting that the inferior portion of the kidney capsule will curve away from the chest wall, while the diaphragm curves toward the chest wall.

which is typically found on the anterolateral chest wall of a supine patient. In a supine patient, the operator should first identify lung sliding with the high-frequency linear transducer on the midclavicular line of the inferior thorax and slide the transducer in a cephalad direction to identify the most apical area of loss of lung sliding.

Lung and Pleural Biopsy

Only pulmonary parenchymal lesions abutting the pleural line are accessible via transthoracic ultrasound–guided biopsy. Evaluate for the absence of lung sliding, suggestive of focal pleurodesis, in the area of possible needle insertion with the goal of decreasing the chances of a postprocedure pneumothorax. Use of a linear transducer is recommended for performing pleural biopsies.

NEEDLE TRAJECTORY

A safe needle trajectory requires avoidance of the subdiaphragmatic organs, heart, vasculature, and visceral surface of the lung when performing a lung biopsy. Positive identification of the diaphragm is critical to avoid hepatic or splenic injury. A possible error of

inexperienced operators is misidentifying the hyperechoic, curvilinear capsule of the kidney as the diaphragm, sometimes called a "pseudo-diaphragm". This only occurs in the setting of ascites separating the kidney capsule from the liver or spleen causing the liver or spleen to look like consolidated lung tissue sitting within a presumed pleural effusion. One way to differentiate the capsule of the kidney and the diaphragm is to note that the inferior portion of the diaphragm extends laterally to the chest wall, whereas the inferior kidney capsule curves medially (Fig. 11.2; Video 11.7).

Intercostal Vessels

The anticipated needle trajectory should be evaluated with a high-frequency linear transducer using color or power Doppler to exclude tortuous or collateral intercostal vessels (Fig. 11.3). Intercostal vessels are commonly exposed in the intercostal space in the first 6 cm lateral to the spine and in elderly patients (Fig. 11.4, Videos 11.8 and 11.9).[7,8] Tilt the transducer 45-60 degrees on the chest wall to align the ultrasound beam as parallel as possible to the direction of bloodflow of the intercostal vessels. Adjust the color Doppler gain to avoid a false-negative assessment. Before inserting a

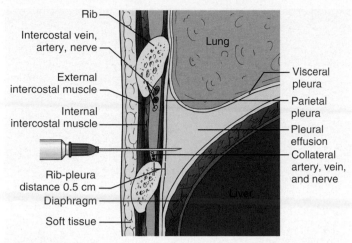

Figure 11.3 Chest Wall Anatomy.

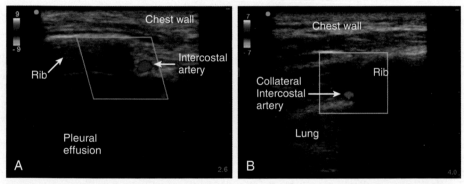

Figure 11.4 Intercostal Artery. (A) Intercostal artery on the inferior rib margin seen with color flow Doppler. (B) A collateral intercostal artery is detected on the superior rib margin using color flow Doppler.

needle in the anterior chest or paravertebral area, review any prior imaging (CT or magnetic resonance imaging [MRI]), with special emphasis on the location of cardiac structures and large vessels.

Depth of Needle Insertion

Measuring the distance between the skin surface and parietal pleura allows the operator to anticipate the needle insertion depth before penetrating into the pleural space. A minimum pleural effusion depth of 1.5 cm is recommended to perform a thoracentesis safely (Fig. 11.5).[9-11] When performing biopsies of lung or pleural-based lesions, measurement of the diameter of the target lesion in multiple planes should be performed. Operators must be aware that transducer pressure on the skin

will result in underestimation of depth measurements, often called compression artifact. Therefore skin pressure should be released prior to freezing the image and measuring depths.[5]

Angle of Needle Insertion

The angle of needle insertion must replicate the angle of the transducer used to identify the best trajectory for pleural access. When marking a site for needle insertion, the operator should make a conscious effort to memorize the transducer angle. Failure to insert the needle along the desired trajectory is a common source of error for not reaching the visualized fluid at the anticipated depth and can lead to major complications, such as vascular injury or organ perforation.

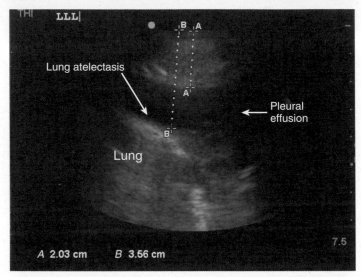

Figure 11.5 Depth of Pleural Effusion. Measurement of the distance between the parietal and visceral pleura. A minimum pleural effusion depth of 1.5 cm is recommended for thoracentesis.

Confirmation of Guidewire or Catheter Position

Ultrasound can be used to confirm the position of the guidewire or catheter in the pleural space in cases where the inserted location is uncertain (Fig. 11.6; Videos 11.10 and 11.11).[12] In cases of pneumothorax, the catheter cannot be visualized beyond the chest wall owing to the presence of intrapleural air. When performing biopsies, evaluation of the biopsy site after the procedure may be useful in ruling out postprocedure bleeding or pneumothorax (see below).[13]

Thoracentesis

Use of ultrasound guidance is recommended for thoracentesis due to the increased rate of procedural success and reduced risk of complications.[14-23] The high success rates and safety rely on eliminating inadvertent attempts to drain effusions when no or minimal fluid is present and the proper identification of intrathoracic organs and vascular structures.

The most common complications of thoracentesis include pneumothorax, pain, shortness of breath, cough, bleeding, and vasovagal reaction. Other complications that have been described are reexpansion pulmonary edema, inadvertent liver or splenic injury, hemothorax, infection, subcutaneous emphysema,

air embolism, and chest wall or subcutaneous hematoma. Most importantly, the use of ultrasound guidance significantly reduces the rates of traumatic pneumothorax, with odds ratios ranging from 0.3 to 0.8 compared with landmark-based thoracentesis.[16-23]

Ultrasound guidance for therapeutic thoracentesis appears to almost eliminate needle trauma as the immediate cause of postprocedural pneumothorax in spontaneously breathing and mechanically ventilated patients.[14,15,24,25] Pneumothorax in this setting has been reported to be associated with unexpandable lung, often referred to as pneumothorax ex vacuo.[26] The use of pleural manometry during thoracentesis may identify cases of unexpandable lung.

Selection of a suitable needle insertion site requires demonstration of pleural fluid immediately adjacent to the parietal pleura and sufficient distance from the diaphragm and lung throughout the respiratory cycle. The diaphragm, liver, and spleen should be identified unequivocally. A minimum pleural effusion depth of 1.5 cm is recommended to perform a thoracentesis safely.[9-11] The distance from the upper margin of the rib to the parietal pleura is approximately 5 mm, regardless of the chest wall thickness. If the needle lumen is suspected to be occluded by blood clot or solid debris during drainage, the needle can be flushed by injecting a small amount of sterile saline.

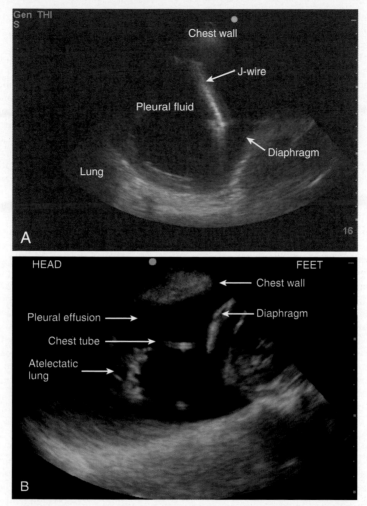

Figure 11.6 Guidewire (A) and chest tube (B) confirmation in the pleural space.

Real-time visualization of needle insertion during thoracentesis is not generally performed because it adds complexity and may interfere with maintaining the proper needle insertion angle.[9] However, experienced providers may use real-time visualization to obtain a diagnostic sample when a pleural fluid collection is small, loculated, or otherwise difficult to access.

After pleural fluid return is achieved and if a large-volume drainage is indicated, the needle is withdrawn once a guidewire is inserted with subsequent placement of a pleural drainage catheter using the Seldinger technique. When only a diagnostic thoracentesis is needed, a sufficient quantity of pleural fluid can be withdrawn into a 30- to 60-mL syringe using

an 18- to 20-gauge needle without insertion of a catheter. During a therapeutic drainage, the operator may use ultrasound to assess the volume of residual pleural fluid before removing the drainage catheter (Video 11.12). Lung sliding should be documented before and after the procedure to exclude an immediate post-procedure pneumothorax (Video 11.13).

Chest Tube Placement

Indications for ultrasound-guided chest tube placement include pleural infection, hemothorax, malignant pleural effusion, chemical pleurodesis, and pneumothorax. Placement of a small-bore catheter (14 Fr) using a modified-Seldinger technique is effective for the clinical scenarios mentioned previously except hemothorax, for which a large-bore catheter (32 Fr) is recommended. In the case of malignant pleural effusions, a tunneled pleural drainage catheter (15.5 Fr) may be used for repeated drainage. The approach described previously is used for site marking for chest tube placement (see earlier, "Techniques").

The insertion of chest tubes for pneumothorax deserves special attention. Ultrasound can guide catheter insertion for pneumothorax when a lung point is clearly visualized. When located, inserting a small thoracostomy tube using Seldinger technique over the area of absent lung sliding is safe and effective. It is important to recognize that the distance between the parietal and visceral pleura cannot be visualized in the presence of intrapleural air. Therefore needle advancement should be halted immediately upon return of air, typically 5 mm deep to the rib. A high-frequency linear transducer is used to clear the specific site of catheter insertion by making sure that loss of lung sliding is seen at that site, and the same transducer can be used to monitor for resolution of the pneumothorax after chest tube insertion.[27] Subcutaneous emphysema in the chest wall precludes the use of ultrasound. In contrast to drainage catheter insertion for a pleural effusion, the guidewire will not be visualized on ultrasound due to the intrapleural air. Caution is advised to avoid serious visceral pleural injury when a large bulla is suspected or a small pneumothorax is present. Review of prior CT chest imaging is paramount.

Medical Thoracoscopy (Pleuroscopy)

Ultrasound can identify a safe trocar insertion site for thoracoscopy. In patients with a pleural effusion, a low-frequency transducer is used to identify an optimal trocar insertion site after the patient has been placed in a lateral decubitus position. Applying the principles described earlier (see the section "Techniques") will increase the chances of adequate visualization of the pleural cavity and minimize risk of visceral injury.[28] When there is no pleural fluid or focal pleurodesis, a high-frequency linear transducer can be used to identify a pleural space where there is lung sliding, and a trocar can be safely inserted.[29]

Transthoracic Biopsy Procedures

Ultrasound-guided needle biopsy is suitable for peripheral lung lesions abutting the pleura, anterior mediastinal masses, and pleural lesions. When performing transthoracic biopsy procedures, real-time needle visualization is recommended (Video 11.14). Regarding the type of needle biopsy, use of a coaxial needle has the advantage of performing a single puncture of the visceral pleura, allowing multiple passes with both fine-needle aspiration and cutting needles (Tru-Cut™ core biopsy needle) as indicated. A needle guide may be used to stabilize the needle during real-time visualization (see Fig. 11.1); however, a disadvantage is that needle guides limit the ability to change the needle angle.[10] Vascularity of the target lesion can be evaluated with color Doppler using a high-frequency transducer. When increased vasculature is seen within a lesion, both capillary technique to obtain a sample and avoidance of the vessels are recommended to prevent blood contamination of the sample. When suction is applied to obtain a sample, release the negative pressure prior to withdrawing the needle to avoid contaminating the sample or aspirating the biopsy sample into the syringe.

LUNG BIOPSY

Only pulmonary lesions abutting the pleura and visualized throughout the respiratory cycle are accessible for ultrasound-guided biopsy (Fig. 11.7; Video 11.15). There are two advantages of using ultrasound guidance over CT guidance for biopsy of peripheral lung lesions. First, ultrasound can easily differentiate solid from liquid tissue in partially necrotic lesions. During the procedure, the biopsy needle can be directed toward solid (more echogenic) areas of the lesion to improve histologic yield.[30] Second, ultrasound can easily identify areas of focal pleurodesis adjacent to the lesion, decreasing the risk of iatrogenic pneumothorax. The use of contrast enhancement in ultrasound-guided lung biopsies has been reported extensively.[31,32] This technique helps differentiate areas of atelectasis or pneumonia (pulmonary arterial blood supply, early contrast enhancement); tumor (bronchial artery supply, late contrast enhancement); and tissue necrosis, fluid collection, or embolism (absence of contrast) (Fig. 11.8; Video 11.16).[33] Compared to unenhanced

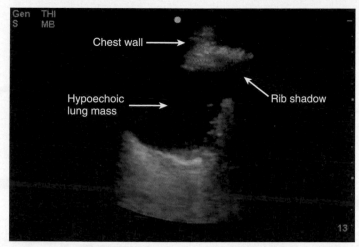

Figure 11.7 Lung Mass. A moderate-sized, hypoechoic peripheral lung mass is seen abutting the chest wall.

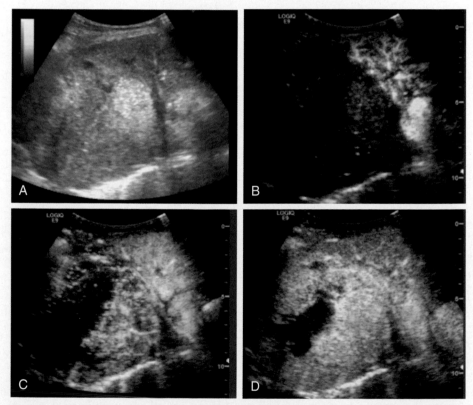

Figure 11.8 Contrast-Enhanced Lung Ultrasonography. (A) A two-dimensional unenhanced ultrasound image. (B) Early contrast-enhancement is seen with atelectatic lung. (C) Late contrast enhancement is seen with lung tumor. (D) An area unenhanced by contrast suggests necrosis. (Reprinted with permission of the American Thoracic Society. Copyright © 2016 American Thoracic Society. The American Journal of Respiratory and Critical Care Medicine is an official journal of the American Thoracic Society.)

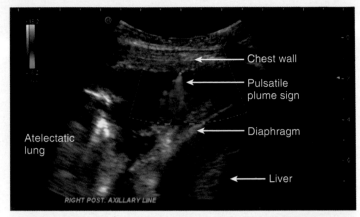

Figure 11.9   Pulsatile Plume Sign. Color flow Doppler reveals injury to an intercostal artery at the biopsy site. (Reprinted with permission of the American Thoracic Society. Copyright © 2016 American Thoracic Society. The American Journal of Respiratory and Critical Care Medicine is an official journal of the American Thoracic Society.)

images, the use of contrast improves the diagnostic yield of biopsies (94% vs. 78%).[31]

LUNG ABSCESS DRAINAGE

Only after failure of conservative management of a lung abscess (long-term broad-spectrum antibiotics and spontaneous drainage via the airways) is a more invasive management strategy considered. For patients who are not surgical candidates and have a lung abscess larger than 4 cm abutting the pleura, percutaneous transthoracic drainage guided by ultrasound is a treatment option.[34] Complications related to percutaneous transthoracic drainage are low, including contamination of a sterile pleural space and development of a bronchopleural fistula. The risk of these complications can be reduced by using a high-frequency linear transducer to select a needle insertion site without lung sliding (i.e. an area of focal pleurodesis adjacent to the lung abscess).[35]

ANTERIOR MEDIASTINAL BIOPSY

Masses in the anterior mediastinum may be accessible to ultrasound-guided biopsy provided that the lung is displaced sufficiently to create an sonographic window through the anterior rib cage. Vascular structures should be ruled out along the needle trajectory by using a high-frequency linear transducer with color Doppler. Careful review of any prior CT scans should be performed during preprocedural preparation. A core biopsy using a cutting needle is usually needed to biopsy anterior mediastinal masses unless metastatic carcinoma is suspected, in which case fine-needle aspiration may be sufficient.[36,37]

PLEURAL BIOPSY

A high-frequency linear transducer may detect abnormal areas of the pleura, such as pleural thickening or nodularity. Ultrasound-guided pleural biopsy has a higher diagnostic yield as compared with random pleural biopsy.[38] In cases of mesothelioma, a biopsy sample demonstrating tissue invasion is required; if the patient is not a candidate for pleuroscopy, ultrasound-guided biopsy may be considered as the initial diagnostic procedure.[39] In such cases, a core biopsy using a cutting needle to demonstrate chest wall invasion is crucial. This is achieved by a partial withdrawal of the coaxial needle into the rib interspace before discharging the cutting needle. The cutting aspect of the needle is oriented caudally, away from the neurovascular bundle. After the samples have been taken, the operator may consider reassessment of the biopsy site using color Doppler with a high-frequency linear transducer to rule out a "pulsatile plume sign," a rare complication indicating an active intercostal artery injury has occurred with subsequent hemorrhage into the pleural space (Fig. 11.9; Video 11.17).[13]

PEARLS AND PITFALLS

- Despite the availability of bedside ultrasonography, pleural and lung interventions may not be possible in cases of severe obesity and subcutaneous emphysema.
- Distances from the skin surface to the parietal and visceral pleura can be readily measured with ultrasound. When a needle is being inserted over a rib, the needle will have to be advanced about 5 mm from the upper margin of the rib to enter the pleural space. A minimum pleural effusion depth of 1.5 cm measured at end-inspiration is recommended to perform thoracentesis.

- Color Doppler assessment with a high-frequency linear transducer over the intended needle trajectory is a valuable technique to minimize potential risk of vascular injury to intercostal vessels.
- Visualization of the guidewire with ultrasound is recommended to confirm proper placement before inserting a large-diameter dilator or catheter.
- Proper correlation of ultrasound findings with prior computed tomography scans is essential, especially for procedures in close proximity to large vessels or organs.
- Only lung lesions abutting the pleura are suitable for ultrasound-guided biopsy.

CHAPTER 12

Dyspnea and Pulmonary Embolism

Christopher Dayton ■ Lewis A. Eisen

KEY POINTS

- Providers must readily recognize the five main discriminating artifacts produced by lung and pleural ultrasound: lung sliding, A-lines, B-lines, consolidation, and pleural effusion.
- Algorithms based on the presence or absence of lung ultrasound artifacts allow providers to systematically approach and accurately diagnose patients with acute dyspnea and respiratory failure.
- Point-of-care ultrasound is a useful bedside tool to diagnose and determine the severity of acute pulmonary embolism.

Background

Physical examination and chest radiography have limited diagnostic accuracy in determining the etiology of acute dyspnea.[1] Ultrasound of the thorax has proven to be a more accurate bedside tool that can rapidly detect the presence or absence of pulmonary pathologies, including alveolar/interstitial syndrome,[2] pleural effusion,[3] pneumothorax (PTX),[4-6] and consolidation.[7-12] Specific extrapulmonary ultrasound examinations can provide further discriminatory power as certain causes of respiratory failure have multiorgan effects. The systematic use of ultrasound to evaluate the lungs, heart, inferior vena cava (IVC) and deep veins of the extremities has significant potential to facilitate timely diagnosis and management of patients with acute dyspnea and respiratory failure.[13-19] This chapter refers to evaluation of the right ventricle (RV), IVC, and lower extremity veins for deep venous thrombosis (DVT) discussed in later chapters (see Chapters 16, 17, and 34).

Pulmonary Embolism

Pulmonary embolism (PE) is a cause of acute dyspnea that is associated with a high mortality if untreated (30%) or if treatment is delayed.[20,21] Diagnostic testing for acute PE is typically pursued with a computed tomography (CT) angiogram which is expensive and exposes patients to intravenous contrast and ionizing radiation. As an alternative to CT angiography, a multiorgan ultrasound examination may reveal findings that can help rule in an acute PE: presence of a DVT, subpleural infarctions, RV dilatation, or clot-in-transit.[22-29]

In particular, finding a deep vein thrombosis on ultrasound in a patient suspected of having an acute PE is very specific for a diagnosis of PE.[17,22,26,27] Subpleural infarcts can be visualized with ultrasound represented by triangular or round areas of subpleural consolidation that may or may not be associated with a pleural effusion. These lesions are most commonly found in the lower lobes and provide modest support for a diagnosis of PE.[23-25] Cardiac ultrasound may be performed and provides supportive but not specific evidence of PE when acute RV dilatation or hypokinesis is found.[30,31]

Furthermore, ultrasound can provide some information about the severity of a confirmed PE. Ultrasound detection of RV systolic dysfunction or RV to left ventricle (LV) diameter ratio >0.9 (normal <0.6) is evidence of a submassive PE in a patient with a PE.[32-37] Given the increased morbidity and mortality of a submassive PE with acute RV dysfunction, administration of thrombolytics should be considered.[37] Periodically, a thrombus will be visualized in the IVC or right heart. These "clots-in-transit" are associated with poor outcomes when treated with heparin alone and administration of thrombolytics should be considered.[28,29]

General Principles

A systematic approach to dyspneic patients using lung ultrasound has been previously described (see Chapter 9).[17] An algorithm to interpret patterns found during a systematic multiorgan ultrasound exam in the context of acute respiratory failure is presented here. (Fig. 12.1). Ultrasound findings should always be interpreted in the clinical context of the patient and combined with other clinical data.

Algorithm for Acute Dyspnea

Step 1: Is there lung sliding?
1. If yes, proceed to Step 2.
2. If no, look for B-lines. If no B-lines are present, then look for absence of a lung pulse or presence of a stratosphere (or barcode) sign on M-mode. If found, look for a lung point to rule in PTX. If no lung point is found, consider additional testing with a chest x-ray or CT scan to evaluate for PTX.

Step 2: What is the predominant lung ultrasound pattern?
1. A-line pattern: suggests PE or acute airway obstruction from asthma or chronic obstructive pulmonary disease. If PE is suspected, proceed to PE algorithm
2. B-line pattern: Characterize B-line pattern
   a. Bilateral and uniformly distributed without areas of sparing along with a smooth, thin, sliding pleural line: Pulmonary edema
   b. Unilateral, patchy pattern with irregularly thickened pleura with diminished sliding: Early or atypical pneumonia
   c. Bilateral with areas of sparing and irregularly thickened pleura with diminished sliding: acute respiratory distress syndrome (ARDS)
   d. Supplementary ultrasound imaging: Left ventricular systolic function. Rule out severe mitral or aortic regurgitation, IVC diameter and respiratory variation, and complete lung evaluation for areas of consolidation.
3. Consolidation: Characterize consolidation
   a. Volume loss with either no air bronchograms or static air bronchograms: Atelectasis
   b. Dynamic air bronchograms, normal or expanded lung volume, no lung flapping: Pneumonia
4. Pleural Effusion: Consider as the primary cause of dyspnea if size is moderate to large with lung flapping. Characterize as complex vs. simple

Step 3: Is PE suspected?
1. Estimate risk of PE using available clinical data and prediction rules.
   a. History, clinical impression
   b. Wells score, Pulmonary Embolism Rule-out Criteria rule
   c. Age-adjusted D-dimer
2. A moderate or high probability of PE is present
   a. Perform lower extremity venous compression ultrasound exam to assess for DVT. Consider performing an upper extremity venous compression ultrasound exam based on risk factors and clinical suspicion. If positive for DVT, start treatment for DVT and PE.
   b. Perform supplementary ultrasound examinations.
      1. Lungs: Visualization ≥1 peripheral, focal subpleural consolidations with or without an associated pleural effusion supports but does not definitively diagnose PE.
      2. Heart: Dilation and hypokinesis of the RV are associated with PE that are submassive or massive.
      3. IVC: IVC dilation is a corroborating finding of RV dilation and hypokinesis from increased pulmonary arterial pressure. Clot-in-transit may be seen in the IVC or RV which is associated with poor outcomes and necessitates rapid and definitive treatment with either thrombolysis or thrombectomy.
   c. It is imperative that providers understand that point-of-care ultrasound cannot rule out PE, and therefore dedicated imaging with a CT angiogram or ventilation/perfusion (VQ) scan should be performed when indicated. Consider other causes of acute dyspnea that will present with a relatively normal lung ultrasound examination, including asthma,

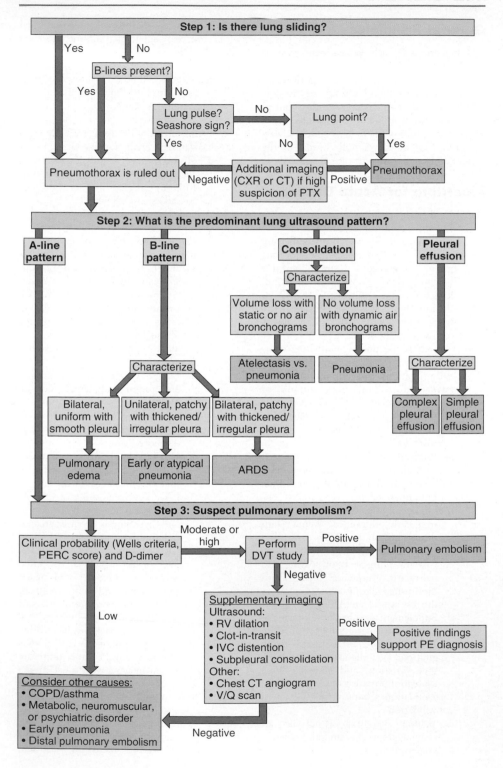

Step 1: Is there lung sliding?

Yes / No

B-lines present?

Yes / No

Lung pulse? Seashore sign? — No → Lung point?

Yes / No / Yes

Pneumothorax is ruled out ← Negative — Additional imaging (CXR or CT) if high suspicion of PTX — Positive → Pneumothorax

Step 2: What is the predominant lung ultrasound pattern?

A-line pattern | B-line pattern | Consolidation | Pleural effusion

Consolidation → Characterize
- Volume loss with static or no air bronchograms
- No volume loss with dynamic air bronchograms

Volume loss with static or no air bronchograms → Atelectasis vs. pneumonia

No volume loss with dynamic air bronchograms → Pneumonia

Pleural effusion → Characterize
- Complex pleural effusion
- Simple pleural effusion

B-line pattern → Characterize
- Bilateral, uniform with smooth pleura
- Unilateral, patchy with thickened/irregular pleura
- Bilateral, patchy with thickened/irregular pleura

Bilateral, uniform with smooth pleura → Pulmonary edema

Unilateral, patchy with thickened/irregular pleura → Early or atypical pneumonia

Bilateral, patchy with thickened/irregular pleura → ARDS

Step 3: Suspect pulmonary embolism?

Clinical probability (Wells criteria, PERC score) and D-dimer

Moderate or high → Perform DVT study — Positive → Pulmonary embolism

Negative

Supplementary imaging
Ultrasound:
• RV dilation
• Clot-in-transit
• IVC distention
• Subpleural consolidation
Other:
• Chest CT angiogram
• V/Q scan

Positive → Positive findings support PE diagnosis

Negative

Low

Consider other causes:
• COPD/asthma
• Metabolic, neuromuscular, or psychiatric disorder
• Early pneumonia
• Distal pulmonary embolism

chronic obstructive pulmonary disease (COPD), neuromuscular diseases causing diaphragmatic weakness, metabolic disorders, and psychiatric illnesses.

Case Studies: The following five case scenarios demonstrate the integration of an algorithmic approach to thoracic ultrasound in the evaluation of patients with acute dyspnea or respiratory failure.

CASE 12.1

CASE PRESENTATION

The rapid-response team is called to evaluate a patient in respiratory distress on the telemetry unit. The patient is a 76-year-old woman with a history of diabetes mellitus and hypertension. She was admitted a week earlier for a non-ST elevation myocardial infarction and congestive heart failure. She underwent cardiac catheterization with stents placed in the right coronary and left circumflex arteries. Left ventricular ejection fraction was estimated as 35%.

Vital signs: T 37°C, pulse 110 (telemetry demonstrated sinus rhythm), blood pressure 103/55, respiratory rate 34, oxygen saturation 92% with nonrebreather mask. Physical examination shows moderate respiratory distress with rapid and shallow breaths and scattered rhonchi at the bases. Heart is tachycardic and regular, and jugular venous distention is present. Extremities have 1+ bilateral pitting edema.

ASSESSMENT

The differential diagnosis for this patient includes pulmonary edema, PE, cardiac tamponade, and pneumonia. The history and physical exam of this patient, including jugular venous distension, suggest pulmonary edema, but chest auscultation is unimpressive for the degree of respiratory distress. While awaiting chest radiography, a lung ultrasound is performed.

Lung ultrasound of the anterior hemithoraces reveals the presence of sliding with A-lines throughout (Fig. 12.2; Videos 12.1 and 12.2). A rapid assessment of the lower extremity veins reveals a noncompressible right common femoral vein consistent with a DVT (Fig. 12.3 and Video 12.3). Bedside cardiac ultrasound shows an apical 4-chamber view with a normal RV:LV diameter ratio <0.6, and no clot-in-transit is noted (Fig. 12.4 and Video 12.4).

CASE RESOLUTION

Lung ultrasound showing absence of B-lines bilaterally, especially in the middle and upper lobes provided evidence that clinically significant pulmonary edema was not present. Other etiologies for acute respiratory distress had to be considered. The bilateral A-line pattern increased the probability that the patient had a PE, bronchoconstriction from COPD or asthma, or a metabolic or neuromuscular disorder. Finding a proximal lower extremity DVT supported a diagnosis of PE. There were no clinical signs of massive or submassive PE and no echocardiographic evidence of acute RV heart failure. The patient was given a bolus of heparin followed by a continuous infusion and aggressive diuresis was avoided based on the ultrasound findings.

CASE PEARLS

- When acute respiratory complaints are accompanied by a normal lung ultrasound exam, providers should consider PE in the differential diagnosis.
- Most PEs originate from the lower extremity veins, and venous branch points are common sites to find DVTs, particularly the common femoral vein-greater saphenous vein junction and trifurcation of the popliteal vein.
- When acute dyspnea is associated with hypotension, providers should consider hemodynamic compromise secondary to massive PE, which will invariably present with a dilated RV. Massive PE is an indication for thrombolytic therapy barring absolute contraindications.
- Be cautious in diagnosing "clot-in-transit" in low-flow states of cardiogenic or obstructive shock. Low-flow states can have the appearance of spontaneous echo contrast or "smoke" creating an appearance of echoes moving within the vessel, albeit not in aggregate and thus does not represent an organized thrombus (Video 12.5).

Figure 12.1 Algorithm for Acute Dyspnea and Pulmonary Embolism. *ARDS*, Acute respiratory distress syndrome; *COPD*, chronic obstructive pulmonary disease; *CT*, computed tomography; *CXR*, chest x-ray; *DVT*, deep venous thrombosis; *IVC*, Inferior vena cava; *PE*, pulmonary embolism; *PERC*, Pulmonary Embolism Rule Out Criteria; *PTX*, pneumothorax; *RV*, right ventricle; *V/Q*, ventilation/perfusion.

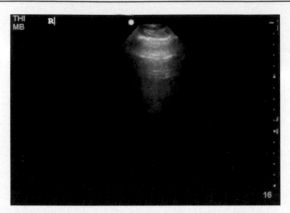

Figure 12.2   Case 1: A-Lines Are Seen in Bilateral Upper Lung Lobes.

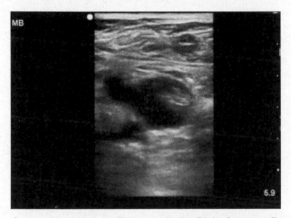

Figure 12.3   Case 1: Deep Venous Thrombus in the Right Common Femoral Vein.

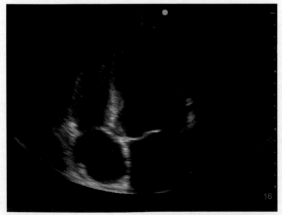

Figure 12.4   Case 1: Normal RV:LV Ratio Is Seen From an Apical 4-Chamber View. *LV*, Left ventricle; *RV*, right ventricle.

CASE 12.2

CASE PRESENTATION

A 72-year-old man presents to the emergency department with dyspnea and acute on chronic renal failure (stage IV chronic kidney disease). He is given an infusion of nitroglycerin and furosemide with some improvement. The nephrology service recommends urgent dialysis for volume overload. During placement of a hemodialysis catheter, the right internal jugular vein is punctured three times before successful cannulation and catheter insertion. While finishing the procedure, the patient develops acute, severe dyspnea.

Vital signs: pulse 144 and regular, blood pressure 182/83, respiratory rate 38, oxygen saturation 92% on a nonrebreather mask. Physical examination shows moderate respiratory distress. Heart sounds are regular and tachycardic. Jugular venous distension is present. Lung exams shows rapid, shallow breathing and lung sounds are difficult to hear due to noise in the emergency department. Lower extremities show 1 + bilateral pitting edema.

ASSESSMENT

After a difficult hemodialysis catheter placement, there is concern for iatrogenic PTX. Another possible etiology for his respiratory decompensation is fluid overload for which hemodialysis is planned. The management of these two conditions differs markedly. Pleural injury leading to PTX or hemothorax requires chest tube placement. In contrast, worsening fluid overload may require noninvasive or mechanical ventilation that could exacerbate an unidentified PTX. Lung ultrasound demonstrates the presence of lung sliding over bilateral anterior lung fields with multiple B-lines with a thin smooth pleural surface

(Fig. 12.5; Videos 12.6 and 12.7). Gross evaluation of the left ventricle demonstrates reduced systolic function (Video 12.8). The IVC is dilated (2.5 cm) and plethoric without respiratory variation (Video 12.9)

CASE RESOLUTION

The presence of bilateral lung sliding immediately ruled out PTX, a diagnosis that can be ruled out as long as a non-A-line pattern is seen. Bilateral B-lines supported the diagnosis of an interstitial syndrome, the most common being cardiogenic pulmonary edema, in particular with the thin, smooth pleural line. A clinical diagnosis of cardiogenic pulmonary edema was further supported by the presence of decreased left ventricular systolic function and a plethoric IVC. The patient was moved to a seated position, nitroglycerin infusion was increased, and noninvasive positive pressure ventilation was started. Symptoms improved while awaiting hemodialysis initiation.

CASE PEARLS

- Presence of either lung sliding, or any non-A line pattern (B-lines, consolidation, or effusion), over the anterior lung fields of a supine patient can rapidly rule out PTX as a cause of respiratory failure.
- The most common cause of bilateral anterolateral B-lines with a thin pleural line is cardiogenic pulmonary edema.
- Prior to attempting central line placement, perform a brief lung ultrasound exam to determine if lung sliding is present preprocedure. Therefore, if lung sliding is absent postprocedure, then the provider knows a PTX is highly likely, especially if accompanied by signs and symptoms.

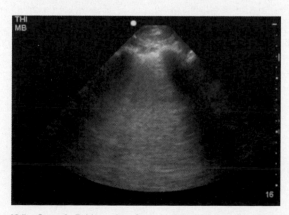

Figure 12.5　Case 2: B-Lines Are Seen in Bilateral Anterior Lung Fields.

CASE 12.3

CASE PRESENTATION

A 68-year-old woman with a history of COPD is admitted to the intensive care unit (ICU) with respiratory distress from a COPD exacerbation. She became progressively more hypercapneic, despite noninvasive ventilation. Rapid sequence intubation is performed with the endotracheal tube visualized passing between the vocal cords, and capnography confirms endotracheal intubation. Postintubation, breath sounds are decreased but present bilaterally. Her saturation is 85% despite an FiO_2 of 100%. Her peak pressure is 40 mm Hg with a plateau pressure of 30 mm Hg. The patient is taken off the ventilator and ventilated manually with 100% oxygen without improvement.

Vital signs: pulse 102 and regular, blood pressure 120/67, oxygen saturation 85% (intubated with bag-valve mask, FiO_2 = 100%). Physical examination shows a sedated and paralyzed patient. Heart sounds are regular and tachycardic. Lungs sounds are faint and equal bilaterally.

ASSESSMENT

This patient is postintubation with elevated peak pressures and desaturation, despite various interventions. Differential diagnosis includes severe aspiration, PTX, suboptimal endotracheal tube placement, atelectasis, and worsening COPD exacerbation. Nebulized bronchodilators are given to relieve any airway obstruction. Chest radiography was ordered while an urgent bedside lung ultrasound exam was performed.

Right lung ultrasound shows sliding with an A-line pattern, consistent with a normally aerated lung (Fig. 12.6 and Video 12.10). Left lung ultrasound shows absence of sliding, presence of lung pulse, and an A-line pattern (Video 12.11). The presence of lung pulse indicates that the visceral and parietal pleura are directly apposed, thus ruling out a significant PTX. The absence of sliding with the presence of lung pulse suggests right mainstem intubation. Minimal movement of the left hemidiaphragm during inspiration further

confirms the presence of right mainstem intubation (Videos 12.12 and 12.13).

CASE RESOLUTION

The endotracheal tube was pulled back 3 cm with improvement of oxygen saturation to 100% and a decrease in peak airway pressures to 25 mm Hg. A chest radiograph later confirmed proper placement of the endotracheal tube just above the carina.

CASE PEARL

- A high-frequency, linear transducer provides excellent visualization of the pleural line when lung sliding is the primary question. The apex of the lung normally exhibits minimal pleural sliding since it is distant from the diaphragm.
- Lack of lung sliding by ultrasound is not specific for PTX. If lung sliding is absent or equivocal and PTX is suspected, search for a lung point to rule in PTX. Other causes of absent lung sliding include pleurodesis (chemical pleurodesis, infectious or inflammatory states, or fibrotic lung diseases), lung volume loss (complete atelectasis, mucous plugging, pneumonectomy), and reduced or absent lung ventilation (apnea, mainstem intubation).
- Similar to other diagnostic tests, it is important to clinically correlate ultrasound findings. Even if PTX is confirmed by finding a lung point, recall that clinical signs will depend on the size of the PTX. For example, a small apical PTX is likely to be asymptomatic and may even be difficult to detect with ultrasound imaging. Conversely, a clinically emergent tension PTX will typically show diffuse lack of sliding. Therefore, if a small apical PTX is identified in a patient with sudden cardiopulmonary collapse, the PTX is unlikely to be the sole etiology and other causes for the sudden change should be sought.

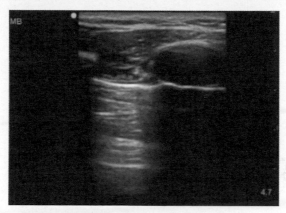

Figure 12.6 Case 3: A-Lines Seen With a High-Frequency Linear Transducer.

CASE 12.4

CASE PRESENTATION

A 65-year-old man recently treated for community-acquired pneumonia is admitted to the ICU on mechanical ventilation for presumptive multilobar pneumonia. History was limited due to his acute dyspnea and respiratory failure. The radiology report of his admission chest x-ray states, "well-positioned endotracheal tube, pulmonary venous congestion with bilateral infiltrates, and small pleural effusions." The patient is placed on broad-spectrum antibiotics and requires vasopressors to maintain his blood pressure. His arterial oxygenation (PaO$_2$) is 60 mm Hg with an FiO$_2$ of 60% and positive end-expiratory pressure at 14 cm H$_2$O. He is not stable for transport to obtain a CT scan of the chest.

Vital signs: pulse 124 and regular, blood pressure 102/63, oxygen saturation 95%. Physical examination shows the patient is sedated and intubated. Heart sounds are regular and tachycardic. Lung exam shows decreased breath sounds in the right base with rales anteriorly. On the left chest, rales are heard from the base to midlung field.

ASSESSMENT

This patient has significant hypoxemia. Bilateral infiltrates on chest x-ray could represent ARDS, diffuse pulmonary edema, or lobar consolidations with contribution from pleural effusions or atelectasis. Given the limitations of a portable, supine chest x-ray, an ultrasound of the thorax is performed.

Lung sliding and A-lines are seen bilaterally in the upper lobes (Fig. 12.7; Videos 12.14 and 12.15). A left pleural effusion is seen with multiple septations suggesting an infectious etiology (Fig. 12.8 and Video 12.16). Ultrasound of the right lower lobe reveals a consolidated lung consistent with pneumonia and a small pleural effusion. Dynamic air bronchograms are seen on inspiration (Fig. 12.9 and Video 12.17).

CASE RESOLUTION

Thoracentesis was performed on the left hemithorax. Laboratory analysis was consistent with empyema, and a chest tube was placed. Antibiotics were continued. Oxygen and vasopressor requirements subsequently decreased.

CASE PEARLS

- Chest radiography cannot accurately discern lung and pleural conditions that cause opacification of the lower hemithoraces along the diaphragm, whereas ultrasound can rapidly differentiate the most common etiologies: pneumonia vs. pleural effusion.
- Ultrasound has demonstrated similar diagnostic accuracy as CT scans for several pulmonary conditions, especially characterization of pleural effusions as simple vs. complex with or without septations. Initially, septations are generally only detectable by ultrasound.

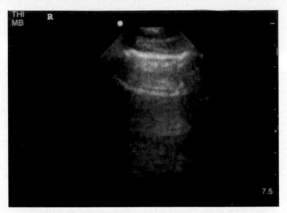

Figure 12.7 Case 4: A-Lines Are Seen in Bilateral Upper Lung Lobes.

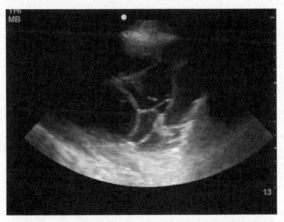

Figure 12.8 Case 4: Complex, Septated Left-Sided Pleural Effusion.

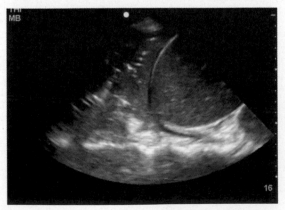

Figure 12.9 Case 4: Consolidated Right Lower Lobe With Air Bronchograms and a Small Pleural Effusion.

CASE 12.5

CASE PRESENTATION

A 35-year-old man with a history of diabetes mellitus is brought to the Emergency Department with lethargy and respiratory distress. The patient's wife reports a history of malaise, epigastric abdominal pain, and vomiting for 1 day. Vitals: 101°F, pulse 132, blood pressure 103/48, respiratory rate 40 with oxygen saturation 100% on 5 L/min nasal cannula. Physical examination shows a man in moderate to severe respiratory distress. He opens his eyes to stimuli and only responds with one-word answers. Heart sounds are regular and tachycardic without any murmurs. Lungs sounds are clear bilaterally. Abdominal exam is soft with mild epigastric tenderness to palpation. No lower extremity edema is present.

ASSESSMENT

The patient presents with findings of respiratory distress, fever, tachycardia, lethargy, and borderline hypotension (mean arterial pressure = 66). Upon presentation, the differential diagnosis is broad and includes sepsis secondary to pneumonia or other infectious source, PE, and diabetic ketoacidosis. As the team obtains IV access and sends labs, a point-of-care ultrasound exam is performed.

Bilateral anterior, lateral, and posterior lung fields reveal the presence of lung sliding with A-lines (Fig. 12.10; Videos 12.18 and 12.19). Note that single B-lines in the lower lobes can be a normal finding. Because PE is a diagnostic consideration, bilateral lower extremity compression ultrasound exams of the deep veins are performed, and results are negative (Video 12.20). Additional ultrasound imaging of his heart and IVC demonstrate a hyperdynamic LV, an RV:LV diameter ratio <0.9, an IVC that collapses completely on inspiration, and no evidence of clot-in-transit (Fig. 12.11 and Videos 12.21–12.23).

CASE RESOLUTION

The patient's fingerstick glucose was significantly elevated at >600 mg/dL. Additional lab studies showed an arterial blood gas pH of 6.95, serum bicarbonate of 14 with an elevated anion gap, and positive serum ketones. A respiratory Polymerase Chain Reaction (PCR) panel was positive for influenza B. He was resuscitated aggressively with IV fluids, started on an insulin drip and antivirals, and admitted to the hospital.

CASE PEARLS

- In patients with respiratory distress, when point-of-care ultrasound does not find evidence of pneumonia, atelectasis, pulmonary edema, pleural effusion, pneumothorax, or PE, providers should consider metabolic, neuromuscular, or psychiatric illnesses in the differential diagnosis.
- Point-of-care ultrasound imaging cannot rule out a diagnosis of PE. In cases where an alternative diagnosis does not surface, then additional diagnostic testing, most often a CT angiogram or V/Q scan, should be obtained to rule out PE.

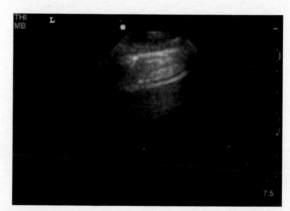

Figure 12.10   Case 5: Bilateral Anterior, Lateral, and Posterior Lung Fields Show A-Lines.

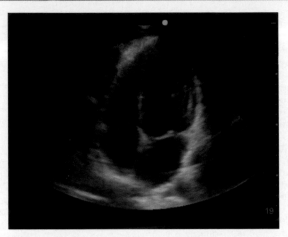

Figure 12.11   Case 5: Normal RV:LV Ratio in an Apical 4-Chamber View. *LV*, Left ventricle; *RV*, right ventricle.

CHAPTER 13

Overview

Kirk T. Spencer

KEY POINTS

- Goal-directed echocardiography can improve medical decision making or alter time to initiation of appropriate treatment, especially in patients who are unstable, have heart failure, or have indeterminate volume status.
- After limited training, providers can accurately assess left ventricular systolic function, right ventricular size and function, pericardial effusion, and inferior vena cava size and respiratory variation.
- Training in focused cardiac ultrasound should include three core components: didactic education, hands-on imaging practice, and image interpretation experience.

Background

Ultrasound is more portable and less expensive than other modalities (computed tomography [CT], magnetic resonance imaging [MRI], nuclear perfusion) used to image the heart. The simplified operation, substantially smaller size, and reduced cost of portable ultrasound devices have appealed to physicians from diverse specialties, leading to their widespread adoption for the assessment of cardiac and hemodynamic questions at the bedside.[1,2] Although a wide variety of terms have been used to refer to this technology (Table 13.1), the concept is to perform a goal-directed, bedside examination of the cardiovascular system using ultrasound to answer specific, clinically-driven questions. Additional distinctions of point-of-care cardiac ultrasound are highlighted in Table 13.2.

Indications and Applications

A point-of-care cardiac ultrasound examination should be conducted in conjunction with other bedside measures, such as physical examination and laboratory data, to formulate a diagnostic impression and guide appropriate management.

The specific cardiac views to acquire differ depending on clinical need. Device capabilities and provider skills for both image acquisition and interpretation are the major considerations when defining which cardiac abnormalities can reliably be detected. A standard comprehensive echocardiogram has 60 views, takes 45 minutes to complete, and requires 3 to 6 months of training to perform and interpret competently.[3,4] Conversely, a point-of-care cardiac ultrasound exam calls on the provider

TABLE 13.1   Terms for Point-of-Care Cardiac Ultrasound

Term	Acronym in Use
Basic Critical Care Echocardiography	BCCE
Bedside cardiac ultrasound	
Cardiac limited ultrasound	
Cardiopulmonary limited ultrasound exam	CLUE
Directed bedside echocardiography	
Focus assessed transthoracic echocardiography	FATE
Focused bedside echocardiography	
Focused echocardiography	
Focused cardiac ultrasound/ultrasonography	FoCUS, FOCUS, FCU
Focused rapid echocardiographic exam	FREE
Goal-directed echocardiography	GDE
Hand-carried cardiac ultrasound	
Hand-carried echocardiography	
Handheld cardiac ultrasound	HCU
Handheld echocardiography	
Pocket cardiac ultrasound	
Pocket echocardiography	
Point-of-care cardiac ultrasound/ultrasonography	PoCUS, POCUS
Point-of-care echocardiography	

TABLE 13.2   Key Features of a Point-of-Care Cardiac Ultrasound Examination

- Performed at the bedside
- Adjunct to physical examination
- Problem-oriented
- Limited in scope
- Simplified protocol
- Dynamic protocols (vary by clinical problem and training of provider)
- Time-sensitive
- Repeatable
- Interpretation of specific parameters (not comprehensive evaluation of all findings)
- Real-time interpretation
- Discrete qualitative interpretation (present/absent; normal/moderate or more deviation from normal)
- Actionable results for clinical decision-making
- Facilitated early diagnosis/triage/management

Point-of-care cardiac ultrasound allows the detection of findings that are occult to bedside physical exam, like pericardial effusion, or simply difficult to detect with traditional bedside tools, like left ventricle [LV]) dysfunction. Most studies have concentrated on diagnostic accuracy to detect specific abnormalities compared with a gold standard. Prior reports have shown reduced use of other imaging tests when goal-directed echocardiography is used in the intensive care unit (ICU) setting.[5,6] Future studies should identify the settings in which point-of-care cardiac ultrasound facilitates improved health outcomes.

UNSTABLE PATIENTS

One of the earliest documented benefits of point-of-care cardiac ultrasound was demonstrated in patients with penetrating chest trauma.[7,8] In hemodynamic instability, an exam can be performed rapidly at the bedside and clearly adds to the traditional clinical evaluation of patients.[9-11] The use of goal-directed echocardiography during the initial evaluation of patients with hemodynamic instability is rapidly becoming the standard of care in ICUs. Specific ultrasound protocols have been developed to standardize and expedite the assessment of hypotensive patients.[12-14] Incorporation of a goal-directed echocardiography protocol in the evaluation of patients with

to become proficient in a limited number of high-yield views that can be performed quickly and require limited training. Awareness of the differences between comprehensive standard echocardiography and goal-directed echocardiography is a prerequisite for safe, competent, and responsible cardiac ultrasound use.

undifferentiated hypotension results in a more accurate physician impression of final diagnosis.[15,16] In critically ill patients, goal-directed echocardiography has been shown to improve the bedside assessment of volume status and LV systolic function.[17-21] In hemodynamically unstable patients, a cardiac assessment can guide management with regard to volume repletion, diuresis, and initiation and titration of vasoactive medications.[22] Cardiac ultrasound can also identify findings suggestive of hemodynamically important pulmonary embolism at the point of care.[23] During cardiopulmonary resuscitation, cardiac ultrasound is often used to evaluate for cardiac standstill when a decision must be made whether to cease or continue resuscitative efforts (see Chapter 23).[24-26] It is critical that when ultrasound is used in cardiac arrest, it not interfere with or delay cardiopulmonary resuscitative efforts and that it be performed either during pulse checks or using goal-directed transesophageal echocardiography after securing the airway (see Chapter 21).[25]

DECOMPENSATED HEART FAILURE

In patients with acute decompensated heart failure (ADHF) and/or cardiogenic shock, physicians who have had proctored hands-on point-of-care cardiac ultrasound training can readily distinguish patients with normal versus reduced LV systolic function.[27,28] It is clear that cardiac ultrasound is superior to physical examination, electrocardiography (ECG), chest x-ray, and blood chemistries for the detection of LV systolic dysfunction (LVSD) in patients with ADHF.[27] Although patients with heart failure will eventually benefit from a comprehensive echocardiogram, a point-of-care exam provides immediate knowledge of LV systolic function, which allows both the initiation of appropriate therapies and avoidance of contraindicated therapies. Early use of point-of-care cardiac ultrasound during the hospitalization of ADHF patients predicts diuretic responders better than renal function or brain natriuretic peptide,[29] and its application at discharge has been shown to predict hospital readmission more powerfully than clinical and laboratory variables.[30] Data suggest that length of stay and hospital readmissions may be reduced when cardiac ultrasound is routinely integrated into the care of hospitalized patients with ADHF.[31,32]

VOLUME STATUS

Assessment of volume status is routine in patients with cardiorespiratory failure. Identification of volume depletion in a hypotensive patient or volume excess in a dyspneic patient can facilitate diagnosis and treatment. It is clear that body habitus limits the evaluation of jugular venous pressure (JVP), and JVP is often poorly assessed even when clearly visible. Ultrasound assessment of the inferior vena cava (IVC) is both more feasible and accurate than physical exam in detecting elevated central venous pressure.[33] IVC size and collapsibility correlate with central venous pressure and can assist in the management of both fluid administration and diuresis. In an outpatient setting, discrepancies between clinical and sonographic assessments of volume status are common, but ultrasound has been shown to be superior at predicting adverse cardiac events.[34]

SCREENING

Because cardiac ultrasound will identify cardiac pathology with greater accuracy than physical examination, it can potentially be used to screen for asymptomatic cardiac abnormalities. LVSD is ideal for screening. It is a prevalent problem (occurring in 2%–4% of the general population), frequently asymptomatic and occult to physical examination, readily detectable with ultrasound, and has effective therapies even in the preclinical stage.[35,36] Several studies have demonstrated the feasibility of using cardiac ultrasound for identifying LVSD when screening asymptomatic patient populations.[37-41] A cost analysis study suggested that, rather than screening all patients directly, the application of cardiac ultrasound in patients with an abnormal B-type natriuretic peptide (BNP) or ECG was the most cost-effective strategy for identifying asymptomatic LV dysfunction.[42] Cardiac findings of great prognostic importance, including left ventricular hypertrophy (LVH) and left atrial (LA) enlargement, have been successfully detected in screening studies using point-of-care cardiac ultrasound.[40,43,44]

Studies have demonstrated the value and clinical impact of point-of-care cardiac ultrasound across a broad array of specialties and settings. Anesthesiologists have identified important cardiac findings that alter management in patients screened in the preoperative period,[45-47] and there have been similar

TABLE 13.3　Evidence-Based Targets for a Point-of-Care Cardiac Ultrasound Examination

Target	References	Assessment	Level of Evidence
LV systolic function	19,21,28,37,39,56–64	Normal/reduced/severely reduced	++++
LV size	72,74	Normal/enlarged	++
LVH	75–77	Normal/mild/severe	++
RV size	23,59,64,75	Normal/enlarged (increased RV/ LV ratio)	+++
LA size	57,72	Normal/enlarged	++
Pericardial effusion	57–60,64,72,75	Absent/present/large	++++
IVC size/collapse	17,20,33,60,64,75,78,79	Small/collapsible Large/noncollapsible	+++
Gross structural valve abnormalities	2	Abnormal	++
Large intracardiac masses	2	Abnormal	++

IVC, Inferior vena cava; *LA*, left atrium; *LV*, left ventricle; *LVH*, left ventricular hypertrophy; *RV*, right ventricle.

findings in medical clinic encounters.[48,49] In more resource-limited settings, the superior diagnostic accuracy of cardiac ultrasound versus auscultation in identifying rheumatic heart disease has been shown to be highly advantageous.[50-55]

Literature Review

Providers can use cardiac ultrasound to identify the presence or absence of specific findings using a rapid bedside examination protocol after limited training. The ability of a point-of-care cardiac ultrasound exam to assess LV systolic function has been well studied. Physicians with limited ultrasound training can detect LVSD with sensitivities of 73% to 100% and specificities of 64% to 96%.[19,21,28,37,39,56-64] Several studies have demonstrated that parasternal imaging alone is adequate for the subjective assessment of LV systolic function even though apical abnormalities may not be appreciated.[27,39,65,66]

For cardiac imaging, there is a general consensus that a limited number of views is adequate to assess the diagnostic targets, including the subcostal four-chamber, subcostal IVC, parasternal long-axis, parasternal short-axis, and apical four-chamber views.[1,2,67-69] The parasternal short- and long-axis views are easier to master than apical or subcostal views.[70] Parasternal views consistently provide more interpretable images than apical views because parasternal landmarks are more reliable and parasternal views are less dependent on patient positioning and body habitus. Less experienced

providers prefer the parasternal window for the assessment of LV systolic function.[71] Nonexpert sonographers can obtain adequate parasternal views nearly twice as often as adequate apical views.[72]

Several cardiac diagnoses can be made from a point-of-care cardiac ultrasound examination (Table 13.3). Providers should pursue proficiency in identifying abnormalities that (1) are pertinent to their clinical practice, such as the evaluation of RV size by critical care physicians; (2) are within their individual image acquisition and image interpretation expertise; (3) have high value when used in combination with physical examination and other clinical data; (4) can be acquired quickly to manage time-sensitive clinical presentations, making a 2- to 5-minute protocol ideal; (5) are frequently encountered in clinical practice, as maintenance of competence is difficult with rare findings; and (6) have evidence-based data supporting accurate diagnosis by providers with limited training in echocardiography.[1,2,67-69,73]

Some of the cardiac diagnoses that meet these criteria are listed in Table 13.3. A general consensus exists that patients should be referred for comprehensive echocardiography to detect abnormalities beyond the scope of a point-of-care cardiac ultrasound exam or suspected undetected cardiac pathologies.[2,10] The use of quantitative spectral Doppler techniques generally requires additional training. Some users will be motivated to pursue such training; however, the majority of users will be able to answer their clinical questions using the targets outlined in Table 13.3.

When it is used by physicians without formal echocardiographic training, point-of-care cardiac ultrasound is superior to physical examination for the detection of cardiac abnormalities including LV enlargement, LVSD, LA enlargement, LV hypertrophy, pericardial effusion, and RA pressure elevation.[27,33,74,75,80,81] After brief training, use of bedside ultrasound has been shown to greatly improve the clinical diagnoses of medical students and junior physicians over diagnoses made using physical examination, history, and ECG findings.[61]

Limitations

Smaller ultrasound devices cannot create the same image quality as a full-platform ultrasound machine (see Chapter 50). However, pocket and hand-carried devices have been miniaturized to improve portability, costs, and availability. This compromise results in loss of some functionality and screen size which may limit the interpretation of more nuanced or detailed findings. In an effort to simplify operation, some devices only have controls for depth and gain adjustment, omitting image enhancement capabilities found on higher-end devices. As point-of-care cardiac ultrasound relies largely on qualitative assessments, the absence of calculation packages and other tools for quantitative analysis is generally not an important limitation.

Some pathologies, regardless of the provider's level of training, are generally considered the domain of the cardiologist-echocardiographer, such as congenital heart disease and prosthetic valves.

Training

Several studies have demonstrated acceptable accuracy of nonexpert providers performing cardiac ultrasound exams.[17–21,23,27,28,33,37–39,56–61,63,64,73–78,82] The heterogeneity of these studies makes it difficult to draw specific conclusions about training. Training protocols have differed with respect to trainee experience, ultrasound devices, duration of training, imaging protocols, and clinical settings.

A structured training program is the best approach for providers to acquire with the necessary knowledge and technical skills. Studies with novice providers have shown an acceptable skill level to perform and interpret cardiac ultrasound exams after 20 to 30 repetitions,

if the scope of image acquisition and interpretation is limited to parasternal views.[70,83,84] For apical imaging, more extensive training is required and the number of studies for competency appears to be more than 45.[64,70]

Although there is general agreement that proficiency should be determined by competency-based assessments before being used in patient care, no validated tools exist to determine competency.[2] Most guidelines and training requirements are based on time (hours or months) in training and number of ultrasound exams performed, which are used as surrogates of competency.[10,85–88] Unfortunately the correlation is weak between the number of studies interpreted/months of training and the provider's interpretation accuracy.[89] The correlation between number of exams performed with image acquisition skills is better, which supports training programs with significant hands-on imaging practice. Despite these limitations, there is general agreement that a number of supervised and unsupervised studies should be logged before a competency assessment is performed.[2] The number of supervised exams needed will depend on the number of pathologies the provider desires to diagnose in clinical practice and the number of views required to reliably evaluate these diagnoses. Image acquisition skills are learned more slowly than image interpretation skills.[64,70,83]

Didactic education should cover ultrasound physics and normal cardiac anatomy from standard ultrasound views. The ultrasound appearance of common abnormalities within the provider's scope of practice should be reviewed. Hands-on practice should proceed within a reasonable period of time after didactic education, as significant delays can be deleterious to skill acquisition.[83]

The standard cardiac acoustic windows, imaging planes, transducer manipulation, and basic anatomy can be learned using simulation and practice on live models[90,91]; however, proctored scanning in patient-care settings provides invaluable experience. A randomized medical student education study demonstrated superior image acquisition skills when proctored by a sonographer versus self-directed simulation-based training.[92] Although independent imaging practice is valuable, all learners need adequate proctored scanning practice. Providers should acquire skills using the same device that will be used in clinical practice, or one with similar capabilities. Thus, training on stable outpatients using a high-end, full-platform ultrasound machine does not prepare a provider to image critically ill patients using a small portable ultrasound machine.

It is essential to review images because hands-on training does not expose learners to all the pathologies and normal variants seen in clinical practice. Selected images can be reviewed in didactic sessions or self-directed educational modules. The breadth of cases reviewed should be modified based on the clinical setting, scope of practice, and diagnoses likely to be encountered.

Like many skills in medicine, ultrasound skills diminish notably with nonuse.[93] Maintaining competence in point-of-care cardiac ultrasound requires an ongoing commitment to scanning patients and interpreting images.

CHAPTER 14

Cardiac Ultrasound Technique

Scott Millington

Background

A point-of-care cardiac ultrasound examination can be an invaluable clinical tool in the hands of experienced providers. Because cardiac ultrasound requires assessment of both structure and function, the highest quality images should be acquired for optimal assessment. In order to be confident in the interpretation of cardiac ultrasound exam findings, views from two or more imaging planes should be obtained. Although a significant investment of time is required, providers from different disciplines and levels of experience can master the techniques described in this chapter.[1-7]

Novice ultrasound users can find solace in that provider skills and confidence generally increase rapidly after learning the basic transducer positions. Novice users can become comfortable with cardiac ultrasonography with adequately supervised and structured practice. Training traditionally focuses on achieving proficiency in five core cardiac views: parasternal long-axis, parasternal short-axis (mid-ventricular level), apical 4-chamber, subcostal 4-chamber, and subcostal inferior vena cava (IVC) views.[8-10]

Anatomy: Imaging Windows, Planes, and Views

An *imaging window* refers to an anatomic position on the body where an ultrasound transducer is placed to visualize specific structures. In transthoracic echocardiography, there are three standard imaging windows: parasternal, apical, and subcostal windows (Fig. 14.1).

An *imaging plane* refers to an anatomic plane (sagittal, coronal, or transverse) along which the ultrasound beam is aligned. All anatomic structures, unless they are perfectly spherical, have a long and short axis.[11] Imaging planes are named in relation to the axes of the heart in cardiac ultrasound, and four planes are conventionally described: long-axis, short-axis, 4-chamber, and 2-chamber. The long-axis plane bisects the heart vertically from the left ventricular apex to the aortic valve (AV) at the base of the heart. The short-axis plane is perpendicular to the long axis and generates cross sections of the ventricles. Similar to the long-axis plane, the 4-chamber plane extends from the apex to base of the heart but bisects the tricuspid valve (TV) and mitral valve (MV). The 2-chamber plane is perpendicular to the 4-chamber plane (Fig. 14.2). Between the long and short axes of

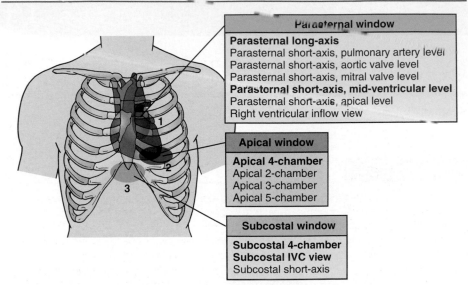

Figure 14.1 Standard Transthoracic Cardiac Imaging Windows. For transthoracic cardiac imaging, three standard cardiac windows are used: *(1)* parasternal, *(2)* apical, and *(3)* subcostal. From each imaging window, several different imaging views can be obtained that are named according to the cross-sectional plane. The five key cardiac views are bolded. *IVC*, Inferior vena cava.

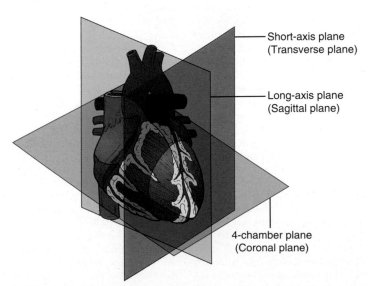

Figure 14.2 Cardiac Imaging Planes. Four standard cardiac imaging planes are conventionally described: long-axis, short-axis, 4-chamber, and 2-chamber (not shown). The long-axis plane bisects the heart longitudinally from the left ventricular apex to the aortic valve. The short-axis plane is perpendicular to the long-axis plane and bisects the hearts transversely. The 4-chamber plane extends from the apex to the base of the heart, bisecting the mitral and tricuspid valves.

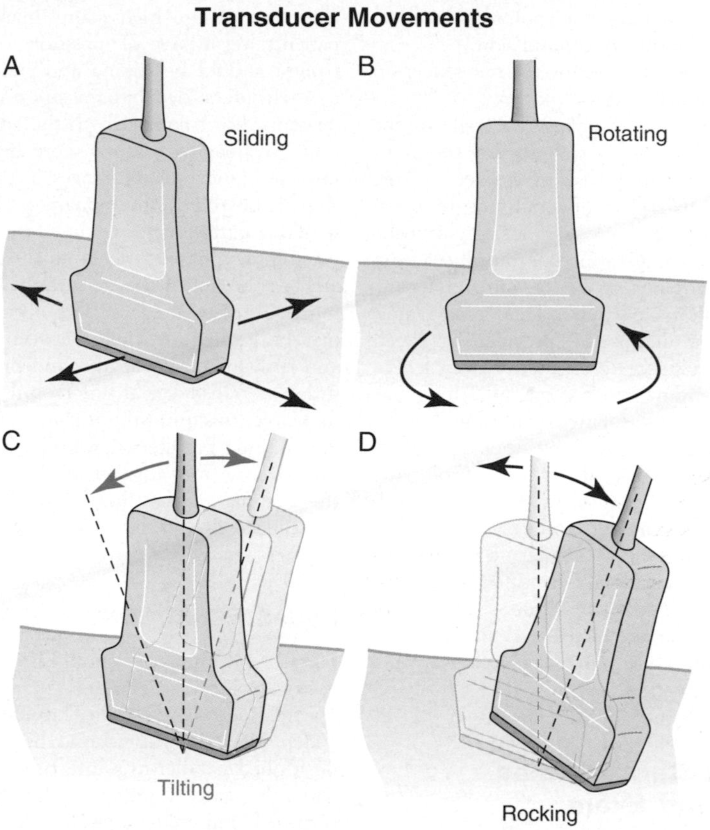

Transducer Movements

Figure 14.3 Transducer Movements. Sliding is relocation of the transducer on the skin surface. Rotating refers to twisting the transducer along its central axis, like a corkscrew. Tilting refers to changing the angle of the imaging plane to obtain serial cross-sectional images. Rocking refers to aiming the ultrasound beam toward or away from the transducer orientation marker to center the image on the screen.

the heart, an infinite number of oblique planes exist that are not conventionally named.

Combining imaging windows and planes gives rise to *imaging views*. Imaging views are standard cross sections of the heart obtained from specific windows. Within each imaging window, there are several different views that can be acquired along the different imaging planes. Imaging views are named according to the window and plane. For example, in the parasternal window the two principal views are the parasternal long-axis view and parasternal short-axis view.

The human thorax, with its bony ribs and air-filled lungs, is a naturally challenging environment to image with ultrasound. Despite these barriers, the fundamental transthoracic cardiac ultrasound views are attainable in most patients from the parasternal, apical, and subcostal windows; each of these windows

is explored in detail in this chapter. Specific clinical questions may occasionally require use of other windows to obtain views that are not part of a standard point-of-care exam, such as suprasternal views to evaluate the aortic arch. Inability to acquire satisfactory images occurs in a minority of patients, and a transesophageal echocardiogram may be indicated for an adequate assessment of the heart (see Chapter 20).[12]

Transducer Movements

Understanding the conventional nomenclature to describe transducer movements is important for communicating with colleagues and training new users. There are four primary movements of the transducer: sliding, rotating, tilting, and rocking (Fig. 14.3).[11,13]

1. *Sliding* refers to relocating the transducer on the skin surface; it is the process of

physically moving the point of contact between the transducer and skin.

2. *Rotating* refers to twisting the transducer on its central axis, like a corkscrew.

3. *Tilting* refers to changing the angle of the imaging plane while maintaining the point of contact with the skin surface. Tilting allows visualization of serial cross-sectional images of a structure from a single acoustic window, such as tilting the transducer from the cardiac base to apex to acquire serial parasternal short-axis views. This "cross-plane" movement allows the provider to sweep through a structure of interest from left to right, or from cranial to caudal. Tilting may also be called sweeping or fanning.

4. *Rocking* refers to aiming the ultrasound beam either toward or away from the transducer orientation marker while maintaining the point of contact with the skin surface. Rocking is similar to tilting but in a perpendicular plane of motion. This "in-plane" movement allows centering of the image on the screen and allows visualization beyond the current field of view in a specific direction.

Point-of-Care Cardiac Ultrasound Exam

The number of possible cardiac imaging views can seem limitless at first glance, but the quantity of conventionally defined views is limited. From the conventional imaging windows, as many as 16 traditional imaging views can be obtained with a comprehensive transthoracic echocardiogram. From a point-of-care perspective, mastery of five imaging views will allow the vast majority of clinically relevant questions to be addressed:

1. Parasternal long-axis view (PLAX)
2. Parasternal short-axis, midventricular level view (PSAX)
3. Apical 4-chamber view (A4C)
4. Subcostal 4-chamber view (S4C)
5. Subcostal IVC view (IVC)

Parasternal Window

IMAGING WINDOW

Cardiac ultrasound exams traditionally begin in the parasternal window. An important advantage of the parasternal window is the ability to acquire high-quality images in most patients regardless of position. Ideally, the patient should be supine and can be rotated to a left lateral decubitus position to bring the heart in direct contact with the anterior chest wall. An imaging window more inferiorly may provide higher quality images in patients with chronic obstructive pulmonary disease.

The parasternal window is imaged by placing a phased-array transducer immediately to the left of the sternum in the third or fourth intercostal space. The optimal window may be located anywhere between the second and fifth intercostal spaces, and providers may slide the transducer an intercostal space above or below to acquire the highest quality image. An optimal parasternal window has the least interference from adjacent ribs and lung. Once the optimal window has been identified, the transducer should be held in place without sliding.

PARASTERNAL LONG-AXIS VIEW

For a PLAX, the probe should be adjusted with the transducer orientation marker pointing toward the patient's right shoulder (Fig. 14.4; Video 14.1). The ultrasound beam should be positioned parallel to a line running from the patient's right shoulder to left hip. Images obtained represent anatomic cross sections through the long axis of the heart from the cardiac apex to base.

The right ventricle (RV) is seen anteriorly, at the top of the screen. While holding the transducer steady, visualize the aortic and mitral valves and center the ultrasound beam over the LV. An ideal view is obtained when both the AV and MV are clearly visualized in the same plane and the ultrasound beam is centered along the long axis of the left ventricle (LV). Slight rotation and tilting of the transducer opens the left ventricular cavity to its fullest extent, avoiding the tendency to foreshorten the cavity. This common error can result in overestimation of LV systolic function and underestimation of LV cavity dimension. If a good-quality image cannot be achieved, consider sliding the transducer up or down one intercostal space and beginning anew. Alternatively, the patient may be positioned in a left lateral decubitus position. Finally, cooperative patients can be asked to consciously regulate their respiratory cycle, ideally by having them hold their breath at end-expiration.

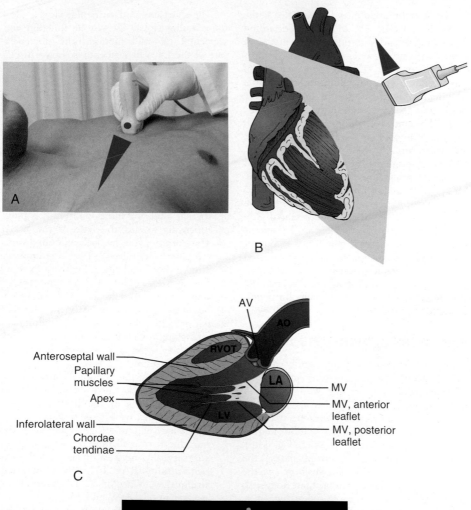

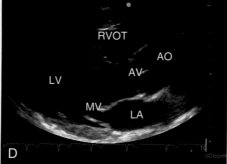

Figure 14.4 Parasternal Long-Axis View. (A) Transducer position. (B) Imaging plane. (C) Cross-sectional anatomy. (D) Ultrasound image. *AO*, Aorta; *AV*, aortic valve; *LA*, left atrium; *LV*, left ventricle, *MV*, mitral valve; *RVOT*, right ventricular outflow tract.

Key structures that must be identified in the PLAX include the AV, MV, LV, pericardium (both anterior and posterior to the heart), right ventricular outflow tract (RVOT), left ventricular outflow tract (LVOT), and portions of the ascending and descending thoracic aorta. The depth should be adjusted to visualize the descending thoracic aorta in the far field.

In the context of point-of-care ultrasound, the PLAX is used primarily to assess LV size and function, AV, MV, and left atrial size. Although imaging is limited to visualization of the anteroseptal and inferolateral LV walls, LV systolic function can be accurately assessed in this view. Pericardial effusions can also be detected, especially when circumferential. Providers cannot reliably comment on RV size or function because only a small cross section of the RVOT is seen; however, a severely dilated RV can be reliably detected. The PLAX provides a basic assessment of the AV and MV and allows evaluation for dynamic obstruction at the level of the LVOT.

PARASTERNAL SHORT-AXIS VIEW

The most effective way to rapidly acquire a high-quality PSAX view is to start with a high-quality PLAX. Starting with the transducer centered over the MV in a PLAX, the transducer is then rotated 90 degrees clockwise to point the transducer orientation marker toward the patient's left shoulder (Fig. 14.5). Care should be taken to avoid sliding the transducer into a different position on the chest. Using two hands can facilitate a smooth transition from a long-axis to a short-axis view, with one hand rotating the transducer and the other hand stabilizing the transducer on the skin surface.

Five different imaging planes can be achieved in the parasternal short-axis view. For purposes of point-of-care ultrasound, the midventricular level is favored by most providers for its reliable portrayal of global LV systolic function. A midventricular parasternal short-axis view is achieved when both papillary muscles are visualized in cross section and appear symmetric, as shown in Fig. 14.5. It is important to rotate the transducer sufficiently to obtain a true cross-sectional image of the LV cavity that appears circular. An oval-shaped LV cavity indicates off-axis imaging or foreshortening, which can lead to erroneous interpretation of LV systolic function.

The short-axis midventricular view is ideal for assessing global LV systolic function and segmental LV wall motion. The nomenclature of the LV wall segments is shown in Fig. 14.6. This view also helps assess the shape and function of the interventricular septum in the context of RV dilatation and dysfunction. Large- or moderate-sized circumferential pericardial effusions are also well visualized.

The other short-axis planes, beyond the midventricular plane, may be useful in specific clinical contexts and are listed in anatomic sequence, from the cardiac base to the apex (Fig. 14.7):

1. *Pulmonary artery level:* From the midventricular level, the ultrasound beam is tilted superiorly toward the base of the heart. The correct plane has been acquired once the pulmonary valve (PV), main pulmonary artery (MPA), and ascending aorta in short axis are seen (Video 14.2). In rare cases of acute pulmonary embolism (PE), a thrombus may be seen in the MPA or proximal left or right pulmonary arteries. Pulmonary regurgitation velocities may be used to estimate the mean and diastolic pulmonary artery pressures.

2. *AV level:* From the pulmonary artery level, the transducer is tilted slightly inferiorly, toward the apex of the heart. An ideal image includes a short-axis view of the AV, which may require a slight rotation of the transducer until all three AV cusps appear symmetrically. An ideal image includes the right atrium (RA), TV, RVOT, and left atrium (LA) (Video 14.3). This view allows assessment of the AV and TV.

3. *MV level:* When rotating from a parasternal long-axis to short-axis view, the distinct "fish mouth" appearance of the MV is usually seen first (Video 14.4). This view allows assessment of MV anatomy, but in acutely ill patients this view has limited utility. LV systolic function may be underestimated compared to the midventricular level due to restriction from the MV annulus.

4. *Midventricular, papillary muscle level:* This view yields the most useful clinical information in the vast majority of acutely ill patients. Both papillary muscles are symmetrically seen in cross section in the center of the circular left ventricular cavity (Video 14.5). Motion of the individual LV chamber wall segments is best assessed at this level as well as overall LV systolic function.

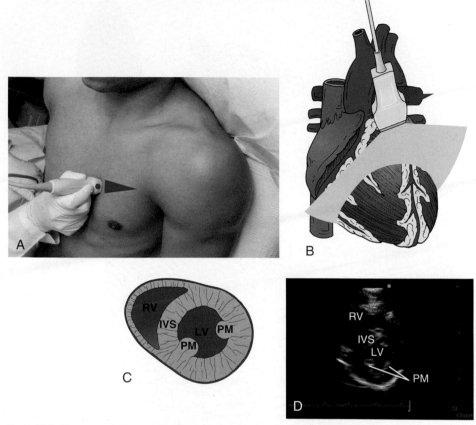

Figure 14.5 Parasternal Short-Axis View. (A) Transducer position. (B) Imaging plane. (C) Cross-sectional anatomy. (D) Ultrasound image. *IVS*, Interventricular septum; *LV*, left ventricle; *PM*, papillary muscle; *RV*, right ventricle.

5. *Apical level:* This short-axis view is obtained by tilting the transducer to aim the ultrasound beam inferiorly, toward the apex of the heart. The LV apex is visualized sequentially starting from the midpapillary muscle level and moving inferiorly (Video 14.6). LV systolic function may be overestimated compared to the midventricular level. In rare cases, an LV apical thrombus may be seen.

Apical Window

IMAGING WINDOW

In the traditional cardiac imaging sequence, the apical window follows the parasternal window. In general, acquiring adequate quality images from the apical window is more challenging than from the parasternal or subcostal windows. Ideally, patients should be positioned in a left lateral decubitus position, or at least supine with some leftward rotation. In the critically ill, who may not tolerate being repositioned, apical views may still be achieved, although with some reduction in image quality. In obese or mechanically ventilated patients, acquiring interpretable apical images may not always be possible.

APICAL 4-CHAMBER VIEW

Positioning the transducer over the LV apex is critical for accurate imaging from the apical window, and its position can vary significantly between patients. In general, the apex is located just inferolateral to the left nipple in men and underneath the inferolateral quadrant of the left breast in women. One approach is to slide

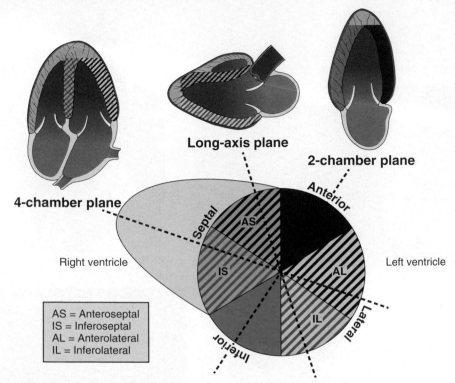

Long-axis plane

2-chamber plane

4-chamber plane

Right ventricle

Left ventricle

AS = Anteroseptal
IS = Inferoseptal
AL = Anterolateral
IL = Inferolateral

Figure 14.6 Left Ventricular Wall Segments and Imaging Planes. The left ventricle is divided into three sections along its long axis (basal, midcavity, and apical sections). The basal and midcavity sections have six segments (anterior, anterolateral, anteroseptal, inferior, inferolateral, inferoseptal walls), whereas the apical section has four segments (septal, inferior, lateral, anterior walls).

the transducer inferolaterally on the chest from the parasternal short-axis position toward the apex. Alternatively, identify the spleen first and then slide the transducer cephalad to the apex. Once the LV apex is visualized, the transducer is tilted steeply to aim the ultrasound transducer face toward the patient's right shoulder. The transducer orientation marker should be pointed to the patient's left side (Fig. 14.8).

The transducer should be rocked to align the interventricular septum in a vertical position in the center of the screen. The transducer may need to be slightly rotated so the LV and RV cavities are visualized in a true longitudinal cross-section. Subtle adjustments of transducer position may be required to optimize the view of the LV cavity, specifically to avoid foreshortening. Foreshortening commonly occurs in the apical window when the transducer is not over the true apex and the heart appears short and globular, rather than long and oval. An ideal apical 4-chamber view is presented in Fig. 14.8

and Video 14.7; note the LV, RV, LA, and RA can all be seen clearly in addition to the MV and TV.

The apical 4-chamber view is part of a standard point-of-care cardiac ultrasound exam and can provide a tremendous amount of clinical information. This view allows assessment of RV systolic function and size relative to the LV. The MV and TV can be evaluated, and pericardial fluid can also be detected. Adequate assessment of global LV systolic function is usually possible, although only the anterolateral and inferoseptal walls are visualized. Although not part of a standard point-of-care exam, additional apical views can provide a more complete evaluation of the heart (Fig. 14.9):

1. *Apical 4-chamber view:* This is the basic view from the apical window, as described above (Video 14.7).

2. *Apical 2-chamber view:* Starting from an apical 4-chamber view, the transducer is rotated 90 degrees counterclockwise. The

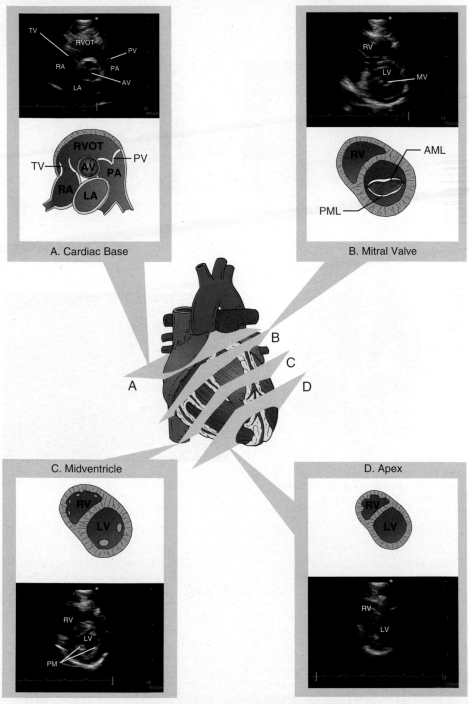

Figure 14.7 Parastornal Short-Axis Imaging Planes and Cross-Sectional Anatomy at Different Levels.
(A) Cardiac base—pulmonary artery and aortic valve levels. (B) Mitral valve. (C) Midventricle. (D) Apex.
AML, Anterior mitral leaflet; *AV,* aortic valve; *LA,* left atrium; *LV,* left ventricle; *PA,* pulmonary artery; *PML,* posterior mitral leaflet; *PV,* pulmonary valve; *RA,* right atrium; *RV,* right ventricle; *RVOT,* right ventricular outflow tract; *TV,* tricuspid valve.

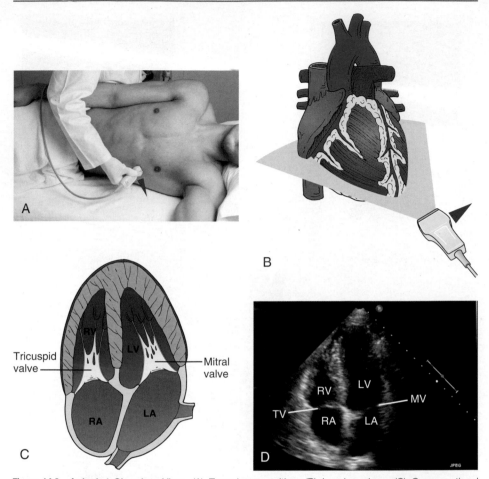

Figure 14.8   Apical 4-Chamber View. (A) Transducer position. (B) Imaging plane. (C) Cross-sectional anatomy. (D) Ultrasound image. *LA*, Left atrium; *LV*, left ventricle; *MV*, mitral valve; *RA*, right atrium; *RV*, right ventricle; *TV*, tricuspid valve.

ideal view demonstrates only the LV, MV, and LA (Video 14.8). If any part of the RV or LVOT is in view, then the transducer is underrotated or overrotated, respectively. This view allows for assessment of regional LV function, specifically with respect to the anterior and inferior LV walls.

3. *Apical 3-chamber view:* Starting from the apical 2-chamber view, the transducer is rotated an additional 30 degrees counterclockwise. The ideal view demonstrates the LV, MV, and LA, with the LVOT and AV now appearing at the 5 o'clock position (Video 14.9). This view allows assessment

of regional LV function, specifically of the inferolateral and anteroseptal LV walls.

4. *Apical 5-chamber view:* Starting from the apical 4-chamber view, the transducer is tilted 20 to 30 degrees anteriorly, to aim the ultrasound transducer face toward the chest wall. The ideal view demonstrates the same four chambers as the apical 4-chamber view (LV, RV, LA, and RA) but with the addition of the LVOT and AV at the 7 o'clock position (Video 14.10). This view provides additional information about the AV and is used to measure stroke volume or cardiac output using spectral Doppler (see Chapter 21).

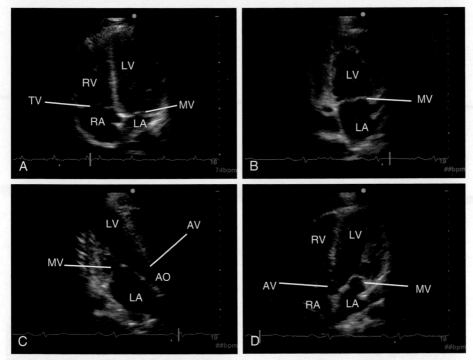

Figure 14.9   Apical Views in Different Planes. (A) 4-Chamber. (B) 2-Chamber. (C) 3-Chamber. (D) 5-Chamber. *AV*, Aortic valve; *LA*, left atrium; *LV*, left ventricle; *MV*, mitral valve; *RA*, right atrium; *RV*, right ventricle; *TV*, tricuspid valve.

Subcostal Window

IMAGING WINDOW

In the point-of-care ultrasound context, the subcostal window can provide high-yield information rapidly, especially in acutely ill patients. The subcostal window offers several advantages:

1. Supine positioning is favorable for subcostal imaging.
2. Surface landmarks are reliable, permitting rapid image acquisition in most cases.
3. In emergent situations, such as during cardiac arrest, the subcostal area is generally otherwise unoccupied and imaging from here minimizes interference with resuscitative efforts.
4. In patients with hyperinflated lungs due to chronic lung disease or mechanical ventilation, downward displacement of the heart leads to improved image quality from the subcostal window.
5. Pericardial tamponade and severe RV dysfunction, two conditions that may require urgent intervention, can often be diagnosed effectively from the subcostal window.
6. Hypovolemia and LV systolic dysfunction, two common clinical conditions, can frequently be diagnosed from the subcostal window.

The transducer is placed immediately below the xiphoid process in the midline with the transducer orientation marker pointed to the patient's left side. The transducer should be pressed down firmly, almost flattened under the xiphoid process. In some patients, a significant amount of pressure is required, and patients should be warned about the potential discomfort. The ultrasound transducer face should be aimed upward toward the heart and left shoulder. If the provider is having difficulty visualizing the heart in this window, patients can bend their knees to relax abdominal wall musculature or perform a brief end-inspiratory breath hold to transiently shift the heart

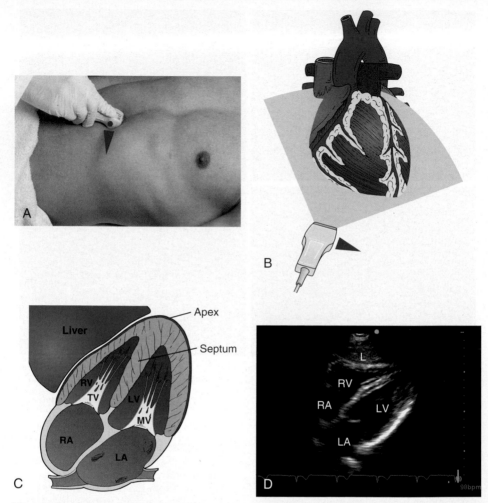

Figure 14.10   Subcostal 4-Chamber View. (A) Transducer position. (B) Imaging plane. (C) Cross-sectional anatomy. (D) Ultrasound image. *L*, Liver; *LA*, left atrium; *LV*, left ventricle; *MV*, mitral valve; *RA*, right atrium; *RV*, right ventricle; *TV*, tricuspid valve.

inferiorly. If bowel or stomach gas impedes image acquisition, the operator can slide the transducer toward the patient's right, abutting the transducer to the right costal margin where it meets the xiphoid process, and use more of the liver as an acoustic window.

SUBCOSTAL 4-CHAMBER VIEW

Once the heart is in view in the subcostal window, subtle transducer manipulation can help acquire an optimal 4-chamber view. Ideally, the RV, LV, RA, LA, and pericardium

should be visualized in cross section along the long axis of the heart (Fig. 14.10, Video 14.11).

The subcostal 4-chamber view allows assessment of RV systolic function and visualization of the RV free wall, which is limited in other views. RV and LV chamber sizes can be compared; however, RV size in this view can be underestimated since the imaging plane is through the inferior portion, rather than middle, of the RV. The subcostal window has high sensitivity for detection of pericardial effusions and diastolic collapse of the RV in cardiac tamponade. In many patients, reasonable visualization of

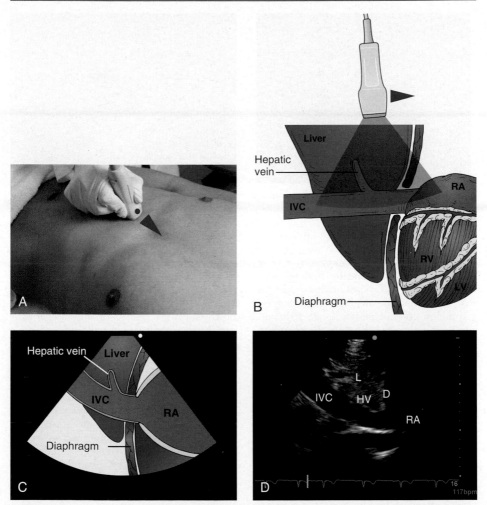

Figure 14.11   Subcostal Inferior Vena Cava View. (A) Transducer position. (B) Imaging plane. (C) Cross-sectional anatomy. (D) Ultrasound image. *D*, Diaphragm; *HV*, hepatic vein; *IVC*, inferior vena cava; *L*, liver; *LV*, left ventricle; *RA*, right atrium; *RV*, right ventricle.

the LV can be achieved, similar to an apical 4-chamber view. A subcostal 4-chamber view allows rapid assessment of global LV systolic function and is usually sufficient to guide management in emergent situations.

INFERIOR VENA CAVA VIEW

From the subcostal window, a longitudinal view of the IVC can be obtained (see Chapter 17). A subcostal IVC view is obtained by starting with a subcostal 4-chamber view, rotating the transducer 90 degrees counterclockwise

to point the transducer orientation marker cephalad, rocking the transducer to aim the transducer face posteriorly, and then tilting the transducer to align the ultrasound beam with the IVC (Fig. 14.11, Video 14.12). Subtle manipulation of the transducer is required to center the ultrasound beam over the IVC and visualize a true longitudinal cross-section of the IVC with the RA-IVC junction on the screen. The IVC's maximal diameter and respiratory variation is measured just distal to the hepatic vein–IVC junction, or 2 cm from the IVC-RA junction.

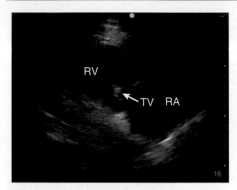

Figure 14.12 Parasternal Right Ventricular Inflow View. *RV*, Right ventricle; *TV*, tricuspid valve; *RA*, right atrium.

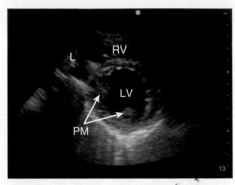

Figure 14.13 Subcostal Short-Axis View. *L*, Liver; *LV*, left ventricle; *PM*, papillary muscle; *RV*, right ventricle.

An ideal subcostal IVC long-axis view shows the hepatic vein(s) emptying into the IVC, along with the IVC itself draining into the RA. Visualizing the RA-IVC junction avoids a common error of mistaking the abdominal aorta for the IVC. Although the abdominal aorta is commonly more calcified, pulsatile, surrounded by retroperitoneal fat, and located left of the IVC, it is often mistaken for the IVC during a rapid bedside evaluation by novice providers.

Additional Cardiac Views

PARASTERNAL RIGHT VENTRICULAR INFLOW VIEW

From a PLAX, a right ventricular (RV) inflow view is obtained by tilting the transducer to aim the ultrasound transducer face toward the patient's right hip. The ideal RV inflow view allows visualization of the RV, RA, and TV without any portion of the LV (Fig. 14.12, Video 14.13). This view permits visualization of the posterior leaflet of the TV and assessment of tricuspid regurgitation (TR). If a portion of the LV is seen, the septal leaflet may be mistaken for the posterior leaflet. In patients with TR, spectral Doppler can be used to measure the pressure gradient across the valve to estimate the pulmonary artery systolic pressure.

SUBCOSTAL SHORT-AXIS VIEW

A subcostal short-axis view is similar in appearance and clinical utility to the parasternal short-axis view. Acquisition of a short-axis view, either from the parasternal or subcostal window, is recommended for a complete hemodynamic assessment. The subcostal short-axis view is particularly useful in patients who have obstructive lung disease or are mechanically ventilated, as these conditions tend to degrade parasternal image quality.

From the subcostal 4-chamber view, the transducer is rotated 90 degrees counterclockwise to point the transducer orientation marker toward the patient's head. Upon rotation of the transducer, the first structure to be visualized will be the base of the heart, similar to the pulmonary artery level or the AV level in the parasternal window. To obtain a midventricular view at the level of the papillary muscles, tilt the transducer to aim the ultrasound transducer face toward the apex (Fig. 14.13, Video 14.14).

Similar to the parasternal short-axis view, the subcostal short-axis view can be used to assess global LV systolic function and segmental LV wall motion. Interventricular septal dynamics and circumferential pericardial effusions can also be seen.

SUPRASTERNAL WINDOW

Although suprasternal imaging is not routinely performed, the suprasternal window allows visualization of the aortic arch, which may be relevant for rapid detection of acute aortic pathologies in the point-of-care context. The patient is positioned supine with the neck extended. The transducer is placed in the suprasternal notch with the transducer orientation marker pointed to the patient's left shoulder.

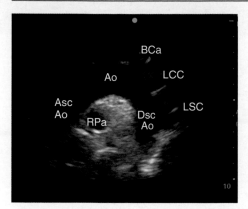

Figure 14.14 Suprasternal Long-Axis View. *Ao,* Aortic arch; *Asc Ao,* Ascending aorta; *BCa,* brachiocephalic artery; *Dsc Ao,* descending aorta; *LCC,* left common carotid artery; *LSC,* left subclavian artery; *RPa,* right pulmonary artery.

The transducer is tilted inferiorly to aim the transducer face toward the mediastinum. The transducer need to be rotated 10 to 20 degrees counter-clockwise to align the ultrasound beam longitudinally with the aorta. A suprasternal long-axis view allows visualization of the aortic arch and portions of the ascending and descending aorta. The right pulmonary artery is seen in cross section below the arch of the aorta (Fig. 14.14 and Video 14.15). To corroborate findings from the long-axis view, a suprasternal short-axis view can be obtained by rotating the transducer 90 degrees clockwise to visualize the aortic arch in cross-section.

PEARLS AND PITFALLS

The near limitless degrees of freedom associated with cardiac ultrasound imaging may seem overwhelming but the vast majority of common clinical questions can be answered by focusing on the five core views: parasternal long- and short-axis, apical 4-chamber, subcostal 4-chamber, and subcostal IVC. After providers have mastered cardiac image acquisition, they may begin to integrate their findings with the clinical presentation of a patient to guide clinical management. Interpretation and integration of common and important findings are emphasized in Chapters 15 to 19.

- Novice providers should focus on mastering the five core cardiac views. Additional views can be learned as experience accrues based on the common clinical questions that may arise in a specific patient population.
- Start by practicing the basic cardiac image acquisition skills on non-obese, stable, and cooperative patients from whom high-quality images can be easily obtained.
- Patient positioning is important in cardiac ultrasound imaging. Acquisition of interpretable images from the parasternal and apical windows is best performed in a left lateral decubitus position, whereas a supine position is needed for the subcostal window.
- Once a view of the heart is first captured, only subtle transducer manipulation is needed to optimize the image. Radical transducer movements often result in loss of the entire view, which is a common error committed by novice providers.
- Cardiac sonographers can be a valuable resource for novice providers to improve their cardiac image acquisition skills. Providers that are struggling to master the five core cardiac ultrasound views should consider supervised practice with an experienced cardiac sonographer.
- Integration of point-of-care cardiac ultrasound into the clinical care of real patients is the most difficult phase and should be done progressively under the supervision of an experienced provider. Quality assurance is essential to protect patient safety.

CHAPTER 15

Left Ventricular Function

Robert Arntfield ■ Stephen D. Walsh ■ Pierre Kory ■ Nilam J. Soni

KEY POINTS

- A qualitative determination of left ventricular systolic function can sufficiently guide point-of-care decisions and can be accurately performed by providers after brief, focused training in cardiac ultrasound.
- Qualitative assessment of left ventricular systolic function is categorized as hyperdynamic, normal, reduced, or severely reduced based on evaluation of endocardial excursion, myocardial thickening, and septal motion of the anterior leaflet of the mitral valve.
- Determination of left ventricular diastolic function, regional wall motion abnormalities, and hemodynamic calculations can be performed at the bedside but require additional training beyond what is required for gross interpretation of LV systolic function.

Background

Left ventricular (LV) systolic dysfunction can cause or significantly complicate acute illness. In undifferentiated shock, point-of-care LV assessment has been shown to increase accuracy in diagnosis and treatment decisions using a qualitative approach to classify LV systolic function. Physicians from a broad range of medical specialties can perform ultrasound imaging of the LV after participating in focused training in cardiac image acquisition and interpretation.[1-12]

Left Ventricular Systolic Function

Under normal conditions, the left ventricle is the largest and most muscular chamber of the heart and can be readily assessed from standard transthoracic cardiac ultrasound windows. The most common views include the parasternal long-axis (PLAX), parasternal short-axis, apical four-chamber, and subcostal four-chamber views. An organized approach to cardiac image acquisition is needed for efficient application at the point-of-care (see Chapter 14).

Traditional quantitative methods of determining LV function, including Simpson's biplane method or fractional area of change, are not commonly utilized in point-of-care cardiac ultrasound. These methods require additional training, are time-consuming, prone to error, and do not necessarily lead to higher accuracy in assessing LV systolic function.[13] Therefore, point-of-care cardiac ultrasound has embraced a qualitative approach for determining LV systolic function.

Numerous studies have demonstrated the feasibility and accuracy of point-of-care cardiac ultrasound using a qualitative approach to guide management of acutely ill patients.[1-7] Many studies have demonstrated a visually estimated left ventricular ejection fraction (LVEF) is comparable to a quantitative, calculated LVEF using comprehensive echocardiography as the gold standard. When visually estimating LV systolic function, attention is paid to all LV segments with particular focus on three cardinal characteristics (Fig. 15.1):

1. *Endocardial excursion.* Does the endocardium move symmetrically toward the center of the LV chamber during systole?
2. *Myocardial thickening.* Does the myocardium increase in thickness by approximately 40% in all LV segments during systole?
3. *Septal motion of the anterior mitral valve leaflet tip (E-point septal separation* in classic

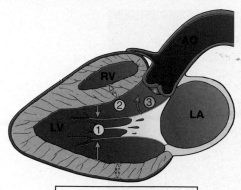

1 - Endocardial excursion
2 - Myocardial thickening
3 - Septal motion of anterior
    leaflet of mitral valve

Figure 15.1   Determination of Global Left Ventricular *(LV)* **Systolic Function.** LV systolic function is visually estimated by assessing endocardial excursion, myocardial thickening, and septal motion of the anterior mitral valve leaflet (E-point septal separation). Endocardial excursion is movement of the endocardium toward the center of the LV chamber during systole. Myocardial thickening is symmetrical muscle thickening by at least 40% of all LV segments. The anterior leaflet tip of the mitral valve normally approaches within 1 cm of the septum. *AO,* Aorta; *LA,* left atrium; *LV,* left ventricle; *RV,* right ventricle.

echocardiography nomenclature). Does the anterior mitral valve leaflet tip come within 1 cm of the septum, which corresponds with an LVEF greater than 40%?

This approach easily permits broad classification of LV systolic function into four discrete categories: (1) normal, (2) hyperdynamic, (3) reduced, and (4) severely reduced LV systolic function. With the focus on broad gradations of LV systolic function, this qualitative schema has the inherent benefits of being intuitive to use and clinically relevant to integrate into patient care.

NORMAL LEFT VENTRICULAR SYSTOLIC FUNCTION

In patients with normal LV systolic function, the myocardium can be seen thickening in all segments with the endocardium moving toward the center of the LV chamber in systole. In views where the mitral valve is seen, the leaflet tips can be seen approaching the

walls of the LV (Fig. 15.2). It is important to remember that the LV empties incompletely under normal conditions. The diameter of the mid-LV chamber measured at the endocardial borders decreases by approximately 30% to 40% during systole, leaving on average between 30% and 50% of blood volume in the LV at end-systole (Fig. 15.3, Videos 15.1 and 15.2).

HYPERDYNAMIC LEFT VENTRICULAR SYSTOLIC FUNCTION

Identifying a hyperdynamic LV can be useful in the assessment of unexplained hypotension or acute dyspnea, most often representing hypovolemia or severe peripheral vasodilation (e.g., septic illness). In such settings, endocardial excursion and myocardial thickening of the LV is increased, leading to total or near-total end-systolic obliteration of the LV cavity (Fig. 15.4 and Videos 15.3 and 15.4). Although a hyperdynamic LV frequently suggests hypovolemia and/or vasodilation, other etiologies that can severely decrease preload or afterload should be considered, many of which will have accompanying abnormal findings easily gleaned from a multi-system point-of-care ultrasound (POCUS) exam. Examples include massive pulmonary embolism, severe mitral regurgitation, or cardiac tamponade. Furthermore, high-output cardiac failure due to various etiologies, such as thyrotoxicosis, anemia, or infection, can also be considered.

REDUCED AND SEVERELY REDUCED LEFT VENTRICULAR SYSTOLIC FUNCTION

As outlined above, grading of LV systolic function is common in POCUS and focuses on a qualitative approach with discrete gradations of LV function. For a dysfunctional LV, decreased function is typically described as either reduced or severely reduced and can be derived from assessing three key parameters: (1) endocardial excursion, (2) myocardial thickening, and (3) mitral valve excursion.

Diminished endocardial excursion and myocardial thickening are somewhat intuitive to interpret as representing reduced LV systolic function, but mitral valve excursion in the assessment of LV systolic function *(E-point septal separation)* warrants some explanation. Conceptually, as the pathologic LV dilates, the mitral valve leaflets become tethered by the

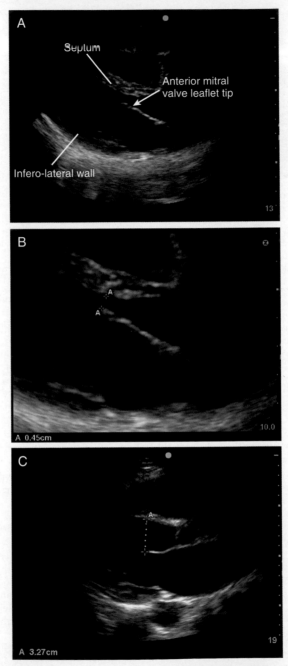

Figure 15.2 Normal Septal Motion of the Anterior Mitral Valve Leaflet. (A) Normal approximation of the anterior mitral valve leaflet tip toward the interventricular septum is shown in early diastole from a parasternal long-axis view, and (B) a zoomed view measuring the distance (0.45 cm in this case). (C) Decreased mitral valve excursion is seen with severely reduced left ventricular systolic function (3.27 cm in this case).

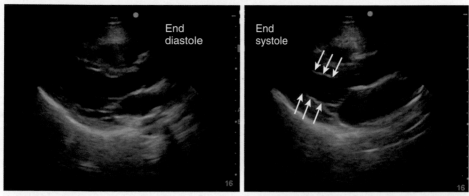

Figure 15.3   Normal Endocardial Excursion and Myocardial Thickening. Normal excursion of endocardium (arrows) and myocardial thickening of the septal and inferior left ventricular walls is seen during systole.

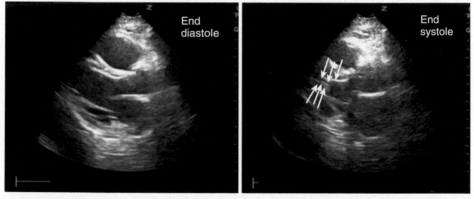

Figure 15.4   Hyperdynamic Left Ventricular Systolic Function. Increased myocardial thickening and endocardial excursion (arrows) is seen during systole from a parasternal long-axis view, with obliteration of the left ventricular cavity.

fixed length of their taught chordae tendineae. Such tethering at end-systole, coupled with a low stroke volume that leads to reduced filling of the LV in diastole, results in limited opening of the anterior leaflet of the mitral valve. This is best appreciated from the PLAX view (Fig. 15.5 and Video 15.5). A qualitative estimate of greater than 1 cm distance from the tip of the anterior mitral valve leaflet to the septal wall at full opening can diagnose reduced LV systolic function with an EF less than 40% with a sensitivity, specificity, and accuracy of 69%, 91%, and 89%, respectively.[14] This type of assessment has been shown to be easy to implement at the bedside after brief training.[6,14] It is important to remember that detection of LV systolic dysfunction by POCUS requires thoughtful integration into clinical management, as its impact and relevance to any given patient or disease state will vary by individual.

Reduced LV systolic function exhibits less endocardial excursion, less myocardial thickening, and diminished approximation of the anterior mitral valve leaflet tip to the septum compared to normal (Video 15.6). When the LV systolic function becomes severely reduced, very limited endocardial excursion and severely diminished thickening of the myocardium are appreciated. The mitral valve opens minimally due to a very limited inward flow from the left atrium and tethering of the mitral valve by the dilated LV chamber (Video 15.7).

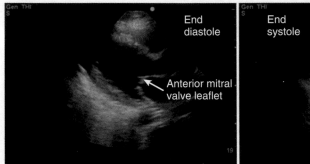
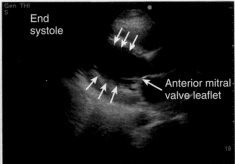

Figure 15.5   Reduced Left Ventricular Systolic Function. Increased distance between the anterior mitral valve leaflet and septum, as well as diminished endocardial excursion (arrows) and myocardial thickening, is seen from a parasternal long-axis view.

Assessment of Left Ventricular Function From Common Views

PARASTERNAL LONG-AXIS VIEW

Cardiac ultrasound imaging traditionally starts from the parasternal window. The PLAX view visualizes the LV through the anteroseptal and inferolateral walls, with the apex commonly out of view (Fig. 15.6). The PLAX view can be easily learned and reliably acquired, and this single view is used as part of a rapid screening examination.[7,12] Being perpendicular to the endocardium, this view lends itself well to assessing myocardial thickening and endocardial excursion of the LV walls (Video 15.8), as well as excursion of the anterior leaflet of the mitral valve. The anterior leaflet tip should nearly contact the septum in diastole when LV systolic function is normal; however, if structural valve disease is present, such as aortic regurgitation or mitral stenosis, the excursion of the anterior mitral valve leaflet cannot be used to assess LV systolic function in these relatively uncommon circumstances. When LV systolic function is reduced, the distance between the septum and anterior mitral valve leaflet increases as the LV dilates and diastolic filling is diminished (see Fig. 15.5).

An important pitfall in acquiring PLAX views is off-axis imaging. If the LV chamber is captured obliquely, the diameter of the LV may be falsely narrowed and can falsely mimic hyperdynamic LV function (Video 15.9). Table 15.1 outlines common pitfalls in assessing LV systolic function from different views. Examples of normal (see Videos 15.1 and 15.8),

hyperdynamic (see Videos 15.3 and 15.10), reduced (see Videos 15.6 and 15.11), and severely reduced (see Videos 15.7 and 15.12) LV systolic function from the PLAX view are provided.

PARASTERNAL SHORT-AXIS VIEW

Parasternal short-axis views (PSAX) are obtained by rotating the transducer 90 degrees clockwise from a PLAX view. PSAX views show cross sections of the LV from base to apex (see Chapter 14, Figure 14.7). Unlike other views, the PSAX allows visualization of all four LV walls simultaneously, making a true global approximation of LV systolic function intuitive and feasible (Fig. 15.7 and Video 15.13). Normally, all four LV walls should be seen contracting toward the center of the LV cavity in a PSAX view. When assessing LV systolic function, the PSAX view at the midventricular (papillary muscle) level is preferred because assessing LV systolic function at the mitral valve level is subject to underestimation (Video 15.14), whereas the apical level is subject to overestimation of LV systolic function (Video 15.15). Because of the circular nature of the LV in short-axis, providers can focus their eyes on the center of the LV cavity and assess the movement of all LV walls toward the center. Some providers may go as far as to place a finger in the center of the LV cavity while performing their visual, qualitative assessment. Examples of normal (see Video 15.13), hyperdynamic (Video 15.16), reduced (Video 15.17), and severely reduced (Video 15.18) LV systolic function from the parasternal short-axis view are shown.

Providers using POCUS may also detect gross regional wall motion abnormalities in

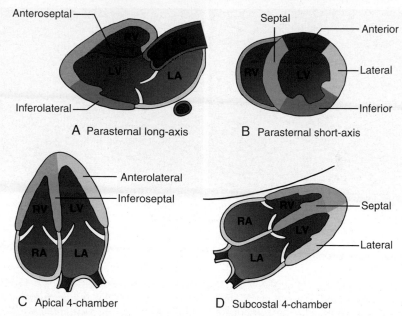

Figure 15.6 Left Ventricular Walls From Common Cardiac Views. (A) The parasternal long-axis view visualizes the anteroseptal and inferolateral walls. (B) The parasternal short-axis view allows circumferential visualization of the left ventricle to assess regional wall motion of the septal, inferior, lateral, and anterior walls. (C) The apical 4-chamber view allows visualization of the inferoseptal and anterolateral walls. (D) The imaging plane of the subcostal 4-chamber view can vary, but in general, the septal and lateral walls are visualized. *AO,* Aorta; *LA,* left atrium; *LV,* left ventricle; *RA,* right atrium; *RV,* right ventricle.

TABLE 15.1   **Common Pitfalls in Assessing Left Ventricular Systolic Function**

View	Pitfall: Potential Overestimation of LV Systolic Function	Pitfall: Potential Underestimation of LV Systolic Function
Parasternal long-axis	Off-axis, oblique plane through LV Sigmoid septum Severe hypertrophy/hypertrophic cardiomyopathy	Regional wall motion abnormality Valvular disease (decreased mitral valve excursion due to severe aortic insufficiency or mitral stenosis)
Parasternal short-axis	Apical level view	Mitral valve level view
Apical 4-chamber	Foreshortened LV due to off-axis imaging	Regional wall motion abnormality
Subcostal 4-chamber	Foreshortened LV due to off-axis imaging	Regional wall motion abnormality
All views	Hypotension/decreased afterload	Tachyarrhythmia

LV, Left ventricle.

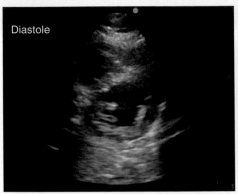
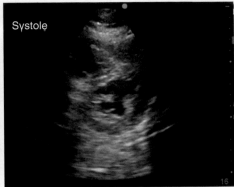

Figure 15.7 Parasternal Short Axis View. The circumferential nature of the parasternal short-axis view at the midventricular level shows the left ventricular walls at end-diastole and end-systole, allowing interpretation of global left ventricular systolic function.

the PSAX view (see Fig. 15.6, Video 15.19), although accuracy and integration of these findings typically require additional experience. Point-of-care providers must remain cognizant of the intended scope of their study and individual skill set.

APICAL 4-CHAMBER VIEW

The apical 4-chamber (A4C) view also provides information about LV systolic function, as it cuts through the inferoseptal and anterolateral walls of the LV from the apical window (see Fig. 15.6). Because the ultrasound beam is more parallel to the axis of these walls, visualization of endocardial resolution may be diminished compared to the more perpendicular ultrasound beam alignment of parasternal views. If an A4C view is obtained from a rib interspace that is too cephalad, the heart and LV will be foreshortened, which may lead to overestimation of LV systolic function. Similar to the PLAX view, only two walls of the LV are seen, and corroborating views are always recommended to assess for regional wall motion abnormalities. Less commonly, another pattern of asymmetrical contraction may be seen from the A4C view due to stress-induced cardiomyopathy (Takotsubo cardiomyopathy). This pattern of contraction shows a dilated apex and normal to hyperdynamic contraction of the LV base. Prompt recognition at the bedside can result in more efficient diagnosis and treatment of this increasingly appreciated phenomenon.[15] Examples of normal (Video 15.20), hyperdynamic

(Video 15.21), reduced (Video 15.22), and severely reduced LV systolic function (Video 15.23) from an A4C view are shown.

SUBCOSTAL WINDOW

The subcostal 4-chamber (S4C) view is relatively easy to acquire by placing the transducer in the subxiphoid space and utilizing the liver to provide an acoustic window (see Chapter 14). Because only the septal and lateral LV walls are visualized in the far field, the S4C view is often more challenging to use to confidently categorize LV function (see Fig. 15.6). The S4C view should be used in isolation only to grossly estimate LV systolic function in emergency situations, such as severe hypotension or during cardiac arrest. Examples of normal (Video 15.24), hyperdynamic (Video 15.25), reduced (Video 15.26), and severely reduced (Video 15.27) LV systolic function from the S4C view are shown.

When providers are restricted to imaging from the subcostal window, as is common in critically ill patients, particularly those with hyperinflated lungs or undergoing active cardiopulmonary resuscitation, the subcostal short-axis view may be invaluable to provide a corroborating view of the LV. To obtain this view, the transducer is rotated counterclockwise to point the transducer marker toward the head of the patient. A short-axis view of the LV at the papillary muscle level can be acquired and interpreted similar to the PSAX view as discussed above (Fig. 15.8 and Video 15.28).

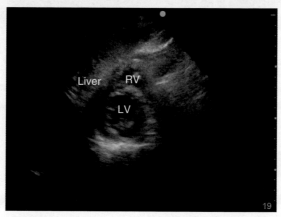

Figure 15.8 Subcostal Short-Axis View (Midventricular Level). The subcostal short-axis view provides a corroborating view of gross left ventricular systolic function, in addition to the subcostal 4-chamber view, especially when limited to imaging from only the subcostal window. *LV,* Left ventricle; *RV,* right ventricle.

PEARLS AND PITFALLS

- Accuracy of image interpretation depends on the acquisition of high-quality images. Interpretation of off-axis images often leads to overestimation of left ventricular (LV) systolic function that can negatively affect the clinical management of acutely ill patients.
- The parasternal long-axis (PLAX) and apical 4-chamber (A4C) views visualize only the LV anteroseptal and inferolateral, and anterolateral and inferoseptal walls, respectively, which can lead to underestimation of LV systolic function if a regional wall motion abnormality is present. Thus, the parasternal short-axis (PSAX) is unique in that it can supplement other cardiac views by providing a circumferential view of all LV walls.
- Several PSAX planes exist, but the midventricular, papillary muscle level is the highest yield view for global LV systolic function determination in the point-of-care setting.
- Mitral valve excursion is an excellent adjunct to include in evaluation of LV systolic function and is best appreciated from the PLAX view. If the anterior leaflet tip of the mitral valve comes within 1 cm of the septum, LV ejection fraction can be considered to be greater than 40%.
- Excursion of the anterior mitral valve leaflet tip may be reduced due to reasons unrelated to LV systolic function, including mitral valve stenosis or aortic regurgitation. Conversely, in acute LV dysfunction (e.g., myocardial infarction) mitral valve excursion may be preserved. Thus, using mitral valve excursion alone to estimate LV systolic function can be misleading and should always be integrated with the interpretation of myocardial thickening and endocardial excursion.
- When the subcostal window is the only available window, adding the subcostal short-axis view to the subcostal 4-chamber (S4C) view can greatly assist in determination of LV systolic function. From the S4C view, rotate the transducer counterclockwise with the transducer marker pointing cephalad to capture a subcostal short-axis view.

CHAPTER 16

Right Ventricular Function

James F. Fair III ■ Robert Arntfield

KEY POINTS

- The objective of point-of-care right ventricular assessment is to evaluate for acute right heart failure caused by an increase in pulmonary artery pressure or direct right ventricular injury.
- Right ventricular failure can be rapidly recognized using point-of-care ultrasound through a qualitative analysis of right ventricular size, function, and interventricular septal kinetics.
- Quantitative measures, including tricuspid annular plane systolic excursion and right ventricular systolic pressure, may be used to objectively trend responses to therapeutic interventions.

Background

The left ventricle (LV) has historically been the focus of hemodynamic and echocardiographic evaluation of the heart. More recently, the importance of right ventricular (RV) function has been recognized, and guidelines have emerged describing standard ways to assess normal RV dimensions and function.[1,2]

Evaluation of RV function is essential to help diagnose and manage shock and respiratory failure in acutely ill patients. Conditions that may cause acute RV failure, either through sudden pulmonary hypertension (e.g., pulmonary embolism [PE], mechanical ventilation, acute respiratory distress syndrome [ARDS]) or through primary RV failure (e.g., trauma or infarction) should be considered, depending on clinical circumstances.

Assessment of RV function and early identification of acute right heart failure is essential when managing patients in shock. In addition to guiding decisions about inotropic support and fluid resuscitation, RV structure and function has been shown to be of prognostic value in those with left heart failure,[3] acute PE,[4] ARDS,[5] and severe sepsis.[6] In patients with septic shock, RV size can guide fluid resuscitation. Volume loading of a dysfunctional RV with interventricular septal bowing can further compromise LV filling, leading to worsened LV output and a progressive shock state.[7]

In patients with suspected PE who are in circulatory failure, one study has suggested that upwards of 90% of patients with PE as the cause of their shock will have features of RV failure on point-of-care cardiac ultrasound.[8] For those with established PE without shock, if signs of RV failure are demonstrated by ultrasound, there is elevated risk of serious adverse events including enduring pulmonary hypertension. Thus, characterizing the RV is an important contributor in clinical decision-making for those with suspected or confirmed PE.[9]

In patients with respiratory failure, point-of-care cardiac ultrasound can diagnose and assess the severity of pulmonary hypertension to guide ventilator management decisions. For example, in patients with ARDS, indiscriminate increases in positive end-expiratory pressure (PEEP) will create an elevation in RV afterload, potentially yielding a drop in overall cardiac output. Such heart-lung interactions may lead to worsening shock states in those with compromised RV function. While titrating positive pressure ventilation, providers must balance the benefits of increasing alveolar recruitment with potential harms of increasing RV overload. Serial echocardiographic monitoring of RV size and morphology during ventilator adjustments in patients with high levels of PEEP or high airway pressures is feasible and well characterized.[10]

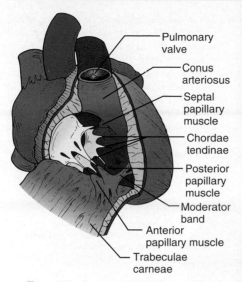

Figure 16.1 Anatomy of the right ventricle.

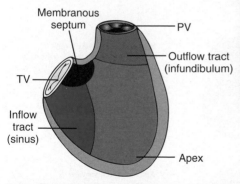

Figure 16.2 Sections of the Right Ventricle: Inflow Tract (Sinus), Apex, and Outflow Tract (Infundibulum). *PV*, Pulmonic valve; *TV*, tricuspid valve.

Anatomy

The right ventricle is located in the mediastinum behind the middle to lower part of the sternum. It is positioned anterior to the LV, and the RV chamber is divided anatomically into three parts: an inflow tract (sinus), outflow tract (infundibulum), and apex. Even though the apex is heavily trabeculated, the main contributors to RV systolic function are the inflow and outflow tracts (Figs. 16.1 and 16.2). During systole, muscles of the inflow tract primarily contract to elevate RV pressure, and muscles of the outflow tract stretch to modulate pressure and prolong systole.

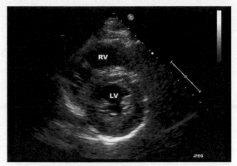

Figure 16.3 Shape of Right Ventricle *(RV)*. Normal crescent-shaped RV as seen from a parasternal short-axis view. *LV*, Left ventricle.

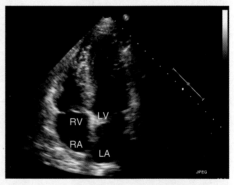

Figure 16.4 Shape of Right Ventricle (RV). Normal triangular-shaped RV as seen from an apical 4-chamber view. *LA*, Left atrium; *LV*, left ventricle; *RA*, right atrium.

RV contraction is complex and occurs in phases. First, the trabeculated inflow tract contracts longitudinally, shortening the distance from base to apex. Second, the RV free wall contracts radially toward the interventricular septum, shortening the circumference of the chamber. Last, torsion from contraction of the left ventricular base and apex pulls the right ventricle to contract similarly.[11]

The RV free wall is normally thinner than the LV free wall because the RV pumps blood into the pulmonary vasculature, which has lower resistance compared to the systemic circulation. The normal RV chamber size is approximately two thirds the size of the LV chamber. The RV has a crescent shape when viewed in transverse cross section from a parasternal short-axis view (Fig. 16.3) and a triangular shape when viewed in a coronal plane from an apical 4-chamber (A4C) view (Fig. 16.4).[11]

Assessment of Right Ventricle From Common Views

The RV is best visualized using the standard echocardiography views that are discussed in Chapter 14. Because of its complexity in structure and function, the RV should be assessed from all available cardiac views. Interpretation of RV size and function from the most common cardiac views includes the following (Fig. 16.5):

1. *Parasternal long-axis view:* Visualization of the proximal RV outflow tract and RV free wall is seen in the near field (see Fig. 16.5A). In a normal heart, the RV will appear to be roughly the same size as the ascending aorta and the left atrium (known as the "rule of thirds"). This view may reveal an underfilled LV due to minimal RV output (Video 16.1). Gross distortions in RV size or function may be suspected from this view but must be confirmed by additional views before making any important clinical decisions.

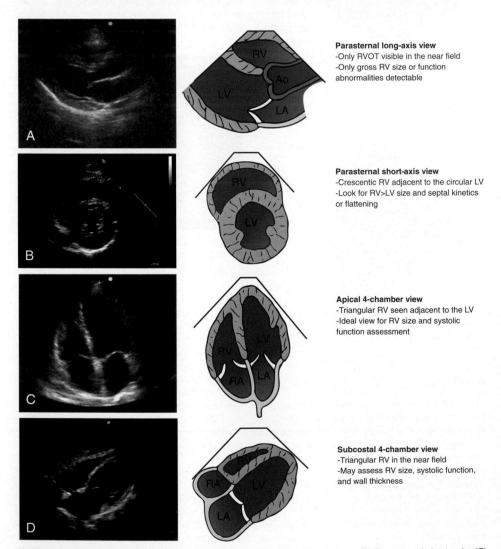

Parasternal long-axis view
-Only RVOT visible in the near field
-Only gross RV size or function abnormalities detectable

Parasternal short-axis view
-Crescentic RV adjacent to the circular LV
-Look for RV>LV size and septal kinetics or flattening

Apical 4-chamber view
-Triangular RV seen adjacent to the LV
-Ideal view for RV size and systolic function assessment

Subcostal 4-chamber view
-Triangular RV in the near field
-May assess RV size, systolic function, and wall thickness

Figure 16.5 **Standard Right Ventricle *(RV)* Views.** (A) Parasternal long-axis. (B) Parasternal short-axis. (C) Apical 4-chamber. (D) Subcostal 4-chamber. *Ao,* Aorta; *LA,* left atrium; *LV,* left ventricle; *RA,* right atrium; *RVOT,* right ventricular outflow tract.

2. *Parasternal short-axis view (midventricular level):* Normally, the crescent-shaped RV sits next to the circular LV in this view. This view allows direct comparison of the RV size relative to the LV size (see Fig. 16.5B). An assessment of the interventricular septum and its kinetics is particularly valuable in this view. Altered septal kinetics are seen with RV pressure overload ranging from a septal "bounce" to a flattened septum (see "Interpretation" below).

3. *Apical 4-chamber view (A4C):* This is the most informative single view for global RV assessment. With a side-by-side comparison of the RV and LV, the relative RV size can be easily interpreted when an on-axis image is acquired (see Fig. 16.5C). The interventricular septum is also visualized allowing interpretation of septal kinetics. The RV systolic function is usually qualitatively estimated, but a quantitative estimate may be calculated (see discussion of tricuspid annular plane systolic excursion [TAPSE] below). Alignment of blood flow parallel to the ultrasound beam in this view is ideal for Doppler flow evaluation of the tricuspid valve for determination of pulmonary pressures.

4. *Subcostal 4-chamber view (S4C):* The RV is seen as a triangular chamber adjacent to the liver in the near field (see Fig. 16.5D). Like the A4C view, the S4C view provides a side-by-side comparison of size and function of the RV and LV. As long as the operator guards against off-axis imaging, which is a common pitfall in this view, the S4C view can be valuable to evaluate the RV when an A4C view cannot be obtained. Because the RV free wall is nearly perpendicular to the ultrasound beam, this view can provide excellent visualization of the RV endocardium and is ideal to assess RV wall thickness—a finding that can help differentiate acute from chronic RV disease.

Interpretation of Right Ventricular Size and Function

Point-of-care evaluation of the RV is often performed in patients with acute circulatory dysfunction or respiratory failure. In these patients, RV evaluation is focused on assessing the presence or absence of right heart failure.

Acute right heart failure commonly results from either direct RV tissue damage or a sudden increase in resistance of the pulmonary circulation (acute cor pulmonale). Direct RV tissue damage typically occurs from infarction or blunt trauma, whereas acute cor pulmonale typically results from a massive or submassive PE, ARDS, severe hypoxia, metabolic derangements, or mechanical ventilation with high airway pressures.[12,13]

In addition to acute RV failure, many other important diagnostic findings may be obtained from a detailed RV evaluation. Some applications, such as characterization of tricuspid regurgitation (TR) severity, determination of RV systolic pressure, or evaluation for endocarditis are more nuanced and require additional training to attain proficiency.

Assessment of the RV should be performed systematically to look for characteristic signs of RV stress or failure. The constellation of findings described below varies between patients depending on the etiology and chronicity of disease, physiologic adaptation, and therapies initiated.

1. **RV size:** The RV free wall musculature is relatively weak and, in acute RV failure, the chamber dilates. The most common and practical approach to determine RV enlargement is to perform a direct side-by-side comparison of RV and LV size. RV size assessment is most intuitively done from the A4C view but can also be appreciated from the S4C view. In the A4C view, the transducer should be oriented to appropriately visualize the lateral free wall of the RV and acquire the largest possible RV chamber width (Fig. 16.6 and Video 16.2, Video 16.3). A qualitative assessment of RV size is most commonly performed using the following parameters in end-diastole (Fig. 16.7):
   a. Normal RV size: less than 2/3 LV size.
   b. Moderate dilation: RV size greater than 2/3 LV size.
   c. Severe dilation: RV size greater than LV size.[14]

   Another important finding is identifying the dominant chamber at the apex. The RV becomes the dominant apical chamber as it dilates and displaces the LV, which is seen best in the A4C view (Fig. 16.8 and Video 16.4). As the RV dilates, as seen from the short axis, it assumes a more circular shape (Fig. 16.9 and Video 16.5). In the A4C view, RV dilation distorts the chamber from a

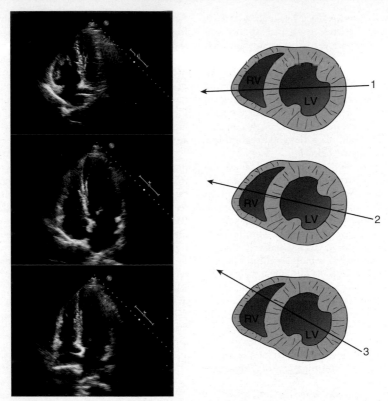

Figure 16.6   Off-Axis Views of Right Ventricle *(RV)*. An optimal apical 4 chamber view should demonstrate all 4 chambers in the same plane with the septum vertical in the middle of the screen. The RV size should be assessed with the transducer centered and equally bissecting the right and left ventricles (line 2). Rotating the transducer over the apex can make the RV size look falsely enlarged (line 1) or falsely reduced (line 3). *LV,* Left ventricle.

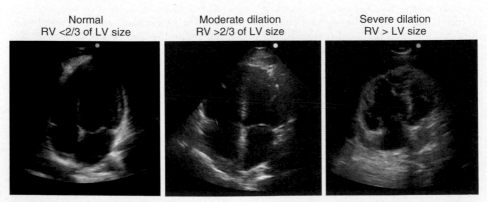

Figure 16.7   Right Ventricle *(RV)* **Dilation.** Normal, moderately dilated, and severely dilated right ventricle from an apical 4-chamber view. *LV,* Left ventricle.

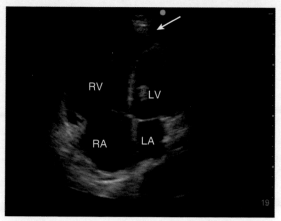

Figure 16.8 Apical Domination. An enlarged right ventricle (RV) displaces the left ventricle (LV) to dominate the apex as shown in an apical 4-chamber view (*arrows* denote RV occupying the apex). *LA*, Left atrium; *RA*, right atrium.

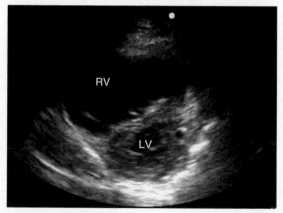

Figure 16.9 Dilated Right Ventricle (RV). Dilated RV with a round shape, rather than a typical crescentic shape in a parasternal short-axis view. *LV*, Left ventricle.

normal triangular shape to a more ovoid shape (Fig. 16.10 and Video 16.6).

2. **RV wall thickness:** Distinguishing between acute right heart failure (e.g., massive PE) and chronic right heart failure (e.g., from chronic obstructive pulmonary disease or COPD) is often clinically important for diagnosis and management. While PE can only be definitively diagnosed by CT angiogram of the chest or echocardiography showing clot-in-transit, RV wall thickness can provide important supporting information about the chronicity of the right-sided heart failure. As RV pressure increases, the RV hypertrophies over time and increased RV wall thickness suggests a more chronic

process. Measuring wall thickness is best performed at end-diastole from a S4C view, with care taken to avoid including trabeculations. The normal width of the RV free wall should be less than 5 mm.[1,15] An RV wall thickness in excess of 1 cm strongly suggests a chronic process (Fig. 16.11 and Video 16.7). Of note, having chronic RV disease does not exclude the possibility of an acute event superimposed on chronic RV failure. Further, acute increases in RV wall thickness can occur within 48 hours of acute, sudden increases in pulmonary artery pressure (e.g., acute PE), and echocardiography cannot differentiate an acute versus chronic increase in these circumstances.

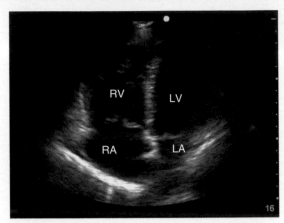

Figure 16.10   Dilated Right Ventricle *(RV)*. Dilated RV with an oval shape, rather than a typical triangular shape in an apical 4-chamber view. *LA*, Left atrium; *LV*, left ventricle; *RA*, right atrium.

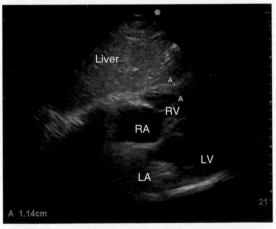

Figure 16.11   Right Ventricle *(RV)* Hypertrophy. Increased right ventricular wall thickness of 1.1 cm (normal <5 mm) at end-diastole in a subcostal 4-chamber view of a patient with chronic pulmonary hypertension. *LA*, Left atrium; *LV*, left ventricle; *RA*, right atrium.

Thus, assessing RV wall thickness may be most helpful to diagnose an acute process in patients with RV failure and a normal wall thickness (<5 mm).

3. **Interventricular septum:** The shape and movement of the interventricular septum provide valuable information about pressure in the RV. The septum is best seen in parasternal short-axis and A4C views. Normally, the LV is circular with the interventricular septum concave toward the LV chamber in systole and diastole (Fig. 16.12A and Video 16.8). When pressure rises in the RV, the normally rounded septum flattens and is pushed towards the LV. Septal

flattening signifies that the pressure in the RV is greater than the LV at that point in the cardiac cycle. This can occur in systole, diastole, or both. Septal flattening is more commonly seen in diastole alone, since it requires chronic, severe pulmonary hypertension for an RV to be capable of generating systemic range pressures during systole. Flattening of the septum during diastole is called paradoxical septal movement, and a septal "bounce" may be seen. (Videos 16.9 and 16.10). Progressively increasing pressure leads to flattening of the septum with sustained pressure elevation throughout the cardiac cycle.[16] Septal flattening is

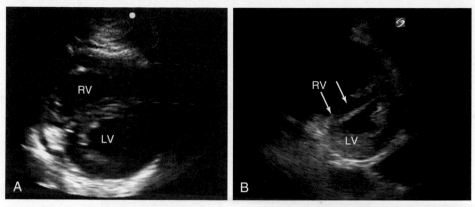

Figure 16.12   Interventricular Septum. Comparison of a normal interventricular septum (A) and a flattened septum bowing into the left ventricle in a patient with right ventricular failure (B) from a parasternal short-axis view. *LV,* Left ventricle; *RV,* right ventricle.

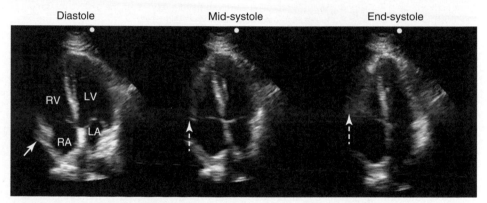

Figure 16.13   Right Ventricle *(RV)* Systolic Function. RV primarily contracts longitudinally which is seen as the tricuspid annulus moves toward the apex during systole from an apical 4-chamber view *(arrow)*. *LA,* Left atrium; *LV,* left ventricle; *RA,* right atrium.

particularly well appreciated from a parasternal short-axis view where the normally circular LV becomes "D" shaped (see Fig. 16.12B and Video 16.11).

4. **RV systolic function:** Two-dimensional echocardiographic methods of assessing RV systolic function remain relatively crude compared to newer three-dimensional or MRI techniques.[17] The RV primarily contracts longitudinally, from base to apex with vertical movements, in contrast to the radial, concentric contractions of the LV (Fig. 16.13 and Video 16.12). RV systolic function is evaluated by examining the dynamics of the RV free wall and the tricuspid valve annulus, which are best seen in either an A4C or S4C view. Similar to determination of LV systolic function, a

qualitative method is routinely used for point-of-care evaluation of RV systolic function. A visual estimation is used to categorize RV systolic function as normal or having a mild (Video 16.13), moderate (Video 16.14), or severe (Videos 16.15 and 16.16) decrease in systolic function based on subjective evaluation.

Although no quantitative method is universally accepted to assess RV systolic function, a method known as the TAPSE is the most widely used echocardiographic method. It is the ease and speed of determining TAPSE that has led to its widespread adoption. TAPSE measures the longitudinal excursion of the lateral tricuspid annular plane during systole from an A4C view. To measure TAPSE, M-mode is employed

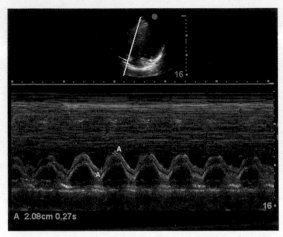

Figure 16.14 **Tricuspid Annular Plane Systolic Excursion (Tapse).** M-mode image of TAPSE measurement from an apical 4-chamber view. The repeating sawtooth pattern represents the systolic movement of the tricuspid annulus. TAPSE is the height in millimeters (20 mm in this case).

by aligning the cursor line to cut through the lateral tricuspid annulus. This results in a time-motion image of the characteristic annular movement in systole (Fig. 16.14). Normal range for TAPSE is greater than 22 to 24 mm, and decreased RV systolic function is defined as TAPSE less than 17 mm.[1,2] Though TAPSE may not be considered essential in all cases of RV assessment, its relative ease allows quantitative trending of systolic function after hemodynamic interventions and may provide prognostic value for those with acute RV failure from PE.[18]

5. **Estimating pulmonary artery pressures:** Determining the presence and severity of pulmonary hypertension may add important information to the global assessment of the RV. Elevated RV afterload may be an acute physiologic process (e.g., in massive PE), a chronic process (e.g., in COPD or sleep apnea) or due to a primary disorder of the pulmonary vasculature (e.g., idiopathic pulmonary arterial hypertension). The most widely adopted echocardiographic method to estimate pulmonary artery pressure is by determining right ventricular systolic pressure (RVSP). Though requiring some comfort with spectral Doppler techniques, RVSP is widely used for its noninvasiveness compared to right heart catheterization, the gold standard, and repeatability, allowing trending in response to therapeutic interventions. RVSP may guide RV afterload

management strategies from ventilator settings in the intensive care unit (ICU) to vasodilator doses in a pulmonary hypertension clinic.

Determining RVSP is a two-step process using the formula: RVSP = (Pressure gradient [PG] between RV and RA) + RA Pressure. First, the RV–RA PG is calculated. To do this, TR is required and should be identified using color flow Doppler from the view that maximally measures the TR jet, most commonly the A4C view in a goal-directed echocardiogram. A continuous wave Doppler sample gate is then placed through the TR jet yielding a spectral Doppler wave-form (Fig. 16.15 and Video 16.17) The peak velocity of the TR jet is then measured, and by using the modified Bernoulli equation (Pressure = $4V^2$), the ultrasound will determine the PG. The second step of this process is to estimate the RA pressure and add the RA pressure to the PG. The RA pressure is estimated in a spontaneously breathing patient by visualizing the inferior vena cava (IVC) in long-axis during respiration (see also Chapter 17). If the IVC is greater than 2.1 cm and less than 50% collapsible with respirations, it has relatively high pressure and is assigned a value of 15 mm Hg. (Video 16.18) If the IVC is less than 2.1 cm and collapsible greater than 50%, then it has relatively low pressure and is assigned a value of 3 mm Hg. (Video 16.19) If it is any combination in between, then it is given a value of 8 mm Hg.[19]

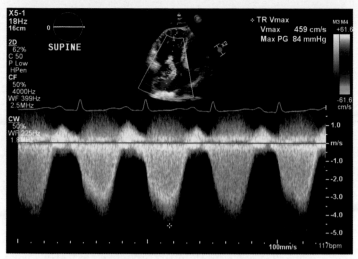

Figure 16.15 Tricuspid Regurgitation Measurement. Continuous wave spectral Doppler waveform showing the peak velocity and pressure gradient measurement.

For those receiving positive pressure ventilation, the IVC diameter correlates linearly with RA pressure, but there is minimal respirator variation of IVC size.[20] Practically, unless the IVC is small (<1 cm), most providers will use a broadly inclusive RA pressure range of 10 to 20 mm Hg for determining RVSP in patients on mechanical ventilation.

Other common findings when assessing the RV include indwelling catheters and leads from pacemakers or implantable defibrillators (Fig. 16.16 and Video 16.20). Visualization of the RV may be helpful to guide placement of pulmonary artery catheters or temporary pacemakers in emergency situations (Video 16.21).

The RV is heavily trabeculated compared to the LV. Appearance of additional muscle densities, including a prominent linear structure known as the moderator band, are normal findings in the apex of the RV and should not be mistaken for pathologic findings. Table 16.1 summarizes the findings and pitfalls of RV assessment.

PEARLS AND PITFALLS

• The right ventricle (RV) may be difficult to visualize because of its location under the sternum. When parasternal or apical windows are challenging to acquire,

the subcostal window is an excellent alternative.
• The crescentic, triangular-shaped RV is distinct from the circular, ovoid-shaped left ventricle (LV). The RV wraps around the LV, and off-axis imaging of the RV from any plane can falsely increase or decrease the RV size. Always tilt or fan the transducer through the RV to capture the largest RV diameter before making any assessment about its size or function.
• In mechanically ventilated patients, high airway pressures, especially excessive PEEP, may worsen or induce acute RV failure.
• In patients with RV failure and a wall thickness of less than 0.5 cm, the RV dysfunction is likely acute.
• Sufficient TR must be present and the continuous wave Doppler cursor line must be aligned parallel to the regurgitant jet to accurately determine right ventricular systolic pressure (RVSP).
• When acute RV failure is identified in patients with shock, providers can use ultrasound to decide whether fluid resuscitation or administration of inotropes and diuretics is the most appropriate next step in clinical management.

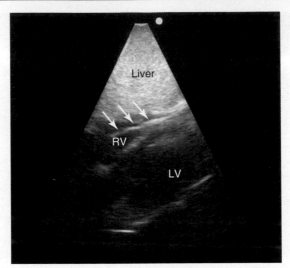

Figure 16.16   Pacemaker. Hyperechoic pacemaker wire *(arrows)* is seen in the right ventricle *(RV)* from a subcostal 4-chamber view. *LV,* Left ventricle.

TABLE 16.1   **Summary of Right Ventricular Assessment**

Characteristic	Findings in RV Failure	Best View(s)	Pitfall(s)
RV size	RV >2/3 of LV size (moderate dilation) RV >LV size and apex dominated by RV (severe dilation)	Apical 4-chamber or subcostal 4-chamber	Off-axis imaging may underestimate RV size (see Fig. 16.6 and Video 16.2)
RV shape	Loss of crescentic shape (short-axis view) and triangular shape (4-chamber view)	Parasternal short-axis Apical 4-chamber or subcostal 4-chamber	Off-axis imaging may obscure findings
RV wall thickness	Generally <0.5 cm in acute failure Chronic failure may be >1 cm	Subcostal 4-chamber	Cannot exclude acute on chronic RV failure Avoid measuring trabeculations
Interventricular septum	Paradoxical septal motion (mild) Septal flattening (moderate to severe)	Parasternal short-axis	Paradoxical septal motion not specific to RV failure Off-axis imaging can falsely give appearance of flattened septum
RV systolic function	Diminished longitudinal contraction of RV or TAPSE <17 mm	Apical 4-chamber or subcostal 4-chamber	Poor imaging of RV free wall is common
RV systolic pressure	>35 mm Hg is pathologic, but pressures may drop during failure	Apical 4-chamber	Measurements not parallel to flow underestimate velocity

LV, Left ventricular; *RV,* right ventricular; *TAPSE,* tricuspid annular plane systolic excursion.

CHAPTER 17

Inferior Vena Cava

Matthew D. Tyler ■ Robert Arntfield ■ Aviral Roy ■ Haney Mallemat

KEY POINTS

- The inferior vena cava (IVC) is readily visualized using point-of-care ultrasound and can guide fluid management decisions when taken in context of cardiac and lung findings on ultrasound.
- Correct interpretation of changes to the IVC requires a thorough understanding of hemodynamics and respiratory physiology.
- Patients with cardiac tamponade will have a plethoric, dilated IVC, and absence of this finding can rapidly rule out tamponade in patients with a pericardial effusion.

Background

A point-of-care ultrasound examination of the inferior vena cava (IVC) offers a rapid, non-invasive determination of right atrial pressure and, in some instances, can guide determining volume status and volume responsiveness. Image acquisition and interpretation can be mastered after a brief, focused training and various training protocols have been shown to be effective for providers from diverse medical specialties.[1] Despite the relative ease in image acquisition, interpretation of IVC findings is nuanced, requiring thorough knowledge of its validated uses, its limitations, and integration with other clinical data.

Anatomy

The IVC is located to the right of the aorta and courses from the retroperitoneal space through the liver and diaphragm to connect with the right atrium (RA) (Fig. 17.1). The IVC appears as a large, intrahepatic vessel with thin walls from the subcostal cardiac window and under normal physiologic conditions typically demonstrates respirophasic variation in its diameter (Video 17.1). The IVC is a capacitance vessel and is therefore sensitive to changes in intrathoracic and intraabdominal pressures. In spontaneously breathing patients, when the intrathoracic pressure becomes negative during inspiration, a decrease in the IVC diameter is seen. In patients passively receiving positive-pressure ventilation, the intrathoracic pressure increases with the delivery of a breath causing an increase in the IVC diameter (Figs. 17.2 and 17.3). Conditions such as chronic pulmonary hypertension, right heart dysfunction, and tricuspid valve regurgitation can alter the normal size and respirophasic variation of the IVC.[2,3] Additionally, the size of the IVC may be influenced by noncardiac factors, including venous return from the splanchnic circulation, diaphragm excursion during breathing, and elevated intraabdominal pressure.[4,5]

Indications and Applications

The most common clinical indications for assessing the IVC with ultrasound are summarized in Table 17.1.

Ultrasound of the IVC has traditionally been used to help guide fluid management decisions in hypotensive patients being resuscitated.[6-8] Specifically, the IVC maximum diameter and degree of collapsibility during the respiratory cycle may influence a clinician's decision to infuse or withhold fluids. Though this practice is widely used, there is conflicting

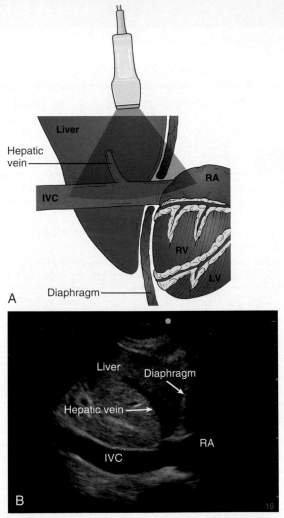

Figure 17.1 Inferior Vena Cava (IVC) Anatomy. A long-axis view (A) and image (B) of the IVC from the subcostal window bisects the right atrium, diaphragm, and liver. *LV,* Left ventricle; *RA,* right atrium; *RV,* right ventricle.

evidence in the literature for the accuracy and generalizability of these techniques (see "Image Interpretation," later).

IVC ultrasound can be used to approximate the central venous pressure (CVP).[9,10] Despite its frequent use in many clinical settings, CVP itself has not been shown to be predictive of volume responsiveness.[11] The CVP does have some applicability in more advanced echocardiography, including estimation of pulmonary arterial pressure.

The echocardiographic features of pericardial tamponade (right atrial and ventricular collapse, spectral Doppler inflow variations, M-mode techniques) require experience to accurately acquire and interpret (see Chapter 18). However, due to the elevation in CVP that occurs in the context of a hemodynamically significant circumferential pericardial effusion, assessment of the IVC carries great value in this scenario. When tamponade is present, the IVC will be dilated and plethoric. If the IVC

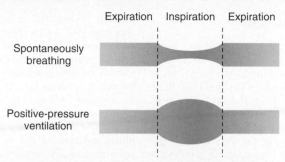

Figure 17.2 Respirophasic Variation of the Inferior Vena Cava (IVC). During inspiration, the IVC collapses with spontaneous breathing and distends with passive positive pressure ventilation.

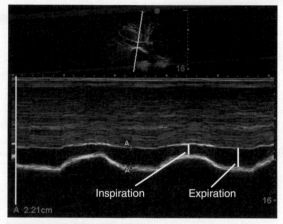

Figure 17.3 M-Mode With Respirophasic Variation. Normal respirophasic variation of the inferior vena cava is seen using M-mode in a spontaneously breathing patient.

TABLE 17.1   Indications for Inferior Vena Cava Ultrasound

Indication	Notes
Central venous pressure	Approximation in spontaneously breathing patients
Pericardial effusion	Nondilated IVC can rule out tamponade physiology
Right heart failure	Dilated IVC seen in cor pulmonale and severe tricuspid regurgitation
	Cannot use IVC to infer CVP or volume responsiveness
Device placement confirmation	Identify correct placement of venous devices, including extracorporeal membrane oxygenation (ECMO) catheters and femoral transvenous pacemakers
Volume responsiveness	Limited utility

CVP, Central venous pressure; *IVC,* inferior vena cava.

collapses during the respiratory cycle, then tamponade can be ruled out.[12]

The size and collapsibility of the IVC may help providers determine the necessary amount of fluid to remove in patients undergoing hemodialysis or those with acute decompensated heart failure. IVC findings may help determine if fluid removal has been adequate and may be a useful adjunct to the patient's dry weight.[13-17]

Image Acquisition

In adults, any low-frequency ultrasound transducer can be used to visualize the IVC, either a phased-array, curvilinear, or micro-convex transducer. Phased-array transducers are most commonly used to image the IVC. Two techniques to image the IVC have been described.

1. Subcostal cardiac window

A long-axis view of the IVC at the right atrial junction from the subcostal window is the recommended view based on reliability and reproducibility (see Chapter 14).[18,19] A phased-array transducer is placed in the subcostal window with the transducer orientation marker pointing cephalad (Fig. 17.4). A technique to ensure visualization of the IVC is to start with a subcostal 4-chamber view, focusing on the RA, and then rotate the transducer counterclockwise to align the ultrasound beam along the course of the IVC. An ideal long-axis view of the IVC should demonstrate the IVC entering the RA and a segment of a hepatic vein joining the IVC. Identifying both the RA-IVC junction and hepatic vein(s) helps to avoid mistaking the IVC for the neighboring aorta (Video 17.2). The pulsatile, thicker-walled aorta can be visualized by tilting the transducer

medially (Video 17.3). It is imperative to visualize the IVC longitudinally with the transducer centered on its long axis to assess the true diameter and collapsibility accurately. Off-axis imaging generates an oblique view of the vessel, resulting in a falsely small diameter, the so-called "cylinder effect" (Fig. 17.5). Once a long-axis view of the IVC with the RA-IVC junction is acquired, very fine adjustments by tilting and rotating the transducer should be performed to ensure alignment of the beam over the IVC at its largest diameter.

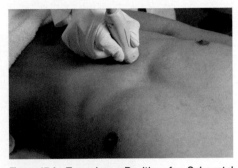

Figure 17.4 Transducer Position for Subcostal Inferior Vena Cava (IVC) View. A subcostal long-axis view of IVC is acquired with the transducer marker pointed cephalad.

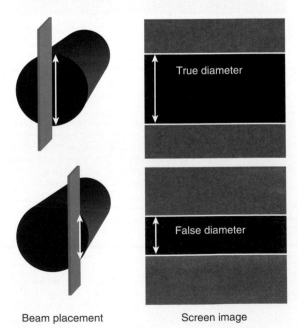

Beam placement   Screen image

Figure 17.5 Cylinder Effect. Imaging the inferior vena cava in an off-axis, oblique plane will falsely narrow the diameter (cylinder effect) which can be seen with any cylindrical structure.

2. Transhepatic coronal view

The liver parenchyma provides an excellent acoustic window to visualize the IVC and can be used when a subcostal IVC view is not obtainable (e.g., pregnancy, postoperative wounds, dressings, bowel gas, patient discomfort). The transducer is placed on the mid-axillary line with the transducer orientation marker pointed cephalad. Tilting the transducer posteriorly (i.e., to aim the ultrasound beam posteriorly) captures a long-axis view of the IVC passing through the liver and diaphragm. The aorta is seen deep to the IVC in this view (Figs. 17.6 and 17.7 and Videos 17.4 and 17.5).

To quantitatively measure the IVC diameter and changes with respiration, the image should be frozen and calipers used to measure the diameter perpendicular to the long axis of the vein approximately 2 cm from the RA-IVC junction.[20] This location has been shown to have good inter-rater reliability and is readily reproducible.[21] Once the largest diameter is measured, the cine function can be used to scroll frame by frame to find the smallest IVC diameter within the same respiratory cycle. M-mode may also be used to follow the variation of the IVC diameter during the respiratory cycle (Fig. 17.8). Ensure that the M-mode sampling plane is perpendicular to the IVC to avoid falsely elevated IVC dimensions.

Image Interpretation

Interpretation of IVC size and collapsibility varies depending on the clinical scenario. The four most common clinical questions that IVC ultrasound may be used to address are:
1. Volume responsiveness
2. Tamponade physiology
3. CVP estimation
4. Device placement

VOLUME RESPONSIVENESS

When assessing for volume responsiveness, an important consideration is the mechanism by which the patient is breathing, which can be broadly classified as:
1. Spontaneous ventilation—breathing spontaneously with or without the help of an invasive or noninvasive ventilator.

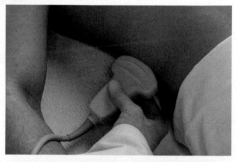

Figure 17.6 Transducer Position for Transhepatic Inferior Vena Cava (IVC) View. A transhepatic coronal view of the IVC is acquired on the mid-axillary line with the transducer notch pointed cephalad. A phased-array or a curvilinear transducer (as shown here) may be used.

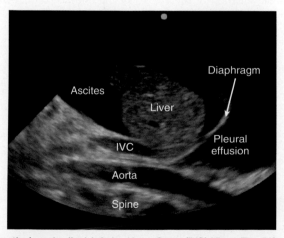

Figure 17.7 Transhepatic Longitudinal Inferior Vena Cava *(IVC)* View. The IVC, aorta, and spine are seen deep to a cirrhotic liver in a patient with ascites and right pleural effusion. Note: the radiology convention (screen marker to the left) was used in this case.

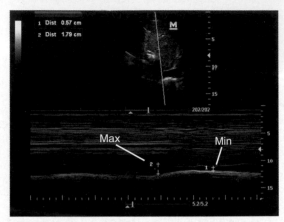

Figure 17.8　Inferior Vena Cava (IVC) Respirophasic Variation. This M-mode image of IVC demonstrates respirophasic variation in a spontaneously breathing patient. The maximum and minimum diameters are measured using calipers.

2. Passive ventilation—mechanically ventilated with no spontaneous breathing effort.

Spontaneous Ventilation

There is considerable uncertainty about the utility of evaluating the IVC for preload responsiveness in spontaneously breathing patients. Several small studies have concluded that measuring IVC index (Diameter$_{max}$ − Diameter$_{min}$/Diameter$_{max}$), the IVC$_{max}$ diameter, or IVC$_{min}$ diameter could be used to determine which patients may be fluid responsive, albeit with only modest accuracy.[1,22-26] However, there are also multiple studies that demonstrate no correlation between the variation of the IVC diameter and fluid responsiveness, leading many to believe that it should not be used in isolation in spontaneously breathing patient (Fig. 17.9).[27-33]

Given the conflicting data presented in literature, there is no consensus on the percentage collapse obtained by IVC ultrasound that can be recommended as a cut-off for administering a fluid bolus to increase cardiac output. Conversely, many experts believe extremes of IVC diameter alone may be useful to guide management; however, the heterogeneity of variables affecting cardiac output has made testing this hypothesis with high quality research challenging. Thus, it is our position that in shock states, near-total collapsibility or small IVC size (<1 cm) suggest preload sensitivity but should be integrated with other clinical data and ultrasound findings of the heart and lungs.

Passive Ventilation

Mechanically ventilated patients who are passive (i.e., not triggering any breaths) have standardized loading conditions on their IVCs and therefore have long been regarded as the ideal patients for assessing fluid responsiveness using the IVC (Fig. 17.10, Video 17.6). This population has been studied with older, small studies showing a correlation between fluid responsiveness and an IVC *distensibility* index (IVC$_{max}$ diameter − IVC$_{min}$ diameter / IVC$_{max}$ diameter) of greater than 12% to 18%.[34-37] These patients also had to meet strict enrollment criteria, including ventilating tidal volume of ≥8 cc/kg and a regular cardiac rhythm. Some newer studies have demonstrated that the IVC distensibility index may not be as reliable as once thought in determining which patients may be fluid responsive.[29,33,38-41] Further, few ICU patients (2%) meet all of these criteria at any one time, compared with up to 39% of operating room patients.[42,43] Regardless, IVC distensibility remains a physiologically sound and clinically specific concept.

Similar to the IVC collapsibility index, the distensibility index is only one component of an overall evaluation of a hypotensive patient. Using the above cited literature as a guide, we modestly offer the conclusion that an IVC distensibility index ≥12% to 18% *may* indicate a patient will benefit from intravenous fluids, whereas an IVC distensibility index ≤12% to 18% *may* indicate a patient will not benefit from intravenous fluids. When the IVC is

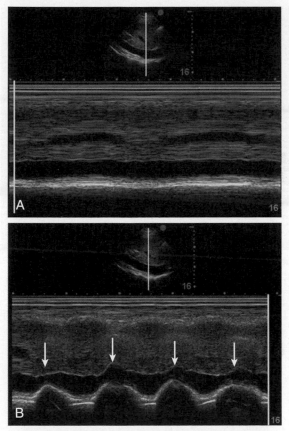

Figure 17.9 Inferior Vena Cava (IVC) Variation With Spontaneous Ventilation. These M-mode images were obtained from the same patient moments apart with different respiratory effort. (A) Rapid, shallow breathing, exerting little influence on IVC size. (B) Rapid, deeper breaths creating significant collapse and variation of IVC size *(arrows)*. This example highlights the difficulty in standardizing IVC assessment in spontaneously breathing patients.

small (<1 cm diameter) or completely collapses with respiration, fluid resuscitation can be clinically justified in most patients (Fig. 17.11, Videos 17.7 and 17.8).

In contrast to the IVC, the superior vena cava (SVC) has shown increasing reliability via its respirophasic changes in response to ventilation in predicting volume responsiveness.[41,44] Assessment of the SVC is restricted to transesophageal echocardiography and, whereas its use and availability at the point-of-care are increasing (see Chapter 20), its application is not yet routine.

Lastly, passive leg raise maneuver and stroke volume variation from the left ventricular outflow tract are compelling adjuncts to any assessment of preload sensitivity. These techniques are more labor intensive, but we encourage fluency in these concepts for providers who routinely encounter this clinical scenario (see Chapter 21).

TAMPONADE PHYSIOLOGY

When a pericardial effusion is detected and cardiac tamponade is suspected, IVC ultrasound can serve as a sensitive screening tool to determine whether pressure within the pericardial sac exceeds right atrial and CVP.

A patient with a pericardial effusion and a plethoric IVC (defined by less than 50% collapse after deep inspiration), has a 97% sensitivity for a diagnosis of tamponade; however, specificity is only 40% (Video 17.9).[12] Thus, if

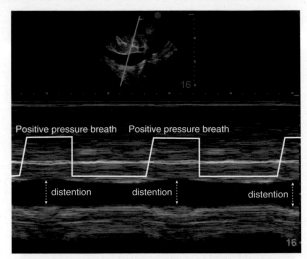

Figure 17.10   Inferior Vena Cava Variation With Passive Ventilation. M-mode image showing lack of respirophasic variation in a mechanically ventilated patient who is passive on the ventilator.

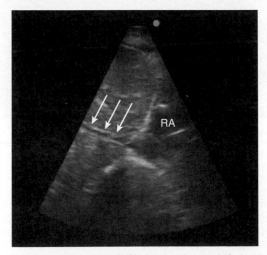

Figure 17.11   Collapsed Inferior Vena Cava (IVC). Small, collapsed IVC, (*arrows*). *RA*, Right atrium.

a diagnosis of tamponade is being considered, it may be effectively ruled out by demonstrating IVC collapse of 50% or more with deep inspiration without having to pursue more sophisticated echocardiographic techniques (Fig. 17.12). The combination of a dilated IVC and pericardial effusion indicates that cardiac tamponade may be present, although a dilated IVC is not specific for tamponade (Fig. 17.13 and Video 17.10). If a clinical diagnosis cannot

be made, consultation or comprehensive echocardiography should be obtained.

ESTIMATING CENTRAL VENOUS PRESSURE

IVC diameter and collapsibility have long been used by cardiologists to estimate the CVP. Determining the CVP can be useful when used with other advanced echocardiographic

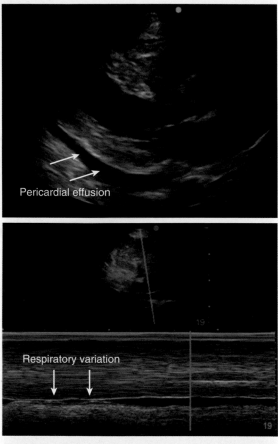

Figure 17.12   Pericardial Effusion Without Tamponade. A moderate pericardial effusion is seen along with a small, collapsible inferior vena cava. Except in rare situations (post-procedural or loculated pericardial effusions), this combination of findings rules out pericardial tamponade.

TABLE 17.2   **Inferior Vena Cava Diameter and Collapsibility and Central Venous Pressure**

IVC Diameter and Collapse (%)	Central Venous Pressure (Mean) (mm Hg)
Normal: ≤2.1 and >50%	0–5 (mean 3)
Intermediate:	5–10 (mean 8)
≤2.1 cm and <50% collapse or	
>2.1 cm and >50% collapse	
High: >2.1 and <50%	10–20 (mean 15)

IVC, Inferior vena cava.
See references 48, 49, 50.

measurements to calculate pulmonary arterial pressures (see Chapter 16). The utility of CVP to assess volume status and guide fluid management, however, is controversial and has its limitations.[45-47] Guidelines for estimating CVP based on IVC diameter and collapsibility are presented in Table 17.2.[48-50] It is important to note these measurements have been validated in awake and spontaneously breathing patients and not in ventilated patients.

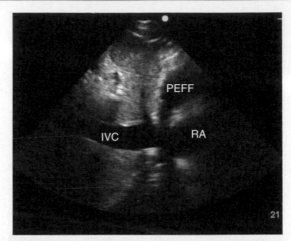

Figure 17.13   Dilated Inferior Vena Cava *(IVC)* and Pericardial Effusion. A dilated IVC with a pericardial effusion *(PEFF)* is consistent with but not specific for cardiac tamponade. *RA*, Right atrium.

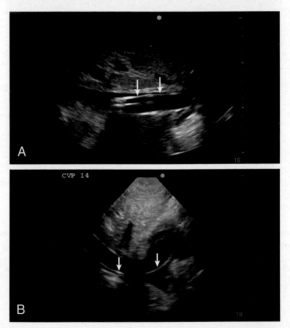

Figure 17.14   Devices in Inferior Vena Cava (IVC). (A) An Avalon catheter *(arrows)* is used in veno-venous extracorporeal membrane oxygenation. The catheter is placed in the right internal jugular vein and passes through the superior vena cava, right atrium, and into the IVC. (B) A femorally inserted transvenous pacemaker wire is seen *(arrows)* in the IVC entering the right heart.

DEVICE PLACEMENT

Various devices used in critical care (e.g., femorally inserted temporary pacemakers, bicaval veno-venous catheters for extracorporeal membrane oxygenation [ECMO], IVC filters, etc.) are inserted through the IVC (Fig. 17.14). Using the same techniques described above, providers can assess for successful placement during the procedure, or inadvertent dislodgement or migration after the procedure (Videos 17.11 and 17.12).

PEARLS AND PITFALLS

- Distinguish the abdominal aorta from the inferior vena cava (IVC). The IVC can be tracked to the right atrium after it traverses through the liver. The aorta lies to the left of the midline and has thicker walls, is pulsatile, and is surrounded by a fat layer.
- When assessing the diameter of the IVC, it is important to acquire the widest diameter and be aware of the cylinder effect: off-axis, oblique scanning of the vein leads to underestimation of the maximum diameter.
- Assess the IVC diameter and respiratory variation 2 cm from the RA-IVC junction or just caudal to the insertion of a hepatic vein. If using M-mode, make sure the sampling line is perpendicular to the IVC walls.
- IVC ultrasound should be used cautiously in the evaluation of a patient's volume status and potential fluid responsiveness.
- A dilated, noncollapsible IVC has high sensitivity for cardiac tamponade, and IVC ultrasound can be used to rule out tamponade physiology when the IVC is collapsible.
- Estimation of CVP can be determined by IVC diameter and collapsibility: IVC > 2.1 cm with < 50% collapse = CVP 10–20 (mean of 15) mm Hg; IVC ≤ 2.1 cm with > 50% collapse = CVP 0–5 (mean 3) mm Hg.

CHAPTER 18

Pericardial Effusion

Shane Arishenkoff ◼ Maili Drachman ◼ John Christian Fox

KEY POINTS

- Pericardial effusions can be rapidly and accurately detected by providers with focused training in point-of-care ultrasonography.
- 2D echocardiographic findings of cardiac tamponade generally appear along a continuum of hemodynamic compromise, from a dilated inferior vena cava to right atrial systolic collapse to right ventricular diastolic collapse.
- Use of ultrasound guidance for pericardiocentesis reduces the risk of complications and improves procedure success rates.

Background

With the increased adoption of point-of-care cardiac ultrasound, pericardial effusions are more readily and frequently identified. In addition to being able to identify pericardial effusions, clinicians who use point-of-care ultrasound must be clinically skilled in assessing the hemodynamic importance of their echocardiographic findings.

Pericardial effusions are defined as the presence of fluid in the pericardial space that exceeds 50 mL and may be caused by malignancy, uremia, trauma, infection, and rheumatologic diseases. Although the prevalence of pericardial effusions in the general population is not known, data suggests that up to 13.6% of patients with otherwise unexplained dyspnea presenting to an emergency department have pericardial effusions of varying clinical significance.[1]

When considering a life-threatening pericardial effusion in the form of tamponade, physical exam findings, such as Beck's triad (hypotension, jugular venous distension, and muffled heart sounds), are not specific and may be more reliable in trauma patients with rapid accumulation of fluid.[1,2] Few applications of emergency point-of-care ultrasound are more time sensitive and potentially lifesaving as cardiac ultrasound to detect tamponade.[3] It is well documented that focused cardiac ultrasound performed by appropriately trained noncardiologists with varying scopes of practice[4-6] can reliably diagnose pericardial effusions with greater than 95% accuracy compared with comprehensive transthoracic echocardiography.[7,8] Once a pericardial effusion is identified, the reproducibility of point-of-care ultrasound is of particular value, allowing frequent reassessment for changes in size and hemodynamic impact. If a pericardial effusion is found, the next steps are to assess its size, hemodynamic importance, and possible associated diseases.[9]

Image Interpretation

The pericardium is a dense, fibrous double-layered membrane that completely encircles the heart and a few centimeters of the proximal aorta and pulmonary arteries. The dense parietal pericardial tissue is highly echogenic and is easily recognized as the sonographic border of the heart. The pericardial sac is a space contained between the visceral and parietal pericardium.

A normal heart contains approximately 10 mL of serous fluid in the pericardial sac. This small amount of fluid is occult on ultrasound, and the parietal and visceral layers of pericardium are seen as one hyperechoic layer adjacent to the myocardium. Pericardial effusions are most often seen as an anechoic band

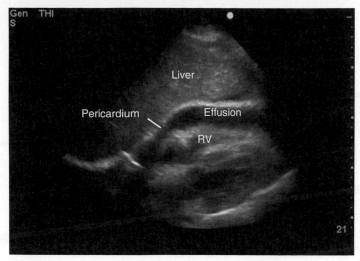

Figure 18.1 Pericardial Effusion (Subcostal View). A small pericardial effusion is seen separating the pericardial layers between the liver and the right ventricular *(RV)* free wall from a subcostal 4-chamber view.

that encircles the heart and separates the parietal pericardium from the heterogeneous, gray myocardium. In general, if a pericardial effusion is only visible in systole, the effusion is less than 50 mL and represents a clinically insignificant effusion.[9] Although a very small amount of fluid can be normal, distinguishing the origin (physiologic vs. pericardial disease) is not routinely possible with ultrasound. In high-risk clinical circumstances where trivial effusions may be harbingers of important, evolving pericardial disease (e.g., in penetrating trauma or after a cardiac procedure), even a very small effusion should be considered pathologic until proven otherwise, and frequent reassessment of the effusion is essential.

Free-flowing pericardial fluid initially accumulates posteriorly and is identified in the most dependent area of the pericardial sac. In the subcostal 4-chamber view, an effusion is seen as an anechoic stripe between the right ventricular free wall and the pericardium adjacent to the liver (Fig. 18.1 and Video 18.1). In the parasternal long-axis and short-axis views, pericardial effusions are seen posterior to the left ventricle but anterior to the descending thoracic aorta (Fig. 18.2 and Video 18.2). As the volume of pericardial fluid increases, the effusion becomes circumferential (Fig. 18.3). After cardiac surgery or percutaneous cardiac procedures, or in patients with recurrent

pericardial disease, pericardial fluid may be loculated or clotted, and does not flow freely with changes in patient position. Recognition of a loculated pericardial effusion is important because hemodynamic compromise can occur with even a small amount of fluid through direct chamber compression (Video 18.3). Additionally, pericardial effusions can develop septations, which are most often associated with infectious effusions (Fig. 18.4 and Video 18.4).

Pericardial Effusion Mimickers

A number of conditions can mimic pericardial effusion and must be distinguished from true effusions. First, epicardial fat interposed between the two layers of pericardium may be misdiagnosed as a pericardial effusion because both fluid and fat can appear anechoic or hypoechoic within the pericardial space. There are three important characteristics that can be applied to help distinguish fat from true pericardial fluid. First, compared to fluid, fat appears more gray or echogenic in appearance, rather than anechoic (Video 18.5). Second, an effusion, unless it is loculated, which is relatively rare, will typically collect in the most dependent pericardial space (posteriorly in a supine patient). Hence, isolated pericardial

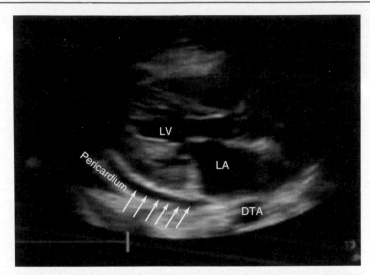

Figure 18.2   Pericardial Effusion (Parasternal View). Posterior accumulation of a small pericardial effusion in the far field *(arrows)* seen from a parasternal long-axis view. *DTA,* Descending thoracic aorta; *LA,* left atrium; *LV,* left ventricle.

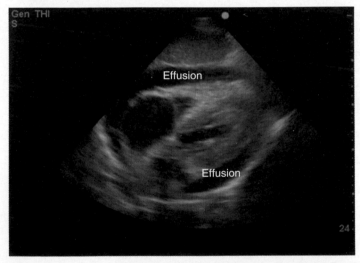

Figure 18.3   Circumferential Pericardial Effusion. Moderate to large circumferential pericardial effusion in a subcostal 4-chamber view.

separation anteriorly is most likely to be a fat pad (Fig. 18.5 and Video 18.6). Lastly, fat is most bountiful in the right atrioventricular sulcus and along right ventricular free wall, with minimal presence over the left ventricle.[9]

Effusions containing pus, fibrin, thrombus, or cellular debris from malignancy may appear more echogenic and can be overlooked as myocardium or adjacent lung tissue (Fig. 18.6 and Video 18.7). Second, a pleural effusion can be mistaken for a pericardial effusion. In a parasternal long-axis view, both effusions are seen as anechoic areas posterior to the left atrium and left ventricle but can be distinguished based on their relationship to the descending thoracic aorta (DTA). A pericardial

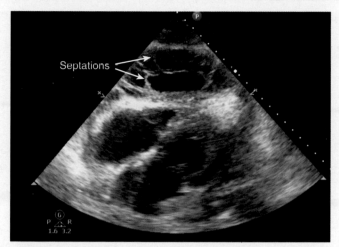

Figure 18.4 Septated Pericardial Effusion. A large pericardial effusion with septations is seen from a subcostal 4-chamber view in a patient with methicillin-resistant *Staphylococcus aureus* (MRSA) sepsis.

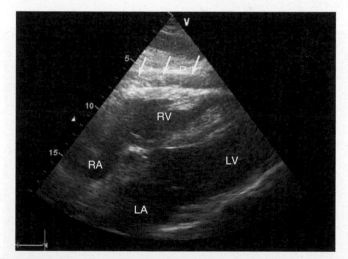

Figure 18.5 Epicardial Fat Pad. An epicardial fat pad *(arrows)* is shown in a subcostal 4-chamber view. Key features include echodensities visible in the fat layer as well as absence of a circumferential fluid collection. *LA,* Left atrium; *LV,* left ventricle; *RA,* right atrium; *RV,* right ventricle.

effusion traverses anterior to the DTA, whereas a left pleural effusion is seen posterior to the DTA (Figs. 18.7 and 18.8 and Videos 18.8 and 18.9). If the DTA is not well seen, an effusion should be confirmed from parasternal short-axis and subcostal views, or a dedicated left pleural view can also be obtained. Lastly, in certain views, providers must be vigilant not to mistake peritoneal fluid for pericardial fluid. Because the subcostal cardiac imaging plane crosses the upper abdomen, ascites may be misinterpreted as pericardial fluid in this view (Fig. 18.9 and Video 18.10). The absence of circumferential fluid around the heart, and acquiring corroborating cardiac and abdominal ultrasound views, can avoid this pitfall.

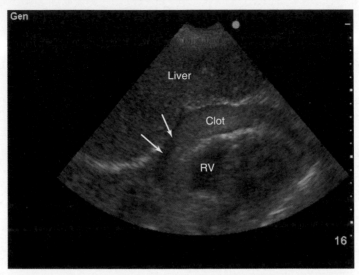

Figure 18.6   Pericardial Clot. Pericardial blood clot is seen from a subcostal 4-chamber view. Mixed echo densities are common in complex effusions. *Arrows* point to some anechoic effusion (blood) that has not clotted. *RV,* Right ventricle.

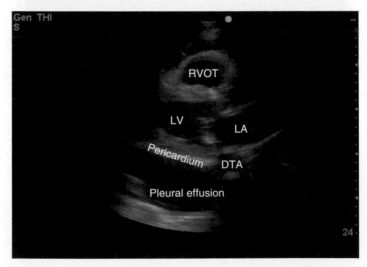

Figure 18.7   Pericardial Versus Pleural Effusions. A large left pleural effusion without a pericardial effusion is seen in a parasternal long-axis view. The anechoic space representing the pleural fluid does not track anterior to the descending thoracic aorta *(DTA)*, distinguishing it from a pericardial effusion. *LA,* Left atrium; *LV,* left ventricle; *RVOT,* right ventricular outflow tract.

Pathologic Findings

Hemodynamic effects of fluid in the pericardial space depend on both the volume and rate of fluid accumulation, as well as the patient's intravascular volume status. A slowly expanding pericardial effusion (e.g., malignant effusion) can become quite large (>2000 mL) with little increase in pericardial pressure (Video 18.11), whereas rapid accumulation of even a small volume of fluid (50–100 mL) can lead to a marked increase in pericardial pressure (e.g., myocardial perforation during placement of a pacemaker lead) (Fig. 18.10). Other important

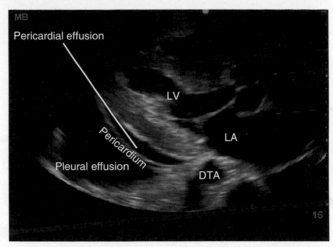

Figure 18.8 Pericardial and Pleural Effusion. A parasternal long-axis view demonstrates both a pericardial effusion and left pleural effusion. Pericardial effusions are distinct because they track anterior to the descending thoracic aorta (DTA), while left pleural effusions are only posterior to the DTA. *LA*, Left atrium; *LV*, left ventricle.

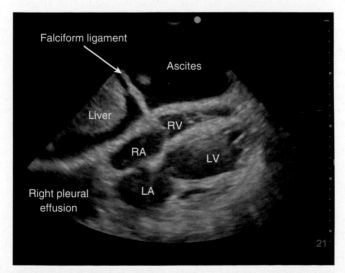

Figure 18.9 Pericardial Effusion Versus Ascites. Ascites with no pericardial effusion is seen from a subcostal 4-chamber view. Attention to the falciform ligament and the absence of circumferential fluid around the heart can help avoid this pitfall. Note a right pleural effusion is also present. *LA*, Left atrium; *LV*, left ventricle; *RA*, right atrium; *RV*, right ventricle.

factors that determine the hemodynamic consequences of pericardial fluid accumulation include pericardial fluid characteristics (serous vs. blood), anatomic distribution (loculated vs. circumferential), integrity of the pericardial layers (inflamed, neoplastic, invasion, fibrous), volume status of the patient, and the size, thickness, and function (pulmonary hypertension) of the underlying cardiac chambers.[10]

PERICARDIAL EFFUSION SIZE

Several scales for quantifying the volume of a pericardial effusion have been described.

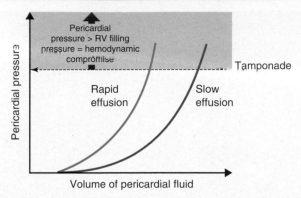

Figure 18.10   Pericardial Fluid Accumulation. Relationship of pressure within the pericardium versus pericardial effusion volume. Rapidly accumulating pericardial effusions cause a sudden rise in pericardial pressure leading to cardiac tamponade at smaller volumes, while slowly accumulating effusions cause a gradual rise in pericardial pressure leading to tamponade at much higher volumes. *RV,* Right ventricle.

Although size does not routinely predict hemodynamic importance, large effusions are a major risk factor for poor prognosis and will generally require closer attention and more frequent intervention. In addition, the size of a pericardial effusion can be helpful in identifying its etiology. For instance, a large effusion without inflammatory signs or tamponade is more likely to be chronic and idiopathic with a likelihood ratio of 20.[11] To this end, having a common language when describing effusion size is of value. The taxonomy outlined below is most commonly used and reflects the widest dimension of pericardial fluid that is measured at end-diastole (Fig. 18.11):

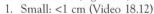

1. Small: <1 cm (Video 18.12)
2. Moderate: 1–2 cm (Video 18.13)
3. Large: >2 cm (Video 18.14)

CARDIAC TAMPONADE

When evaluating a patient for cardiac tamponade, it is fundamental to remember that tamponade is a clinical diagnosis. Tamponade physiology occurs when the pressure within the pericardium exceeds the pressure of one or more cardiac chambers, resulting in impaired cardiac filling and a corresponding drop in cardiac output (Fig. 18.12). Cardiac tamponade should be suspected clinically in any hemodynamically unstable patient with a nontrivial, circumferential pericardial effusion (Video 18.15). It is important to recognize that tamponade physiology may be evident on ultrasound prior to deterioration of vital signs and

can potentially identify a worsening condition prior to hemodynamic instability. Cardiac ultrasound findings of tamponade include collapse of the right atrium (RA) during ventricular systole, collapse of the right ventricle (RV) during ventricular diastole, and a dilated inferior vena cava (IVC) due to reduced right-sided filling (Table 18.1). Once a meaningful pericardial effusion is identified, the simplest and most contributory echocardiographic next step is to examine the IVC for its diameter and collapsibility. A dilated IVC carries a 97% sensitivity for tamponade.[15] Thus, if the IVC is not dilated or demonstrates good respiratory variation, cardiac tamponade is extremely unlikely to be present. This negative predictive value of a normal IVC can be extremely helpful to rule out tamponade in clinical situations where an effusion is present but may be a distractor from a more plausible cause of illness. A dilated IVC, on the other hand, is not specific for tamponade; however, when concern for cardiac tamponade is present, it lends physiologic support to this diagnosis.

In cardiac arrest, cardiac tamponade is a potentially reversible cause of pulseless electrical activity (PEA) that can be detected by emergency cardiac ultrasound.[16] The incidence of pericardial effusion in patients with PEA who demonstrate cardiac contractility has been reported to be as high as 67%.[17] Cardiac ultrasound during cardiac arrest is particularly useful because PEA and near-PEA are electrical rhythms that are indistinguishable without direct visualization of the heart (see Chapter 23).

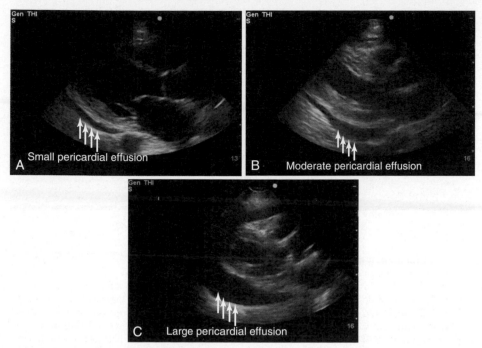

Figure 18.11   Pericardial Effusion Size. Small (A), moderate (B), and large (C) pericardial effusions *(arrows)* seen from a parasternal long-axis view.

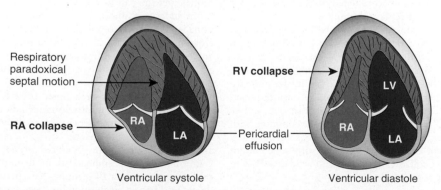

Figure 18.12   Cardiac Chamber Collapse. Effects of elevated pericardial pressure on both the right atrium and the right ventricle. Each chamber is subject to collapse during its respective diastolic phase when chamber pressure is lowest. *LA,* Left atrium; *LV,* left ventricle; *RA,* right atrium; *RV,* right ventricle.

TABLE 18.1   Cardiac Ultrasound Findings in Cardiac Tamponade

- **Circumferential pericardial effusion:** usually moderate to large, except for loculated effusions
- **RA systolic collapse:** inversion of the RA free wall for greater than a third of ventricular systole has a sensitivity of 94% and a specificity of 100% for the diagnosis of tamponade[11]
- **RV diastolic collapse:** sensitivity 60%–90%; specificity 85%–100%[12]
- **Reciprocal respiratory variations in ventricular volumes:** in the apical 4-chamber view, an increase in RV volume with inspiration (shift in septal motion toward the LV in diastole and toward the RV in systole) and a decrease during expiration (normalization of septal motion) can be appreciated[13]
- **Plethora of the inferior vena cava (IVC):** a dilated inferior vena cava with <50% inspiratory decrease in diameter that is measured 1–2 cm distal to the IVC–RA junction (sensitivity 97%, specificity 40%)[14]

IVC, Inferior vena cava; *RA,* right atrium; *RV,* right ventricle.

A late finding seen in large pericardial effusions is a "swinging heart" inside the pericardial cavity (Video 18.16), responsible for the celebrated electrocardiogram (ECG) finding of electrical alternans. Other ultrasound findings consistent with cardiac tamponade include respiratory variation of transvalvular inflow variation (>60% for tricuspid and >30% for mitral) using pulsed-wave Doppler, exaggerated diastolic reversal of blood flow in the hepatic veins during expiration,[9] and reduced early diastolic tissue Doppler velocity. These techniques are generally considered to be reserved for advanced echocardiographers.

Certain findings may be misinterpreted as cardiac tamponade in patients with pericardial effusions who have some degree of RA/RV collapse: (1) normal ventricular or atrial systole are easier to appreciate in the presence of pericardial fluid and can be misinterpreted as RA/RV collapse, (2) slight diastolic "notching" of the RV wall which is common with pericardial effusions, and (3) RA collapse may occur in hypovolemic states with concomitant IVC collapse, as opposed to a dilated IVC in tamponade.

Pericardial Drainage

Cardiac tamponade is a true cardiac emergency requiring rapid diagnosis and treatment. When clinical signs suggest a hemodynamically significant effusion, treatment should begin immediately with expansion of intravascular volume and consideration of the temporary usage of vasoactive drugs if the patient is hypotensive.[18,19] These temporizing interventions are only a prelude to definitive, procedural treatment. Removal of pericardial fluid can be divided into surgical and percutaneous interventions. Surgical drainage is preferred in traumatic hemopericardium and purulent pericarditis[20] and has traditionally involved the creation of pericardial windows, pericardiopleural fistulae, or pericardiectomies. However, with the exceptions of penetrating trauma and loculated effusions, including postoperative tamponade, the standard of care for management of cardiac tamponade has shifted to percutaneous techniques over the past two decades.[21]

In addition to those effusions causing tamponade, pericardial drainage is indicated for effusions greater than 20 mm by ultrasound[22] and may be performed in smaller effusions for diagnostic purposes, such as pericardial fluid cytology and epicardial or pericardial biopsy. With the exception of emergency pericardiocentesis, relative contraindications include uncorrected coagulopathy, anticoagulant therapy, thrombocytopenia (platelets <50,000/mm^3) and small, posterior, or loculated effusions. Caution should be emphasized in hemopericardium due to aortic dissection where pericardiocentesis has, in small numbers, been shown to worsen outcomes.[23]

The procedural success rate for ultrasound-guided pericardiocentesis is 97% with an overall complication rate of 4.7%.[24] It should be emphasized that ultrasound guidance is the standard of care in pericardiocentesis. Complication rates of landmark-based pericardiocentesis are substantially higher, with morbidity reaching 20%[25] and mortality reported as high as 6%.[26-28] When ultrasound guidance is used to perform pericardiocentesis, the rate of major complications, including cardiac perforation resulting in death or immediate cardiac surgical intervention, pneumothorax, and intercostal artery laceration, is 1.2%. The minor complication rate, including transient chamber penetrations and supraventricular tachyarrhythmias, is 3.5%. Success rate with ultrasound guidance is high (93%) in patients with anterior effusion greater than 10 mm, whereas the success rate is only 58% with small, posterior effusions.[24] Innovative techniques, including the use of endobronchial and endoscopic ultrasound, to guide pericardiocentesis have been recently described and may become more common.[29,30]

The technique of ultrasound-guided pericardiocentesis is neither strictly defined nor standardized, and the subcostal, apical, or parasternal window can be used to access the pericardial space. The subcostal approach is the most common and often easiest in the majority of patients. In terms of safety, the needle entry site and trajectory should be determined by ultrasound. The location with the largest fluid collection and thinnest chest wall should be marked. Real-time ultrasound guidance to track the needle tip is challenging and often requires a two-person technique with one provider standing at the apex holding the transducer and a second provider advancing the needle via a subcostal approach.

In addition to locating the optimal needle insertion site, cardiac ultrasound can help determine the needle insertion depth to drain a pericardial effusion and monitor drainage during the procedure. In a subcostal approach, a long 16- to 18-gauge angiocatheter is inserted between the xiphoid process and left costal margin at a shallow angle (<30 degrees) to pass under the costal margin. The needle is aimed toward the left shoulder and advanced slowly while continuously aspirating the syringe. Once the pericardium is pierced and fluid is aspirated, a one-time therapeutic drainage can be performed or a pigtail catheter can be inserted over a guidewire for prolonged drainage.[23] It is crucial to confirm needle location within the pericardial space prior to dilating the tract and inserting a pericardial drain. Confirmation can be achieved by administering agitated saline or reinjecting a few milliliters of effluent using a three-way stopcock. Visual confirmation with ultrasound can be achieved by seeing turbulent flow or bubbles within the pericardial space (Fig. 18.13 and Video 18.17). Visualization of bubbles in the LV cavity (Fig. 18.14 and Video 18.18) should prompt withdrawal, re-angling of the needle, and surgical consultation.

For prolonged drainage, an indwelling pigtail catheter can be left in the pericardial space until less than 25 to 30 mL of fluid is drained in a 24-hour period. Insertion of a pericardial catheter for extended drainage has evolved to become standard of care. Recurrence rates of pericardial effusion are lower with insertion of a pericardial catheter versus percardiocentesis alone (23% vs. 65%), and surgical intervention has similarly low recurrence rates.[24]

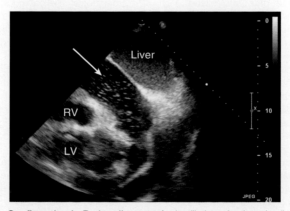

Figure 18.13 Needle Confirmation in Pericardiocentesis. Instillation of agitated saline into the pericardial space *(arrow)* confirms proper needle location during pericardiocentesis seen from an off-axis subcostal 4-chamber view. *LV,* Left ventricle; *RV,* right ventricle.

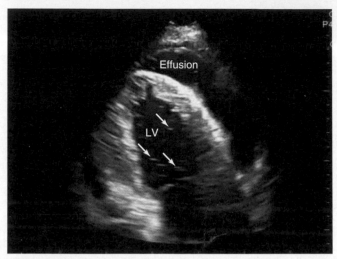

Figure 18.14   Needle Penetration Into Left Ventricle. Visualization of bubbles in the left ventricle while injecting agitated saline *(arrows)* reveals inadvertent deep penetration of the needle tip into the left ventricle *(LV)* during pericardiocentesis.

PEARLS AND PITFALLS

- Differentiating pericardial from pleural effusions: Pericardial effusions are usually circumferential. From a parasternal long-axis view, pericardial effusions are anterior to the descending thoracic aorta (DTA), whereas pleural effusions are posterior to the DTA. If a pleural effusion is suspected, a dedicated view of the left pleural space should be obtained.
- Differentiating pericardial effusion from epicardial fat pad: Fatty tissue will appear hypoechoic but will often have some echogenicity, as opposed to the majority of effusions which are anechoic. Effusions almost always collect posteriorly initially; if the echo-free space is found only anteriorly, the structure is most likely an epicardial fat pad. When in doubt, corroborating views from different cardiac windows should be obtained.
- Loculated pericardial effusions: After surgical or percutaneous procedures, or in patients with recurrent pericardial disease, pericardial fluid may be loculated. Recognition of a loculated effusion is especially important because hemodynamic compromise can occur with even a small volume of loculated fluid and may require transesophageal echocardiography for further evaluation.
- Echogenic pericardial effusion: If pericardial fluid has substantial pus, fibrin, blood, or cellular debris, it can appear comparatively echogenic and can be mistaken for myocardium or adjacent tissues.
- Cardiac tamponade is a clinical diagnosis: The patient's medical history, vital signs, physical exam, and cardiac ultrasound findings must all be considered when declaring a diagnosis of cardiac tamponade.
- A dilated inferior vena cava (IVC) has high sensitivity (97%) for cardiac tamponade: When the IVC is not dilated (<2.5 cm) or shows respiratory variation, providers can have a high degree of confidence that tamponade is not present.
- Right atrial collapse due to hypovolemia: RA collapse may be seen in patients with hypovolemia who do not have cardiac tamponade. An important distinguishing point is the IVC in hypovolemic patients will be collapsed.

CHAPTER 19

Valves

Ahmed F. Hegazy

KEY POINTS

- Basic cardiac valve assessment can be performed with two-dimensional ultrasound and color flow Doppler.
- Severe aortic or mitral regurgitation can be detected with bedside ultrasound, which is critical to recognize in patients with acute circulatory or respiratory failure.
- A complete valvular assessment requires advanced training and warrants consultation for comprehensive echocardiography.

Background

Detecting gross valvular pathology is an important aspect of point-of-care cardiac ultrasound. Patients presenting with undifferentiated cardiorespiratory failure should be examined for acute valvular pathology at the bedside. A basic point-of-care ultrasound valvular assessment includes a two-dimensional (2-D) visual inspection of valve structure and a color flow Doppler interrogation, as well as assessment of atrial and ventricular size and function. Conditions in which a point-of-care valve assessment can guide patient management include unexplained pulmonary edema, heart failure, septic shock, and ventilator dependence. Contraindications to extracorporeal circulatory support (e.g., ruling out aortic insufficiency for intra-aortic balloon pumps and venoarterial extracorporeal membrane oxygenation [ECMO]) can also be excluded using point-of-care ultrasound.

Guidelines from the American Society of Echocardiography (ASE) and European Association of Echocardiography (EAE) describe in detail the echocardiographic assessment of native valve regurgitation, stenosis, and prosthetic valve dysfunction.[1-7] A comprehensive assessment of native valve regurgitation integrates multiple quantitative, semiquantitative,

and qualitative measures to grade severity. Although an integrated quantitative assessment of the mitral valve is more accurate and reflects long-term outcomes and mortality,[8] such assessments require both time and expertise. Interobserver agreement using quantitative parameters is low, even among experienced echocardiographers.[9] Thus, currently some authors describe the process of accurate quantification of valvular regurgitation as more of an art than a science.[10] Further, quantitative assessments rarely add to the acute management of massive regurgitation that is readily apparent by a qualitative assessment.[11] The expertise, equipment, and time required to perform a detailed valvular assessment is therefore beyond the scope of point-of-care ultrasound.

A document summarizing point-of-care cardiac ultrasound competencies for basic and advanced skill sets in critical care has been published.[12] A focused cardiac valvular assessment primarily uses 2-D visual inspection and color flow Doppler to screen for severe aortic or mitral regurgitation (MR). Untreated acute severe valvular regurgitation has an unacceptably high mortality rate. If valvular regurgitation is identified, chronicity is difficult to determine without prior imaging.[11] Because the essence of point-of-care valve assessment is to expeditiously identify abnormalities that may be affecting the patient's hemodynamics, classifying severity of regurgitation is important. Severe valvular regurgitation begets early action, whether it is consultation for urgent comprehensive echocardiography, mechanical support, or surgery. Thus, a helpful framework for interpretation is to dichotomously categorize regurgitant valvular lesions as "severe," capable of causing or complicating acute illness, versus "nonsevere" for all other gradations of valvulopathy. If evaluation for severe versus nonsevere regurgitation is indeterminate in an acutely ill patient, then prompt comprehensive echocardiography may be warranted. It is important to note that some severely regurgitant lesions are immutably chronic and may not warrant urgent intervention.

General Considerations

TWO-DIMENSIONAL IMAGING

A 2-D inspection of the valve and its surrounding anatomic scaffolding should be performed in multiple views. If an abnormality is detected, the provider should note the exact location (i.e., leaflet involved), suspected process (e.g., endocarditis, ischemia, dilation), and mechanism of dysfunction (e.g., prolapse, flail, restriction, perforation).[5,6] Assessment of prosthetic valve function and pathology requires expert level skill in echocardiography.

Calcifications, vegetations, thickening, flail leaflets, and tethering can all be discerned with a 2-D evaluation.[1] A major structural defect should prompt the provider to consider the presence of a severe lesion. Infective endocarditis cannot be ruled out with point-of-care cardiac ultrasound considering that comprehensive, full-platform echocardiography is falsely negative in 15% of patients.[7] Vegetations typically arise on the lower-pressure side of a valve and may be detected if destructive or large.

Finally, it is imperative to recognize adaptive responses of cardiac chambers to valve abnormalities. Assessing atrial and ventricular size can help determine severity, as well as chronicity. The left ventricle (LV) and left atrium (LA) are often not dilated with acute left-sided valvular regurgitation. However, differentiating acute versus chronic regurgitation is challenging, requires review of previous echocardiograms, and often requires advanced echocardiographic skills.

SCOPE OF EXAMINATION

Compared with other domains of point-of-care cardiac ultrasound, such as assessment of the right ventricle, left ventricle, and inferior vena cava, valvular assessments are less often actionable. Thus, a point-of-care exam is goal-directed to identify severe mitral or aortic regurgitation (AR) that, if undetected and unmanaged, may lead to critical illness or death.[12] Acute severe AR from aortic dissection, endocarditis, or trauma, and acute severe MR from ischemia or endocarditis must be recognized in a timely fashion. Tricuspid regurgitation (TR) is also readily identifiable and may support underlying diagnoses, such as pulmonary hypertension, pulmonary embolism, or endocarditis.

Valvular stenosis may be suspected based on 2-D evaluation but requires expertise to accurately assess severity and is a less time-sensitive diagnosis in general. Characterization of stenotic valves relies on spectral Doppler and is therefore considered a skill more suitable for advanced echocardiographers.

COLOR FLOW DOPPLER

Color flow Doppler is the main modality used for a rapid assessment of valvular regurgitation. Providers must be aware of important considerations and common pitfalls when using color flow Doppler. Understanding key concepts, such as pulse repetition frequency, Nyquist limit, and aliasing, are requisite starting points before using color flow Doppler (Fig. 19.1 and Table 19.1; see also Chapters 2 and 5).

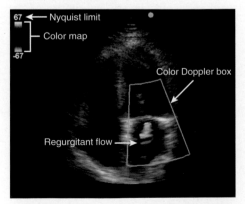

Figure 19.1 Color Doppler. The screen displays the Nyquist limit, color map, and color box overlying the mitral valve with a regurgitant jet in the left atrium.

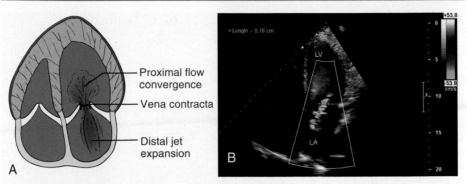

Figure 19.2   Vena Contracta Width. (A) Schematic demonstrating the location of vena contracta width measurement. (B) Apical 4-chamber view showing vena contracta width determination of 0.78 cm consistent with severe mitral regurgitation. *LA,* Left atrium; *LV,* left ventricle.

TABLE 19.1   **Terminology for Color Flow Doppler**

Term	Definition
Pulse repetition frequency (PRF)	The PRF (pulses per second) is how frequently the transducer sends and receives a signal and is determined by flow velocity and image depth. If a second pulse is sent before the first is received, the transducer cannot discriminate between the reflected signals from both pulses and ambiguity (aliasing) occurs.
Nyquist limit	Nyquist limit is the upper limit velocity of blood flow that the machine can accurately display with color flow Doppler before aliasing occurs and is the PRF divided by 2.
Aliasing	When the velocity of blood flow exceeds the Nyquist limit, the machine is unable to accurately display the direction or speed of blood flow.
Color map	A color map defines the color and brightness assigned to the direction and velocity of flow, respectively. Typical convention is *blue* for blood flowing *away* from the transducer and *red* for blood flowing *toward* the transducer. Velocities are encoded by the hues of blue or red; brighter hues signify faster velocities, whereas duller hues signify slower velocities.

The following recommendations can help optimize the performance and accuracy when assessing regurgitation with color flow Doppler[1,6,13]:

- Minimize imaging depth
- Narrow image sector size
- Adjust color gain appropriately
- Align the imaging plane to be parallel with blood flow
- Set the Nyquist limit to 50 to 70 cm/sec
- Use the smallest color box that reasonably includes the valve and receiving chamber

Color flow Doppler identifies regurgitant flow and assesses severity based on size of the color jet. An additional parameter that can help grade severity of regurgitation is measurement of vena contracta width (VCW) of the color flow Doppler jet. The VCW is the narrowest diameter of the regurgitant color flow Doppler jet and reflects the effective regurgitant orifice area (EROA). The VCW is measured perpendicular to the color flow jet in the neck between the proximal flow convergence (PFC) and distal jet expansion (Fig. 19.2 and Video 19.1). It is a measurement largely independent of driving pressures and flow rates for fixed orifices; however, its accuracy with multiple jets is uncertain.[5,6,13]

SPECTRAL DOPPLER

Spectral Doppler includes pulsed-wave and continuous-wave Doppler which offers a quantitative, but time-consuming, approach to valvular and hemodynamic assessment. These techniques can be applied at the point of care after additional training. Parameters, such as flow reversals, antegrade flow density and velocity, pressure half-time (PHT), and deceleration time (DT), are all spectral Doppler-derived parameters that assist in grading severity of a valve lesion but are beyond the scope of this chapter.[1,7,5,6,14]

Pathologic Findings

MITRAL REGURGITATION

MR is back flow of blood into the LA due to incomplete closure of the mitral valve leaflets during systole. The degree of regurgitation is primarily affected by the regurgitant orifice area but is also influenced by the duration of systole and LA–LV pressure gradient.[12] MR can be due to intrinsic valvular pathology (primary MR) or functional (secondary MR) where the mitral valve is structurally normal.[13]

TWO-DIMENSIONAL FINDINGS

Visually inspecting valve morphology in 2-D mode is the first step of any valvular assessment. The importance of this visual 2-D assessment cannot be overemphasized. Morphological assessment of the mitral valve is usually conducted from the parasternal long-axis (PLAX), apical 4-chamber, and subcostal 4-chamber views. The mitral valve leaflets are normally observed to be thin and pliable and they open fully in diastole. During systole, the valve closes and coaptation should be observed as the leaflet tips fully approximate each other. Morphological abnormalities on 2-D inspection include leaflet thickening, calcification, presence of vegetations, and leaflet perforation (Video 19.2).[1] Leaflet coaptation abnormalities include prolapsed and flail leaflets (Fig. 19.3 and Video 19.3), in addition to leaflet restriction. In the presence of LV dilation and chordal stretch, functional MR can occur with leaflet tenting and malcoaptation (Video 19.4).[6] A hypertrophic septum can potentially cause left ventricular outflow tract (LVOT) flow acceleration and entrainment of the tip of the anterior leaflet of the mitral valve in the LVOT during systole. This entrainment phenomenon is also called systolic anterior motion and can produce a dynamic LVOT obstruction, a condition which should be treated with fluid loading and/or beta blockade as appropriate given the increased mortality associated with this finding, particularly in patients with septic shock[15] (Videos 19.5 and 19.6). Anterior mitral valve leaflet entrainment can be observed on 2-D inspection and should be investigated if

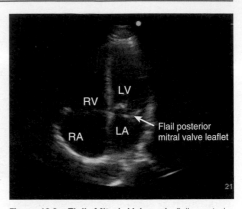

Figure 19.3 Flail Mitral Valve. A flail posterior mitral valve leaflet is seen coapting behind the anterior mitral valve leaflet in an apical 4-chamber view. This valve apparatus failure is consistent with severe mitral regurgitation. *LA,* Left atrium; *LV,* left ventricle; *RA,* right atrium; *RV,* right ventricle.

the interventricular septum appears abnormally thick.[16]

Analysis of the LV and LA size and function is important to contextualize the time course of mitral valve disease. In long-standing chronic MR, a slow increase in LA size and compliance is seen to accommodate the regurgitant volume. The LV may also dilate due to chronic volume overload. In acute or subacute MR, the short time course will not allow for a gradual increase in chamber size and compliance. Acute MR will therefore usually result in acute pulmonary edema, with a normal LA and LV size on 2-D assessment (Video 19.7).[6]

COLOR FLOW DOPPLER FINDINGS

Color flow Doppler is the primary method of detecting and grading MR. Standardized qualitative and quantitative values help determine if MR is severe (Table 19.2).[1,17] Of the findings listed in Table 19.2, jet area determination using color flow Doppler is employed most frequently given its relative simplicity, even though jet area determination is imperfect due to effects of LA size, loading conditions, and LV function.[4,12] Whereas nonsevere MR (Fig. 19.4 and Video 19.8) may be hemodynamically important in some patients, severe MR is important in all patients and must be readily identified (Fig. 19.5 and Video 19.9).

Jet direction can provide clues to the pathology and etiology of MR. Centrally directed jets

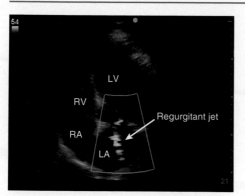

Figure 19.4 Nonsevere Mitral Regurgitation. A small regurgitant jet is seen in the left atrium consistent with nonsevere mitral regurgitation from an apical 4-chamber view. *LA,* Left atrium; *LV,* left ventricle; *RA,* right atrium; *RV,* right ventricle.

are often seen in functional, or secondary MR (see Fig. 19.1 and Video 19.10). A common cause of functional MR is left ventricular systolic dysfunction and LV dilation. Eccentric jets (Fig. 19.6 and Video 19.11) usually occur with asymmetric leaflet dysfunction in primary MR. As a general rule, a hypermobile (prolapsed or flail) leaflet causes a regurgitant jet directed away from that leaflet, whereas a restricted leaflet causes a jet directed towards the affected side.[6] Leaflet prolapse is commonly seen with myxomatous degeneration of the mitral valve. Flail leaflets are typically observed with papillary muscle rupture in the setting of myocardial infarction. Leaflet restriction, with an eccentric

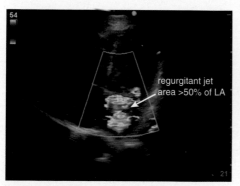

Figure 19.5 Severe Mitral Regurgitation. An apical 4-chamber view showing a color jet filling greater than 50% of the left atrium which is consistent with severe mitral regurgitation. *LA,* Left atrium.

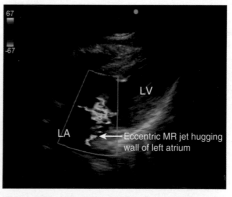

Figure 19.6 Eccentric Mitral Regurgitation. An eccentric mitral regurgitant jet wrapping around the left atrium is seen from a subcostal 4-chamber view. Regardless of the regurgitant jet area, an eccentric jet is an indication of severe mitral regurgitation. *LA,* left atrium; *LV,* left ventricle.

TABLE 19.2 Severe Mitral Regurgitation Findings

2-Dimensional Ultrasound	Color Flow Doppler	Spectral Doppler (Advanced)
• Severe valve lesions (primary: flail leaflet, ruptured papillary muscle, severe retraction, large perforation; secondary: severe tenting, poor leaflet coaptation)	• Central jet area occupies >50% of left atrium • Vena contracta width is ≥0.7 cm (>0.8 for biplane)[a] • Eccentric jet swirling in left atrium	• Regurgitant volume ≥60 mL • Regurgitant fraction ≥50% • Systolic flow reversal in pulmonary veins • E-wave dominant (>1.2 m/sec) • Effective regurgitant orifice area ≥0.4 cm^2

[a]Average of apical 4-chamber and apical 2-chamber views.
From Zoghbi WA, Adams D, Bonow RO, et al. Recommendations for Noninvasive Evaluation of Native Valvular Regurgitation: A Report from the American Society of Echocardiography Developed in Collaboration with the Society for Cardiovascular Magnetic Resonance. *J Am Soc Echocardiogr.* 2017;30(4):303–371. doi:10.1016/j.echo.2017.01.007.

jet towards the affected leaflet, can be encountered in multiple conditions These conditions include papillary muscle dysfunction in the setting of regional LV ischemia and rheumatic mitral valve disease. However, if the rheumatic disease process affects both leaflets equally, the jet can be central.[4] Leaflet destruction from endocarditis typically has an unpredictable direction of the regurgitant jet (Videos 19.12 and 19.13).[7]

Aortic Regurgitation

AR can result from pathology of either the aortic valve or aortic root. Etiologies for acute AR include infective endocarditis, chest trauma, and acute aortic dissection. Other causes of AR include inflammatory diseases, connective tissue disease, and congenital conditions, including bicuspid aortic valve.[1]

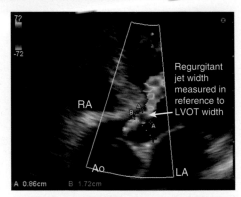

Figure 19.7 Aortic Regurgitation Jet Width. A zoomed image of the aortic valve from an apical 5-chamber view shows the regurgitant jet occupying 50% of the width of the left ventricular outflow tract. *Ao,* Aorta; *LA,* left atrium; *LVOT,* left ventricular outflow tract; *RA,* right atrium.

TWO-DIMENSIONAL FINDINGS

The aortic valve's anatomy and movements are usually best seen in the parasternal long-axis and short-axis views at the aortic valve level. From these views, providers may be able to detect a dilated aortic root (Video 19.14), bicuspid valve, and large vegetations (Video 19.15). Infrequently, a dissection flap may be seen, but the sensitivity of even comprehensive transthoracic echocardiography to detect aortic dissection is low.[18] The vegetations associated with endocarditis of the aortic valve leaflets should not be confused with Lambl's excrescence (Video 19.16) or Arantius' nodules, which are normal findings.[19]

It is essential to assess for left atrial and ventricular adaptation in response to AR. Chronic volume overload secondary to AR causes dilation of the LV (Video 19.17). Although ventricular function is normal initially, left ventricular dysfunction ensues progressively.[4] In patients with acute AR, the left ventricular end-diastolic pressure rises dramatically, and a noncompliant ventricle is subjected to acute volume overload (Video 19.18). Acute worsening of chronic regurgitation would produce similar findings, although often with greater symptom burden.[11]

COLOR FLOW DOPPLER FINDINGS

Color flow Doppler can detect the presence of AR and help determine its severity. Common views for use of color flow Doppler evaluation

are the apical 5-chamber view (Fig. 19.7) for its favorable Doppler alignment with the aortic valve and the PLAX view for its excellent axial resolution of the aortic valve, LVOT, and aorta (Fig. 19.8). Criteria for severe AR are listed in Table 19.3.[1]

Tricuspid Regurgitation

The tricuspid valve's anterior leaflet is the largest of its three leaflets. These leaflets are normally thinner than the mitral valve. The tricuspid valve should always be evaluated in context with right ventricular size and function. Functional TR due to right ventricular pressure or volume overload is more common than structural TR due to pathology of the valve (Video 19.19). Etiology of structural TR includes endocarditis, rheumatic heart disease (with associated mitral and aortic valve disease), myxomatous degeneration, Ebstein anomaly, carcinoid syndrome, and trauma (Video 19.20).[4]

TWO-DIMENSIONAL FINDINGS

Evaluation of the tricuspid valve is similar to the mitral valve. A 2-D view of the right heart from subcostal and apical 4-chamber views may reveal flail leaflets, vegetations, and prolapse, as well as severe tenting and coaptation defect of the valve suggestive of functional TR.

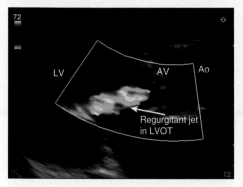

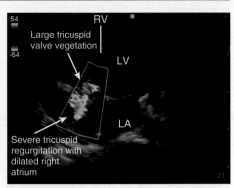

Figure 19.8 Aortic Regurgitation. The aortic valve *(AV)* with regurgitant flow into the left ventricular outflow tract *(LVOT)* is shown from a parasternal long-axis view. Ao, Aorta; *LV,* left ventricle.

Figure 19.9 Severe Tricuspid Regurgitation. Apical 4-chamber view demonstrating severe tricuspid regurgitation due to infective endocarditis. Note the large vegetation, severe right atrial enlargement, and small pericardial effusion. *LA,* Left atrium; *LV,* left ventricle; *RV,* right ventricle.

TABLE 19.3 **Severe Aortic Regurgitation Findings**

2-Dimensional Ultrasound	Color Flow Doppler	Spectral Doppler (Advanced)
• Severe valve lesion (abnormal/flail, or wide coaptation defect)	• Large central jet area; variable in eccentric jets • Jet width/LVOT diameter ≥65% • Jet area/LVOT area >60% • Vena contracta width >0.6 cm	• Pressure half-time steep and <200 msec • Prominent holodiastolic flow reversal • Regurgitant volume ≥60 mL • Regurgitant fraction ≥50% • Effective regurgitant orifice area ≥0.3 cm^2

LVOT, Left ventricular outflow tract.
From Zoghbi WA, Adams D, Bonow RO, et al. Recommendations for Noninvasive Evaluation of Native Valvular Regurgitation: A Report from the American Society of Echocardiography Developed in Collaboration with the Society for Cardiovascular Magnetic Resonance. *J Am Soc Echocardiogr.* 2017;30(4):303–371. doi:10.1016/j.echo.2017.01.007.

COLOR FLOW DOPPLER FINDINGS

Color flow Doppler can detect presence of severe TR (Fig. 19.9 and Videos 19.21–19.25).[1] Findings supporting the diagnosis of severe TR include a central jet occupying greater than 50% of the right atrial area, a VCW ≥0.7 cm, or presence of an eccentric jet hugging the right atrial wall. Table 19.4 lists the defining features of severe TR.[1]

Stenotic Valvular Lesions

Stenotic valves generally have several abnormal findings on 2-D examination with ultrasound. In general, a normal morphologic appearance rules out any clinically significant stenosis.

Stenotic valves commonly show diminished mobility, thickening, and calcifications (Figs. 19.10 and 19.11 and Video 19.26). In addition, the upstream chambers tend to dilate or hypertrophy in response to the increased workload caused by the stenosis.[2] For a point-of-care cardiac ultrasound evaluation, it is reasonable to subjectively assess valves for findings suggestive of stenosis. A qualitative point-of-care inspection of valves may also provide diagnostic information when aiming to rule out significant aortic stenosis. An aortic valve that appears normal morphologically and displays normal leaflet mobility rules out severe aortic stenosis.[20] If valvular stenosis is suspected, a comprehensive echocardiogram using Doppler and quantitative methods should be obtained.

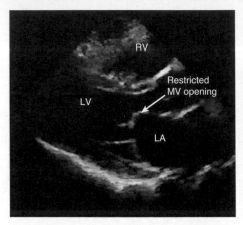

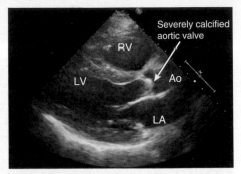

Figure 19.11 Severe Aortic Stenosis. Severely calcified aortic valve in a patient with severe aortic stenosis seen in a parasternal long-axis view. *Ao,* Aorta; *LA,* left atrium; *LV,* left ventricle; *RV,* right ventricle.

Figure 19.10 Rheumatic Mitral Stenosis. Diminished mitral valve opening with the characteristic "diastolic doming" or "hockey stick" pattern suggestive of rheumatic mitral stenosis seen in a parasternal long-axis view. *LA,* Left atrium; *LV,* left ventricle; *MV,* mitral valve; *RV,* right ventricle.

TABLE 19.4   Severe Tricuspid Regurgitation Findings

2-Dimensional Ultrasound	Color Flow Doppler	Spectral Doppler (Advanced)
• Severe valve lesions (flail leaflet, large perforation, or leaflet retraction with poor coaptation)	• Large central jet, or eccentric wall-impinging jet of variable size • Central jet occupying >50% of right atrium[a] • Vena contracta width ≥0.7 cm[a]	• Regurgitant volume ≥45 mL • Systolic flow reversal in hepatic vein • Tricuspid inflow E-wave dominance (>1 m/sec) • Effective regurgitant orifice area >0.4 cm^2

[a]Setting the Nyquist limit to 50 to 70 cm/sec.
From Zoghbi WA, Adams D, Bonow RO, et al. Recommendations for Noninvasive Evaluation of Native Valvular Regurgitation: A Report from the American Society of Echocardiography Developed in Collaboration with the Society for Cardiovascular Magnetic Resonance. *J Am Soc Echocardiogr.* 2017;30(4):303–371. doi:10.1016/j.echo.2017.01.007.

PEARLS AND PITFALLS

• The scope of a point-of-care valve assessment should focus particularly on detection of severe mitral, aortic, and tricuspid valve regurgitation.
• Performing a 2-D visual inspection of valve morphology is an imperative first step in assessing valve abnormalities.
• A morphologically normal valve with normal leaflet opening and mobility rules out clinically significant stenosis.
• Color flow Doppler is the most basic and widely used technique used to identify and determine severity of regurgitation.
• Understanding the physics of color flow Doppler and its limitations is essential for safe and effective use of this imaging modality. To optimize color flow Doppler imaging, adjust the ultrasound settings: shallow depth, appropriate gain, narrow sector, and smallest possible color Doppler box oriented as parallel as possible to blood flow.
• Review of prior echocardiogram results is invaluable to differentiate acute,

acute on chronic, or chronic valvular regurgitation when no obvious chamber enlargement is present. Left atrial and ventricular dilation suggest chronic regurgitation of the mitral and aortic valves, respectively.
- Hemodynamic significance of a valve lesion does not always match the echocardiographic severity and vice versa.
- If image resolution is excellent, the vena contracta width is a useful, adjunctive approach to determine severity of regurgitation of the mitral valve (≥ 7 mm = severe) and aortic valve (>6 mm = severe).

CHAPTER 20

Transesophageal Echocardiography

Brian M. Buchanan ■ Hailey Hobbs ■ Robert Arntfield

KEY POINTS

- Transesophageal echocardiography (TEE) yields more reliable acoustic windows and higher quality images than transthoracic echocardiography (TTE).
- For those competent in point-of-care cardiac ultrasound, interpretation of TEE images is a transferable cognitive skill that can be rapidly learned.
- The 28 views of a comprehensive TEE are not generally required for a goal-directed, point-of-care TEE. A goal-directed TEE with four views is a suitable starting point and is sufficient to rapidly identify life-threatening pathology in a hemodynamically unstable patient.
- Point-of-care TEE has unique value in cardiac arrest where it may assist in diagnosis, management, and prognosis without threat of interrupting high-quality chest compressions.

Background

Point-of-care transesophageal echocardiography (POC-TEE) is of particular value in instances where a transthoracic approach may be limited by anatomy or clinical condition, such as obesity, lung hyperinflation, subcutaneous emphysema, or cardiac arrest.[1-3]

High-quality TEE images can be reliably acquired such that diagnostic superiority over TTE has been demonstrated in multiple clinical scenarios, including hemodynamic instability, prediction of volume responsiveness, intra-cardiac shunts, thoracic aortic dissection, and post-cardiac surgery.[4-8]

Despite its reliability and high diagnostic yield in critical illness, TEE uptake at the point-of-care is still considered novel. Barriers to widespread adoption include transducer cost, inter-disciplinary politics, and lack of training standards for POC-TEE.

TRAINING

There are some unique training considerations when it comes to POC-TEE. TEE was historically a tool of cardiologists, but published guidelines and consensus statements support use by physicians specializing in anesthesiology, emergency medicine, and critical care, especially for resuscitation.[3,6,9-13] International training standards in critical care echocardiography have further subdivided POC-TEE into basic and advanced critical care echocardiography.[14] Perioperative TEE performed by cardiac anesthesiologists during cardiac surgery requires a distinct body of knowledge, rigorous training, and certification that is distinct from POC-TEE.

Though interpretation of images is generally transferable across both transthoracic echocardiography (TTE) and TEE, TEE requires additional training in spatial orientation,

TABLE 20.1 **Basic and Advanced Indications for Point-of-Care Transesophageal Echocardiography**

Basic Applications	Advanced Applications
Shock	Advanced hemodynamics *(heart-lung interactions, stroke volume, diastology)*
Cardiac arrest	Procedural guidance *(ECMO, pacemaker, line placement)*
Volume status	Endocarditis
Pericardial effusion	Advanced valvular assessment
Severe valvulopathy	Acute aortopathy *(aortic dissection)*
	Perforated foramen ovale/shunts
	Cardiac source of embolism *(left atrial appendage)*

ECMO, Extracorporeal membrane oxygenation

probe insertion, and manipulation techniques. Unlike TTE, the invasive nature of TEE precludes training on normal subjects. As an alternative, high fidelity simulation offers a supplementary opportunity to practice both probe insertion and manipulation.[9,15] Simulation has been shown to rapidly accelerate training to attain competence in multiple disciplines.[16-19]

The number of required studies to achieve competence in POC-TEE across subspecialties is evolving. One expert consensus in critical care suggests 35 fully supervised TEEs to obtain competence in advanced critical care echo, but this number can be made lower if simulation is used in training.[16,19,20,21]

INDICATIONS

The leading indications for POC-TEE are similar to those of TTE, including the assessment of volume status, biventricular function, pericardium, and left-sided valves. In selected cases, providers with advanced training can perform more advanced applications (Table 20.1). The choice to use POC-TEE is typically driven by poor quality or indeterminate information from a point-of-care TTE examination or when TTE may be less feasible due to clinical logistics, such as during cardiopulmonary resuscitation (CPR) or surgery.

CONTRAINDICATIONS

Absolute contraindications to TEE include perforated esophagus or stomach; esophageal tumor, stricture, or diverticulum; active gastrointestinal (GI) bleeding; and recent esophageal or upper GI surgery. Relative contraindications are outlined in Table 20.2.[22] If the patient or

TABLE 20.2 **Contraindications to Transesophageal Echocardiography**

Contraindications to TEE		
Absolute	1.	Gastrointestinal (GI) pathology *(perforated viscus, active upper GI bleeding, recent upper GI surgery)*
	2.	Esophageal pathologies *(stricture, tumor, perforation, diverticulum, esophagectomy, esophago-gastrectomy, recent esophageal surgery)*
Relative	1.	GI pathology *(recent upper GI Bleed, peptic ulcer disease, esophagitis, dysphagia, GI surgery, symptomatic hiatal hernia)*
	2.	Esophageal pathologies *(Mallory-Weiss Tear, scleroderma, esophageal varices)*
	3.	Cervical spine disease *(atlantoaxial joint disease, severe arthritis)*
	4.	Prior head/neck/chest radiation
	5.	Coagulopathy, thrombocytopenia

TEE, Transesophageal echocardiography.
From Hilberath JN, Oakes DA, Shernan SK, et al. Safety of transesophageal echocardiography. *J Am Soc Echocardiogr.* 2010;23(11):1115–1127. doi:10.1016/j.echo.2010.08.013.

family is unable to provide a reliable history, the medical records should be reviewed for any contraindications. Ultimately, like any procedure, the risks and potential benefits must be weighed.

COMPLICATIONS

TEE has a low complication rate and a well-established safety profile.[4,21-24] Adverse events and complications of TEE are largely dependent on security of the airway, pharmacological sedation, contraindications, and provider experience. The overall complication rate ranges from 0.03% for important esophageal trauma to less than 2.3% for minor oropharyngeal bleeding when TEE is utilized in patients who are fully anticoagulated.[21,24-26]

In the case of POC-TEE, most patients are critically ill and usually intubated, significantly mitigating the risks associated with airway security. Sedation-induced hypotension and apnea may require transient vasopressors and change in ventilation strategy, respectively. Oropharyngeal and esophageal injuries associated with probe insertion or manipulation are infrequent,[4,22] but range from minor (self-limited oropharyngeal bleeding) to major complications (esophageal perforation). Although the risk of esophageal perforation is a source of anxiety for some, it occurs infrequently (0.01%–0.03% of TEE exams) across broad populations.[21,22] A list of TEE complications is shown in Table 20.3.

TABLE 20.3 Complications Resulting From Transesophageal Echocardiography

Complications	
Oropharyngeal	Lip laceration, dental injury, perforation of hypopharynx, accidental tracheal intubation, major bleeding
Esophageal	Odynophagia, dysphagia, laceration, or perforation
Gastric	Gastric laceration or perforation, hemorrhage
Other	Airway compromise, thermal injury, pressure necrosis, bronchospasm, laryngospasm, dysrhythmia, anesthetic induced hypotension

See references 6, 21, 22, 24, 25.

Anatomy: Imaging Windows, Planes, and Views

The esophagus yields an expansive acoustic window alongside the heart and great vessels, with no intervening bone, muscle, or substantial soft tissue. This close proximity to the heart affords the use of high frequency ultrasound transducers capable of producing images of higher quality than TTE.

The two principle acoustic windows of TEE are the midesophageal (ME) and transgastric (TG) windows. The ME window is located at approximately 30 to 35 cm of insertion depth. The left atrium closely approximates the esophagus and is in the near field of all ME views. Further advancement of the probe past the gastroesophageal junction yields the TG window. Individual variations in anatomy require focusing on the images obtained, rather than adhering strictly to probe insertion depths and transducer angles. Similar to TTE, understanding the anatomical relationships of the heart and great vessels in long and short axes is essential to acquire specific views. See Chapter 14 for more details on standard cardiac imaging planes.

Standard TEE imaging views are named according to the acoustic window and cross-sectional imaging plane (Fig. 20.1). With the probe inserted at approximately 30 to 35 cm in the ME position and the transducer angle at 0 degrees, the heart is seen in a coronal plane. This position displays the 4-chamber view by TEE, a mirrored view of the apical 4-chamber view by TTE. Within this one acoustic window, there is potential to generate innumerable views of different structures along a full 180-degree spectrum. As such, providers must focus on goal-directed questions and views when using POC-TEE.

Image Acquisition

PROBE INSERTION TECHNIQUES

TEE probe insertion is an endoscopic skill that warrants unique consideration among point-of-care ultrasound (POCUS) techniques. In most scenarios that merit POC-TEE, the patient will be sedated with a secured airway. The probe should be in an unlocked position and never be manipulated forcefully. The probe tip has a thermometer designed to alert the provider of high temperatures for potential risk of thermal

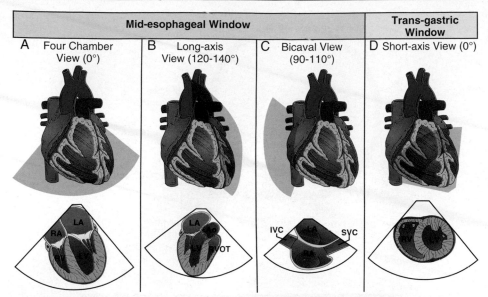

Figure 20.1   Transesophageal Echocardiography (TEE) Imaging Planes & Views. The standard cardiac imaging planes to acquire TEE views are shown. The 4 main point-of-care TEE views are the midesophageal 4-chamber (A), long-axis (B), and bicaval (C) views, and the transgastric short-axis view (D). *Ao,* Aorta; *CS,* coronary sinus; *IVC,* inferior vena cava; *LA,* left atrium; *LV,* left ventricle; *RA,* right atrium; *RV,* right ventricle; *RVOT,* right ventricular outflow tract; *SVC,* superior vena cava. (Modified from Otto, CM. *Textbook of Clinical Echocardiography.* 6th ed. Philadelphia, PA: Elsevier; 2018; Figures 3-1 – 3-17.)

injury. After applying sufficient lubrication, the probe is inserted with passive or active ante-flexion as it passes through the pharynx and hypopharynx. The most common insertion pitfall is straying from midline, which may result in wedging the probe in the pyriform fossa. We recommend a jaw thrust maneuver routinely to facilitate insertion. Rarely, a laryngoscope may be required.

TRANSDUCER MOVEMENTS

Transducer movements with TEE are unique. The transducer head is located in the GI tract, whilst the provider must maneuver the probe using the probe controls outside of the body (Fig. 20.2). Probe and transducer manipulation is described as four different actions (Fig. 20.3 and Video 20.1).

1. Advancement and withdrawal: The probe can be advanced and withdrawn from the esophagus to the stomach. The names of all TEE views start with the imaging window in the GI tract, such as ME long-axis view or TG short-axis view. When advancing or withdrawing the probe, the probe's flexion must be in a neutral and unlocked position.

2. Anteflexion and retroflexion: The larger control wheel flexes the probe tip anteriorly (anteflexion) or posteriorly (retroflexion) along the anterior-posterior axis.

3. Probe rotation: The entire probe can be rotated within the esophagus with the reference point being the anterior face of the probe. Large rotational movements are needed to image structures outside the central thorax, such as the descending thoracic aorta and vena cava, whereas minor rotation will fine tune the image to focus on specific areas.

4. Lateral flexion: Manipulation of the smaller, outer control wheel on the handle flexes the probe tip laterally to the right or left. In practice, this control is seldom used, but can occasionally be useful in optimizing the imaging or Doppler plane.

5. Imaging plane: Almost all TEE probes have two small buttons on the side of the probe handle to electronically steer and toggle the imaging plane from a neutral position

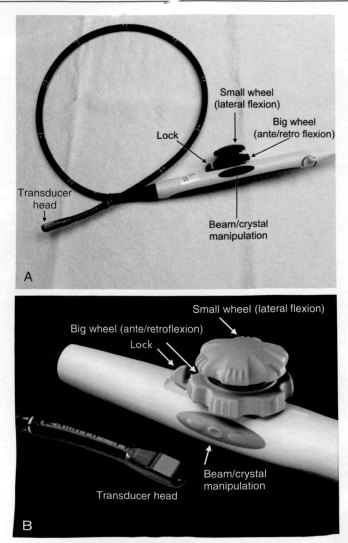

Figure 20.2   Transesophageal Echocardiography (TEE) Probe. (A) A TEE probe has a handle, body, and tip. (B) Probe controls are located on the handle. The large wheel controls anteflexion/retroflexion, whereas the small wheel controls lateral flexion.

0 degrees all the way to 180 degrees in an axial plane.

Imaging Protocol

POC-TEE is implicitly a goal-directed examination and will rarely require all 28 views of a comprehensive TEE. The clinical questions being posed and provider training determine the views acquired. Although there are a few different TEE protocols,[27-29] we recommend that novice POC-TEE operators initially learn four basic views. These four views are reliable for the scope of basic POC-TEE (left ventricular function, right ventricular function, pericardium, and volume status) and introduce the operator to the mechanical and cognitive skills of TEE. This focused four-view protocol closely parallels fundamental views of TTE (Table 20.4).

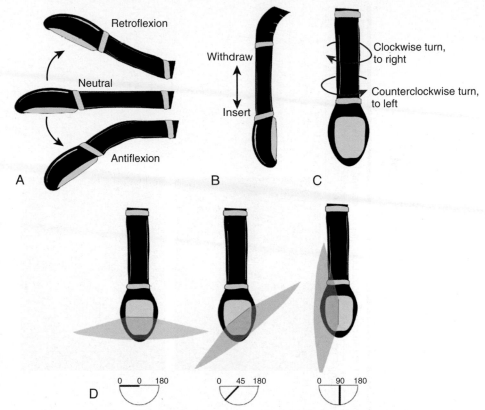

Figure 20.3   Manipulation of the TEE probe. The four main motions of the TEE manipulation are (A) ante-flexion and retroflexion, (B) insertion and withdrawal, (C) rotation, and (D) omniplane angulation. (From Lang et al. ASE's Comprehensive Echocardiography Second Edition, Saunders/Elsevier, 2016. Figure 11-1.)

MIDESOPHAGEAL 4-CHAMBER VIEW

With the probe in the ME position and an imaging plane of 0 degrees, the ME 4-chamber view is acquired (Video 20.2). The imaging plane traverses from the esophagus posteriorly (near field) to the mediastinum anteriorly (far field). If the apex of the left ventricle (LV) is foreshortened, gently retroflex the probe within the ME until the LV appears ovoid.

MIDESOPHAGEAL LONG-AXIS VIEW

From the ME window with the imaging plane set at 120 to 140 degrees, the ME long-axis view can be obtained (Video 20.3). The ME long-axis view is the TEE counterpart to the parasternal long-axis from TTE.

MIDESOPHAGEAL BICAVAL VIEW

The long axis of the superior and inferior vena cavae correspond to an imaging plane of 90 to 110 degrees in the ME window. As the cavae are located to the right of midline, the probe itself must be manually rotated along its own axis in a clockwise direction. (Video 20.4).

TRANSGASTRIC SHORT-AXIS VIEW (PAPILLARY MUSCLE LEVEL)

Starting from the ME position with the imaging plane set at 0 degrees, the probe is advanced into the stomach. Once the probe enters the stomach, it is anteflexed to obtain a TG short-axis view at the papillary muscle level (Video 20.5).

TABLE 20.4   Basic Transesophageal Echocardiography Views, Corresponding Transthoracic Echocardiography Views, and Common Applications

TEE Views	Corresponding TTE Views		Applications
Midesophageal 4-chamber		Apical 4-chamber	• LV function • RV size and function • Aortic, mitral, tricuspid valves • Pericardial effusion
Midesophageal long-axis		Parasternal long-axis	• LV function • Aortic and mitral valve • LVOT and ascending aorta • Pericardial effusion

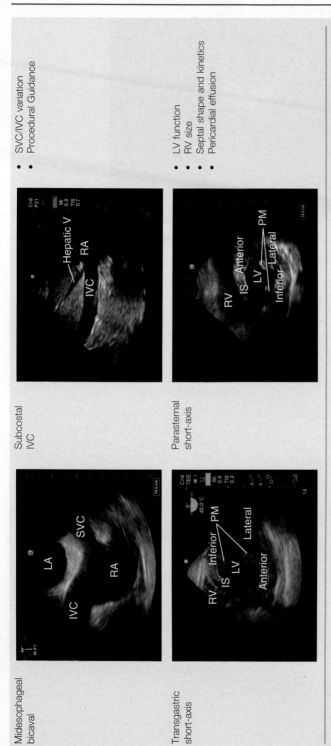

Midesophageal
bicaval

Subcostal
IVC

- SVC/IVC variation
- Procedural Guidance

Transgastric
short-axis

Parasternal
short-axis

- LV function
- RV size
- Septal shape and kinetics
- Pericardial effusion

Ao, Aorta; IS, interventricular septum; IVC, inferior vena cava; LA, left atrium; LV, left ventricle; LVOT, left ventricular outflow tract; MV, mitral valve; PM, papillary muscles; RA, right atrium; RV, right ventricle; SVC, superior vena cava; TEE, transesophageal echocardiography; TTE, transthoracic echocardiography; TV, tricuspid valve.

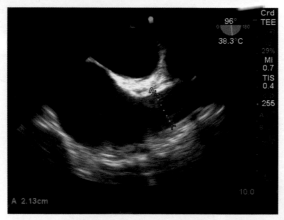

Figure 20.4 Superior Vena Cava Measurement. A midesophageal bicaval view is shown here with calipers across the superior vena cava measuring a diameter of 2.13 cm.

Selected Applications

The cornerstone of point-of-care cardiac ultrasound, whether TTE or TEE, is the assessment of LV function, RV function, pericardial effusion, and volume status in patients with hemodynamic or respiratory compromise. However, the superior image quality, indwelling location, and novel views of TEE enable operators to answer clinical questions that may not be possible with TTE.

VOLUME STATUS ASSESSMENT

TEE affords unobstructed views of the great vessels not visible on TTE, including the superior vena cava (SVC) (Fig. 20.4). Using the ME bicaval view, the M-mode cursor is placed perpendicular to the SVC to measure its widest possible diameter (Fig. 20.5 and Video 20.6). The magnitude of respirophasic variation of the SVC can be determined using the SVC collapsibility index [SVCCI (%) = Max−Min/Max diameter × 100].[30] In a general ICU population, respirophasic variation of the SVC has demonstrated better diagnostic accuracy than inferior vena cava (IVC) or pulse pressure variation to predict volume responsiveness.[7,30,31]

In applying the SVC findings, a few important values are worth mentioning. A 21% change in SVC with respiratory cycle can be used as a dynamic indicator of volume responsiveness with 81–84% specificity in a general ICU population (Fig. 20.5). Higher specificity

of 90% can be achieved using a cutoff value of 31% change. On the contrary, the sensitivity of SVC variation to rule out volume responsiveness is best with a change of less than 4% with each respiratory cycle.[1,7]

CARDIOPULMONARY RESUSCITATION

POC-TEE is particularly useful in cardiac arrest, offering threefold diagnostic, therapeutic and prognostic information to guide management. Goal-directed intra-arrest POC-TEE may rapidly identify the cause of the arrest with minimal interference to the resuscitative team. In particular, avoiding transthoracic imaging prevents direct interference with the provision of chest compressions.

The ME 4-chamber view is the initial view acquired during cardiac arrest allowing assessment of the LV, RV, pericardium and quality of CPR (Fig. 20.6). TEE enables a comprehensive hemodynamic interrogation of cardiac arrest mechanics, including an assessment of inciting causes and cardiac activity during pulse checks. Case series have identified a therapeutic impact for TEE changing cardiac arrest management in 31% to 67% of cases.[5,9,32]

Finally, detection of cardiac activity with TEE during pulse checks can help guide prognostication. Cardiac activity seen by ultrasound during pulse checks is associated with a significantly higher chance of immediate survival and return of spontaneous circulation (ROSC), whereas absence of any myocardial activity has

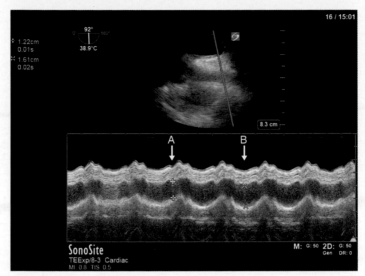

Figure 20.5 Superior Vena Cava (SVC) Variation With M-Mode. Measurement of SVC variation during inspiration (A) and expiration (B) reveals a 24% change (1.61 cm – 1.22 cm × 100% = 24%).

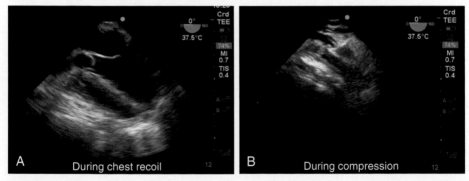

Figure 20.6. Midesophageal 4-Chamber View During Cardiac Arrest. The heart is seen during chest recoil (A) and during active compressions (B).

predicted far inferior outcomes (Videos 20.7 and 20.8; see also Chapter 23).[33]

PROCEDURAL GUIDANCE

High-quality images yielded by TEE may guide a variety of procedures. Invasive procedures, including placement of extra-corporeal membrane oxygenation (ECMO) cannulae, intra-aortic balloon pumps, pulmonary artery catheters, and transvenous pacemakers can be dynamically guided with direct visualization with TEE.[34-36]

The ME bicaval view is particularly valuable for procedures. This view provides a long-axis

view of the SVC where guidewires, catheters, and cannulae can be directly visualized. By advancing the probe in the same 90-degree, sagittal imaging plane, the IVC can be visualized in a long-axis plane from a TG window (Video 20.9).[34,35]

POST-STERNOTOMY SHOCK

After sternotomy, TEE is routinely indicated for shock assessment as most transthoracic cardiac windows are obscured due to dressings, chest tubes, and positive pressure ventilation. Although the unique anatomical and surgical questions related to post-sternotomy assessment may frequently call for an advanced echocardiographer, the scope of a basic POC-TEE user, especially in the assessment of pericardial or mediastinal tamponade, may reveal the etiology and guide immediate management of shock in these patients. (Video 20.10).

FUTURE DIRECTIONS

The increasing accessibility of POC-TEE has brought a series of changes to the way circulatory failure is being managed in acute care environments. Areas of future growth include expansion of POC-TEE protocols, routine adoption in bedside ECMO cannula insertion,[36] rapid identification of aortic dissection in emergency departments,[8,37] application of transesophageal lung ultrasound,[38] and development of small indwelling TEE probes for continuous monitoring.[39-42]

PEARLS AND PITFALLS

- Naso- and orogastric tubes and thermometers can introduce air in between the TEE probe and esophageal mucosa, precluding the acquisition of high-quality images. Removal of these devices should be considered prior to probe insertion.
- Providers should review the patient's chart for contraindications prior to performing TEE. Absolute contraindications to TEE include esophageal pathologies (strictures, tumor, diverticulum, esophagectomy, esophagogastrectomy, recent esophageal surgery) and gastrointestinal pathologies (perforated viscus, active upper gastrointestinal bleeding, recent upper gastrointestinal surgery).
- In certain acutely ill patients, the presence of a relative contraindication may be outweighed by the potential diagnostic benefit of POC-TEE.
- The wealth of anatomic information afforded by POC-TEE can be overwhelming to novices learning this skill. Starting with a four-view protocol enables providers to focus their attention on life-threatening pathologies.
- In cardiac arrest, the midesophageal 4-chamber view should be the first view acquired. TEE may identify reversible causes of cardiac arrest without interrupting CPR compared to transthoracic imaging, and may guide management and prognostication.

CHAPTER 21

Hemodynamics

Gulrukh Zaidi ■ Vincent I. Lau ■ Paul Mayo

KEY POINTS

- Critical care echocardiography is an essential skill for frontline providers to aid in the diagnosis and management of patients with circulatory failure.
- Several spectral Doppler techniques can be applied in critically ill patients to perform a quantitative hemodynamic assessment.
- Stroke volume determination is a common hemodynamic technique that can help determine preload sensitivity.

Background

Point-of-care cardiac ultrasound or critical care echocardiography (CCE) is a useful diagnostic and monitoring tool for frontline providers. CCE has a robust and growing body of evidence, including guidelines for provider training. Basic CCE uses two-dimensional (2D) transthoracic imaging to perform a goal-directed examination aimed at answering common clinical questions. Basic CCE is a key components of point-of-care ultrasonography, as it allows immediate and serial qualitative assessments of cardiac function. Quantitative hemodynamic assessments include measurement of intra-cardiac pressures and flows that require the use of spectral Doppler techniques. Use of spectral Doppler requires additional training because of the quantitative nature and potential for significant error. As an introduction to hemodynamic assessment, this chapter will focus on the two most common topics: measurement of left ventricular (LV) stroke volume (SV) and identification of preload sensitivity.

Doppler Principles

Doppler ultrasound is used to measure the velocity and direction of blood flow in the cardiac chambers and blood vessels by utilizing the Doppler effect. Comprehensive knowledge of Doppler principles is requisite to performing quantitative hemodynamic measurements, and key principles are reviewed in Chapter 2. Before using Doppler ultrasound, providers must be familiar with pulsed-wave Doppler (PWD) and continuous-wave Doppler (CWD); pulse repetition frequency (PRF) and aliasing; and the effects of blood flow direction and Doppler interrogation.

Left Ventricular Stroke Volume

Knowledge of SV and cardiac output (CO) is valuable for providers managing circulatory failure. The SV measurements can guide diagnosis, influence management decisions, and allow trending of therapeutic interventions. Traditionally, SV was only obtainable through invasive monitoring, typically restricted to the intensive care unit (ICU) or operating room, but with the increasing availability of point-of-care ultrasound, trained providers may perform quantitative hemodynamic assessments in nearly any setting. The measurement of left ventricular stroke volume (LV SV) requires acquisition of high-quality 2D cardiac views and knowledge of potential pitfalls when using Doppler ultrasound.

187

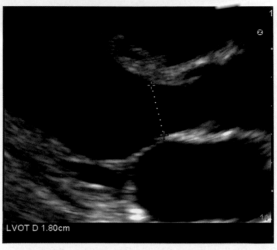

Figure 21.1 **Left Ventricular Outflow Tract (LVOT) Dimension.** Measure of LVOT diameter by zooming in to the base of the aortic valve from a parasternal long-axis view. LVOT area = $(1.8 \text{ cm}/2)^2 \times 3.14 = 2.5 \text{ cm}^2$.

STEP 1: MEASUREMENT OF LEFT VENTRICULAR OUTFLOW TRACT

Accurate measurement of the left ventricular outflow tract (LVOT) diameter is critical for two reasons. First, transthoracic echocardiography tends to underestimate the measurement.[1,2] Second, when calculating SV, the LVOT radius is squared, leading to significant error if an inaccurate measurement is obtained.

To measure the LVOT diameter, the provider must first acquire a high-quality parasternal long-axis view focusing on the LVOT and aortic valve (AV). Ideally, capture the plane that bisects the right coronary cusp hinge point anteriorly and the interleaflet triangle between the left and noncoronary cusps posteriorly.[3] Zoom in to the AV for greatest accuracy in measurement, and freeze the image to view the AV maximally opened in mid-systole. Use the machine calipers to measure the diameter of the LVOT at the base of the AV (Fig. 21.1). Divide the diameter in half to obtain the radius of the LVOT, and calculate the cross-sectional area of the LVOT[4]:

$$\text{LVOT area} = 3.14 \times (\text{Radius of LVOT})^2$$

Normally, the LVOT diameter in adults varies between 1.8 and 2.2 cm and correlates to some extent with body habitus. As a reference, the measured LVOT area should be within 2 mm of the predicted LVOT diameter based on body surface area: $\text{LVOT}_{predicted}$ (mm) = (5.7 × BSA) + 12.1.[3]

STEP 2: MEASUREMENT OF VELOCITY TIME INTEGRAL

First, the operator must obtain a high-quality apical 5-chamber view. From an apical 4-chamber view, the transducer is tilted 10 to 20 degrees aiming the ultrasound beam toward the anterior chest wall to visualize the LVOT and AV. Focus on the LVOT, and optimal visualization of the LVOT may require an off-axis apical 5-chamber view. Place the pulsed-wave Doppler sample volume gate in center of the LVOT (Fig. 21.2). The resultant tracing is of the LVOT systolic flow velocity (Fig. 21.3). Trace the systolic velocity flow curve, and the machine's cardiac software will calculate the area under the curve to yield the velocity time integral (VTI). The VTI is measured in centimeters and represents the distance blood is propelled forward from the LVOT to the aorta with each cardiac contraction.

STEP 3: CALCULATION OF STROKE VOLUME

The following formula is used to calculate the LV SV:

$$\text{LV SV (cm}^3) = \text{LVOT area (cm}^2) \times \text{LVOT VTI (cm)}$$

The equation is based on the concept that a volume of blood in the shape of a cylinder is pushed from the LVOT into the aorta during systole. The SV represents the volume

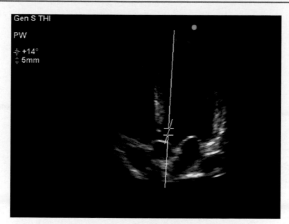

Figure 21.2 Left Ventricular Outflow Tract (LVOT) Velocity. The pulsed-wave Doppler sample volume gate is positioned in the center of the LVOT in an apical 5-chamber view to obtain the velocity time integral for stroke volume determination.

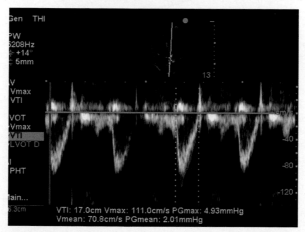

Figure 21.3 Velocity Time Integral (VTI). The VTI function calculates the area under the curve of the left ventricular outflow from an apical 5-chamber view.

of the cylinder whose base is the LVOT cross-sectional area, and height is the LVOT VTI (Fig. 21.4). The VTI represents the distance that this cylinder of blood travels with each LV contraction. An example of these three steps to calculate the SV can be seen in Fig. 21.5 and Video 21.1. The cardiac software included with most ultrasound machines will calculate the LV SV once the LVOT diameter and VTI have been entered. LV SV measured with this technique is accurate compared to thermodilution measurement.[5] However, providers should be aware of some common pitfalls of this technique:

1. A high-quality 2D image of the LVOT must be acquired to accurately measure the LVOT diameter. Because the LVOT radius is squared, any errors in measurement of the LVOT diameter multiplicatively affect the accuracy of the final SV calculation. Obtaining 2 to 3 measurements and using the mean value can mitigate this error. Generally, the LVOT diameter is more often underestimated when measured with transthoracic echocardiography.

2. Like all Doppler measurements, the LVOT VTI is angle dependent and requires adequate visualization of the LVOT. Providers should manipulate the 2D image in order to achieve an optimal Doppler intercept angle. Further, respiratory movement may cause the heart to move in and out of the

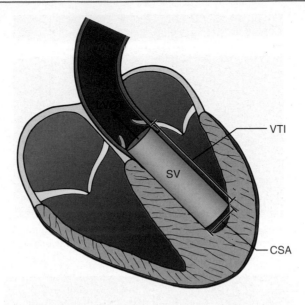

Figure 21.4   Stroke Volume *(SV)*. The SV is a volume of blood in the shape of a cylinder. The height of the cylinder is the velocity time integral *(VTI)*, and the base is the cross-sectional area *(CSA)* of the left ventricular outflow tract *(LVOT)*. By multiplying these two values together (base × height), the SV is calculated.

imaging plane leading to erroneous Doppler flow measurements.

3. The Doppler sample volume gate should be placed sufficiently proximal to the AV to avoid velocity acceleration effect that would cause overestimation of the LVOT VTI. If the AV closure signal is apparent on the VTI curve, the sample volume gate is too close to the AV (Fig. 21.6).

4. If the patient has an irregular heart rhythm, such as atrial fibrillation, LV SV will vary with changes in LV filling time. Obtaining several measurements (≥5 with atrial fibrillation) and using the mean value will generate the average LV SV.

In addition to using the LVOT VTI to calculate the LV SV, it can be used as a semi-quantitative tool for:

1. *Rapid detection of reduced SV.* Measurement of the LVOT VTI can serve as a rapid assessment to detect reduced LV SV. If VTI is in the normal range (18 to 22 cm), then hemodynamic failure is not associated with a reduction in LV SV. If there is major reduction in VTI, a quantitative calculation of LV SV may be required in order to determine if the oxygen delivery (DO_2) is reduced to a dangerous extent.

2. *Preload sensitivity.* The LVOT VTI and peak velocity correlate with the SV, and both of these measurements have utility for determination of preload sensitivity.

Clinical application of the LV SV measurement:

1. *LV ejection fraction has limited correlation with LV SV.* Patients with a small, hyperdynamic LV often have a high ejection fraction but reduced LV SV. On the contrary, patients with a severe dilated cardiomyopathy and reduced ejection fraction may have a normal LV SV. In patients with hemodynamic failure, providers can measure both the LV SV and ejection fraction to guide their clinical decision-making.

2. *Serial measurement of LV SV.* When an intervention to increase LV SV is initiated, serial measurements of LV SV provide immediate data about the effectiveness of the intervention. For example, if an inotrope is started to augment CO, the provider can measure LVOT VTI serially as the drug is titrated in defined increments.

3. *Calculation of cardiac output.* The LV SV is required for calculation of CO which can be accomplished by multiplying the SV by the patient's heart rate: CO = SV × heart rate.

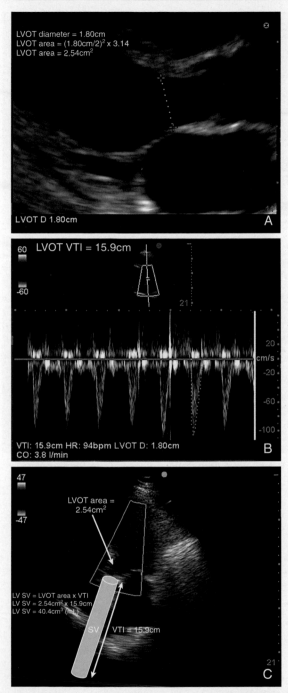

Figure 21.5   Stroke Volume Calculation. (A) First, the left ventricular outflow tract (LVOT) diameter is measured from a zoomed parasternal long-axis view. (B) Second, the pulsed-wave Doppler sample gate is placed in the LVOT below the aortic valve and the velocity time integral (VTI) is measured (15.9 cm in this case). (C) Third, the VTI is multiplied by the LVOT area to calculate the stroke volume: LV SV = 2.54 cm² × 15.9 cm = 40.4 cm³ or mL.

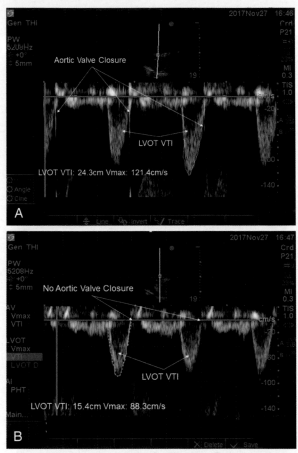

Figure 21.6 Correct Pulsed-Wave (PW) Doppler Sample Gate Placement. (A) Incorrect placement of the PW Doppler sample gate too close to the aortic valve (AV) results in overestimation of the left ventricular outflow tract (LVOT) velocity time integral (VTI) due to flow acceleration through the AV. The presence of an AV closure signal indicates the PW Doppler sample gate is too close to the AV. (B) Absence of aortic valve closure artifact confirms correct placement of the PW Doppler sample gate in the LVOT. Avoidance of aortic valve flow acceleration reduces the LVOT VTI measurement from 24.3 cm to 15.4 cm in this patient.

4. *Valvular assessment.* Measurement of LV SV, LVOT VTI, and LVOT peak velocity are frequently indicated for advanced, quantitative assessment of valvular stenosis and regurgitation.

5. *Preload sensitivity.* The LV SV may be used for determination of preload sensitivity as discussed below.

Assessment of Preload Sensitivity

Assessment of preload sensitivity (also called volume responsiveness) is a routine question in the resuscitative setting. The importance of this clinical question has been increasingly recognized as the peril of excessive volume resuscitation has been shown to increase mortality in critically ill patients.[4,6]

In cases where volume resuscitation is indicated by clinical findings (hemorrhage, gross hypovolemia, etc.) there is little role for echocardiography in immediate decision-making. In the more common scenario, where clinical and laboratory findings are more ambiguous, point-of-care ultrasound and echocardiography can guide clinical decision-making. In the absence of contraindications to volume loading based on initial ultrasound assessment (dilation of the right ventricle, reduced LV systolic function, profuse bilateral B-lines on lung ultrasonography), the provider will find value in proceeding with advanced techniques to determine whether volume expansion will augment LV SV and CO. Three results are possible:

1. High probability of preload sensitivity: Volume resuscitation is indicated.
2. Low probability of preload sensitivity: Volume resuscitation is not indicated.
3. Indeterminate result: Decision for volume resuscitation requires additional data or may be based on clinical gestalt.

Unfortunately, even with advanced techniques, ultrasonography may yield an indeterminate result. Review of the literature shows that establishing firm cutoff values for any commonly utilized techniques results in a significant number of false positives and false negatives.[7] Alternatively, providers can use a "gray zone" approach, where values in the extremes are considered diagnostic, but otherwise, values are considered to be indeterminate and clinical judgment is required. In the early literature, absolute cutoff values were the norm, but more recent literature contradicts this approach.[7]

Analysis of the respirophasic variation of the SV, LVOT VTI, or LVOT peak velocity have utility for assessment of preload sensitivity based on the well validated use of respirophasic variation of pulse pressure measured from the arterial wave form.[8,9] Assessing for respirophasic variation of arterial pulse pressure is a surrogate for detecting respirophasic SV variation but when using Doppler echocardiographic techniques, the SV variation, can be measured directly. Quantitative SV calculation is not required, as the LVOT VTI or LVOT peak velocity are directly proportional to SV, given that the LVOT diameter remains constant throughout the cardiac cycle. Respirophasic variation of SV greater than 12% indicates that a patient has a high probability of being preload sensitive (i.e., SV and presumably CO will rise with volume resuscitation).[10] For respirophasic SV variation to be useful, the operator must be aware of some important caveats of this approach:

1. The patient is on mechanical ventilator support with a tidal volume (TV) of at least 8 cc/kg (ideal body weight). When assessing for preload sensitivity, TV may need to be increased briefly from the standard 6 cc/kg.
2. The patient should be completely passive with the ventilator and not making any spontaneous respiratory effort.

3. The patient is in regular sinus rhythm with a heart rate to respiratory rate ratio greater than 3.6.
4. Although initial reports identified a cutoff value of 12% as indicative of preload sensitivity, the respirophasic variation is better interpreted using a "gray zone" approach as discussed previously (i.e., the greater percentage change in SV, LVOT VTI, or LVOT peak velocity, the greater probability that the patient is preload sensitive).
5. Providers include assessment of RV function in their analysis of respirophasic variation of SV, as the presence of RV failure is another cause for significant respirophasic variation that contraindicates volume resuscitation.
6. Respirophasic variation of SV may change in conjunction with changes of TV and positive end-expiratory pressure (PEEP). Increases in TV and PEEP can increase respirophasic variation of SV. Therefore, serial measurements should be made using the same TV and PEEP.
7. Many patients on mechanical ventilation do not fulfill requirements (items 1-6 listed above) for measurement of respirophasic variation of SV, LVOT VTI, or LVOT peak velocity.[11]

An alternative method of determining preload sensitivity is the passive leg raising (PLR) technique. To start, the patient is positioned in the semi-Fowler position (head of bed at 30 degrees). The LVOT VTI is measured. The patient is then placed in a supine position and both legs are raised to 45 degrees. This results in rapid blood redistribution into the thoracic compartment. One minute later, the LVOT VTI is again measured (see eFig. 21.8). Significant increase in VTI or SV indicates preload sensitivity. Initial reports identified a cutoff value of 14% as an indication of preload sensitivity,[11] but recent reports indicate that a "gray zone" approach is more appropriate. An advantage to PLR is that it has been validated in patients with spontaneous respiratory effort and in patients with atrial fibrillation, provided several LVOT VTI measurements are averaged together.[12] The change in SV can also be measured using a variety of noninvasive monitoring devices, if echocardiographic imaging is not possible. Additionally, respirophasic variation of the brachial artery peak velocity correlates with radial artery pulse pressure variation.[13] This offers an alternative method to identify preload sensitivity, although with the same limitations of measuring the LVOT VTI.

Several other echocardiographic techniques to assess preload sensitivity have been described.[14] Respirophasic variation of superior vena cava (SVC) size has similar utility for identification of preload sensitivity[15] but requires use of transesophageal echocardiography (see Chapter 20). One study comparing various echocardiographic indices found respiratory variation of LVOT peak velocity greater than 18% and SVC variation greater than 31% were specific for predicting fluid responsiveness in ventilated patients.[7]

Providers without training or equipment with Doppler capability can incorporate 2D measurement of the IVC size and dynamics into their assessment of preload sensitivity (see Chapter 17).[16]

Training

Although we contend that competence in basic CCE is an essential skill for frontline providers, competence in advanced CCE may not be required and should be determined by a provider's practice requirements. Providers may choose to become skilled at a limited number of Doppler measurements, such as LVOT VTI and its derivatives. A smaller group may be interested in comprehensive mastery of advanced CCE to achieve a skill level similar to cardiology-trained echocardiographers with a focus on critical care applications. Competence in advanced CCE requires comprehensive study of Doppler ultrasound, as Doppler measurements are fraught with potential error. Mastery of basic level echocardiography is, by comparison, relatively straightforward.

The National Board of Echocardiography and the major professional societies of critical care medicine have developed a national level certification in advanced CCE.[17] This includes a written board examination and a process to ensure the candidate is competent in bedside image acquisition, image interpretation, and clinical integration relevant to advanced CCE. Certification requirements are modeled on the international consensus statement on training standards for advanced CCE that is the basis for the European Diploma of Echocardiography developed by the European Society of Critical Care Medicine.[18]

PEARLS AND PITFALLS

- Measurement of left ventricular (LV) stroke volume (SV) allows calculation of variables, including cardiac output and peripheral oxygen delivery, that are key to guiding fluid resuscitation of patients with hemodynamic failure.
- Measurement of the respirophasic variation of SV, LV outflow tract (LVOT) velocity time integral (VTI), or LVOT peak velocity can be used to identify preload sensitivity of patients in shock. Instead of using specific cutoff values to determine preload sensitivity, providers can use a "gray zone" approach to interpret changes.
- In order to use the LVOT VTI to characterize preload sensitivity, several criteria are required:
  - Patient is on ventilatory support without spontaneous respiratory effort, tidal volume is set at 8 cc/kg (ideal body weight), and without high positive end-expiratory pressure level.
  - Patient is in a normal sinus cardiac rhythm with heart rate/respiratory rate greater than 3.6 and without right ventricular dysfunction.
- The passive leg raising technique can be used in patients with spontaneous respiratory effort and atrial fibrillation in order to evaluate for preload sensitivity.
- Poor alignment of the Doppler sample volume gate with the direction of blood flow will result in underestimation of LV SV. The LVOT VTI can be measured by either transthoracic echocardiogram (TTE) (apical 5-chamber or 3-chamber view) or transesophageal echocardiogram (TEE) (transgastric long-axis view at 120 degrees or deep transgastric long-axis view at 0 degrees). In general, whichever view affords the most favorable Doppler angle should be selected to provide the most accurate result. Additionally, placement of the pulsed-wave Doppler sample volume gate too close to the AV will result in an overestimation of LV SV due to flow acceleration.
- Inaccurate measurement of LVOT diameter will result in a grossly inaccurate measurement of LV SV because the LVOT radius is squared in the calculation. Using an average of two to three independent measurements can improve accuracy.

CHAPTER 22

Hypotension and Shock

Mangala Narasimhan ■ Viera Lakticova

KEY POINTS

- Point-of-care ultrasound is a noninvasive, reliable tool to rapidly and accurately assess hemodynamically unstable patients at the bedside.
- Hypovolemic, cardiogenic, obstructive, and distributive shock can be readily differentiated using established point-of-care ultrasound protocols.
- Goal-directed, serial point-of-care ultrasound examinations can be performed to monitor critically ill patients in shock.

In hemodynamically unstable patients, point-of-care ultrasound allows providers to rapidly differentiate the etiology of shock at the bedside and monitor response to therapies. Selecting and delivering life-saving interventions to reverse shock is entirely dependent on identifying the underlying etiology; for example, massive fluid resuscitation required in hypovolemic shock would cause immediate decompensation if delivered to a patient with acute cor pulmonale, or inotropic therapy initiated in a volume-depleted patient could likewise end in death. The majority of point-of-care cardiac ultrasound exams in critically ill shock patients consist of five standard assessments that allow for accurate classification and initiation of appropriate therapy[1]:

1. Left ventricular size and function
2. Right ventricular size and function
3. Pericardial effusion
4. Intravascular volume status
5. Gross valvular abnormalities

Various protocols have been published describing a point-of-care ultrasound approach to patients in shock. The five standard assessments described previously comprise the goal-directed echocardiography (GDE) approach but are also core components of other shock protocols, including the Rapid Ultrasound in Shock (RUSH) and Sonography in Hypotension and Cardiac arrest (SHoC) protocols.[1-3] The RUSH and SHoC protocols combine the same principles of GDE with other diagnostic ultrasound exams. RUSH and SHoC protocols include evaluation of the heart (parasternal and subcostal cardiac views, and subcostal inferior vena cava [IVC] view) and a whole body ultrasonography approach to the thorax, abdomen, and lower extremities for pneumonia, pleural effusion, pneumothorax, peritoneal free fluid, abdominal aortic aneurysm, disorders of the kidneys and bladder, and lower extremity deep venous thrombosis.[2,3] Other protocols have been published that include similar cardiac evaluation as the GDE, RUSH, and SHoC protocols.[3,4] The key ultrasound findings to evaluate patients in shock are summarized in Table 22.1.

TABLE 22.1   **Shock Evaluation With Point-of-Care Ultrasound**

	Hypovolemic Shock	Cardiogenic Shock	Obstructive Shock	Distributive Shock
Cardiac exam	**LV:** - Hyperdynamic function - End-systolic effacement (PLAX, PSAX)	**LV:** - Severely reduced function (all views) - Dilated chamber	**LV:** *Tamponade*: - Hyperdynamic function - Pericardial effusion with RA systolic and RV diastolic collapse	**LV:** - Hyperdynamic or normal function (early sepsis) - Hypocontractile function (late sepsis)
	RV: - Normal/small size (A4C)	**RV:** - Possible dilated chamber **Valves:** - Possible severe MR or AR detected by color flow Doppler - Possible AS by 2D exam	**RV:** *Pulmonary Embolism*: - Dilated, strained RV (A4C, S4C) - D-shaped septum (PSAX)	**RV:** - Normal/small size
Pulmonary exam	**Lungs:** - A-line predominance	**Lungs:** - B-line predominance	**Lungs:** *Pneumothorax*: - Lung sliding absent in pneumothorax - A-line predominance	**Lungs:** - Possible pneumonia (consolidation pattern or focal B-lines)
	Pleura: - No pleural effusion	**Pleura:** - Possible bilateral pleural effusions	**Pleura:** *Pulmonary Embolism*: - Possible Small pleural effusion, small sub-pleural consolidations (infarcts)	**Pleura:** - Possible pleural effusion (pneumonia, empyema)
IVC exam	Collapsed IVC	Distended IVC	Distended IVC	Normal/collapsed IVC
Supplementary exams	**Abdomen:** - Abdominal aortic aneurysm - Aortic dissection - Intra-abdominal hemorrhage (FAST exam) **Vascular:** - Collapsed veins (internal jugular, femoral veins)	**Abdomen:** - Peritoneal fluid in chronic right or left heart failure	**Vascular:** *Tamponade*: - Distended IJ vein *Pulmonary Embolism*: - LE DVT study	**Abdomen:** - Possible peritoneal fluid (peritonitis)

2D, 2-Dimensional; *A4C*, apical 4-chamber view; *AR*, aortic regurgitation; *AS*, aortic stenosis; *DVT*, deep venous thrombosis; *FAST*, focused assessment with sonography in trauma; *IJ*, internal jugular; *IVC*, inferior vena cava; *LE*, lower extremity; *LV*, left ventricle; *MR*, mitral regurgitation; *PE*, pulmonary embolism; *PLAX*, parasternal long-axis view; *PSAX*, parasternal short-axis view; *RA*, right atrium; *RV*, right ventricle; *S4C*, subcostal 4-chamber view.

CASE 22.1

CASE PRESENTATION

A 59-year-old man with a history of coronary artery disease and myocardial infarction presented to the emergency department (ED) with lightheadedness and near syncope. Vital signs: temperature 38°C, pulse 122 bpm, blood pressure 86/40 mm Hg, respiratory rate 28 per minute, oxygen saturation 88%.

Physical exam: Lethargic, moderate respiratory distress, dry mucous membranes, unable to complete full sentences, tachycardic without murmur, faint crackles in bilateral bases, no peripheral edema.

Initial testing was significant for leukocytosis, elevated lactate, and pyuria on urinalysis. Chest x-ray revealed bilateral interstitial opacities with an oxygen saturation of 88% on a 100% non-rebreather mask. ECG revealed a left bundle branch block. Initial troponin was normal.

ASSESSMENT

Sepsis was suspected as the underlying cause of patient's hypotension and lethargy based on the presence of fever and pyuria. The chest radiograph was attributed to development of acute respiratory distress syndrome given the patient's volume depletion without peripheral edema. Intravenous fluid resuscitation was initiated, but neither blood pressure nor clinical exam improved after 2 L of intravenous fluids. The critical care team was consulted and performed a focused cardiac and lung ultrasound exam that revealed the following:

- Left ventricle (LV) size and function: LV dilated with severely reduced function (reduced endocardial excursion, reduced myocardial thickening, and limited septal motion of the anterior leaflet of the mitral valve) (Fig. 22.1 and Video 22.1).
- Right ventricle (RV) size and function: Limited assessment, RV seen only in parasternal long-axis view; however, appears mildly enlarged, possibly hypocontractile from this view.
- Inferior vena cava (IVC) size and collapsibility: Dilated to almost 3 cm, noncollapsible (Fig. 22.2 and Video 22.2).
- Pericardial effusion: Absent.

- Valvular function: Moderate mitral regurgitation (MR) seen on color flow Doppler (Fig. 22.3 and Video 22.3).
- Lung ultrasound: Anterior lung zones with confluent B-lines with smooth, thin pleura that are sliding (Fig. 22.4 and Video 22.4).

The severely reduced global LV function suggested a possible primary cardiac cause of hypoperfusion. The bilateral anterior lung zones with confluent B-lines and a smooth, thin, sliding pleural line is consistent with hydrostatic pulmonary edema with a pulmonary artery occlusion pressure greater than 18 mm Hg.[5] The dilated IVC provides further evidence of elevated cardiac filling pressures. Absence of severe MR confirmed acute cardiogenic shock from LV failure as the primary cause. Dobutamine infusion, diuresis, and anticoagulation were initiated with improvement in dyspnea, urine output, and mental status. Repeat troponin was elevated, and urgent cardiac angiography revealed an occluded left anterior descending artery that was treated with angioplasty and stent placement.

CASE RESOLUTION

Cardiogenic shock presents with signs of a low cardiac output, usually oliguria, cool extremities, decreased mental status, and hydrostatic pulmonary edema. Patients without a history of congestive heart failure warrant further investigation for an acute inciting event. The treatment of cardiogenic shock should be directed at reversing the underlying cause, most commonly ischemia, infarction, or acute on chronic LV failure. Diuretic and/or inotropic therapy with dobutamine should be initiated to support perfusion. Response to therapy can be confirmed and monitored noninvasively with serial repeat bedside ultrasound exams to assess LV systolic function and interstitial pulmonary edema.

CASE PEARLS

- The presence of bilateral B-lines over the anterior and lateral lung zones and a thin, smooth, sliding pleura are diagnostic of hydrostatic pulmonary edema.
- Screening of the mitral valve for severe MR with color flow Doppler should be performed in any patient with hydrostatic pulmonary edema and shock.

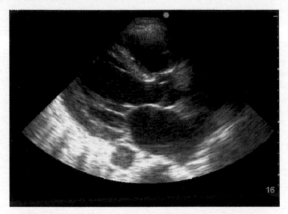

Figure 22.1   Case 22.1—Parasternal Long-Axis View.

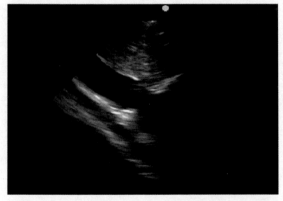

Figure 22.2   Case 22.1—Subcostal Inferior Vena Cava (IVC) View With a Dilated IVC.

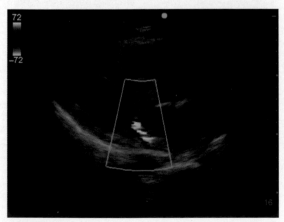

Figure 22.3   Case 22.1—Parasternal Long-Axis View With Color Flow Doppler Revealing Moderate Mitral Regurgitation.

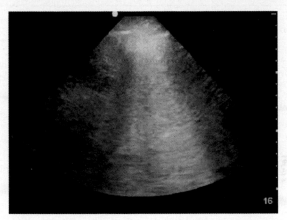

Figure 22.4 Case 22.1—Lung Ultrasound (Upper Lobes) With Confluent B-Lines Bilaterally.

CASE 22.2

CASE PRESENTATION

A 43-year-old woman with a history of asthma and recent ankle surgery presented to the emergency department (ED) with progressively worsening dyspnea over the prior 2 weeks, noting a lack of response to the new bronchodilators that were prescribed by her doctor. Vital signs: pulse 130 bpm, blood pressure 80/42 mm Hg, respiratory rate 30 per minute, oxygen saturation 94% on a non-rebreather mask.

Physical exam: Patient appeared fatigued, slightly lethargic with mildly labored breathing. Her lungs were clear anteriorly with an occasional faint wheeze heard posteriorly. The remainder of the physical exam was normal with the exception of left leg edema distal to the calf.

Initial testing with arterial blood gas revealed severe hypoxemia with a mild respiratory alkalosis. Chest x-ray was normal.

ASSESSMENT

Based on her severe hypoxemia and normal chest x-ray, an acute pulmonary embolism (PE) as the cause of her shock and respiratory distress was strongly suspected. While awaiting a computed tomography (CT) angiogram of the chest, a bedside ultrasound exam was performed to investigate the cause of her respiratory failure. During the ultrasound examination, her blood pressure dropped, leading to cardiac arrest. Bedside ultrasound exam revealed the following:

- Left ventricle (LV) size and function: Hyperdynamic function with a "D"-shaped septum on parasternal short-axis views, consistent with acute cor pulmonale with underfilling of LV (Fig. 22.5 and Video 22.5).
- Right ventricle (RV) size and function: Severely dilated RV noted in both apical 4-chamber and parasternal short-axis views. Apex of heart is dominated by the RV and is contracting well, despite the akinesis of the RV free wall (McConnell's sign) (Fig. 22.6 and Video 22.6).
- Inferior vena cava (IVC) size and collapsibility: Diameter dilated to almost 3 cm, noncollapsible.
- Pericardial effusion: No effusion is seen in any view.
- Valvular function: Valve structure is grossly normal; color flow Doppler revealed no appreciable mitral regurgitation (MR).
- Lung ultrasound: Lung ultrasound showed a predominant A-line pattern with visible lung sliding seen over both anterior chest walls (Fig. 22.7 and Video 22.7).
- Lower extremity compression ultrasound exam for deep venous thrombosis (DVT): Visible echogenic thrombus is seen within the common femoral vein consistent with presence of DVT (Fig. 22.8 and Video 22.8)

The normal aeration pattern throughout both lungs excluded any interstitial process as the cause of dyspnea. Bilateral A-line pattern with normal lung sliding in a patient with acute respiratory failure narrows the differential diagnosis to two main possibilities: obstructive airway disease (asthma/chronic obstructive pulmonary disease) or PE.[5,6] This patient had risk factors for both asthma and PE. The cardiac ultrasound exam

Continued

CASE 22.2—cont'd

revealed a dilated RV with septal bowing producing a D-shaped LV indicative of combined volume and pressure overload of the right heart, or cor pulmonale.[7,8] Acute pressure overload results in RV enlargement with a relatively thin RV wall, normally measuring <5 mm in thickness. Chronic RV pressure strain causes RV hypertrophy, often with RV wall thickness >1 cm. This patient had a dilated RV with a thin wall suggesting an acute process. The apical 4-chamber (A4C) view shows the apex is primarily formed by the RV, a highly abnormal finding, which is further evidence of acute RV pressure overload. Furthermore, the RV apex is contracting well, whereas the midchamber RV free wall is akinetic (McConnell's sign)—an indicator of RV pressure overload that is strongly associated with acute PE, as well as RV infarction.[9,10]

Lower extremity compression ultrasound exam was a supplementary exam in this patient with high suspicion of PE. The right common femoral vein had partially occlusive echogenic material within the vein, diagnostic of thrombus.

CASE RESOLUTION

Based on her clinical history and point-of-care ultrasound findings, she was presumptively diagnosed with an acute PE. Cardiopulmonary resuscitation was initiated with infusion of tissue plasminogen activator (t-PA). A return of spontaneous circulation was documented within 4 to 5 minutes of initiating resuscitation.

CASE PEARLS

- A-lines are seen when air is just below the parietal pleura (as in pneumothorax) or deep to the visceral pleura (normal aeration pattern). The location of air is deduced by lung sliding presence (normal aeration) or absence (pneumothorax).
- Acute right heart pressure overload results in RV dilation with a relatively thin RV free wall, normally measuring <5 mm in thickness. Chronic RV pressure overload results in increased RV wall thickness that is often >1 cm.

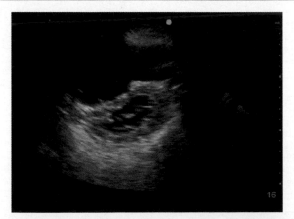

Figure 22.5 Case 22.2—Parasternal Short-Axis View With a Dilated Right Ventricle and "D"-Shaped Septum.

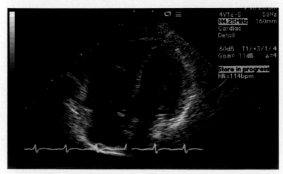

Figure 22.6 Case 22.2—Apical 4-Chamber View Reveals a Dilated Right Ventricle.

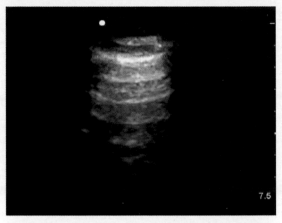

Figure 22.7   Case 22.2—Lung Ultrasound (Upper Lobes) With A-Lines Bilaterally.

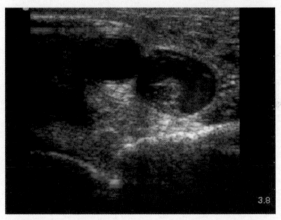

Figure 22.8   Case 22.2—Right Lower Extremity Ultrasound of the Femoral Vein Shows Echogenic Thrombus in the Vein.

CASE 22.3

CASE PRESENTATION

A 49-year-old man with an implanted cardiac defibrillator placed for an unexplained cardiac arrest 10 years earlier presented to the emergency department (ED) with weakness, malaise, and dyspnea developing over 3 days. The patient reported participating in a weekend hiking trip 2 weeks ago.

Vitals signs: temperature 37.7°C, pulse 150 to 160 bpm, blood pressure 88/40 mm Hg, respiratory rate 30 per minute, oxygen saturation 92% on a non-rebreather mask.

Physical exam: The patient was slightly diaphoretic with labored breathing. Breath sounds were coarse bilaterally. Tachycardia with a systolic murmur loudest at the apex was noted. His lower extremities showed no signs of edema or cyanosis. A few scratches were noted on his legs, and the extremities were cool to touch.

Initial testing began with an electrocardiogram revealing supraventricular tachycardia (SVT) without ischemic changes. Portable chest x-ray suggested mild pulmonary vascular congestion without pleural effusions or opacities. Electrolytes and blood gas analysis revealed an acute lactic acidosis, and his white blood count was mildly elevated at 11,400.

Continued

CASE 22.3—cont'd

ASSESSMENT

Based on his low blood pressure, SVT, leukocytosis, and low-grade temperature, sepsis was suspected. He was given an infusion of 3 L of intravenous fluid. Only a minimal response was observed in his blood pressure (90/60 mm Hg). A bedside ultrasound exam for evaluation of the patient's shock state was performed:

- Left ventricle (LV) size and function: Hyperdynamic function with end-systolic effacement of LV cavity was seen in all cardiac views (Figs. 22.9 and 22.10; Videos 22.9, 22.10, and 22.11).
- Right ventricle (RV) size and function: Normal RV shape and function, no appreciable dilation noted (Fig. 22.11, Video 22.11)
- Inferior vena cava (IVC) size and collapsibility: Small IVC with pulsatile variation (Fig. 22.12, Video 22.12).
- Pericardial effusion: Absence of pericardial effusion in all views.
- Valvular function: Grossly normal-color flow Doppler revealed no appreciable mitral regurgitation (color Doppler view not shown).
- Lung ultrasound: Scattered areas with nonconfluent B-lines in the left upper lobe and associated with thickened, irregular pleura. A lack of pleural effusion or consolidation was also noted (Figs. 22.13 and 22.14; Videos 22.13 and 22.14).

The scattered appearance of nonconfluent B-lines with an irregular, thickened pleura suggests an inflammatory or infectious cause rather than hydrostatic pulmonary edema that typically presents with uniform, confluent B-lines with a thin, smooth pleura. The lack of pleural effusions further supports a nonhydrostatic cause of the B-line pattern.[5,6] All cardiac views revealed hyperdynamic LV function, the most common cause of which is underfilling or volume depletion. End-systolic effacement in patients with hemodynamic failure indicates the presence of hypovolemic shock, septic shock, or both. These two shock states can be somewhat differentiated by examining the IVC size and collapsibility. The collapsed IVC noted in this case is diagnostic of severe volume depletion. The ejection fraction from the cardiac views is estimated to be >75%, yet cardiac output is significantly reduced due to low stroke volume from a lack of filling. Absence of pericardial effusion rules out tamponade, and the normal RV size, shape, and function rules out RV failure as a cause of shock.[7]

This patient had a collapsed IVC with "pulsatility," a finding seen in severely volume-depleted patients beyond those in which respiratory variation is seen. The near "virtual" size noted at times during the video can help distinguish distributive from hypovolemic shock. In significant hypovolemic shock, such virtual IVCs are seen, whereas in distributive shock, the IVC diameters can be small, normal, or enlarged.[11,12]

CASE RESOLUTION

The focal areas of irregular pleura with B-lines and absent pleural effusion suggested an infectious pulmonary condition.[13] The hyperdynamic LV function with near virtual IVC was consistent with hypovolemia, an indication for additional fluid resuscitation. After more aggressive fluid resuscitation (additional 3 L), the LV function normalized, and the IVC diameter enlarged and became less collapsible. Blood cultures were positive for Gram-positive cocci in all four bottles within the next 12 hours. A transesophageal echocardiogram days later revealed independently oscillating echogenic structures attached to the defibrillator wire within the RV, revealing an infectious source and further diagnostic proof that the lung ultrasound findings were secondary to an inflammatory or infectious etiology. Discrete, small, subpleural consolidations on ultrasound can be specific for thrombotic or septic embolism; however, they were not seen during the lung ultrasound exam in this case. A computed tomography (CT) scan later revealed focal areas of consolidation consistent with septic emboli in the apices (Fig. 22.15).

CASE PEARLS

- Scattered B-lines associated with a thickened, irregular pleura suggest an infectious or inflammatory etiology.
- End-systolic effacement of the LV cavity associated with a virtual IVC is diagnostic of severe hypovolemia contributing to a shock state.

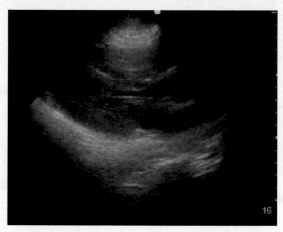

Figure 22.9   Case 22.3—Parasternal Long-Axis View With End-Systolic Effacement of the Left Ventricular Cavity.

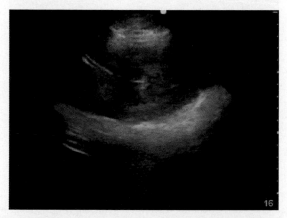

Figure 22.10   Case 22.3—Parasternal Short-Axis View With End-Systolic Effacement of the Left Ventricular Cavity.

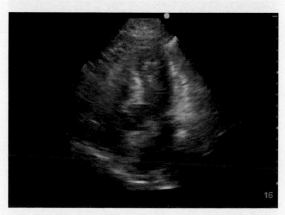

Figure 22.11   Case 22.3—Apical 4-Chamber View With Normal Right Ventricular Size and Shape.

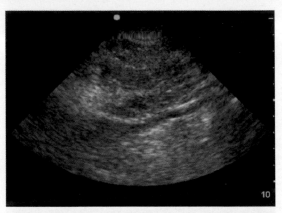

Figure 22.12   Case 22.3—Inferior Vena Cava (IVC) View Shows a Small, Easily Collapsible IVC.

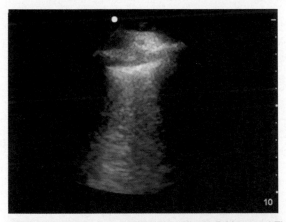

Figure 22.13   Case 22.3—Left Upper Lobe With Nonconfluent B-Lines and Thickened Pleura.

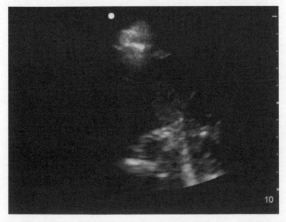

Figure 22.14   Case 22.3—Left Lower Lobe Shows Absence of Pleural Effusion.

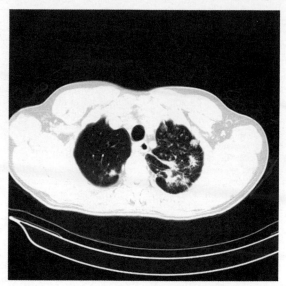

Figure 22.15 Case 22.3—Computed Tomography Scan of Chest Shows Small Areas With Consolidation in the Left Upper Lobe due to Septic Emboli.

CASE 22.4

CASE PRESENTATION

A 72-year-old man with a history of coronary artery disease was noted to have hypotension (70/40 mm Hg) during a routine visit 5 days after a recent coronary artery bypass graft operation. His postoperative course had been uneventful except for the development of atrial fibrillation treated with anticoagulation on day 3. On further questioning, he reported increasing dyspnea, mild cough, and minimal amounts of yellow phlegm. He denied fever or chills but reported generalized weakness. He subsequently developed worsening mental status and decreasing blood pressure (60/40 mm Hg) and was admitted to the hospital.

Vital signs: temperature 37.5°C, pulse 120 bpm, blood pressure 60/40 mm Hg, respiratory rate 24 per minute.

Physical exam: He was generally weak with tachypnea and decreased breath sounds at the left base without rhonchi, crackles, or wheezes. Cardiac exam revealed tachycardia, absent jugular venous distention, and no murmurs.

An ECG showed normal voltage and sinus tachycardia without ischemic changes. Portable chest x-ray showed an enlarged cardiac silhouette that was stable and an increased left basilar opacity suggestive of pleural effusion. Complete blood count showed normal white blood cell count and mild anemia. An arterial blood gas revealed a mixed acute respiratory and metabolic acidosis with an elevated lactic acid level.

ASSESSMENT

The sudden onset of hypotension and dyspnea suggested a differential diagnosis of pericardial effusion with tamponade, pleural effusion from hemothorax, pneumonia, or pulmonary embolism. The patient was given 3 L of normal saline, followed by initiation of norepinephrine due to persistently low blood pressure of 80/40 mm Hg. A bedside ultrasound exam was performed revealing the following:

- Left ventricle (LV) size and function: LV size was normal with normal contractility (myocardial thickening and endocardial excursion of walls in view) (Video 22.15)
- Right ventricle (RV) size and function: RV appeared normal in all views (Fig. 22.16, Video 22.16).
- Inferior vena cava (IVC) size and collapsibility: Dilated to >2 cm, noncollapsible (Fig. 22.17, Video 22.17).
- Pericardial effusion: Absence of pericardial effusion is seen in all views.
- Lung ultrasound: Bilateral anterior upper lobes showed a normal A-line pattern with sliding (Fig. 22.18, Video 22.18). The left lower lobe was significant for a large

Continued

CASE 22.4—cont'd

area of alveolar consolidation, dynamic air bronchograms, and a small pleural effusion (Fig. 22.19 and Video 22.19). Right lower lobe revealed a curtain sign with several B-lines, a finding that can be normal in many patients (Video 22.20).

CASE RESOLUTION

The findings of a "normal" focused cardiac ultrasound exam in this patient with shock is consistent with a diagnosis of distributive or vasodilatory shock after fluid resuscitation. This is the most common constellation of findings seen in septic patients who have been adequately fluid resuscitated, including absence of hyperdynamic LV function and a normal, noncollapsible IVC. This pattern is reassuring to providers, given that other worrisome causes can be ruled out, such as pericardial tamponade or massive pulmonary embolism with RV failure. The absence

of pericardial fluid and normal RV allowed providers to focus on treatment of the left lower lobe pneumonia. Lung ultrasound differentiated the nonspecific left basilar opacification seen on chest x-ray as pneumonia with a small pleural effusion, rather than moderate-sized pleural effusion. Broad-spectrum antibiotics were initiated, and vasopressors were weaned over the subsequent 2 days.

CASE PEARLS

- Septic patients with distributive shock who have received adequate fluid resuscitation typically have a normal focused cardiac ultrasound exam, along with a dilated, noncollapsible IVC.
- Serial ultrasound examinations in shock states can guide fluid resuscitation by monitoring IVC size and collapsibility, LV size, and presence or absence of B-lines.

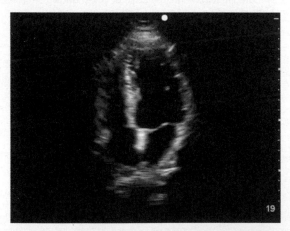

Figure 22.16 Case 22.4—Apical 4-Chamber View With Normal Left and Right Ventricular Size and Function.

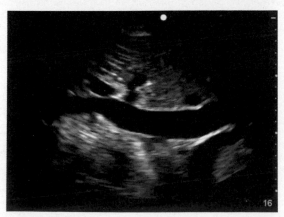

Figure 22.17 Case 22.4—Inferior Vena Cava (IVC) View With a Dilated, Noncollapsible IVC.

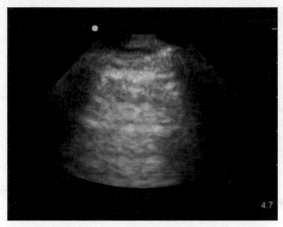

Figure 22.18 Case 22.4—Lung Ultrasound (Upper Lobes) With A-Lines Bilaterally.

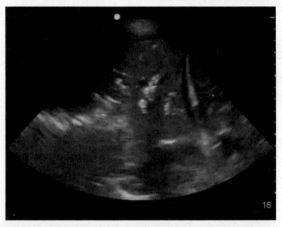

Figure 22.19 Case 22.4—Left Lower Lobe Shows Alveolar Consolidation With Air Bronchograms and Small Pleural Effusion.

CASE 22.5

CASE PRESENTATION

A 63-year-old female was admitted with short-ness of breath thought to be secondary to chronic obstructive pulmonary disease exacerbation. On admission, she was found to be hypercapnic with bilateral decreased breath sounds and mild wheezing. She was placed on noninvasive bilevel respiratory support for increased work of breath-ing. Several hours after her admission, an emergency call is placed for sudden-onset worsening shortness of breath and chest pain.

Vital signs: temperature 37.5°C, pulse 116 bpm, BP of 80/50 mm Hg, respiratory rate 30 per minute, oxygen saturation of 90% on a non-rebreather mask

Physical examination: The patient is awake, alert, and oriented. She is on noninvasive ventilatory support. She is tachypneic and has decreased breath sounds on the right side. No other abnormalities are noted on physical exam.

Her ECG shows sinus tachycardia with no other abnormalities present. She is admitted to the medical ICU for hypoxemic respiratory failure.

ASSESSMENT

A bedside ultrasound exam was performed revealing the following:

- Left ventricle (LV) size and function: LV size and function were normal. Mitral and aortic valves were grossly normal (Video 22.21)

Continued

CASE 22.5—cont'd

- Right ventricle (RV) size and function: RV appeared normal in all views (Video 22.22)
- Inferior vena cava (IVC) size and collapsibility: Normal size and collapsibility (Video 22.23).
- Pericardial effusion: Absence of pericardial effusion is seen in all views (Video 22.24).
- Lung ultrasound: The left anterior lung exam shows normal sliding with an A-line pattern (Video 22.25). The right anterior lung exam shows an A-line pattern but no sliding is seen (Video 22.26). Further ultrasound interrogation on the right anterolateral chest wall reveals a transition point where sliding and absence of sliding is seen in the same field of view, diagnostic of a lung point (Video 22.27).

These findings rule out cardiogenic shock, severe hypovolemic shock, right heart failure, and cardiac tamponade. Careful examination of right lung with ultrasound revealed A-lines but no lung sliding and a lung point on the right anterolateral chest wall. Lung point is the transition point where absence and presence of lung sliding is seen within a single rib interspace, or the transition point where there is and there is not air in between the visceral and parietal pleura. Lung point is 100% specific for pneumothorax.

CASE RESOLUTION

A portable chest x-ray confirmed presence of a right pneumothorax (Fig. 22.20). A chest tube was inserted urgently in the right second intercostal space in the midclavicular line, and her oxygenation improved immediately.

CASE PEARLS

- Lung ultrasound showing an A-line pattern *without* sliding, in the right clinical context, raises high suspicion for pneumothorax. If a lung point is seen, this is confirmatory of pneumothorax and justifies immediate chest tube insertion in an unstable patient.
- Lung ultrasound showing an A-line pattern *with* sliding rules out pneumothorax at the level of interrogation.

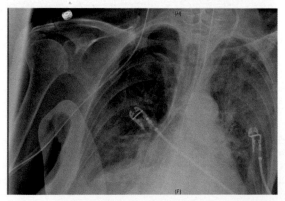

Figure 22.20   Case 22.5—Portable Chest X-Ray Demonstrating a Right-Sided Pneumothorax.

CASE 22.6

CASE PRESENTATION

A 74-year-old male with diabetes, hypertension and coronary artery disease was admitted to the intensive care unit (ICU) for altered mental status. He was intubated for his declining level of consciousness. Encephalitis was suspected and lumbar puncture confirmed a diagnosis of viral encephalitis. His ICU course was complicated by *Candida* fungemia, and he was started on antifungal treatment. A bedside tracheostomy was performed on day 15 of his ICU stay. The tracheostomy procedure was uneventful; however, 45 minutes postprocedure, his vital signs suddenly changed. His BP dropped to 62/42 mm Hg, pulse increased to 120 bpm, and his oxygen saturation decreased to 94%. A postprocedure pneumothorax was suspected and urgent point-of-care ultrasound was performed.

CASE 22.6—cont'd

ASSESSMENT

A bedside ultrasound exam was performed revealing the following:

- LV size and function: LV size was normal but function was hyperdynamic with end-systolic effacement of the LV (Videos 22.28 and 22.29). No valvular dysfunction was seen with color flow Doppler.
- RV size and function: RV size and function appear normal in all views (Video 22.30)
- Inferior vena cava (IVC) size and collapsibility: Small and collapsed, or "virtualized" (Video 22.31).
- Pericardial effusion: Absence of pericardial effusion is seen in all views (Video 22.32).
- Lung ultrasound: The left and right anterior lungs shows normal albeit subtle, sliding with an A-line pattern (Video 22.33).

The apical 4-chamber view showed a normal-sized RV, excluding a hemodynamically significant pulmonary embolism as the cause of the deterioration, and visualization of lung sliding bilaterally excludes the presence of a large pneumothorax causing cardiovascular instability. Thus, acute hypovolemia due to intravascular volume loss was suspected. In the absence of any extrinsic volume loss (e.g., large volume diuresis, bleeding from the trach site, etc.), an ultrasound examination for abdominal or thoracic hemorrhage was undertaken. Evaluation of the abdomen using the focused assessment with sonography in trauma (FAST) exam protocol immediately revealed free flowing fluid (Video 22.34). The echogenic fluid present in abdominal cavity was consistent with intra-abdominal hemorrhage.

CASE RESOLUTION

Volume resuscitation was immediately initiated with blood products. A chest and abdomen angiogram was performed emergently, and surgery and interventional radiology were consulted. The computed tomography (CT) angiogram revealed a splenic artery aneurysm that was bleeding. The patient underwent coiling of the aneurysm. Coiling was successful, but unfortunately, the patient re-bled 24 hours later and required surgical intervention.

CASE PEARLS

- When cardiac ultrasound reveals intravascular volume depletion, broader applications of point-of-care ultrasound to evaluate the lungs, abdomen, and other organs can often identify the underlying etiology.
- In hemodynamically unstable patients, point-of-care ultrasound can rapidly assess patients to guide further workup and initiation of empiric therapies.

CHAPTER 23

Cardiac Arrest

Phillip Andrus ■ Felipe Teran

KEY POINTS

- Point-of-care ultrasound in cardiac arrest can identify patients who have higher rates of survival including those with pseudo-pulseless electrical activity and ventricular fibrillation.
- Treatment of ventricular fibrillation, pericardial tamponade, and tension pneumothorax detected by point-of-care ultrasound during cardiac arrest can be lifesaving.
- Cardiac standstill portends a poor prognosis and can guide cessation of resuscitative efforts.
- Real-time feedback on effectiveness of chest compressions can be obtained with point-of care transesophageal echocardiography during cardiac arrest.

Background

The American Heart Association and the European Resuscitation Council both support the use of ultrasound in cardiac arrest.[1,2] In cardiac arrest, acute care providers regularly use ultrasound to inform the delivery, scope, and limits of resuscitative efforts. Point-of-care ultrasound provides important diagnostic and prognostic information, and guides procedures during cardiac arrest.

Due to the complexity of cardiac arrest care, a defined strategy to incorporate ultrasound into the flow of resuscitation is important. Providers must strategically position themselves at the bedside, select an appropriate transducer, and apply a well-defined algorithm without disruption to cardiopulmonary resuscitation (CPR). The strategy and heuristics of point-of-care ultrasound in cardiac arrest are reviewed in this chapter. For techniques and details of specific ultrasound exams, refer to the appropriate, organ-specific chapter in this textbook.

Diagnostic Approach

During resuscitation of patients with cardiac arrest, the patient's electrical rhythm will direct the care team along prescribed management pathways consistent with advanced cardiac life support (ACLS) guidelines. A focused ultrasound examination allows providers to search for rapidly correctable causes of arrest while CPR is in progress. As more tools such as extracorporeal life support (ECLS) are available to support a patient in arrest, identifying the etiology of arrest using point-of-care ultrasound may prove even more beneficial.[3-5] The role and scope of point-of-care ultrasound in cardiac arrest depends on the underlying cardiac rhythm.

VENTRICULAR FIBRILLATION

If the cardiac rhythm is ventricular fibrillation (or pulseless ventricular tachycardia), immediate defibrillation is indicated, and defibrillation should not be delayed to perform an ultrasound exam. On occasion, focused cardiac ultrasound may detect occult ventricular fibrillation that was mistaken for asystole due to its fine nature.[6] Although this circumstance is rare, recognizing the cardiac ultrasound appearance of ventricular fibrillation may avert an undesirable delay or deferral of defibrillation (Videos 23.1 and 23.2).

TABLE 23.1 **Differential Diagnosis of Pulseless Electrical Activity and Asystole**

H's	T's
Hypovolemia	**Tension pneumothorax**
Hypoxia	**Tamponade (cardiac)**
H⁺ ion (acidosis)	Toxins
Hypo/hyperkalemia	**Thrombosis (pulmonary embolism)**
Hypothermia	**Thrombosis (myocardial infarction)[a]**

[a]After return of spontaneous circulation (ROSC). Ultrasound-definable etiologies are kept in bold.

PULSELESS ELECTRICAL ACTIVITY/ASYSTOLE

Ultrasound has a large role to play when a patient's rhythm is pulseless electrical activity (PEA) or asystole. These cardiac arrest rhythms have a broad differential diagnosis, commonly distilled in a list of five "H's" and "T's" as listed in Table 23.1. Many of these clinical syndromes are rapidly identifiable by point-of-care ultrasound.

Hypovolemia

Hypovolemic arrest should be considered when point-of-care ultrasound reveals a low pre-load state (underfilled inferior vena cava [IVC] or empty left ventricle [LV]) or evidence of volume loss (intra-abdominal or intrapelvic free fluid or abdominal aortic aneurysm). Because of the complex interplay between chest compressions, positive pressure ventilation, and the transmission of these pressures to the IVC during cardiac arrest, accurate interpretation of dynamics of the IVC are generally not possible during cardiac arrest. Thus, in cardiac arrest, generous volume repletion is given in the presence of any collapsed or small caliber IVC (Video 23.3). If hypovolemia is supported by IVC findings, a sonographic search for intra-abdominal fluid can be easily carried out despite ongoing CPR (Videos 23.4 and 23.5). When abdominal free fluid, pelvic fluid, or an abdominal aortic aneurysm is identified as a possible etiology of cardiac arrest (Video 23.6), immediate surgical consultation and administration of blood products may be considered, but prognosis is poor when surgical intervention is indicated for a patient already in arrest.

Tension Pneumothorax

Tension pneumothorax is more commonly seen in trauma patients but may occasionally occur in patients with chronic lung disease or post-procedure. Scanning the pleura for lung sliding should be rapidly performed during a rhythm check, synchronized with delivery of breaths by bag-valve mask (BVM) or a ventilator. Presence of lung sliding excludes pneumothorax reliably at the area of insonation, whereas a loss of lung sliding supports but is not diagnostic of pneumothorax (Video 23.7; see Chapter 10, Pleural Ultrasound Interpretation). In the setting of cardiac arrest, when pneumothorax is either supported by ultrasound or strongly suspected clinically, needle decompression or thoracostomy is indicated.

Cardiac Tamponade

Pericardial effusions appear as anechoic or hypoechoic fluid surrounding the heart. In the arrested patient, even with ongoing CPR, providers can identify the presence or absence of a pericardial effusion (Videos 23.8 and 23.9). The presence of any pericardial effusion during cardiac arrest implicates tamponade as the cause of arrest until proven otherwise. Resuscitative efforts should focus on immediate drainage of the effusion by pericardiocentesis.

Pulmonary Embolism

Evidence of pulmonary embolism (PE) may be seen by point-of-care ultrasound examination during resuscitation. If return of circulation is obtained in a patient with a causative PE, acute right heart strain will typically be seen with a grossly enlarged right ventricle (RV) accompanied by a dilated IVC. During cardiac arrest, however, these right heart findings are non-specific. Sudden reduction in cardiac output due to arrest and subsequent infusion of intravenous fluids during resuscitation can lead to a relatively enlarged RV, a plethoric IVC, and an underfilled LV.[7] However, if thrombus is seen in transit in the atria or ventricles (Video 23.10), or in the femoral or popliteal veins, PE should be suspected as the cause of arrest. Scanning the lower extremity veins for thrombus can be easily performed with ongoing chest compressions (Video 23.11; see also Chapter 34—Lower Extremity DVT). If clinical or ultrasound suspicion for PE is high, then initiating thrombolysis during resuscitation should be considered.[2,8]

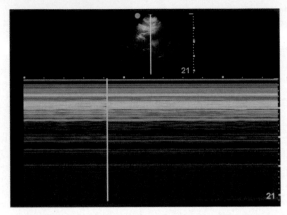

Figure 23.1   Cardiac Standstill. An M-mode image showing cardiac standstill from a subcostal 4-chamber view.

CARDIOPULMONARY RESUSCITATION GUIDANCE

The most important intervention in patients with a nonshockable rhythm during cardiac arrest is the delivery of high-quality chest compressions. Even among providers certified in ACLS, chest compressions are often not performed to recommended standards.[9,10] Efforts to enhance hemodynamic efficacy of CPR through provider feedback have focused on chest compression depth and rate. Point-of-care ultrasound offers the ability to visualize cardiac chambers during chest compressions providing direct feedback on CPR quality.[11,12]

Cardiac output is generated by compression of the ventricles during CPR, according to the cardiac pump theory. When chest compressions are delivered using landmarks recommended by current guidelines, the area of maximal compression has been found to overlie the ascending aorta, aortic root, or left ventricular outflow tract in the majority of cases.[11,13,14] Compressing these structures may actually reduce cardiac output. However, adjusting the site of compressions to maximally compress the LV appears to improve hemodynamics and may lead to higher coronary perfusion pressures, return of spontaneous circulation (ROSC), and survival.[15,16]

Transthoracic echocardiography is not ideally suited to properly assess adequacy of compressions. Transesophageal echocardiography (TEE), however, can reliably provide continuous high-resolution images of the heart along the desired axis of compression. The integration of point-of-care TEE in the emergency department (ED) and intensive care unit (ICU) has raised awareness of CPR quality and influenced the way in which CPR is delivered in these settings (see Chapter 20—Transesophageal Echocardiography).[17]

Prognosis

The most prevalent use of ultrasound in cardiac arrest is determining prognosis. Cardiac standstill, defined as the absence of myocardial activity or endocardial excursion on ultrasound, has an exceedingly poor prognosis (Fig. 23.1 and Video 23.12).[18-20] Valve flutter alone, which may be seen due to fluid shifts or external pressures should not be used as an indicator of cardiac activity. Of the few documented survivors of cardiac standstill, there have been no reports of neurologically-intact survivors.[21,22]

Pulseless patients with electrical activity on the monitor and cardiac activity on ultrasound are said to be in pseudo-PEA (Video 23.13). Greater than 80% of patients thought to be in PEA by clinical assessment alone will have cardiac activity on ultrasound.[23] These patients have been found to be quite distinct from those with PEA without cardiac activity on ultrasound because better outcomes are described.[24-26] In a large observational study of ultrasound findings during cardiac arrest, pseudo-PEA was seen to have the highest association with survival.[22] Identifying this population is clearly high priority when integrating point-of-care ultrasound into resuscitation of cardiac arrest.

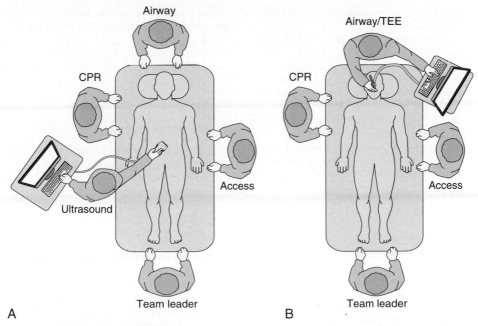

Figure 23.2 Team Member Positions. Positioning of team members during resuscitation while using either transthoracic echocardiography (A) or transesophageal echocardiography (B). *CPR*, Cardiopulmonary resuscitation.

Technique

PROBE SELECTION

Because transthoracic ultrasound imaging during cardiac arrest has several constraints yet must be efficient, a single multifunctional transducer is preferred. With current ultrasound technology, a phased-array transducer with a small footprint is most commonly used, but a micro-convex or curvilinear transducer may be an acceptable alternative. Regardless of the transducer chosen for torso imaging, a high-frequency linear-array transducer is needed for deep venous thrombosis (DVT) scanning and preferred for pneumothorax evaluation.

POSITIONING

In addition to selecting a single transducer, positioning of the sonographer and machine needs to be carefully considered. Resuscitation efforts run most efficiently when team members have designated positions and roles. Ideally, the sonographer should be a separate, dedicated team member, not directly involved in the resuscitation. The sonographer can independently acquire and interpret images to report back to the team leader. When using transthoracic echocardiography, the best position for the sonographer is at the patient's right hip, where the heart, lungs, abdomen, and lower extremity veins can be easily imaged. When using TEE, the ultrasound machine is placed to the left of the head of the bed and the operator is positioned at the head of bed or to the left side of the patient, ensuring that the screen is facing them to facilitate image acquisition and interpretation (Fig. 23.2).

IMAGE ACQUISITION

The quality of images acquired depends on whether chest compressions are ongoing or the team is performing a pulse check. The heart, IVC, abdomen, aorta, and deep veins can be imaged without difficulty during chest compressions. The heart is best imaged in the subcostal or apical 4-chamber views. Restricting cardiac imaging to these views will avoid ultrasound gel spreading to defibrillation pads and interfering with chest compressions or mechanical CPR devices.

Cardiac views should be obtained during both chest compressions and pulse checks. When a chest compression cycle is nearly complete, the sonographer should get into position with the transducer in the best cardiac view to maximize imaging during the compression-free time and minimize any risk of ultrasound-related delay in resumption of chest compressions. Before the pulse check, consider increasing the duration of the video recording setting to >10 seconds in order to capture cardiac images for the entire compression-free period. The stored video clip can be reviewed in detail, if necessary, once chest compressions resume.

If cardiac standstill is identified and resuscitation is terminated, a video clip documenting cardiac standstill should be obtained using either two-dimensional mode (see Video 23.12) or M-mode (see Fig. 23.1). If recording a video clip during a pulse check a retrospective recording mode may be preferred to avoid focusing attention on obtaining images, potentially delaying resumption of chest compressions.

Protocols and Algorithms

A number of protocols and algorithms integrating point-of-care ultrasound with cardiac arrest resuscitation have been designed.[27-29] Some protocols derive from assessment of undifferentiated hypotension and include a comprehensive approach that may not be practicable in cardiac arrest. During resuscitation, the focus should be on high-yield etiologies with an effective intervention, such as cardiac tamponade or pneumothorax. Once ROSC is obtained, a comprehensive ultrasound approach, such as the Rapid Ultrasound for Shock and Hypotension (RUSH) protocol, may reveal an undiscovered etiology of cardiac arrest.[30]

Cardiac arrest ultrasound protocols should account for the physiology of arrest. Because chest compressions should be minimally interrupted during CPR, integrating an ultrasound protocol into resuscitation of patients in cardiac arrest requires dividing views into those that can be performed during chest compressions and those that should be performed during pulse checks. Additionally, TEE may be used to assess depth of chest compressions and guide the site of hand placement to deliver compressions.

The design of a cardiac arrest ultrasound protocol should take into consideration the resources, personnel and equipment available at an institution. An example of an algorithm incorporating this approach is shown in Fig. 23.3.

PEARLS AND PITFALLS

- Identifying ventricular fibrillation
  - Patient with very fine ventricular fibrillation may appear to have asystole on cardiac monitor.
  - Point-of-care ultrasound in these patients will reveal rapid contractions with minimal myocardial wall excursion.
- Avoid confounders of cardiac standstill
  - Mechanical ventilation through lung expansion may transmit movement to the myocardium. Make certain any myocardial motion detected does not coincide solely with ventilation.
  - Valvular motion alone should not be considered a marker of myocardial contraction. Fluid shifts within the vasculature of a patient with no cardiac output may result in movement of the valves.
  - Similarly, fluid swirling in the ventricles may be seen in patients with cardiac standstill. Bubbles injected with intravenous medications may give the impression of significant movement within the heart when there is no myocardial contraction.
- Identifying cardiac tamponade
  - If pericardial effusion is seen in cardiac arrest, assume the patient has pericardial tamponade and proceed to perform emergent pericardiocentesis. Do not delay drainage to correlate right atrial and ventricular movement with the cardiac cycle in a patient with cardiac arrest.
- Choosing a view to image the heart in cardiac arrest
  - The subcostal or apical views are preferred given that compressions will interfere with the parasternal location. Further, ultrasound gel may interfere with CPR if the chest is slippery from gel.

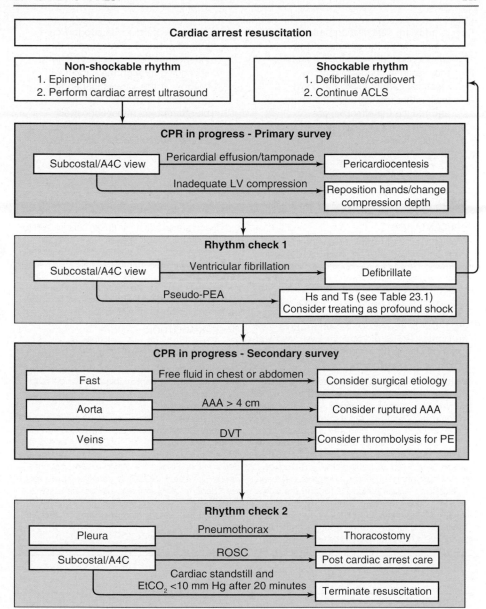

Figure 23.3 Cardiac Arrest Ultrasound Algorithm. *AAA,* Abdominal aortic aneurysm; *ACLS,* advanced cardiac life support; *A4C,* apical 4-chamber view; *CPR,* cardiopulmonary resuscitation; *DVT,* deep venous thrombosis; *EtCO₂,* end-tidal carbon dioxide; *FAST,* focused assessment with sonography in trauma; *LV,* left ventricle; *MI,* myocardial infarction; *PE,* pulmonary embolism; *PEA,* pulseless electrical activity; *ROSC,* return of spontaneous circulation.

- In addition, defibrillation pads are placed on the anterior chest. Ultrasound gel is conductive and may result in conduction of electrical current along the chest wall, rather than through the chest, and reduce the effectiveness of attempts of myocardial defibrillation.

- Advanced cardiac life support care should proceed uninterrupted and independent of a sonographer who is imaging through the subcostal window. If this view is inadequate, an apical 4-chamber view may be attempted. Transesophageal echocardiographic views are superior to both subcostal and apical views.

CASE 23.1

PRESENTATION

A 55-year-old man who was admitted for overnight observation after a cardiac catheterization suddenly becomes unresponsive. The nurse reports the patient was having seizure-like activity and is now obtunded and unresponsive. He has no pulse and the monitor reveals asystole. Cardiopulmonary resuscitation (CPR) is started, one round of medications per advanced cardiac life support (ACLS) protocol are given, and you begin your ultrasound exam.

ULTRASOUND FINDINGS

With CPR in progress, a phased-array transducer is positioned in the subcostal window to obtain a view of the heart (Video 23.14). The view is somewhat limited by chest compressions, but there is no evidence of a pericardial effusion. Next, the transducer is rotated 90 degrees to image the inferior vena cava (IVC; Video 23.15). The IVC is noted to be distended. Sliding over to the right upper quadrant, no free fluid is seen in Morison's pouch (Video 23.16) and the views of the focused assessment with sonography in trauma (FAST) exam are normal. A quick assessment of the aorta shows a normal diameter (Video 23.17). Returning to the subcostal view,

the team prepares for a pulse check. When CPR is held, a fibrillating heart becomes apparent (Video 23.18). The monitor still shows what looks like asystole, but it is clear the patient is in ventricular fibrillation. After defibrillation, a sinus rhythm appears on the monitor, spontaneous circulation returns and you note resolution of the fibrillation on ultrasound (Video 23.19).

CASE RESOLUTION

The patient maintains a sinus rhythm after defibrillation with intermittent ventricular ectopy. The patient is transferred to the intensive care unit (ICU), has an implantable cardiac defibrillator placed by electrophysiology, and recovers uneventfully.

Fine ventricular fibrillation can be mistaken for asystole, and if point-of-care ultrasound reveals ventricular fibrillation or pulseless ventricular tachycardia during a pulse check, immediate defibrillation is indicated. When return of spontaneous circulation (ROSC) is achieved, providers can perform a systematic ultrasound assessment using a shock protocol, such as the Rapid Ultrasound for Shock and Hypotension (RUSH) protocol.

CASE 23.2

PRESENTATION

Cardiopulmonary resuscitation has been underway for several minutes on a 37-year-old woman. During a pulse check, there is scattered organized activity on the monitor, but no carotid pulse can be palpated. She is confirmed to have pulseless electrical activity, and the team focuses on performing high-quality chest compressions. A focused ultrasound exam is performed with ongoing chest compressions.

ULTRASOUND FINDINGS

A subcostal 4-chamber view of the heart reveals a heart with weak but regular contractions (Video 23.20), consistent with pseudo-pulseless electrical activity (PEA). There is no anechoic stripe surrounding the heart, thus ruling out pericardial effusion. Additional ultrasound views are unrevealing, except for a noncompressible left femoral vein consistent with deep venous thrombosis (Video 23.21). Chest

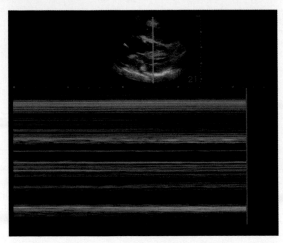

Figure 23.4   Cardiac Standstill. An M-mode image of cardiac standstill from a subcostal 4-chamber view.

CASE 23.2—cont'd

compressions continue while the nurse injects a thrombolytic and starts a heparin infusion. The team is fatiguing as the end-tidal CO_2 reading declines, and during a pulse check, a subcostal 4-chamber view shows cardiac standstill (Video 23.22), and M-mode confirms no cardiac activity (Fig. 23.4).

CASE RESOLUTION

This patient was pronounced dead from a suspected massive pulmonary embolism. Point-of-care ultrasound identified pseudo-PEA and DVT, giving the patient a chance at survival when thrombolytics were administered. After a prolonged resuscitative effort, cardiac standstill was documented by ultrasound, the team determined the patient's arrest was not survivable, and resuscitation was terminated.

Point-of-care ultrasound can identify potentially reversible causes of cardiac arrest, classically taught as the "5 H's and T's" in advanced cardiac life support (ACLS) training, which include pneumothorax, cardiac tamponade, hypovolemia, and DVT/pulmonary embolism. Detection of any of these conditions can guide the team's resuscitative efforts and potentially improve the chances of survival.

CASE 23.3

PRESENTATION

A 46-year-old high school science teacher develops chest pain and collapses. Her students start cardiopulmonary resuscitation (CPR) immediately and call 911. Paramedics establish intravenous access, intubate her, and transport her to the hospital quickly. CPR is continued upon arrival to the emergency department (ED), but after ten minutes, the end tidal CO_2 reading remains low at 9 mm Hg. The cardiac arrest team is equipped with a transesophageal echo transducer and rapidly insert the transducer to guide their intra-arrest management.

ULTRASOUND FINDINGS

A midesophageal long-axis view (Video 23.23) demonstrates excellent compression depth.

However, the point of maximal compression is noted to be over the left ventricular outflow tract and is likely obstructing the outflow that CPR is seeking to generate. The sonographer notifies the team, the team leader directs the providers to move the site of compression lateral and inferiorly along the long axis of the heart. A repeat transesophageal echocardiography (TEE) demonstrates improvement in chest compressions with the left ventricle (LV) being compressed rather than the left ventricular outflow tract (Video 23.24).

CASE RESOLUTION

Shortly after this adjustment is made, the end-tidal CO_2 is noted to rise to 30 mm Hg. A rhythm check reveals sinus tachycardia with palpable

Continued

CASE 23.3—cont'd

carótid pulses. The patient receives postarrest care and is transported to the intensive care unit.

Chest compressions are often not performed to recommended standards, which jeopardizes the effectiveness of CPR. The site of maximal compression is often over the left ventricular outflow tract or ascending aorta which may obstruct outflow. TEE can be used to assess the depth and site of chest compressions and provide immediate feedback to the providers on the quality of chest compressions.

CASE 23.4

PRESENTATION

The rapid response team is called due to a cardiac arrest in a 63-year-old man on chronic hemodialysis who was admitted to the intensive care unit (ICU) for severe hyperkalemia and acute pulmonary edema requiring intubation and mechanical ventilation. On arrival, the patient remains intubated, and the nurse reports having given him one round of epinephrine, calcium, and sodium bicarbonate before return of spontaneous circulation (ROSC) was achieved. He is still hypotensive on the monitor with a blood pressure of 76/44. You start examining him with a subcostal 4-chamber view of the heart.

ULTRASOUND FINDINGS

Upon putting the transducer on the chest, you notice that the patient has a large pericardial effusion, and the right atrial and ventricular free walls are moving abnormally (Video 23.25). You rotate the probe 90 degrees to image the inferior vena cava (IVC) which is dilated and plethoric (Video 23.26). You notify the team leader that the patient has a large pericardial effusion and a plethoric IVC which is consistent with pericardial tamponade.

CASE RESOLUTION

Under ultrasound guidance, a parasternal approach is used to place a pericardial catheter and drain 300 mL of blood from the pericardial space. ROSC is achieved. The cardiothoracic surgeon is notified and the patient is taken to the operating room.

If a pericardial effusion is detected during cardiopulmonary resuscitation (CPR), cardiac tamponade is presumed to be the cause of cardiac arrest, and emergent pericardiocentesis should be performed. Pericardiocentesis is one of the few interventions that can be life-saving and rapidly lead to ROSC during cardiac arrest.

SECTION 4

Abdomen and Pelvis

CHAPTER 24

Peritoneal Free Fluid

Craig Sisson ■ Jessica Solis-McCarthy

KEY POINTS

- Focused abdominal ultrasonography is a sensitive and reliable bedside technique to detect intraperitoneal free fluid, although it cannot differentiate specific types of fluid.
- Ultrasound is the diagnostic modality of choice for the initial screening of unstable blunt trauma patients for peritoneal free fluid.
- Performing abdominal paracentesis with ultrasound guidance has been shown to increase procedural success rates and reduce the risk of complications.

Background

Peritoneal free fluid is divided into intra- and extraperitoneal fluid. Intraperitoneal fluid is located within the peritoneal cavity, whereas extraperitoneal fluid is located outside the peritoneal cavity and is typically referred to as retroperitoneal fluid. In this chapter, we use the term *peritoneal free fluid* to refer to intraperitoneal free fluid.

The gravitationally dependent anatomic locations where peritoneal free fluid preferentially accumulates have been recognized for over a century.[1-3] It has been known that physical examination of the abdomen has low sensitivity for diagnosing intra-abdominal pathologies.[4-8] Providers can use ultrasound to detect small amounts of peritoneal free fluid and guide procedures, most often paracentesis. Free-flowing fluid appears black, or anechoic, on ultrasound imaging (Video 24.1).

Ultrasound cannot precisely differentiate *types* of peritoneal free fluid, such as blood, ascites, urine, or bile. Therefore, historical clues, such as recent trauma or preexisting medical conditions, must be considered when interpreting the presence and significance of peritoneal free fluid.

The minimum amount of fluid in the peritoneal cavity detectable by ultrasound will vary depending on several factors: patient positioning, etiology of fluid accumulation, elapsed time from onset of fluid accumulation, body habitus, quality of images, and provider skill level.[9-13] A range of 100 to 620 mL has been reported as the minimum amount of intraperitoneal free fluid detectable by ultrasound.[14]

Etiologies of peritoneal free fluid can be divided into traumatic and atraumatic causes. In trauma patients, the presence of peritoneal free fluid reflects blood until proven otherwise and is a surrogate marker for solid organ injury.

219

Hemoperitoneum from blunt trauma most commonly originates in the upper abdomen from injury to the spleen or liver.[15] The hepatorenal space is the single most sensitive area for detection of hemoperitoneum secondary to blunt trauma.[16] Atraumatic etiologies of peritoneal free fluid can include emergent causes, such as ruptured ectopic pregnancy, and nonemergent causes, such as chronic ascites due to cirrhosis.

When used for procedural guidance, ultrasound can guide site selection to perform a diagnostic or therapeutic paracentesis. Ultrasound guidance for paracentesis has been shown to improve procedural success rates and decrease reduce the risk of complications, as well as decrease hospital costs and length of stay.[17-19]

Normal Anatomy

Detection of peritoneal fluid by ultrasound requires an understanding of the anatomic spaces where free fluid accumulates in the abdomen. The peritoneal cavity is subdivided into greater and lesser peritoneal sacs. The greater peritoneal sac is further divided into supracolic and infracolic compartments by the transverse mesocolon. Pathologic fluid can pass between the supracolic and infracolic compartments via the paracolic gutters, the peritoneal spaces lateral to the ascending and descending colon.

In the upright and supine positions, the most gravitationally dependent area of the combined *abdomino-pelvic* peritoneal space is the pelvis, specifically caudal to the sacral promontory. In the *abdominal* peritoneal space alone, the hepatorenal space, or Morison's pouch, is the most gravitationally dependent area above the pelvic inlet in a supine position. When fluid accumulation begins in a supine position, fluid gravitates toward the hepatorenal space for three reasons. First, the hepatorenal peritoneal reflection is more posterior relative to other abdominal structures. Second, the lordotic curvature of the lumbar spine and anterior location of the sacral promontory relative to the hepatorenal space prevent free fluid from flowing into the pelvis. Third, the phrenicocolic ligament, a peritoneal reflection in the left upper quadrant, shunts blood from the left upper quadrant toward the hepatorenal space.[20] However, if a patient has been upright, peritoneal free fluid from the abdomen will pool in the pelvis, regardless of the site of origin.

Image Acquisition

A low-frequency curvilinear or phased-array transducer is needed to examine the abdomen and pelvis. Three areas must be evaluated in the assessment for peritoneal free fluid: the right upper quadrant, left upper quadrant, and pelvis. The liver, spleen, and urine-filled bladder, respectively, serve as the acoustic windows to evaluate these areas (Fig. 24.1). An empty or ruptured bladder, subcutaneous emphysema, bowel or stomach gas, wound dressings, and asplenia can reduce the sensitivity of ultrasound to detect peritoneal free fluid from these windows. Placing the patient in a Trendelenburg or reverse Trendelenburg position helps pool peritoneal free fluid in gravitationally dependent areas to increase sensitivity of the examination to detect small volumes of fluid.[13,14,21]

RIGHT UPPER QUADRANT

In the right upper quadrant, three spaces should be visualized: the right subdiaphragmatic space, hepatorenal space, and the inferior pole of the right kidney. Visualizing all three spaces systematically can help avoid missing small collections of fluid. Place the transducer in a coronal plane on the midaxillary line between the 9th and 11th ribs with the transducer orientation marker pointing cephalad and rotated slightly posteriorly (Fig. 24.2). Adjust the transducer position to focus on the potential space between the liver and kidney (hepatorenal space or Morison's pouch) (Fig. 24.3). Tilt the transducer from anterior to posterior through the entire hepatorenal space to visualize the inferior tip of the liver, looking for free fluid. Rock or slide the transducer superiorly to image the right subdiaphragmatic space, and inferiorly to image the inferior pole of the right kidney, which serves as an anatomic marker for the right paracolic gutter (Fig. 24.4; Videos 24.2 and 24.3).

LEFT UPPER QUADRANT

In the left upper quadrant, three spaces should be visualized: the left subdiaphragmatic space (perisplenic space), the splenorenal space, and the inferior pole of the left kidney. In contrast to the right upper quadrant, the left upper quadrant is best visualized with the transducer in a more posterior and superior position due to the location of the spleen. Place the transducer in a coronal plane on the posterior axillary

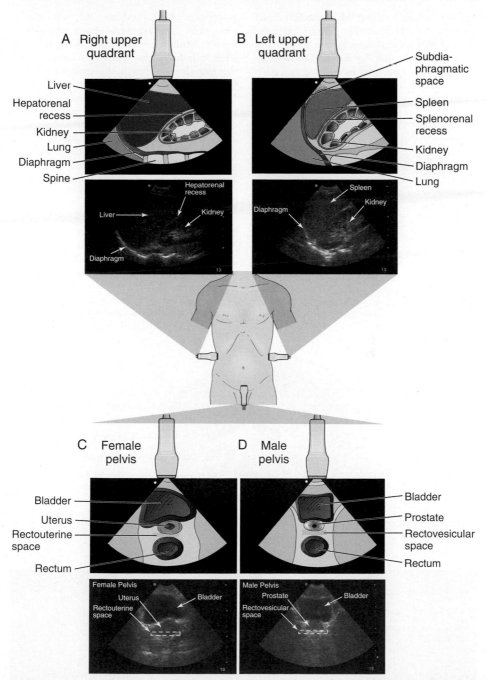

Figure 24.1 Detection of Peritoneal Free Fluid. (A) Right upper quadrant. Visualize the right subdiaphragmatic space, hepatorenal space (Morison's pouch, most important area in the right upper quadrant), and the right inferior pole of the kidney. (B) Left upper quadrant. Visualize the left subdiaphragmatic space (most important area in the left upper quadrant), splenorenal space, and left inferior pole of the kidney. (C) and (D) Pelvic window. Visualize the rectouterine space in females (C) and the rectovesicular space in males (D).

line between the 6th and 9th intercostal spaces with the transducer marker pointing cephalad (Fig. 24.5). Providers usually have to put their "knuckles to the bed" for supine patients. The image may be improved by rotating the transducer 10 to 20 degrees clockwise with the transducer orientation marker pointing slightly

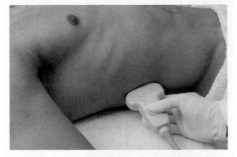

Figure 24.2 Transducer Position in Right Upper Quadrant. Place the transducer on the midaxillary line between the 9th and 11th ribs with the transducer orientation marker pointed cephalad and rotated slightly posteriorly.

posteriorly. First, evaluate the left subdiaphragmatic, or perisplenic space, where fluid is most likely to collect. (Fig. 24.6 and Video 24.4). Similar to the right upper quadrant, tilt the transducer through the perisplenic space from anterior to posterior. In contrast to the hepatorenal space, the splenorenal space is not the preferred location for accumulation of free fluid due to the splenorenal ligaments attaching the spleen, left kidney, and tail of the pancreas. The inferior poles of the left kidney and spleen should be visualized along with the superior portion of the left paracolic gutter.

PELVIS

Peritoneal free fluid in the pelvis accumulates in the rectovesicular space in men and the rectouterine space, or pouch of Douglas, in women (Fig. 24.7). To image the pelvic space, place the transducer in a transverse plane over the pubic symphysis with the transducer marker pointed toward the patient's right. Tilt the transducer inferiorly into the pelvis until

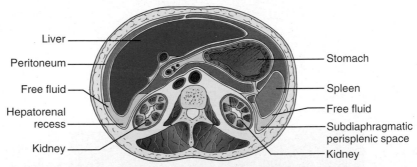

Figure 24.3 Right and Left Upper Quadrant Cross-Sectional Anatomy. Peritoneal free fluid accumulates in the hepatorenal space (Morison's pouch) and perisplenic space.

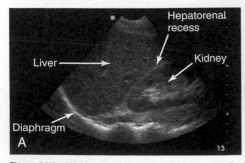
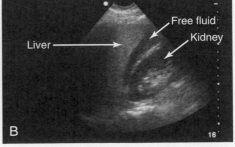

Figure 24.4 (A) Normal right upper quadrant. (B) Peritoneal free fluid in the hepatorenal space in a patient after blunt trauma.

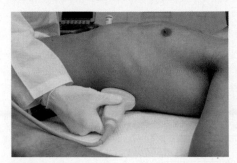

Figure 24.5 Transducer Position in Left Upper Quadrant. Place the transducer on the posterior axillary line between the 6th and 9th ribs with the transducer orientation marker pointed cephalad and rotated slightly posteriorly.

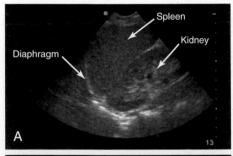

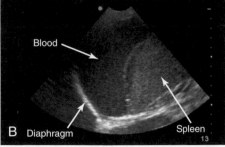

Figure 24.6 (A) Normal left upper quadrant. (B) Peritoneal free fluid in the left subdiaphragmatic space.

the bladder is visualized (Fig. 24.8 and Videos 24.5–24.7). Set the imaging depth to view the bladder in the top one-third to one-half of the screen. Posterior acoustic enhancement is seen deep to the bladder, usually requiring a reduction in the far field gain. It is important to tilt the transducer to visualize the entire bladder from fundus to neck to thoroughly evaluate the rectovesicular or rectouterine space for any free fluid collections (Fig. 24.9; Videos 24.8 and 24.9). Rotate the transducer 90 degrees clockwise to obtain sagittal views of the bladder and

scan the entire bladder from left to right. If the bladder is decompressed, it can be refilled with warm normal saline through the injection port of a urinary catheter with the catheter clamped.

Image Interpretation

In trauma patients, liver or spleen injuries are difficult to visualize, and the presence of peritoneal free fluid is a surrogate marker for solid organ injury. When the source of bleeding is in the upper abdomen, the hepatorenal space is the most sensitive location to detect peritoneal free fluid in supine patients.[16] In the left upper quadrant, free fluid initially accumulates in the left subdiaphragmatic space, whereas in the right upper quadrant, fluid initially accumulates in the hepatorenal space.[20] In the absence of an anatomic obstruction, fluid in the perisplenic space eventually overflows into the more dependent hepatorenal space in the right upper quadrant.

Normally, there is no visible peritoneal free fluid in the abdomino-pelvic cavity in males. In females, a small amount of physiologic fluid may be present in the pelvis. If the volume of pelvic free fluid appears non-trivial or there is strong clinical concern, the source should be investigated. The urgency to evaluate free fluid in the female pelvis depends on the patient's stability and clinical situation.

Generally, all types of peritoneal free fluid, including ascites, blood, bile, lymph, and urine appear black, or anechoic, by ultrasound (see Video 24.1). However, peritoneal free fluid that contains clotted blood, pus, or debris appears more echogenic due to high protein content (Videos 24.10 and 24.11). Solid debris from a ruptured hollow viscus can appear heterogeneously echogenic. Loculations (Videos 24.12 and 24.13) and bowel adhesions to the abdominal wall (Video 24.14) can also be seen.

As fluid accumulates in the abdomen, loops of small bowel begin to float freely and are seen tethered posteriorly by the mesentery (Fig. 24.10 and Video 24.15). The peritoneal space can fill with several liters of fluid, which is accompanied by progressive distention of the abdomen. If the peritoneal free fluid is not removed, intra-abdominal pressure will increase, causing reduced diaphragmatic excursion and potentially causing abdominal hypertension which can lead to abdominal compartment syndrome.

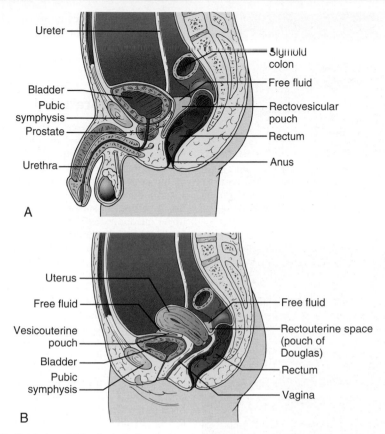

Ureter

Sigmoid colon

Free fluid

Bladder

Pubic symphysis

Prostate

Urethra

Rectovesicular pouch

Rectum

Anus

A

Uterus

Free fluid

Vesicouterine pouch

Bladder

Pubic symphysis

Free fluid

Rectouterine space (pouch of Douglas)

Rectum

Vagina

B

Figure 24.7 Pelvic free fluid collects in the rectovesicular space in males (A) and the rectouterine space (pouch of Douglas) in females (B).

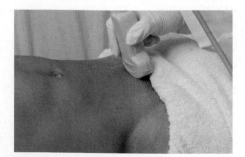

Figure 24.8 Transducer Position for the Pelvis. Place the transducer just above the pubic symphysis and tilt the ultrasound beam inferiorly toward the pelvis.

Pathologic Findings

HEMOPERITONEUM

The extended focused assessment with sonography for trauma (EFAST) examination has evolved to become the standard screening tool for unstable patients with blunt abdominal trauma (see Chapter 33, Trauma). The most sensitive locations to detect small amounts of blood are the hepatorenal space in the right upper quadrant, subdiaphragmatic space in the left upper quadrant, and rectovesicular or rectouterine space in the pelvis. It is important to thoroughly visualize the inferior tips of the liver, spleen, and kidneys, where small amounts of fluid can collect.

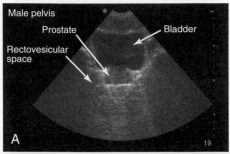

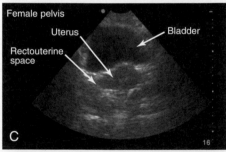

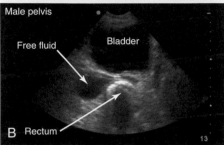

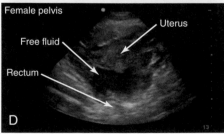

Figure 24.9 Normal (A) and abnormal (B) male pelvis with free fluid collecting in the rectovesicular space. Normal (C) and abnormal (D) female pelvis with free fluid collecting in the rectouterine space (pouch of Douglas).

ASCITES

Ascites is the most common complication of cirrhosis leading to hospital admission,[22] and development of ascites is an important landmark in the natural history of cirrhosis, with 1- and 5-year mortality rates of 15% and 44%, respectively.[23] Ultrasound can differentiate ascites from other common causes of abdominal distention, such as adipose tissue, abdominal wall edema (Video 24.16), and gas-filled loops of bowel (Video 24.17). Ascites volume can be qualitatively categorized as small (Video 24.18), moderate, or large (Video 24.19). In advanced stages of cirrhosis, the liver appears small and fibrotic with increased echogenicity (Video 24.20), and incidental regenerative nodules or masses may be seen (Video 24.21).

Other Pathologies

The vast majority of atraumatic cases of peritoneal free fluid accumulation are due to ascites from cirrhosis. Other causes include right heart failure, renal failure, pancreatitis, and peritoneal dialysis. In females, pathologic conditions related to the ovaries are an important cause of peritoneal free fluid accumulation. A positive pregnancy test without an identifiable intrauterine pregnancy associated with the presence of peritoneal free fluid should be considered an ectopic pregnancy until proven otherwise (see Chapter 29, First Trimester Pregnancy). Other sex-specific causes of peritoneal free fluid include ruptured hemorrhagic ovarian cysts and ovarian malignancies. Malignant ascites can occur with multiple cancers in both sexes. Less common causes of peritoneal free fluid include portal vein, hepatic vein, and inferior vena caval thrombosis.

Paracentesis

Ultrasound guidance has proven to reduce the risk of complications and improve procedural success rates when performing paracentesis.[17-19] Ultrasound is most often used to mark a needle insertion site prior to performing a diagnostic or therapeutic paracentesis. Before performing paracentesis, the bladder should be emptied, either spontaneously or by placement of a urinary catheter, and the patient should be placed in a supine position with the head of the bed elevated 30 to 45 degrees to pool ascites in bilateral lower quadrants.

Using a low-frequency curvilinear or phased-array transducer, scan the lower quadrants of the abdomen in a longitudinal plane with the transducer marker oriented cephalad. Scan lateral to the rectus abdominis muscles to

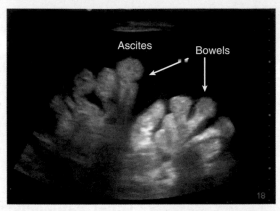

Figure 24.10 Large Volume of Ascites With Free Floating Loops of Small Bowel Tethered by the Mesentery Posteriorly.

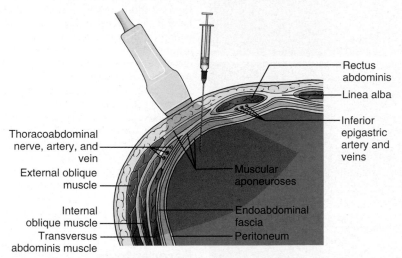

Figure 24.11 Abdominal Wall Cross-Section. The anterolateral muscular aponeurosis of the abdomen wall is the ideal window for paracentesis. Blood vessels of the anterior abdominal wall (inferior epigastric vessels) and lateral abdominal wall (thoraco-abdominal vessels) should be avoided. The lateral abdominal wall has greater adipose tissue and musculature which is not ideal for paracentesis. The avascular linea alba in the midline of the abdomen is an alternative site but the bladder must be decompressed prior to paracentesis.

localize the largest collection of peritoneal free fluid with the greatest distance from nearby organs and the thinnest abdominal wall. Site selection is ideally along the muscular aponeurosis lateral to the rectus abdominis muscles (Fig. 24.11). Medial to the muscular aponeurosis there is greater risk of injury to the inferior epigastric vessels, and laterally the abdominal wall is thicker and there is also risk of injury to vessels (Fig. 24.12). If no peritoneal free fluid is visualized in the lower quadrants, scan the

most gravitationally dependent areas of the abdominopelvic cavity, the right and left upper quadrants and pelvis as described above, to diagnose whether any ascites is present. If only a scant amount of peritoneal free fluid is seen in the lower quadrants, paracentesis cannot be performed safely (Video 24.22).

The abdominal wall has several superficial and deep blood vessels that must be avoided during paracentesis. The inferior epigastric, superficial epigastric, circumflex iliac, and

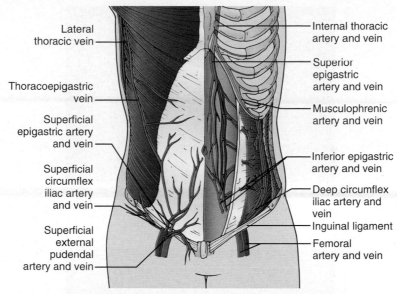

Figure 24.12   Abdominal Wall Vascular Anatomy. Note the location of inferior epigastric, subcostal, circumflex iliac, and thoracoepigastric vessels that should be avoided during paracentesis.

thoracoepigastric arteries and veins are the major blood vessels in the abdominal wall (Fig. 24.12). Selecting a needle insertion site lateral to the rectus abdominis muscles avoids most inferior epigastric vessels, but the exact location, size, and branching of the inferior epigastric vessels varies significantly. For maximal safety, evaluate the needle insertion site with a high-frequency linear transducer using color flow or power Doppler ultrasound to detect any blood vessels that flow through the intended paracentesis site. Place the color flow or power Doppler box on the abdominal wall over the anticipated needle tract (Video 24.23). If blood vessels are detected, slide the transducer a few centimeters laterally and recheck until a site without any visible large blood vessels is identified.

Although ultrasound is most often used to mark a needle insertion site (static guidance), real-time ultrasound guidance can be used to visualize the needle entering the peritoneal cavity when the fluid collection is small or risk of injury to adjacent organs is high. To perform real-time ultrasound-guided paracentesis, cover the transducer with a sterile sheath and place it in the sterile field. A transverse (out-of-plane) or longitudinal (in-plane) approach can be used to track the needle tip under direct visualization. The skin and subcutaneous tissues can

be anesthetized under direct visualization to ensure that you have anesthetized all tissues to the peritoneum (Video 24.24). Similarly, a large-bore needle or needle-catheter is inserted under direct visualization as it enters the peritoneal cavity, and a diagnostic or therapeutic drainage can be performed (Video 24.25).

PEARLS AND PITFALLS

- A fluid-filled stomach can cause a false-positive interpretation of free fluid in the left upper quadrant, especially in urgent or emergent situations (Fig. 24.13).[24]
- Previous abdominal surgeries can alter fluid accumulation in gravitationally dependent areas. It is important to note any surgical scars when performing an abdominal ultrasound exam.
- When fluid surrounding the kidneys does not track into the peritoneum, the presence of retroperitoneal fluid should be considered, particularly from a ureteral injury or abdominal aortic aneurysm. This finding is not sensitive for evaluating retroperitoneal structures, and a computed tomography (CT) scan of the abdomen should be obtained.

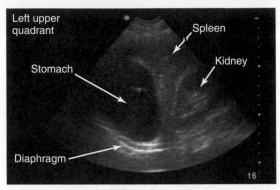

Figure 24.13 **Left Upper Quadrant Window Showing a Fluid-Filled Stomach.** Note that the fluid does not layer under the diaphragm, appears well contained, and the normally round edges of the spleen appear sharp or pointed.

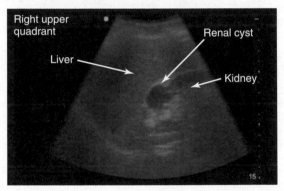

Figure 24.14 **Right Upper Quadrant Renal Cyst Located in the Hepatorenal Space that Could be Mistaken for Free Fluid.**

- Peritoneal free fluid disperses in dependent areas and does not appear well circumscribed, unless adhesions or scarring are present. A working knowledge of abdominal anatomy and its ultrasound appearance will enable providers to differentiate peritoneal free fluid from other structures, such as renal cysts, seminal vesicles, fluid filled viscera and perinephric fat (Fig. 24.14).

- Gas-filled structures, including the stomach, large and small bowels, and subcutaneous emphysema, do not provide adequate windows to visualize underlying organs. For gas-filled loops of small bowel, firm pressure and gentle tilting of the transducer can often shift loops of bowel aside to improve visualization of underlying structures.

CHAPTER 25

Kidneys

Behzad Hassani

KEY POINTS

- The most common indication to perform a point-of-care ultrasound exam of the kidney is to evaluate for hydronephrosis.
- A bladder ultrasound exam should accompany a renal ultrasound exam. A distended bladder due to bladder outlet obstruction is a common cause of hydronephrosis.
- Any suspicious renal mass or lesion detected by point-of-care ultrasound warrants further investigation with diagnostic imaging studies.

Background

Renal ultrasound is an efficient and radiation-free alternative to computed tomography (CT) for the initial workup of low-risk patients who present with acute symptoms ranging from undifferentiated abdominal pain to painless hematuria.[1] Ultrasound is the imaging modality of choice for investigating obstructive uropathy in pregnant and pediatric populations to avoid exposure to ionizing radiation. A recent multicenter, randomized, comparative effectiveness trial compared point-of-care ultrasound (POCUS) versus CT versus radiology-performed ultrasound in the initial emergency department (ED) assessment of patients with suspected nephrolithiasis. No significant differences in patient outcomes (high-risk diagnosis with complications, serious adverse events, pain scores, return ED visits, or hospitalization) were seen between the three groups. However, when POCUS or radiology-performed ultrasound exam was the initial imaging modality, rather than a CT scan, there was reduced cumulative radiation exposure. Additionally, patients in the POCUS versus radiology-performed ultrasound group had a slightly shorter ED length of stay. The study concluded that ultrasonography should be the initial imaging modality in the ED assessment of patients with suspected nephrolithiasis.[2]

Focused renal ultrasound can accurately detect and grade hydronephrosis in the context of obstructive uropathy,[3] directly visualize large obstructing calculi,[4] and characterize renal cysts or solid masses.[5] When clinical suspicion for renal calculus is high, the presence of unilateral hydronephrosis can be considered as de facto evidence of obstructive uropathy due to a calculus. Combining a single plain film of the abdomen (kidneys, ureter, and bladder, or KUB) with an ultrasound exam improves the sensitivity for detecting a calcified stone.[6] Severity of hydronephrosis observed may correlate with the duration of obstruction[7] and possibly with the size of the obstructing calculus.[8] When renal calculus disease is clinically less likely, or an alternate pathology, such as abdominal aortic aneurysm, gallbladder disease, ovarian torsion, or ectopic pregnancy is being considered, the absence of hydronephrosis effectively redirects the workup to other organ systems.

Normal Anatomy

Kidneys are retroperitoneal organs that lie in an oblique longitudinal plane with the inferior pole of each kidney more anterior and lateral compared to its superior pole (Fig. 25.1). Therefore, the transducer must be positioned obliquely to image the kidney along its long axis. The left kidney is located more superiorly

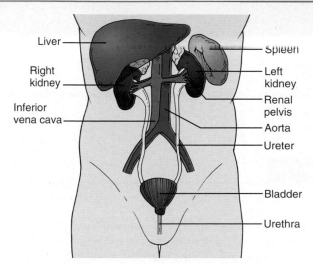

Figure 25.1 Anatomy of the Urinary System.

and posteriorly compared to the right kidney, whereas the right kidney is located more inferiorly and laterally due to the liver. The left kidney is usually visualized through an acoustic window provided by the spleen due to interference by bowel and stomach gas anteriorly. The right kidney is often visualized through an acoustic window provided by the liver. The right kidney is slightly larger than the left kidney, but both kidneys are normally within 2 cm of each other in any dimension.

Kidneys are divided into two distinct anatomic parts: renal parenchyma and renal sinus (Fig. 25.2). Renal parenchyma is further subdivided into renal cortex and medulla. The medulla consists of cone-shaped pyramids. Renal parenchyma surrounds the sinus on all sides except at the hilum. The hilum is where the renal artery, renal vein, and proximal ureter enter the renal sinus. Prominent fatty deposits within the renal sinus give it a hyperechoic appearance and distinguish it from the hypoechoic renal parenchyma. This difference in echogenicity is known as the sonographic double density of the kidney.[5,9]

Image Acquisition

A low-frequency transducer, either phased-array or curvilinear type, provides adequate penetration to image the kidneys. The narrower beam width of a phased-array transducer is ideal for imaging between the ribs, but the wider beam width of a curvilinear transducer allows

visualization of the entire kidney longitudinally in a single view.

When scanning a patient with a suspected renal pathology, consider scanning the unaffected side first to obtain a baseline image to compare with the affected side. To image the right kidney, place the patient in a supine position with the transducer in a coronal plane in the midaxillary line at the level of the xiphoid process. Center the kidney on the screen and rotate the transducer 15 to 30 degrees counterclockwise with the transducer orientation marker ("notch") pointed slightly posteriorly to capture a longitudinal (long-axis) view of the kidney. While holding the transducer in the same location on the skin surface, tilt or fan the transducer anteriorly and posteriorly to assess the entire kidney from its most anterior to posterior surface. Rotate the transducer 90 degrees counterclockwise from the longitudinal view to obtain a transverse (short-axis) view of the kidney. Tilt or fan the transducer superiorly and inferiorly to assess the superior and inferior poles of the kidney (Fig. 25.3)

The left kidney is more posterior and superior than the right kidney. Identify the left kidney with the transducer in a coronal plane on the posterior axillary line. Techniques to improve visualization of the left kidney: (1) move the transducer maximally posterior ("knuckles to the bed"), (2) place the patient in a right lateral decubitus position, or (3) request the patient to perform a breathhold to shift the kidney caudally. Next, rotate the transducer 15

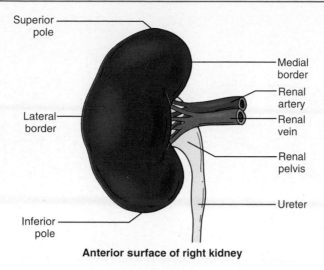

Anterior surface of right kidney

Internal structure of right kidney

Figure 25.2   Cross-Sectional Anatomy of the Kidney.

to 30 degrees clockwise aiming the transducer orientation marker slightly posteriorly to acquire a longitudinal view and then rotate the transducer 90 degrees counterclockwise from the longitudinal view to obtain a transverse view of the kidney.[5,9]

Longitudinal and transverse views of the bladder should be obtained for a complete evaluation of the urinary system (see Chapter 26, Bladder).

Image Interpretation

Gerota's fascia and perinephric fat appear as a hyperechoic band around the kidneys, and the fibrous capsule gives each kidney a hyperechoic outline. Normally, the renal cortex is homogeneously hypoechoic relative to the liver or spleen. The fluid-filled medullary pyramids appear as hypoechoic or anechoic triangular prominences in a semicircular arrangement around the renal sinus. The renal medulla is significantly less echogenic compared to the surrounding cortex.

The renal sinus normally appears hyperechoic due to fat content, and in the absence of hydronephrosis, the sinus appears homogenously hyperechoic with small anechoic pockets of urine (Fig. 25.4 and Video 25.1). The ureter is usually obscured by bowel gas but

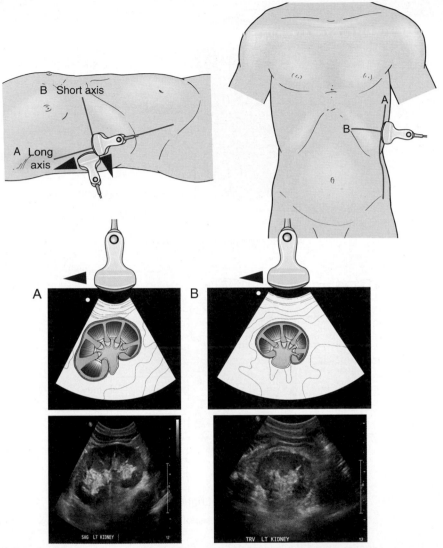

Figure 25.3 Transducer position of longitudinal (long-axis) (A) and transverse (short-axis) (B) views of the kidney.

when distended, the ureter may be visible as a tubular structure extending inferiorly from the renal pelvis.[5,9]

Pathologic Findings

SIZE

Normal kidneys are 9 to 13 cm long, 3 to 7 cm wide, and 3 to 6 cm thick, and normal parenchymal thickness is 1.1 to 2.3 cm.[10] Atrophic kidneys signify chronic kidney diseases and can often be recognized without measuring the actual dimensions. Severely atrophied kidneys are seen with end-stage renal disease and often have small (<5 mm) cortical or medullary simple cysts (Fig. 25.5 and Video 25.2).[11,12]

HYDRONEPHROSIS

Hydronephrosis appears as an anechoic fluid collection within the hyperechoic renal sinus.

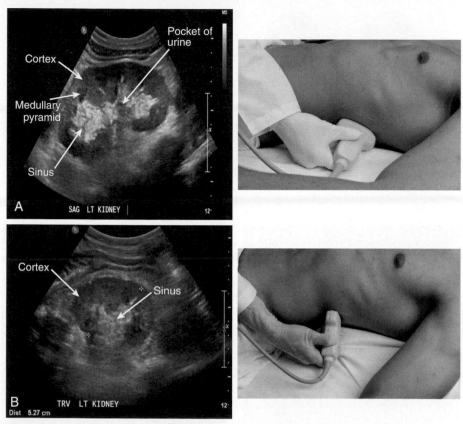

Figure 25.4 Normal kidney in longitudinal (A) and transverse (B) views. Note the prominent, hypoechoic medullary pyramids and hyperechoic renal sinus.

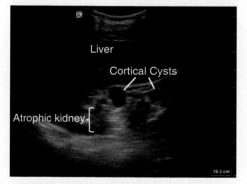

Figure 25.5 Atrophic Kidney. A severely atrophic right kidney with multiple small cysts is seen in a patient with end-stage renal disease.

The severity of hydronephrosis is classified as mild, moderate, or severe (Fig. 25.6)[13] and may correlate with the size of a distal, obstructing renal stone. Many algorithms incorporate the degree of hydronephrosis into clinical decision-making pathways.[1,8,13]

Mild hydronephrosis is defined as enlargement of the calyces with preservation of renal papillae. The renal sinus is normally hyperechoic but becomes anechoic due to central dilation in mild hydronephrosis (Fig. 25.7). As mild hydronephrosis progresses, the degree of central dilation of the renal sinus increases, but the structure of the medullary pyramids is preserved (Fig. 25.8). It is the preservation of medullary pyramidal architecture, not the degree of renal pelvic dilation, that characterizes mild hydronephrosis and differentiates mild from moderate hydronephrosis (Videos 25.3 and 25.4).

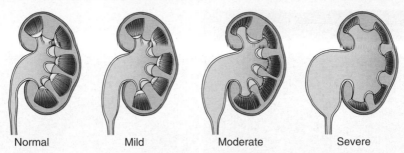

Figure 25.6   Severity of Hydronephrosis. Mild hydronephrosis: enlarged calyces with preservation of renal papillae and pyramids. Moderate hydronephrosis: dilated calyces with obliterated papillae and blunted pyramids. Severe hydronephrosis: calyceal ballooning, complete obliteration of papillae and pyramids, cortical thinning.

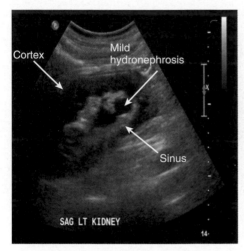

Figure 25.7   Mild Hydronephrosis.

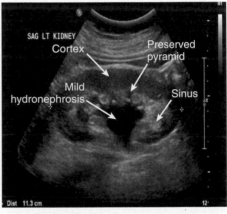

Figure 25.8   Mild Hydronephrosis.

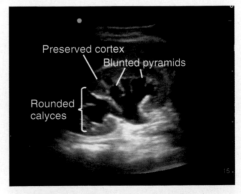

Figure 25.9   Moderate Hydronephrosis.

Moderate hydronephrosis is characterized by rounding of the calyces, obliteration of renal papillae, and blunting of medullary pyramids. Progressive dilation of the calyces leads to glove-like splaying of the renal sinus that has been classically called a "bear-claw" appearance (Fig. 25.9; Videos 25.5 and 25.6). Preservation of the outer cortex is the distinguishing feature between moderate and severe hydronephrosis.

Severe hydronephrosis is defined as calyceal ballooning with variable degrees of cortical thinning. The dilated calyces that characterize moderate hydronephrosis coalesce into a large collection of urine that completely obliterates the renal sinus and medullary pyramids. The renal sinus, which is normally hyperechoic, becomes completely anechoic due to the large, central fluid collection. All that remains of the normal renal architecture is a rim of outer cortex. Total distortion of normal renal architecture is the key distinguishing feature of severe hydronephrosis (Fig. 25.10; Videos 25.7 and 25.8).

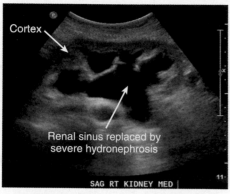

Figure 25.10 Severe Hydronephrosis.

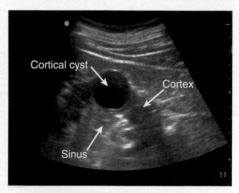

Figure 25.12 Simple Cortical Cyst.

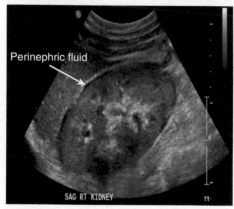

Figure 25.11 Perinephric Fluid. A small amount of perinephric fluid indicative of calyceal rupture and urinary extravasation is seen in a longitudinal view of the kidney.

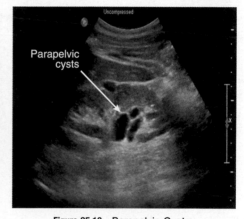

Figure 25.13 Parapelvic Cysts.

A small amount of perinephric fluid due to calyceal rupture and urinary extravasation may be seen with hydronephrosis (Fig. 25.11; Videos 25.9 and 25.10). A urinoma is a collection of perinephric fluid (Video 25.11). Perinephric fluid is associated with significant risk of infection or perinephric abscess formation and requires close follow-up.[1]

Several conditions can mimic the ultrasound appearance of hydronephrosis. The following techniques can help confirm a diagnosis of hydronephrosis: (1) trace the anechoic areas of suspected hydronephrosis to the renal pelvis where the areas should coalesce, (2) scan the kidney in both the longitudinal and transverse planes to thoroughly delineate the architecture of the area of suspected hydronephrosis, and (3) use color flow or power Doppler ultrasound

to differentiate renal vessels from dilated calyces (Video 25.12).[9]

Medullary pyramids may appear anechoic and can be mistaken for collections of urine; however, the triangular pyramids are separated from each other by cortical tissue and should be seen as distinct entities by tilting the transducer. Cortical and parapelvic cysts can also mimic hydronephrosis, but they are distinguished by their smooth walls and spherical shape that is not contiguous with the renal pelvis (Figs. 25.12 and 25.13; Video 25.13).

Renal Calculus

Ultrasound has low sensitivity for visualizing ureteral calculi.[4] Stones may be seen within the renal parenchyma, at the ureteropelvic junction proximally, or at the ureterovesicular junction distally. In general, ureters are obscured by

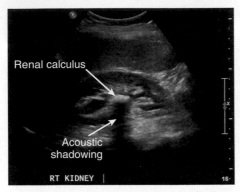

Figure 25.14 Renal Calculus. A large renal calculus with acoustic shadowing is seen in a longitudinal view of the kidney.

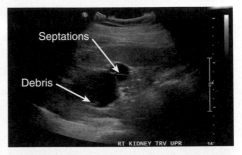

Figure 25.15 Large Complex Cyst. Complex cysts have a heterogeneous appearance with septations, calcifications, or debris.

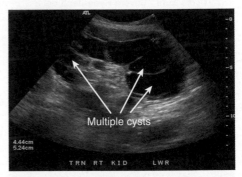

Figure 25.16 Polycystic Kidney Disease. The normal renal architecture is distorted by several cysts of varying sizes.

bowel gas and are difficult to assess as they travel from the kidney to the bladder. Stones are hyperechoic and exhibit acoustic shadowing (Fig. 25.14; Videos 25.14–25.16).

The severity of hydronephrosis may correlate with stone size.[8] Patients with renal colic and moderate or severe hydronephrosis are significantly more likely to have a stone >5 mm than patients with mild or no hydronephrosis.[8] Stones <5 mm generally pass without intervention and stones 5 to 9 mm may pass spontaneously, but stones >1 cm are unlikely to pass and will likely require urologic intervention.[14]

Renal Cyst

Renal cysts are common and usually benign (see Fig. 25.12 and Video 25.17), but renal malignancies may present as complex cysts. To be a benign cyst, all of the following criteria must be met[9]:
1. Thin-walled and smooth, with no septations, internal echoes, or solid elements
2. Round or oval shape that is well demarcated from the adjacent parenchyma and appears homogeneous in all imaging planes
3. Posterior acoustic enhancement must be evident behind the cyst.

If the above criteria are not fulfilled, the presence of a complex cyst (Fig. 25.15 and Video 25.18), renal abscess, or malignancy must be considered and warrants further workup.

Multiple renal cysts are seen in polycystic kidney disease (PCKD) and acquired renal cystic disease (ARCD). PCKD represents an extreme example on the spectrum of renal cystic disease (Fig. 25.16; Videos 25.19 and 25.20). PCKD is characterized by an abundance of irregular cysts of varying size that distort the normal renal architecture bilaterally. These patients often present to acute care settings with flank pain, hematuria, hypertension, and renal failure. ARCD is another condition associated with multiple renal cysts that is present in patients with end-stage renal disease on hemodialysis and is associated with higher risk of renal malignancy. Whereas most patients with chronic kidney disease have bilaterally shrunken and hyperechoic kidneys, those with ARCD have numerous cysts.

Renal Mass

Renal malignancies detected incidentally during abdominal imaging are associated with lower morbidity and mortality rates.[15] Any suspicious mass detected by POCUS warrants further investigation and expert consultation (Fig. 25.17; Videos 25.21 and 25.22).[15] Normal variants that can mimic renal malignancies include prominent columns of Bertin, which are hypertrophied cortical tissue that distort the calyces in the renal sinus (Fig. 25.18).

Renal cell carcinoma is the most common type of renal malignancy in adults. These tumors are notoriously heterogeneous in their sonographic appearance. They can be isoechoic, hypoechoic, or hyperechoic relative to adjacent parenchyma, and they may have a partial cystic appearance that can be mistaken for benign cysts (Videos 25.23 and 25.24). Angiomyolipoma is the most common type of benign tumor of the kidney. These tumors are well-demarcated, hyperechoic masses located within the renal cortex. There is significant overlap in the appearance of angiomyolipomas and echogenic renal cell carcinoma.[5] Therefore, providers using POCUS should obtain additional radiographic imaging and seek expert consultation when incidental masses are detected.

PEARLS AND PITFALLS

- When evaluating the kidneys with ultrasound, start by scanning the asymptomatic kidney to compare it to the symptomatic side.
- When an abnormal finding is suspected, it is imperative to tilt or fan the transducer in a longitudinal plane to evaluate the abnormal structure in multiple planes.
- A bladder ultrasound exam should accompany a renal ultrasound exam. A distended bladder due to bladder outlet obstruction may cause bilateral hydronephrosis, and a repeat renal ultrasound exam should be performed after bladder decompression.
- Hydronephrosis may be under recognized in hypovolemic patients due to transient collapse of the calyces. Reevaluate suspected hydronephrosis after fluid resuscitation in patients with volume depletion.
- Renal blood vessels can be misinterpreted as mild hydronephrosis where they enter and exit the renal sinus. Use color flow or power Doppler ultrasound to differentiate blood vessels from hydronephrosis.

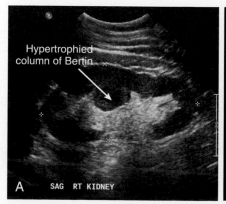

Figure 25.17 Renal Mass. A large, irregularly-shaped renal mass with heterogeneous echogenicity is seen that was diagnosed as renal cell carcinoma after further workup.

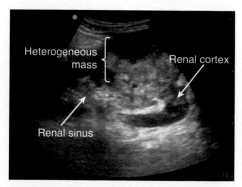
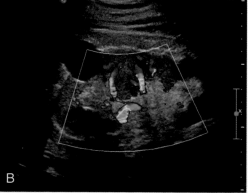

Figure 25.18 Hypertrophied Column of Bertin. Normal cortical tissue protruding into the sinus is seen with two-dimensional imaging (A), and absence of hypervascularity by color flow Doppler confirms this tissue to be a column of Bertin (B). Note the simple cortical cyst.

- Varying degrees of hydronephrosis, most often on the right side, is common in pregnancy and may not be pathologic.
- Unilateral hydronephrosis may be due to external ureteral compression by a mass, retroperitoneal lymphadenopathy, or an obstructing renal calculus.
- Absence of hydronephrosis does not rule out ureterolithiasis because small calculi may not create significant obstruction.
- Renal calculi are common and detection of a nonobstructing parenchymal stone may be unrelated to the patient's clinical presentation.
- All renal masses are malignant until proven otherwise. Detection of a renal mass by point-of-care ultrasound requires further workup with additional radiographic imaging.

Bladder

Behzad Hassani

Background

Bedside ultrasound evaluation of the bladder has several clinical applications. Estimation of bladder volume, confirmation of proper urinary catheter placement, detection of stones, and assessment of ureteral jets in suspected obstructive uropathy are the core indications for point-of-care bladder ultrasound.

Many patients who present with a complaint of urinary retention do not truly have urinary retention.[1] Evaluation of bladder volume based on physical exam is inaccurate in a significant percentage of patients due to body habitus. Bladder ultrasound can precisely determine bladder volume and avoid unnecessary urinary catheterization. When urinary catheterization is necessary, bedside ultrasound can confirm proper placement and functioning of the catheter. In pediatric patients, bladder volume estimation can eliminate unnecessary catheterization,[2] and real-time ultrasound guidance can reduce complications associated with suprapubic bladder aspiration.[3]

Normal Anatomy

The bladder is a triangular organ that is positioned directly posterior and inferior to the pubic symphysis (Fig. 26.1). Ureters enter the trigone of the bladder posteriorly and inferiorly (Fig. 26.2). In males, the prostate encircles the bladder neck caudally and normally measures less than 5 cm in transverse diameter.

Image Acquisition

A curvilinear transducer (3.0–5.0 MHz) is ideal for imaging the bladder. Its mid-range frequency allows for optimal penetration and resolution, and its wider footprint permits visualization of the entire bladder. A fluid-filled bladder readily propagates sound waves, resulting in posterior acoustic enhancement, or hyperechogenicity deep to the bladder. The far-field gain should be decreased to better visualize hypoechoic or anechoic entities deep to the bladder, such as pelvic free fluid.[4]

The bladder is best visualized from a suprapubic approach. With the patient in a supine position, place the transducer in a transverse plane at the superior edge of the pubic symphysis and aim the ultrasound beam caudally (Fig. 26.3A and Video 26.1). Tilt the transducer cranially and caudally to visualize the entire bladder in a transverse plane. Assess the bladder for its degree of distention and for the presence of stones or masses. If the bladder is not filled, the transducer often has to be pointed caudally into the pelvic cavity

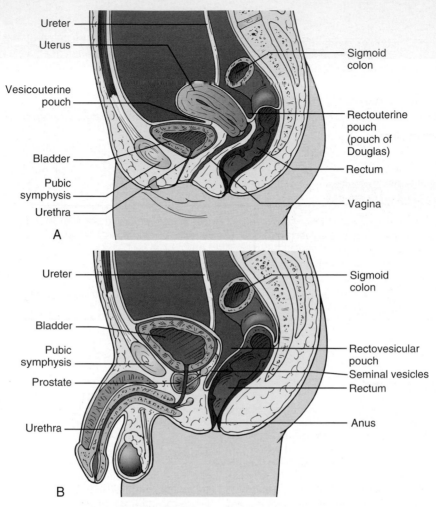

Figure 26.1 Normal Anatomy of the Bladder in a Sagittal Plane. (A) Female pelvis. (B) Male pelvis.

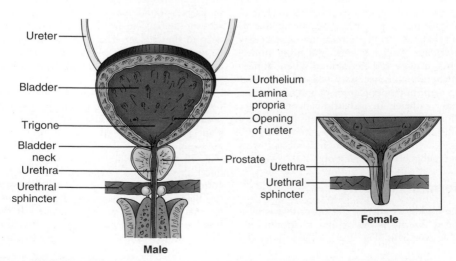

Figure 26.2 Normal Anatomy of the Male and Female Bladder in a Transverse Plane.

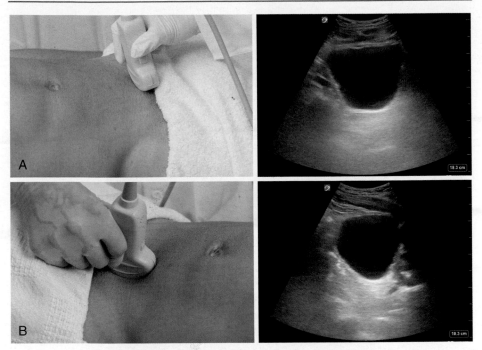

Figure 26.3 Transducer Position. (A) The transducer is placed over the bladder in a transverse plane and tilted caudally to obtain a transverse view. (B) Transducer position to obtain a sagittal view of the bladder.

to identify the bladder. The prostate gland is hyperechoic and can be visualized in a transverse plane deep to the inferior bladder wall. Rotate the transducer 90 degrees clockwise to obtain a longitudinal view of the bladder in a sagittal plane (see Fig. 26.3B and Video 26.2). Scan the bladder thoroughly in a sagittal plane by tilting the transducer to visualize the leftmost and rightmost walls.

In patients with renal colic, visualization of a ureteral jet, or intermittent expression of urine into the bladder, rules out complete obstruction of a ureter. To visualize ureteral jets, scan slowly through the bladder in a transverse plane and focus over the trigone.[4-6] Ureteral jets are best visualized with color flow or power Doppler on a low-flow setting (i.e., low PRF setting). Power Doppler is particularly suited for detecting low-flow states, including ureteral jets. The jets appear as colorful emissions streaming from the base of the bladder toward its center (Fig. 26.4; Videos 26.3 and 26.4). In well-hydrated patients, they appear at regular intervals every 15 to 20 seconds and last less than 1 second.[7] The presence of bilateral ureteral jets in a well-hydrated patient rules out significant obstructive uropathy with high

specificity.[8,9] Ureteral obstruction is suspected when a jet is not visualized on the affected side but is visualized unilaterally on the unaffected side.

Pathologic Findings

URINARY RETENTION

Bladder volume can be estimated using the following formula[10,11]:

$$Bladder\ volume = (0.75 \times width \times length \times height)$$

From a transverse view, the width and anteroposterior dimension (i.e., length) are measured, and from a sagittal view, the superior-inferior dimension (i.e., height) is measured (Fig. 26.5). Past research has demonstrated close correlation between the estimated bladder volume using the above formula and the actual catheterized volume (correlation factor = 0.983).[10] Most point-of-care machines are equipped with built-in functionality to calculate the bladder volume based on the dimensions above.

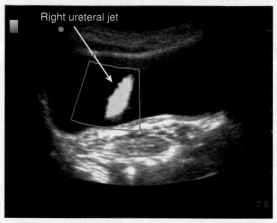

Figure 26.4   Ureteral Jet. A prominent right-sided ureteral jet is seen using power Doppler originating in a transverse view of the bladder.

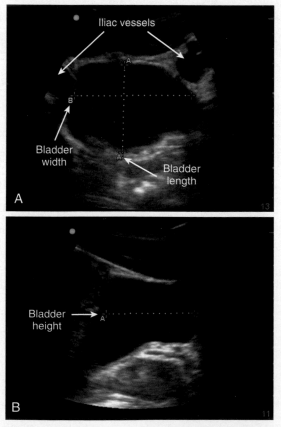

Figure 26.5   Bladder Volume Measurement. (A) Measure the width *(W)* and length *(L)* of the bladder in a transverse plane. (B) Measure the height *(H)* of the bladder in a sagittal plane. Bladder volume is calculated using the following formula: Volume = 0.75 × *W* × *L* × *H*.

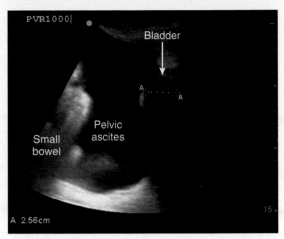

Figure 26.6   Bladder Scanner Error. A bladder scanner cannot differentiate pelvic ascites from urine in the bladder. Only a small amount of urine is present in the bladder, as seen here in a longitudinal view, but the bladder scanner erroneously measured greater than 1 L in this patient.

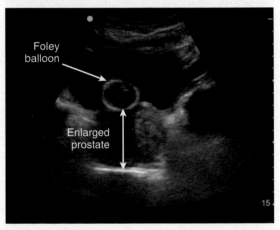

Figure 26.7   Prostatic Hypertrophy. An enlarged prostate gland and bladder with urinary catheter are seen in a transverse view.

It is important to recognize that bladder scanners commonly used to assess bladder volume cannot differentiate pelvic ascites from urine within the bladder. Therefore point-of-care ultrasound should be used to accurately assess bladder volume in patients with ascites (Fig. 26.6).

A qualitative assessment of bladder distention can be performed by noting the location of the bladder dome relative to the umbilicus.[1] Center the bladder dome on the screen in a sagittal plane. The center of the transducer on the skin identifies the location of the dome relative to the umbilicus. The bladder dome extends at least halfway to the umbilicus in the majority of patients with urinary retention (Video 26.5).[1] The presence of urinary retention should prompt a scan of the kidneys to rule out bilateral hydronephrosis (see Chapter 25), a finding that has prognostic implications in the setting of chronic outlet obstruction.

Although bedside transabdominal ultrasound can readily detect prostatic hypertrophy (transverse diameter >5 cm), it cannot distinguish benign hypertrophy from malignancy (Fig. 26.7 and Video 26.6). If clinically indicated, urology consultation and transrectal ultrasound imaging with biopsy may be pursued.

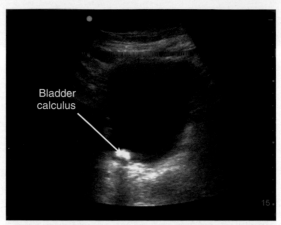

Figure 26.8   Bladder Calculus. A hyperechoic calculus with prominent posterior shadowing is seen in the bladder in a transverse view.

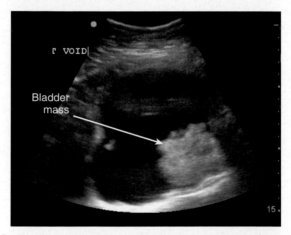

Figure 26.9   Bladder Mass. A large intraluminal bladder mass is seen in a transverse view.

URINARY CATHETER PLACEMENT

Appropriate placement of a urinary catheter in the bladder lumen can be confirmed using ultrasound (Video 26.7). If urine output is low after properly placing a urinary catheter, catheter malfunction can be detected if a large residual volume of urine is visualized (Video 26.8), as well as debris or blood clots that may be obstructing the catheter (Videos 26.9 and Video 26.10).

BLADDER STONES

Bladder calculi are most often seen after successful passage of renal calculi from the ureters into the bladder. Bladder stones may also form de novo secondary to bladder stasis in patients with chronic retention.[4] Bladder stones appear as hyperechoic, mobile entities that demonstrate posterior acoustic shadowing (Fig. 26.8 and Video 26.11).

BLADDER MASS

Bladder masses typically appear either as irregular, echogenic projections from the bladder wall or as foci of increased bladder wall thickness (Fig. 26.9 and Video 26.12).[4-6] Transitional cell carcinoma accounts for the majority of bladder masses. The differential diagnosis of a bladder mass includes malignancy, bladder diverticula, congenital outpouchings of the bladder wall, and bladder wall thickening due to chronic or recurrent cystitis. The bladder wall is normally 3 to 6 mm thick but varies depending on the degree of bladder filling (Video 26.13). Blood clots can be mistaken for a bladder mass, and repeat ultrasound should be performed after adequate continuous bladder irrigation (Video 26.14). Additional imaging and expert consultation are always warranted to further evaluate bladder masses.

PEARLS AND PITFALLS

- To calculate bladder volume accurately, the maximum dimensions should be captured by freezing the image while tilting or fanning the transducer through the bladder. Use the following formula: Bladder volume = (0.75 × width × length × height).
- Free fluid in the pelvis can easily be mistaken for urine in the bladder. Always scan the bladder and surrounding tissues thoroughly in transverse and longitudinal planes. Filling the bladder or identifying an inflated urinary catheter balloon can help distinguish the bladder from pelvic free fluid (Video 26.15).
- Ureteral jets may be infrequent or not visualized in patients due to operator error. Although their presence rules out complete obstruction with high specificity, their absence by ultrasound imaging does not rule in obstructive uropathy.
- Confirmation of proper urinary catheter placement and detection of catheter malfunction are easily accomplished using ultrasound at the bedside.
- Blood clots may appear as bladder masses on ultrasound. Continuous bladder irrigation usually resolves blood clots and afterwards, a thorough investigation can be conducted to evaluate for a mass.

CHAPTER 27

Gallbladder

Daniel R. Peterson

KEY POINTS

- Image acquisition of the gallbladder can be challenging due to variability of gallbladder shape, size, and position.
- Point-of-care ultrasound can detect gallstones, a thickened gallbladder wall, pericholecystic fluid, and a sonographic Murphy's sign to assist in diagnosis of acute cholecystitis.
- A complete biliary ultrasound exam includes measurement of the common bile duct diameter, although a diagnosis of acute cholecystitis can be made without its measurement.

Background

Gallbladder disease is a concern for health care providers from all medical specialties. Disease severity ranges from asymptomatic cholelithiasis to acute cholecystitis to ascending cholangitis. Point-of-care ultrasound (POCUS) is a valuable tool for evaluating patients with right upper quadrant abdominal pain suspicious for gallbladder disease. Advantages of POCUS include avoidance of ionizing radiation, rapid performance, availability in many clinical settings, high sensitivity and specificity for gallbladder disease, and potential reduction in length of stay and cost savings.[1-5]

Several studies have shown that diagnostic accuracy is comparable when a focused gallbladder ultrasound exam is performed by a non-radiologist compared to a comprehensive gallbladder ultrasound exam performed in a radiology suite.[6-10] A recent systematic review found that emergency physician (EP)-performed ultrasound exams for symptomatic cholelithiasis had a sensitivity of 89.8% and a specificity of 88.0%.[5] Furthermore, training of novices to perform limited, point-of-care gallbladder ultrasound exams has been shown to have a steep learning curve with competence attainable without requiring extensive training.[11]

The most important positive findings when performing a point-of-care gallbladder and biliary ultrasound exam are:
- Cholelithiasis
- Sonographic Murphy's sign
- Gallbladder wall thickening
- Pericholecystic fluid
- Common bile duct (CBD) dilation

The presence or absence of gallstones is the first and most important ultrasound finding. Acalculous cholecystitis is uncommon overall but should be considered in hospitalized patients with critical illness. Sonographic Murphy's sign, gallbladder wall thickening, and pericholecystic fluid are all ultrasound features of acute cholecystitis and can be readily detected with POCUS. CBD assessment is technically the most difficult and time-consuming part of the exam. The utility of obtaining CBD measurements when performing point-of-care biliary ultrasound has been called into question in several studies. One retrospective review of 125 pathology-confirmed cases of cholecystitis revealed that all instances of CBD dilation were accompanied by one or more additional sonographic findings of cholecystitis: positive sonographic Murphy's sign, gallbladder wall thickening, pericholecystic fluid, or laboratory abnormalities.[12] A second retrospective review of 777 cases of cholelithiasis and choledocholithiasis showed that isolated CBD dilation without other ultrasound or laboratory abnormalities occurred in only 0.4% of cases.[13] These reviews suggest that CBD visualization confers little additional sensitivity to the point-of-care diagnosis of acute cholecystitis.

A recent study showed that a rapid ultrasound screening exam for gallstones may be sufficient to exclude cholecystitis. Among 164 patients with abdominal pain, the absence of gallstones had a negative predictive value of 100% (95% CI 92.2–100%).[14] Thus, experienced providers can rule out cholecystitis if no gallstones are visualized.

Normal Anatomy

The gallbladder is located in the right upper quadrant of the abdomen along the posterior, inferior edge of the liver (Fig. 27.1). It is pear-shaped and lies along the main lobar fissure between the right and left lobes of the liver. The fundus of the gallbladder is usually the most anterior and inferior structure and is often the first part of the gallbladder visualized with ultrasound. The fundus is continuous with the body and neck that tapers cranially and posteriorly to form the cystic duct (Fig. 27.2). The cystic duct joins the common hepatic duct from the liver to form the CBD.

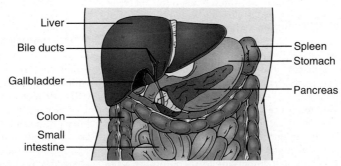

Figure 27.1   Right Upper Quadrant Anatomy. Anatomy of the gallbladder and right upper quadrant.

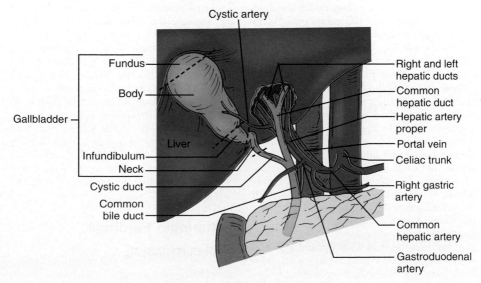

Figure 27.2   Gallbladder Anatomy.

The cystic duct is frequently not visualized with ultrasound and therefore the extrahepatic ductal system is often referred to as the CBD. The CBD continues to the head of the pancreas, where it enters the duodenum through the sphincter of Oddi.

Image Acquisition

Patients are generally in a supine position for most POCUS scanning, including the gallbladder exam. Certain maneuvers can help optimize gallbladder visualization when positioning conscious and cooperative patients. Instructing the patient to hold a deep breath often transiently descends the gallbladder inferiorly into the field of view, or having the patient distend or "puff out" their abdomen will often bring the gallbladder into view while allowing the patient to continue to breathe. Also, turning the patient to a left lateral decubitus position causes the liver and gallbladder to descend below the costal margin and shifts gas-filled loops of the small bowel, enhancing visualization of the gallbladder.

A curvilinear transducer (2 to 5 MHz) is typically used to image the gallbladder. A phased-array transducer may be used as well because its narrower footprint is ideal for imaging in between ribs. It important to use an abdominal exam preset to optimize image resolution. As with all ultrasound scanning, lower frequencies allow deeper penetration into the body, but lower frequencies also have lower resolution. Using the highest possible frequency that provides adequate penetration will maximize resolution when assessing for signs of gallbladder disease.

Start by placing the transducer along the inferior border of the costal margin lateral to the midline on the patient's right side with the transducer marker pointing toward the patient's head. Rock the transducer slightly cephalad (Fig. 27.3). Next, slide the transducer laterally and inferiorly along the costal margin until the gallbladder comes into view. The gallbladder will appear as a hypoechoic oblong or circular structure. Rotate and tilt the transducer with fine movements until the gallbladder is seen along its true long axis. In a longitudinal plane (long-axis view), the relationship between the thick-walled portal vein and gallbladder is often viewed as an "exclamation point" with the hyperechoic main lobar fissure connecting the two structures (Fig. 27.4).

The gallbladder should also be viewed in a transverse plane (short-axis view) by rotating the transducer 90 degrees counterclockwise from the longitudinal plane with the transducer marker pointing to the patient's right (Fig. 27.5). Viewed in a transverse orientation, the gallbladder has a circular shape (Fig. 27.6). It is important to sweep through the entire gallbladder in both transverse and longitudinal planes to ensure complete visualization.

The gallbladder may also be visualized between the ribs of the right anteroinferior chest wall when it is difficult to visualize the gallbladder as previously described. The narrower footprint of a phased-array transducer may be preferred for intercostal imaging to minimize rib shadows. Place the transducer on the right lateral chest wall, in the midaxillary line. From the lateral chest wall, slide the transducer medially between the ribs to first identify the gallbladder and then visualize it in different planes. One limitation of intercostal imaging of the gallbladder is the inability to assess for sonographic Murphy's sign.

Measuring CBD diameter is the most challenging and time-consuming aspect of a point-of-care biliary ultrasound exam as it requires significant training and practice to become proficient. Although its value in diagnosing acute cholecystitis has been challenged (see Background), providers frequently elect to obtain CBD measurements when performing a biliary ultrasound exam. Viewing the gallbladder in a longitudinal plane is helpful to locate and measure the CBD because the CBD is located just anterior to the portal vein (Video 27.1). The portal triad is the area containing the portal vein, CBD, and hepatic artery and is commonly called the "Mickey Mouse" sign (Fig. 27.7). Using the zoom function and color-flow or power Doppler can help distinguish the CBD from the portal vein and hepatic artery. The diameter of the CBD is measured from inner wall to inner wall in either a transverse or longitudinal plane at the point where the hepatic artery courses between the portal vein and CBD, and is normally <6 mm (Fig. 27.8 and Video 27.2).

Pathologic Findings

CHOLELITHIASIS

Gallbladder stones are echogenic, usually mobile structures within the gallbladder that

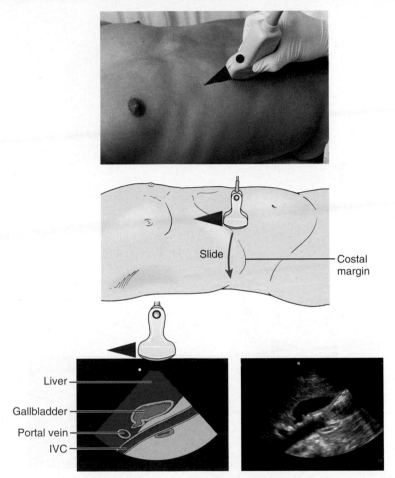

Figure 27.3 Transducer Position for Scanning the Gallbladder in a Longitudinal (Long-Axis) Plane. *IVC,* Inferior vena cava.

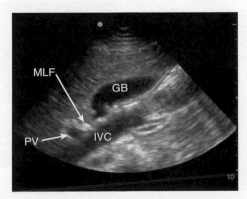

Figure 27.4 Longitudinal (Long-Axis) View of Gallbladder *(GB)*. *IVC,* Inferior vena cava; *MLF,* main lobar fissure; *PV,* portal vein.

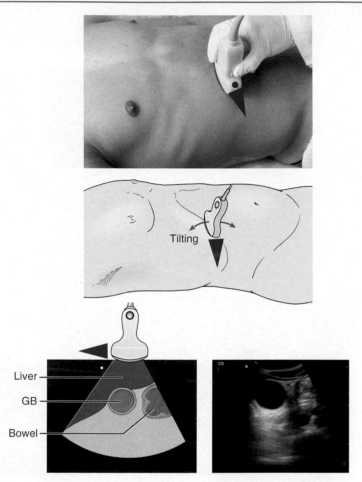

Figure 27.5 Transducer Position for Scanning the Gallbladder *(GB)* in a Transverse (Short-Axis) Plane.

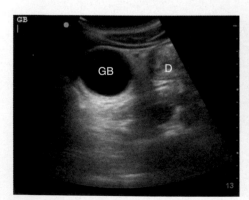

Figure 27.6 Transverse (Short-Axis) View of Gallbladder *(GB)*. *D,* Duodenum.

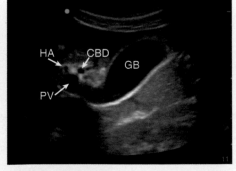

Figure 27.7 Portal Triad in a Transverse Plane With the Gallbladder in a Longitudinal Plane. *CBD,* Common bile duct; *GB,* gallbladder; *HA,* hepatic artery; *PV,* portal vein.

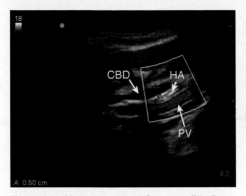

Figure 27.8 Measurement of Common Bile Duct. Color flow Doppler of the portal triad in a longitudinal plane distinguishes the common bile duct *(CBD)* from the hepatic artery *(HA)* and portal vein *(PV)*.

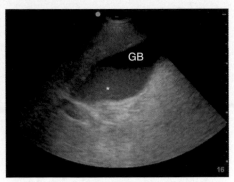

Figure 27.10 Gallbladder Sludge. Biliary sludge *(asterisk)* layering in a gallbladder *(GB)*.

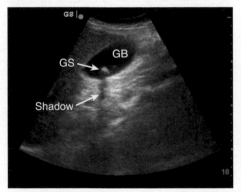

Figure 27.9 Gallstone. A single gallstone *(GS)* within the gallbladder *(GB)* with acoustic shadowing.

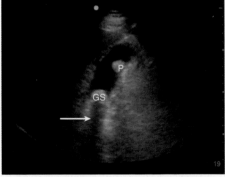

Figure 27.11 Gallbladder Polyp vs. Stone. A polyp *(P)* is seen in the body and a lodged stone *(GS)* in the neck of the gallbladder. Only the stone casts a shadow *(arrow)*.

cast a prominent shadow (Fig. 27.9 and Video 27.3). Stones may be single or multiple and vary considerably in size. Stones in the neck of the gallbladder are less likely to be mobile and more likely to cause symptoms. A gallbladder full of gallstones may only be visualized as an echogenic line with shadowing in the right upper quadrant (wall-echo-shadow sign) (Video 27.4).

Several findings can be mistaken for gallstones, and the two most common findings similar to gallstones are discussed here. Gallbladder sludge is dependent material of variable echogenicity (Fig. 27.10 and Video 27.5). Occasionally, sludge forms into discrete circular structures called tumefactive sludge that can resemble gallstones. An important finding of tumefactive sludge compared to gallstones is the absence of a shadow. It is possible, however, for biliary sludge to cause obstruction and acute cholecystitis. Gallbladder polyps are benign small nodular structures adherent to the gallbladder wall that can be distinguished from gallstones because they are neither mobile nor cast a shadow (Fig. 27.11 and Video 27.6).

ACUTE CHOLECYSTITIS

Cholecystitis is an inflammation of the gall-bladder wall most frequently caused by cystic duct obstruction by a gallstone. The key findings are presence of gallstones, sonographic Murphy's sign, gallbladder wall thickening, and pericholecystic fluid. These findings may present alone or in various combinations, and when considered along with abnormal laboratory findings, a diagnosis of acute cholecystitis can be made.

A sonographic Murphy's sign is elicited by placing pressure with the ultrasound transducer directly over the most anterior portion of the gallbladder. Maximal tenderness directly over the gallbladder compared to other regions of the right upper quadrant is highly predictive of cholecystitis. The combination of gallstones with a positive sonographic Murphy's sign has a positive predictive value >90% for cholecystitis, whereas absence of gallstones with a negative sonographic Murphy's sign has a negative predictive value of 95%.[15]

The gallbladder wall is considered normal if it is ≤3 mm thick. Wall thickness >3 mm is most commonly due to cholecystitis (Fig. 27.12 and Video 27.7).[16] However, false positives for a thickened gallbladder wall include ascites (Video 27.8), congestive heart failure, hepatitis, pancreatitis, hypoalbuminemia, adenomyomatosis, and a nonfasted state (i.e., the gallbladder contracts and wall thickness measurement is not as reliable). It is important to measure wall thickness at the most anterior portion of the gallbladder because acoustic enhancement

of the posterior wall may result in falsely elevated measurements.

Pericholecystic fluid is a feature of cholecystitis in which localized fluid collections are observed adjacent to the gallbladder (Fig. 27.13 and Video 27.9). Careful examination of pericholecystic fluid is warranted to ensure the fluid is not contiguous with the peritoneum as seen with ascites. Edge artifacts, common in biliary ultrasound, represent areas of ultrasound dropout along the curved edge of circular structures and should not be confused with fluid or stones (Fig. 27.14). A ruptured gallbladder presents a challenge because fluid may be observed in the right upper quadrant without identification of the gallbladder.

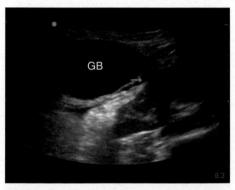

Figure 27.13 Pericholecystic Fluid. Pericholecystic fluid *(arrow)* seen immediately adjacent to the gallbladder *(GB)*.

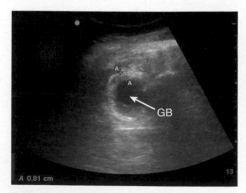

Figure 27.12 Thickened Gallbladder Wall. Gallbladde wall thickening (8.1 mm, normal is ≤3 mm) as seen from a transverse view. *GB*, Gallbladder.

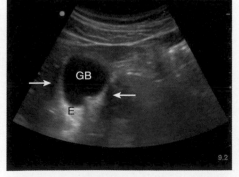

Figure 27.14 Gallbladder Artifacts. Posterior acoustic enhancement *(E)* and edge artifacts *(arrows)* are seen. *GB*, gallbladder.

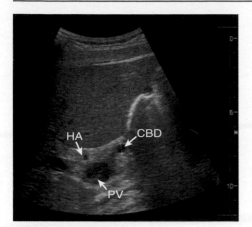

Figure 27.15 Dilated Common Bile Duct *(CBD)*. Short-axis view of the portal triad shows dilated common bile duct CBD (8.4 mm, normal <6 mm). *HA,* Hepatic artery; *PV,* portal vein.

DILATED CBD

Gallstones may also be present in the CBD, termed choledocholithiasis. These stones have either passed through the cystic duct from the gallbladder and became lodged in the CBD or formed in the CBD de novo. Just as with gallbladder stones, they become symptomatic when the stones cause obstruction, resulting in dilation of the CBD and inflammation of the gallbladder. This process can occur in patients after cholecystectomy and can present as acute cholangitis. Thus, measuring the CBD diameter in patients with suspected choledocholithiasis, whether they have a gallbladder or not, is part of a complete biliary ultrasound exam.

The inner diameter of the CBD is considered normal when <6 mm. Obstruction is usually caused by choledocholithiasis or a pancreatic mass and is evidenced by a dilated CBD (Fig. 27.15 and Video 27.2). The upper limit of normal for CBD diameter increases with age; each decade adds a millimeter to the upper limit of normal (e.g., an 8 mm CBD may be normal in an 80-year-old). Patients who are post-cholecystectomy may also have a dilated CBD (up to 10 mm), as it serves as the reservoir for bile.

Acalculous cholecystitis is a less common clinical entity that is characteristically found in critically ill patients in the intensive care unit. It has all the features of acute calculous cholecystitis (positive sonographic Murphy's sign, increased wall thickness, pericholecystic fluid, and a potentially dilated CBD) but without evidence of gallstones.

> **PEARLS AND PITFALLS**
>
> - Techniques to facilitate identification of the gallbladder include:
>   - Patient breathing: Requesting the patient to hold a deep breath or having the patient distend their abdomen often shifts the gallbladder inferiorly into the field of view.
>   - Patient positioning: Moving the patient into a left lateral decubitus position often facilitates visualization of the gallbladder. The liver and gallbladder slide below the costal margin, and gas-filled loops of bowel tend to move aside.
>   - Fasting: If the patient has recently eaten, the gallbladder may be contracted and empty of bile, making it difficult to visualize. If possible, wait several hours and repeat the bedside ultrasound exam with the patient in a fasted state.
>   - Intercostal approach: If the gallbladder cannot be visualized from an infracostal approach due to bowel gas or an elevated hemidiaphragm, an intercostal approach can be used. Place the transducer over the inferior most intercostal space in the midaxillary line and slide the transducer medially until the gallbladder is seen.
> - Recognition of gallstones
>   - Common false positives for gallstones include gallbladder polyps and tumefactive sludge, neither of which cast shadows. Recognition of these mimics can prevent a false-positive diagnosis of cholecystitis.
>   - Small gallstones are more likely to lodge in the neck of the gallbladder and cause cholecystitis than large stones. A shadow may be the only clue to a small, lodged stone.
> - Identification of the common bile duct
>   - Zoom in to the portal triad, and use color flow or power Doppler to help

distinguish the CBD from the portal vein and hepatic artery.
- Fluid in the right upper quadrant
  - Ascites is often visualized in the right upper quadrant, which can mimic pericholecystic fluid and cause thickening of the gallbladder wall.

- Artifacts
  - Edge artifact can be mistaken for pericholecystic fluid or stones.
  - Posterior acoustic enhancement can falsely increase measurement of gallbladder wall thickness, and wall thickness should only be measured of the anterior wall.

CHAPTER 28

Abdominal Aorta

Christopher R. Tainter ■ Gabriel Wardi

KEY POINTS

- Ultrasound is the preferred initial imaging modality for abdominal aortic aneurysm.
- The abdominal aorta should be imaged in two perpendicular planes (transverse and longitudinal) to avoid missing subtle abnormalities. Off-axis imaging can underestimate or overestimate aortic diameter and should be avoided.
- The presence of an intimal flap in the abdominal aorta has a high specificity for thoracic aortic dissection.

Background

The abdominal aorta is a vital retroperitoneal structure with the potential for catastrophic pathology that is often difficult to diagnose. In the words of Sir William Osler, "There is no disease more conducive to clinical humility than aneurysm of the aorta." When a diagnosis of aortic pathology is identified, prompt interventions can improve outcomes for this often time-sensitive presentation.[1]

Abdominal aortic aneurysm (AAA) is the most common aortic abnormality. It may be complicated by thrombosis, dissection of the intimal layer, or rupture, which carries a particularly high mortality of approximately 90%.[2-4] The incidence of AAA increases with age, family history, male gender, peripheral vascular disease, and a history of smoking.[5] The overall prevalence is approximately 4.7% and 3.0% in men and women, respectively,[6] and peak prevalence is 5.9% in men 80 to 85 years old and 4.5% in women greater than 90 years old.[7] Aortic aneurysms account for approximately 15,000 deaths per year in the United States; of these deaths, 9000 are attributable to AAAs. The majority of these deaths occur in men older than 65,[8] with AAAs representing the 15th leading cause of death in Americans between the ages of 60 and 64.[9]

Aortic pathology should be considered in any patient presenting with abdominal discomfort, especially those with known risk factors, classic histories, or exam findings (hypotension, back pain, pulsatile abdominal mass).[5] Of those with ruptured AAAs, it is estimated that nearly 30% were initially misdiagnosed.[3,4] In addition, various recommendations have been made for screening asymptomatic patients, including a grade B recommendation by the US Preventive Services Task Force, which recommends screening all men between the ages of 65 and 75 with a history of smoking.[8]

Use of point-of-care ultrasound is a well-accepted imaging modality to detect and measure AAA.[1] Point-of-care ultrasound has demonstrated high sensitivity (97.5%-100%) and specificity (94.1%-100%) for detection of AAA.[10,11] Aortic diameter measured by point-of-care ultrasound has a strong correlation with measurements by computed tomography (CT), but may slightly underestimate the exact diameter by 2 mm.[1,12]

Normal Anatomy

The abdominal aorta is a retroperitoneal structure that extends from the posterior diaphragm at the 12th thoracic vertebral body where it exits from the thoracic cavity and continues until it bifurcates into the left and right common iliac arteries at the level of the 4th lumbar vertebral body. The normal diameter of

255

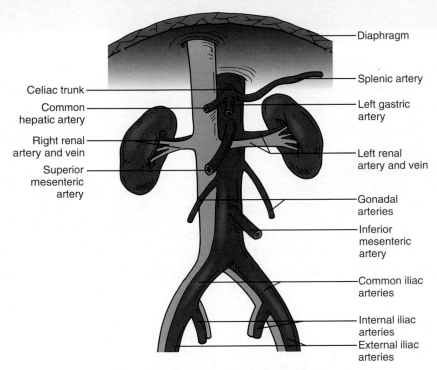

Diaphragm

Splenic artery

Celiac trunk

Common hepatic artery

Left gastric artery

Right renal artery and vein

Superior mesenteric artery

Left renal artery and vein

Gonadal arteries

Inferior mesenteric artery

Common iliac arteries

Internal iliac arteries

External iliac arteries

Figure 28.1   Anatomy of the Abdominal Aorta.

the adult infra-renal aorta is around 2 cm, and a measured diameter greater than 3.0 cm is considered aneurysmal (see the section, "Image Interpretation" below). Descending through the abdomen, the abdominal aorta's major branches include the celiac trunk, superior mesenteric artery, left and right renal arteries, inferior mesenteric artery, and gonadal arteries (Fig. 28.1). Small aortic branches supply the diaphragm, adrenal glands, abdominal wall, and spinal cord.

Image Acquisition

Sonographic visualization of the abdominal aorta is performed using a transabdominal approach to acquire transverse and longitudinal views. Start with the proximal aorta by placing a phased-array or curvilinear transducer (3.5–5 MHz) just below the costal margin in the center of the abdomen with the transducer marker pointing to the patient's right (Fig. 28.2 and Video 28.1). To find the aorta, the spine is a useful landmark. The aorta lies just anterior to the spine, slightly to the left of the midline. The first two major branches of the proximal

aorta are the celiac trunk (Video 28.2) and superior mesenteric artery (Video 28.3). Evaluation of these branches is typically less important when assessing for the simple presence or absence of an AAA, but their identification provides useful landmarks.

Once the aorta is identified in a transverse plane, slide the transducer inferiorly on the abdominal wall, allowing for contiguous imaging of the aorta. With the transducer in a transverse position just above the umbilicus with the ultrasound beam directed posteriorly, the distal aorta is visualized as it divides into the left and right common iliac arteries (Fig. 28.3 and Video 28.4).

After evaluating the aorta in a transverse plane, longitudinal views should be acquired to accurately assess the size of the aorta. Place the transducer over the proximal abdominal aorta, and rotate the transducer clockwise 90 degrees so that the transducer marker ("notch") is pointed toward the patient's head. The celiac trunk and superior mesenteric artery may be visualized when the plane of the ultrasound beam is aligned with these vessels (Fig. 28.4 and Video 28.5).

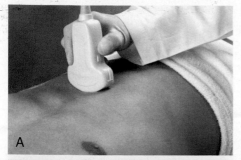

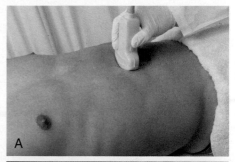

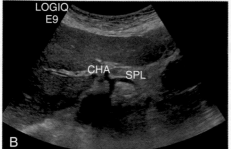

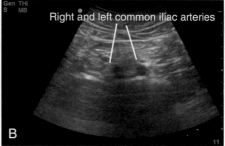

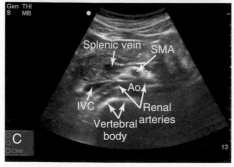

Figure 28.3 Distal Aorta (Transverse View). (A) Transducer position for transverse (short-axis) views of the distal abdominal aorta. (B) Distal aorta is seen dividing into the right and left common iliac arteries from a transverse view.

Figure 28.2 Proximal Aorta (Transverse View). (A) Transducer position for transverse (short-axis) views of the proximal abdominal aorta. (B) Celiac trunk is seen branching into the common hepatic artery *(CHA)* and splenic artery *(SPL)*. (C) Superior mesenteric artery *(SMA)* is seen, along with the left and right renal arteries, branching from the aorta *(Ao)*. Note the position of the splenic vein and inferior vena cava *(IVC)*. A vertebral body is seen posterior to the aorta.

Measurements of the aortic diameter should be obtained in both transverse and longitudinal planes. It is important to measure the aortic diameter with the transducer perpendicular to the aorta to capture a true cross-sectional image because oblique images can underestimate or overestimate the diameter. The diameter of the aorta should be measured proximally and

distally with calipers placed on the outer edges of the aortic walls (Fig. 28.5).

If interpretable images cannot be obtained in the anterior upper abdomen, usually due to bowel gas, drains, or scarring, then an alternate approach is to image the aorta laterally from the left or right flank. With the transducer marker pointing toward the patient's head, place the transducer on the right or left mid-axillary line just below the costal margin to capture longitudinal views of the aorta. Using the spleen as an acoustic window, or presence of ascites or left pleural effusion, can facilitate visualization of the aorta from the left flank (Fig. 28.6 and Video 28.6). From the right flank, a longitudinal view of two tubular, anechoic structures is seen posterior to the liver at the bottom of the image; the near-field structure is the inferior vena cava, and the deeper structure is the abdominal aorta (Fig. 28.7 and Video 28.7). The transducer can be rotated 90 degrees clockwise to obtain transverse views of the aorta, but acquiring transverse images laterally can be challenging due to the depth of the aorta.

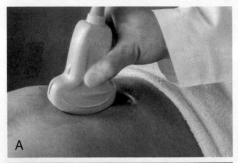

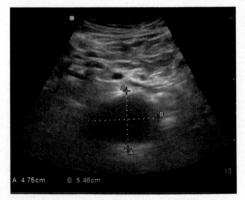

Figure 28.4 Proximal Aorta (Lonitudinal View).
(A) Transducer position for longitudinal views of
the proximal abdominal aorta. (B) Proximal aorta is
seen in a longitudinal plane branching into the celiac
artery and superior mesenteric artery *(SMA)*. The
splenic vein is seen in transverse cross-section as
it crosses over the SMA.

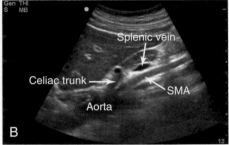

Figure 28.5 Measurement of the Aorta. Calipers
are placed from outer wall to outer wall on the
abdominal aorta to measure its anterior-posterior
and transverse diameters.

If these alternative imaging planes of the
aorta are not possible, there are two techniques
to overcome the obscuration by gas-filled
loops of bowel: (1) repeating the transabdominal study after a time delay may be effective

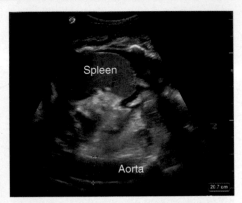

**Figure 28.6 Left Lateral View of the Abdominal
Aorta.** A longitudinal view of the abdominal aorta is
seen from the left flank. The spleen is used as the
acoustic window.

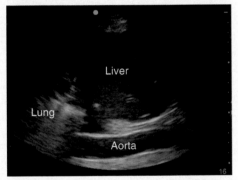

**Figure 28.7 Right Lateral View of the Abdominal
Aorta.** A longitudinal view of the abdominal aorta is
seen from the right flank. The liver is used as the
acoustic window.

in stable patients as the bowels naturally shift
over time; (2) applying firm pressure with the
transducer on the abdominal wall can manually displace loops of bowel.

Image Interpretation

ABDOMINAL AORTIC ANEURYSM

An arterial aneurysm is defined as a permanent full-thickness dilation of an artery having
at least 50% increase in diameter compared
to the expected normal diameter of the artery
in question.[13] For the abdominal aorta, a
diameter greater than 3.0 cm is considered
aneurysmal by convention, and most AAAs
are fusiform rather than saccular. An AAA

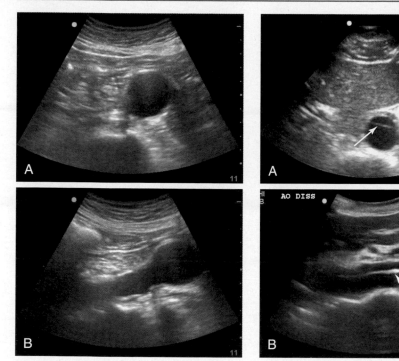

Figure 28.8 Abdominal Aortic Aneurysm. A distal abdominal aortic aneurysm is seen in transverse (A) and longitudinal (B) planes.

Figure 28.9 Abdominal Aortic Dissection. An abdominal aortic dissection with an intimal flap *(arrow)* is seen in transverse (A) and longitudinal (B) planes.

should be imaged in both transverse and longitudinal planes (Fig. 28.8; Videos 28.8 and 28.9).

The rupture risk is directly related to the size of the aneurysm. Small dilations are of less immediate clinical significance, but identification remains important, as these aneurysms should be referred to a vascular surgeon at the time of diagnosis. Shorter surveillance intervals are recommended for larger aneurysms: 12 months for an aortic diameter of 4.0 to 4.9 cm and 6 months for 5.0 to 5.4 cm. Aneurysms with a diameter greater than 5.5 cm should undergo elective repair in patients with acceptable surgical risk.[1] In a patient with acute abdominal or flank pain suspected to be due to an AAA, providers should obtain emergent vascular surgery consultation and/or CT imaging.

AORTIC DISSECTION

Aortic dissection originates from either the ascending (type A) or descending (type B)

thoracic aorta, and can extend distally to the abdominal aorta. Transesophageal echocardiography (TEE) and CT angiography of the aorta remained the preferred modalities to evaluate for thoracic aortic dissection. Although transthoracic echocardiography (TTE) may detect thoracic aortic dissection, its precise role is less well established. Estimates of sensitivity of TTE to diagnose thoracic aortic dissection ranges from 67% to 80%,[14,15] but the presence of an undulating intimal flap portends a very high specificity, approaching 100% (Video 28.10). If there is clinical suspicion of a thoracic aortic dissection and TTE does not confirm the diagnosis, additional testing with either TEE or CT angiography should be pursued to confirm or refute the diagnosis. TEE is one of the preferred modalities to detect a thoracic aortic dissection when trained providers are available (Video 28.11).

An aortic dissection extending to the abdominal aorta can be detected by point-of-care ultrasound when an intimal flap in visualized (Fig. 28.9; Videos 28.12 and 28.13). Color flow

Doppler ultrasound can be used to evaluate a suspected intimal flap (Videos 28.14 and 28.15).

INTRA-AORTIC DEVICE PLACEMENT

Ultrasonography of the aorta can be used to guide placement and confirm the position of intra-aortic devices, including extracorporeal membrane oxygenation (ECMO) cannulas, resuscitative endovascular balloon occlusion of the aorta (REBOA) catheters, or intra-aortic balloon pumps (Video 28.16) (see Chapters 20 and 33).

PEARLS AND PITFALLS

- When the aorta is obscured by bowel gas, applying firm, constant pressure while rocking the transducer can help displace the loops of bowel. The curvilinear probe is particularly useful in this situation. In most cases, a few firm sweeps will displace the loops of bowel and permit visualization of the aorta.
- The aorta can be mistaken for adjacent structures, including the vertebral bodies, para-aortic lymph nodes, and inferior vena cava. The aorta should have pulsatile flow, which can be confirmed by using either color or spectral Doppler ultrasound. Most adjacent structures will not display flow by Doppler, except the inferior vena cava. The inferior vena cava can be differentiated from the aorta by its thin walls, position on the right side of the vertebral bodies, presence of respirophasic variation of flow, and identification of the celiac trunk and superior mesenteric artery arising from the aorta.
- Underestimation of the aortic diameter is more likely to occur in the presence of a mural thrombus, which can be confused with surrounding tissue. To avoid this error, it is important to take the most conservative estimates of aortic diameter by always measuring from the outermost portion of the walls.
- Diametric measurements taken across a cylinder are accurate only if they cross the center of the cylinder and are taken perpendicular to the lumen walls. Measurements between the lumen walls will underestimate the diameter if taken off-center of the cylinder in a longitudinal plane (see cylinder effect, Fig. 17.5), or overestimate the diameter if measured obliquely. In order to increase accuracy, the diameter should always be measured in both transverse and longitudinal planes.

CHAPTER 29

First-Trimester Pregnancy

Starr Knight ■ Nathan Teismann

KEY POINTS

- Point-of-care ultrasound using a transabdominal and transvaginal approach is routinely used to evaluate pregnant patients in the first trimester who are suspected of having an ectopic pregnancy.
- The combination of clinical history, physical examination, serum β-hCG level, and ultrasound findings allows providers to appropriately manage symptomatic first-trimester patients.
- Early pregnancy loss is a common finding in symptomatic first-trimester patients. Generally, this diagnosis should be confirmed by a comprehensive ultrasound exam before discussing treatment options with the patient.

Background

APPLICATIONS AND INDICATIONS

Point-of-care pelvic ultrasound is routinely performed in emergency departments (EDs) and obstetrical clinics for woman with symptoms of abdominal pain or vaginal bleeding in early pregnancy. In these cases, the main diagnostic considerations are (1) a currently viable intrauterine pregnancy (IUP), (2) a failed or nonviable IUP (miscarriage), or (3) an ectopic pregnancy. Along with the results of blood testing and a physical examination, the ultrasound findings are central to the accurate assessment of such patients. In patients not undergoing infertility treatment, the risk of heterotopic gestation is sufficiently low such that the identification of an IUP essentially excludes the diagnosis of ectopic pregnancy.[1]

Patients with an ectopic pregnancy most commonly present with unilateral lower abdominal pain in the first trimester. In cases where the ectopic pregnancy has ruptured, patients may present with acute, diffuse abdominal pain, syncope, hemodynamic instability, or shock. Ectopic pregnancy has been reported to occur in 2% of symptomatic first-trimester patients overall, but the prevalence is much higher in patients presenting to EDs, occurring in 8% to 10% of first-trimester patients.[2,3] In most cases where an ectopic pregnancy is evaluated by point-of-care ultrasound, the diagnosis is made indirectly based on the finding of an empty uterus along with a quantitative β-human chorionic gonadotropin (β-hCG) level above a discriminatory zone of 3000 mIU/mL.[4] However, some cases of ectopic pregnancy may be directly identified by visualization of an extrauterine gestational sac, adnexal ring sign, or extra-ovarian adnexal soft tissue mass. Although a ruptured corpus luteum cyst can cause significant intra-peritoneal bleeding, any pregnant patient in her first trimester with a nontrivial amount of free fluid in the abdomen or pelvis should be considered to have a ruptured ectopic pregnancy until proven otherwise.

LITERATURE REVIEW

Several studies have examined the diagnostic accuracy of point-of-care pelvic ultrasound and its utility in the evaluation of ectopic pregnancy. A 2010 meta-analysis showed that point-of-care pelvic ultrasound displayed excellent accuracy with a sensitivity of 99.3%, a negative predictive value of 99.9%, and a negative likelihood ratio of 0.08, supporting the common practice of using point-of-care pelvic ultrasound to screen patients to exclude ectopic pregnancy.[5] The specificity of ultrasound can vary depending on operator experience, equipment, and whether both transvaginal and transabdominal views are obtained.

Point-of-care ultrasound allows rapid evaluation of symptomatic patients and can be performed around-the-clock by trained providers. A national survey of diagnostic ultrasound usage in EDs revealed that patients with suspected ectopic pregnancy were 50% less likely to receive an ultrasound during evenings and weekends.[6] Furthermore, several studies have shown that the detection of an IUP on bedside ultrasound is associated with increased efficiency, as measured by decreased ED length of stay, especially during off hours.[7-9]

Finally, point-of-care ultrasound allows physicians to evaluate unstable patients rapidly, identify those with hemoperitoneum, and expedite care of those who require operative management for an ectopic pregnancy.[10]

Normal Anatomy

The uterus is a muscular organ that lies in the pelvis between the bladder and the rectum, measuring approximately 7 cm in length and 5 cm in width (Fig. 29.1). The cervix, or inferior portion of the uterus, protrudes into the vagina, and its long axis is generally angled anteriorly relative to the uterus. The part of the uterus superior to the cervix is known as the uterine body, which is normally anteflexed relative to the cervix. The fallopian tubes enter the body of the uterus laterally at the cornua, or uterine horns. The fundus is the portion of the uterus superior to the cornua.

The vesicouterine pouch is the potential space bounded by the bladder and the anterior wall of the uterus. Between the rectum and the posterior wall of the uterus lies the rectouterine pouch, also known as the posterior cul-de-sac or pouch of Douglas. This space is usually filled by loops of small bowel and a trace amount of physiologic free fluid. Pathologic intraperitoneal free fluid can be seen in either space, and in cases of ruptured ectopic pregnancies, it is common for a large amount of intraperitoneal blood to be identified in both the rectouterine and vesicouterine pouches and in the hepatorenal space (Morison's pouch) (see Chapter 24).

In a nulliparous woman, each ovary is located near the lateral wall of the pelvis in the ovarian fossa. This space is bounded superiorly by the external iliac vessels, anteriorly by the broad ligament, and posteriorly by the internal iliac vessels and ureter. It is important to remember that the ovaries are displaced during pregnancy and their position can vary. The normal ovarian size ranges between 2 cm and 4 cm in its largest dimension. The central portion of the ovary (medulla) contains vasculature, and the peripheral portion (cortex) contains follicles and oocytes.

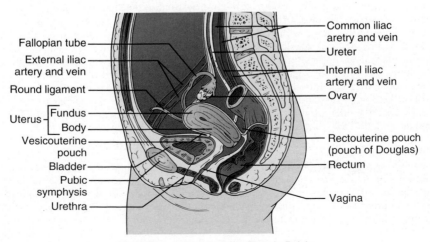

Figure 29.1 Anatomy of the Female Pelvis.

Image Acquisition

TRANSABDOMINAL TECHNIQUE

A curved-array transducer (2–5 MHz) is generally used for transabdominal pelvic scanning (TAS). Most point-of-care machines will have an obstetric preset that uses technical settings optimal for visualizing pelvic structures and for automatic calculation of pregnancy-related measurements. By convention, the screen orientation marker should be located in the upper left side of the screen. The patient should be supine with the lower abdomen exposed. A full bladder is preferred because it provides an acoustic window to visualize the uterus and adnexa. For a transverse view of the uterus, place the transducer immediately above the pubic symphysis with the transducer marker pointing to the patient's right side (Fig. 29.2). A sagittal view is obtained in the same position by rotating the transducer 90 degrees clockwise with the transducer marker pointing cephalad (Fig. 29.3).

In a transverse orientation, the bladder is seen in the near field with the uterus immediately posterior to it (Video 29.1). The ovaries are seen on either side of the uterus, although it is usually not possible to visualize both in a single image. Within the uterus, the myometrium surrounds the endometrium and is less echogenic by comparison. The thickness of the endometrium changes with the menstrual cycle. The endometrium develops a multilayered appearance following menstruation and gradually thickens during the proliferative phase. It thins out again during menstruation, and fluid may be seen in the uterine cavity. The uterus may be interrogated from cervix to fundus by tilting the transducer superiorly and inferiorly with the ultrasound beam aimed into the pelvis.

In a sagittal orientation, the pubic bone may be seen on the top right of the screen casting a shadow into the far field (see Fig. 29.3). The bladder is immediately posterior to the pubic symphysis and appears roughly triangular in shape. The body of the uterus lies posterior to the bladder and can be visualized along with the endometrial stripe, uterine fundus, cervix, and vaginal stripe in this view (Video 29.2). The transducer can be fanned from left to right to obtain multiple cross-sectional views of the uterus. Sliding the transducer to either side and aiming the beam laterally also allows for identification of the ovaries.

Normal ovaries appear spherical or elliptical and are generally isoechoic with scattered

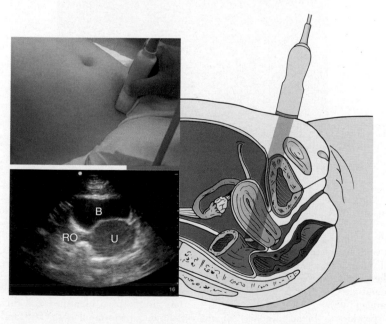

Figure 29.2 Transverse Transabdominal Scanning. *B*, Bladder; *RO*, right ovary; *U*, uterus.

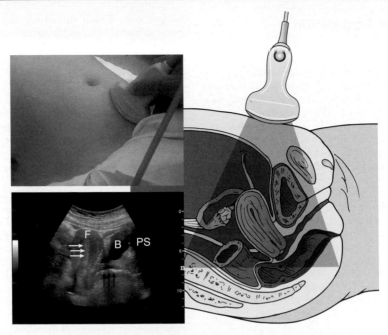

Figure 29.3 Sagittal Transabdominal Scanning. *B*, Bladder; *F*, uterine fundus; *PS*, pubic symphysis; *black arrows*, vaginal stripe; *white arrows*, endometrial stripe.

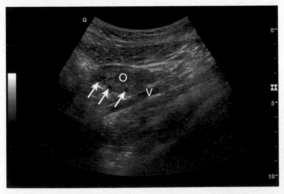

Figure 29.4 Ovary *(O)* (Transabdominal View). *V*, Iliac vein; *arrows*, follicles.

anechoic internal follicles (Fig. 29.4). Ovaries are often difficult to identify on TAS due to overlying bowel gas. The iliac vessels serve as useful landmarks, with the ovaries lying adjacent and just medial to the external iliac vessels. Even in patients who can be imaged easily, the ovaries can be difficult to evaluate on TAS and are best appreciated by transvaginal scanning (TVS).

TAS provides a broad overview of the pelvis and allows visualization of structures in relation to the uterus. In some cases, TAS alone may be adequate to exclude ectopic pregnancy by identifying an IUP. If a gestational sac containing a yolk sac or fetal pole is clearly visualized on TAS, it may not be necessary to undergo TVS. However, it is the experience of the authors that TVS often provides important information even in cases where an IUP has already been identified and thus, we recommend performing both TAS and TVS in most patients.

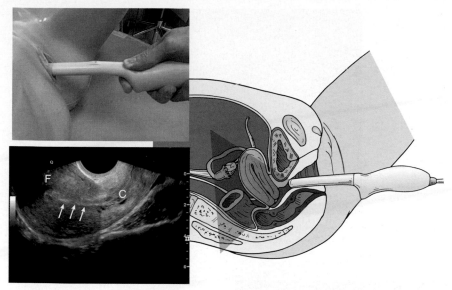

Figure 29.5   Sagittal Transvaginal Scanning. *C*, Cervix; *F*, uterine fundus; *arrows*, endometrial stripe.

TRANSVAGINAL TECHNIQUE

An endocavitary (5–8 MHz) transducer is used for TVS of the pelvis. The patient should be placed in a lithotomy position and encouraged to void before the study. Ultrasound gel is applied to the transducer, which is then covered with a sterile probe cover, and sterile gel is applied atop the cover before insertion in the vaginal canal.

Scanning starts with the transducer marker pointing toward the ceiling, resulting in a sagittal view of the uterus (Fig. 29.5). The decompressed bladder should be used as a landmark for probe insertion: the operator should insert the probe slowly until the bladder is visualized in the near field to the left on the screen. At this point, the uterine fundus should be seen in long axis, and the endometrial stripe can be seen toward the cervix (Video 29.3). Fanning the probe from side to side allows for interrogation of the entire uterus. Visualization of the cervix and the pouch of Douglas is accomplished by aiming the ultrasound beam posteriorly from a midline sagittal position. This area should be examined for the presence of free fluid (Fig. 29.6).

The ovaries can be found on either side of the uterus by tilting the probe laterally toward the pelvic wall. The external iliac vein will generally be seen adjacent to the ovary (Fig. 29.7). Within the ovary, follicles of varying sizes should be visible (Video 29.4). Cysts in the ovaries are common, and polycystic ovaries may be seen (Video 29.5).

Coronal views of the uterus and adnexa are obtained by returning to the midline sagittal position and rotating the transducer counterclockwise 90 degrees so that the transducer marker is pointing toward the patient's right side (Fig. 29.8 and Video 29.6). Normally, only the uterus will be visible, and the provider will have to direct the beam laterally to visualize each ovary. When scanning the ovaries, the ultrasound beam is directed laterally, and an oblique, rather than horizontal, transducer orientation is often preferable as this is typically the best way to visualize the external iliac vessels, the most important landmarks for locating the ovaries.

The utility of TVS lies in the ability to visualize intrauterine contents with high resolution. For example, TVS allows identification of the yolk sac within a gestational sac earlier in pregnancy compared to TAS. Thus, the two techniques are complementary, with TAS providing a broad overview of pelvic contents and TVS providing a focused, high-resolution view of uterine contents.

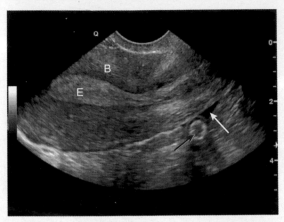

Figure 29.6 Free Fluid in the Pouch of Douglas *(white arrow)* **(Transvaginal Sagittal View).** *B*, Body of uterus; *E*, endometrial stripe; *red arrow*, loop of small bowel.

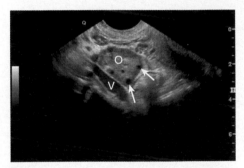

Figure 29.7 Ovary *(O)* **(Transvaginal Sagittal View).** *V*, Iliac vein; *arrows*, follicles.

Image Interpretation

NORMAL FINDINGS

The appearance of a normal pregnancy on ultrasound follows a generally predictable course corresponding with the embryo's gestational age. Thickening of the endometrium is the first sonographic feature seen in pregnancy, but is a nonspecific finding.[11] As the pregnancy progresses, a gestational sac becomes visible (Fig. 29.9 and Video 29.7). This appears as an anechoic, circular or oval structure surrounded by an echogenic ring, the decidua capsularis. Early in pregnancy, it can be challenging to differentiate the true gestational sac of an IUP from other structures of similar appearance, such as a decidual cyst or a collection of fluid within the endometrial canal (i.e., a "pseudogestational sac").[12] The following criteria, which can be remembered by the acronym "FEEDS," are characteristic of a true gestational sac: (1) location in the uterine **F**undus, (2) **E**lliptical or spherical shape, (3) **E**ccentric to the endometrium (i.e., not a collection of fluid within the endometrial canal itself, but implanted adjacently; this is also called the "Intradecidual Sign"[13]) (Fig. 29.10), (4) presence of a **D**ecidual reaction (the ring of tissue immediately adjacent to the gestational sac appears more echogenic than the rest of the uterus; this is also called "Double Decidual sign" [Fig. 29.11]), and (5) a **s**ac diameter >5 mm. In contrast, pseudogestational sacs are composed of fluid secreted by the lining of the endometrium and fill up the potential space of the endometrial canal. They are typically located in the endometrial canal in the body of the uterus, have pointed edges rather than being round and smooth, lack a surrounding decidual reaction, and are typically <5 mm in diameter.

It should be emphasized that although the criteria listed above are *suggestive* of a true gestational sac, definitive proof of an IUP can only be made by *visualization of a yolk sac within an intrauterine gestational sac*.[13,14] The yolk sac appears as a perfectly round, thin-walled echogenic ring with an anechoic center located inside the gestational sac (Fig. 29.12 and Video 29.8). The yolk sac diameter increases in size to a maximum of 6 mm at week 10 and subsequently involutes, disappearing completely by

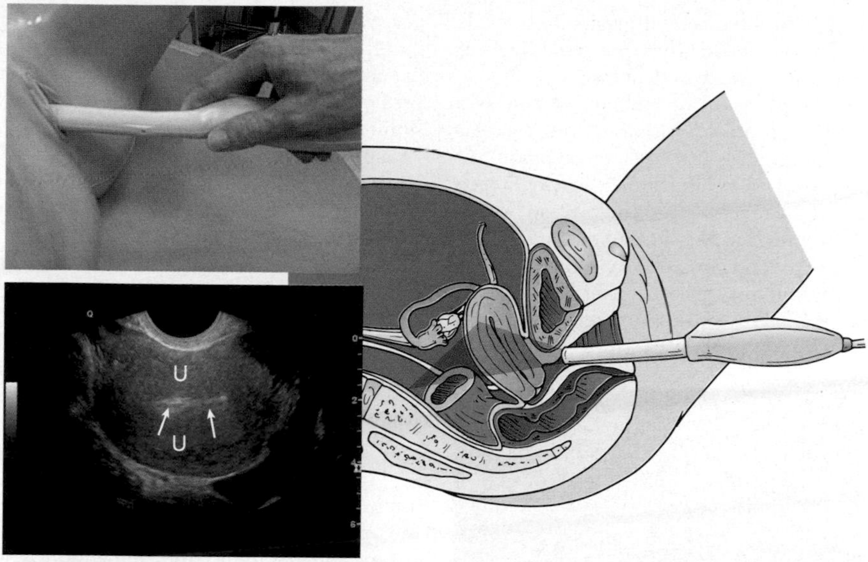

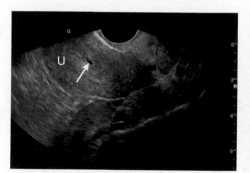

Figure 29.8 Coronal (Transverse) Transvaginal Scanning. *U*, Uterus; *arrows*, endometrial stripe.

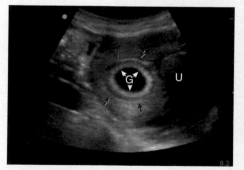

Figure 29.9 Small Gestational Sac *(arrow)* (Transvaginal Sagittal View). *U*, Uterus.

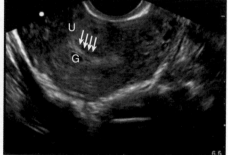

Figure 29.10 Intradecidual Sign. *G*, Gestational sac; *U*, uterus; *arrows*, endometrial stripe.

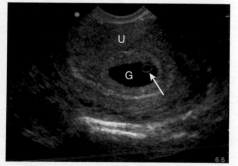

Figure 29.11 Double Decidual Sac Sign. *G*, Gestational sac; *U*, uterus; *red arrows*, outer ring; *white arrows*, inner ring.

Figure 29.12 Gestational Sac *(G)* With Yolk Sac *(arrow)*. *U*, Uterus.

week 12.[15] In most normal pregnancies, a yolk sac will be visualized when the gestational sac is greater than 8 mm in diameter.[16]

The "fetal pole," or embryo, is seen as a small discoid mass adjacent to the yolk sac shortly after the fifth week of gestation. At approximately 6 weeks, cardiac activity is seen within the embryo. The crown-rump length (CRL) represents the longest dimension of the embryo and is used to estimate gestational age in the first trimester (Fig. 29.13). M-mode is used to determine fetal heart rate, which should be between 110 and 175 beats per minute (bpm) in the first trimester (Fig. 29.14).[17] Even in symptomatic first trimester patients, a fetal heart rate within normal range predicts a greater than 90% chance of progression to term.[18-20]

The amnion, seen as a separate anechoic space within the gestational sac, is initially difficult to visualize but is usually apparent by week 7. It should not be confused with a yolk sac (Fig. 29.15). The amnion contains the embryo, and identifying an amniotic sac without an embryo is diagnostic of a failed pregnancy.[21] This is known as an "empty amnion" sign. The chorionic cavity within the gestational sac is eventually obliterated as the amnion expands and fuses with the chorionic margin, a process that is usually completed by week 12.[11]

Finally, the corpus luteum, or a corpus luteum cyst, may be visualized within one of the ovaries (Fig. 29.16 and Video 29.9). The corpus luteum forms from the ruptured follicle after ovulation and functions to support the pregnancy during the first trimester. Clinically, pelvic pain may be experienced if the corpus luteum ruptures, becomes very enlarged (Videos 29.10 and 29.11), or acts as a focus around which the ovary becomes twisted, leading to ovarian torsion.

Of note, an appropriately positioned intrauterine device (IUD) can be seen as a T-shaped, echogenic structure within the body of the uterus (Fig. 29.17 and Video 29.12). In any woman with an IUD and a positive pregnancy test, ectopic pregnancy should be assumed. However, in rare cases, intrauterine

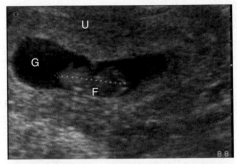

Figure 29.13 Crown-Rump Length. The crown-rump length (CRL) measurement is obtained by using the calipers to measure the longest dimension of the fetus (F). The yolk sac is sometimes seen adjacent to the fetus but should not be included in the measurement. Most machines have a preset function that will calculate the gestational age once the CRL measurement is obtained. In this case, the CRL is 2.72 cm, equivalent to a gestational age of 9 weeks and 4 days. G, Gestational sac; U, uterus.

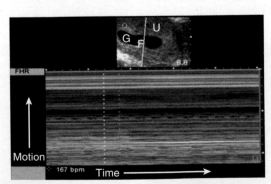

Figure 29.14 M-Mode Used to Measure Fetal Heart Rate. In M-mode, the cursor line should be placed directly over the flicker of cardiac activity within the fetus (F). The small waves repeating at regular intervals correspond to the fetal heartbeat (arrows). Using the measurement function, two cursor lines are placed to mark a cardiac cycle and the machine calculates the heart rate—in this case 167 beats per minute (bpm). G, Gestational sac; U, uterus.

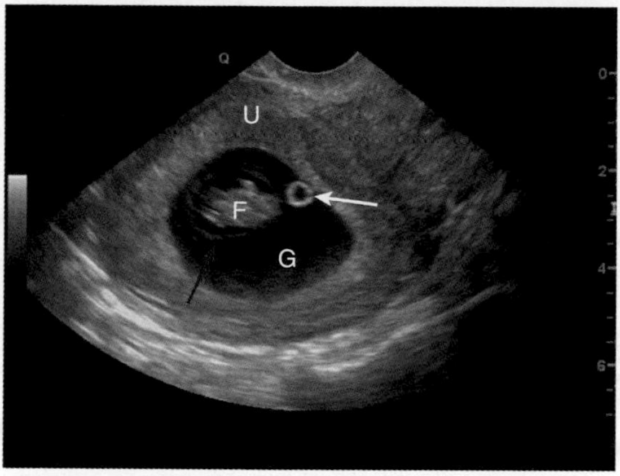

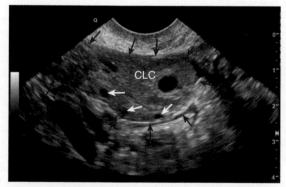

Figure 29.15 Amnion *(red arrow)* and Yolk Sac *(white arrow)* Seen From a Transvaginal View. *F*, Fetus; *G*, gestational sac; *U*, uterus.

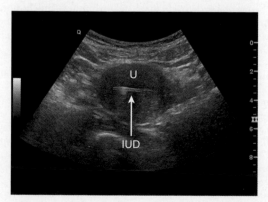

Figure 29.16 Ovary Containing a Corpus Luteum Cyst *(CLC)* From a Transvaginal View. *Red arrows*, Ovarian border; *white arrows*, follicles.

Figure 29.17 Intrauterine device *(IUD)* in the Uterine Cavity Seen From a Transabdominal Transverse View. *U*, Uterus.

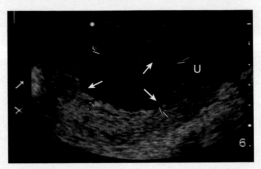

Figure 29.18   Empty Amnion. A large gestational sac *(red arrows)* and empty amnion *(white arrows)*—a sign of pregnancy failure. *U*, Uterus.

pregnancies can also occur even when IUDs are appropriately positioned (Video 29.13).

PATHOLOGIC FINDINGS

Nonviable Pregnancy

Once an IUP has been detected, it is important to assess viability. Generally, a nonviable pregnancy should be considered when the findings do not follow the predicted course described in the previous section. In the past, several signs have been proposed that suggest early pregnancy failure, including gestational sac diameters of various sizes without an embryo (Fig. 29.18),[22] the absence of cardiac activity in an embryo with various CRLs,[23,24] embryonic bradycardia,[17,18,25-29] an irregularly shaped gestational sac,[16] and an abnormally large or small yolk sac.[30]

Clinicians should be aware, however, that normal IUPs can have a widely variable appearance early in their course. Thus, if the pregnancy is desired, there should be no rush to provide surgical or medical treatment for a presumed miscarriage if there is any doubt as to the viability of the pregnancy. Current expert consensus suggests the following as criteria for diagnosing early pregnancy failure: (1) the presence of a gestational sac with a mean diameter of 25 mm or greater with no embryo ("anembryonic gestation"), (2) the presence of an embryo with a CRL of 7 mm or greater without a heartbeat, (3) no embryo with a heartbeat >2 weeks after TVS showed a gestational sac without a yolk sac, (4) no embryo with a heartbeat >11 days after TVS showed a gestational sac with a yolk sac.[4] Generally, definitively diagnosing pregnancy failure falls outside the scope of the point-of-care ultrasound exam, and we

recommend obtaining an expert or diagnostic level ultrasound exam before any surgical or medical management is undertaken.

Subchorionic Hemorrhage

Subchorionic hematoma is commonly seen on ultrasound in women with clinically evident bleeding in early pregnancy. These appear as fluid collections located between the chorionic margin and uterine wall and can vary significantly in shape and appearance. They are crescent-shaped with mixed anechoic and echogenic internal components (Figs. 29.19 and 29.20; Videos 29.14-29.16). It is controversial whether the presence of a subchorionic hematoma has significant prognostic value in terms of pregnancy outcome, but it is generally accepted that very small hematomas in the early first trimester confer little increased risk of miscarriage. Larger hematomas, especially if they occur in the late first or second trimester in women of advanced maternal age, carry a higher risk.[31-33] No specific treatment exists for first-trimester subchorionic hematomas, and acute management in the ED or other acute care settings does not typically change.

Ectopic Pregnancy

In any pregnant patient, ectopic pregnancy should be suspected whenever an IUP is not visualized. Using point-of-care ultrasound, the most common finding is the presence of an empty uterus with a relatively normal appearance. When coupled with a β-hCG level of 3000 mIU/mL or greater, this finding is highly concerning for ectopic pregnancy, regardless of whether the ectopic pregnancy itself can be directly visualized. In this scenario, a comprehensive ultrasound exam should be performed if the patient is stable. Further, any

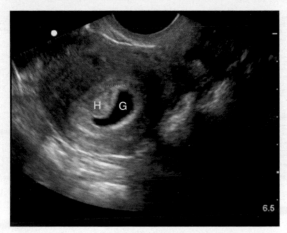

Figure 29.19 Subchorionic Hematoma. A small subchorionic hematoma *(H)* is seen by transvaginal scanning. *G*, Gestational sac.

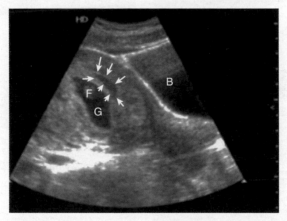

Figure 29.20 Subchorionic Hematoma. A small crescent-shaped subchorionic hematoma *(arrows)* is seen by transabdominal scanning. *B*, Bladder; *F*, fetus; *G*, gestational sac.

significant amount of intraperitoneal free fluid in this setting suggests an acute rupture and should prompt urgent consultation with an obstetrician-gynecologist.

Although it is most common to diagnose an ectopic pregnancy through the indirect means outlined above, familiarity with various sonographic appearances of ectopic pregnancy is recommended for the point-of-care sonographer. In its most basic form, visualization of a gestational sac containing a yolk sac or embryo lying outside of the uterus is definitive evidence of an ectopic pregnancy (Fig. 29.21 and Videos 29.17–29.19). This is an infrequent finding seen in less than 20% of ectopic pregnancies.[34-36]

Identification of a "tubal ring sign" is the next most specific finding. The tubal ring is composed of a ring of trophoblastic tissue with a hypoechoic central cavity that is essentially an extrauterine gestational sac (Fig. 29.22; Videos 29.20 and 29.21). A tubal ring may be confused with a corpus luteum cyst, depending on its proximity to the ovary. It can be differentiated from a cyst by its thick echogenic border and absence of surrounding ovarian tissue.[11] Positive predictive value (PPV) of a tubal ring for ectopic pregnancy is 95%, and it can be found in approximately 20% to 30% of cases.[34-37]

More commonly, an ectopic pregnancy is seen as an irregularly shaped complex adnexal mass that is separate from the ovary (Fig. 29.23

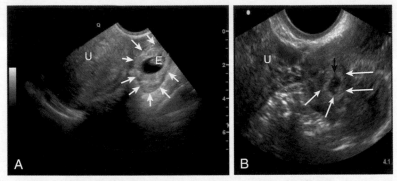

Figure 29.21   Ectopic Pregnancy. (A) An ectopic pregnancy containing an embryo *(E)* in the left adnexal region and (B) an extrauterine gestational sac containing a yolk sac *(red arrow)*. *U,* Uterus; *white arrows,* tubal ring.

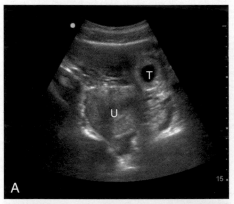

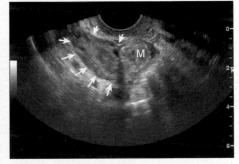

Figure 29.23   Ectopic Pregnancy. A complex adnexal mass *(M)*, which is an ectopic pregnancy, is seen adjacent to the ovary *(arrows)*.

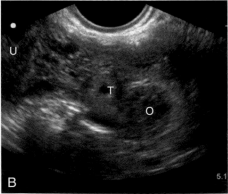

Figure 29.22   Tubal Ring. (A) A tubal ring *(T)* is seen adjacent to the uterus *(U)* and (B) an ovary *(O)*.

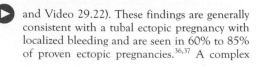

and Video 29.22). These findings are generally consistent with a tubal ectopic pregnancy with localized bleeding and are seen in 60% to 85% of proven ectopic pregnancies.[36,37] A complex adnexal mass is associated with a PPV over 88% for ectopic pregnancy.[38]

As mentioned above, nontrivial pelvic free fluid in the absence of an IUP is highly suggestive of a *ruptured* ectopic pregnancy.[39,40] Fluid can appear entirely anechoic, or it may contain scattered low-level echoes or larger isoechoic components representing clots. The fluid level, as it tracks along the posterior wall of the uterus, can be used to grade the degree of bleeding. Fluid localized to the pouch of Douglas is considered small, fluid that extends to the uterine fundus is moderate, and fluid extending through the peritoneal cavity to Morison's pouch is considered large (Figs. 29.24 and 29.25; Video 29.23). A trace amount of scant anechoic free fluid is nonspecific and may be present with a normal IUP. The likelihood of ectopic pregnancy increases greatly in the presence of moderate or large free fluid, with one study reporting a PPV of 86%.[39]

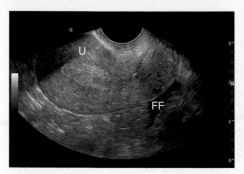

Figure 29.24 Pelvic Free Fluid. A small amount of free fluid *(FF)* is seen in the posterior cul-de-sac. *U*, Uterus.

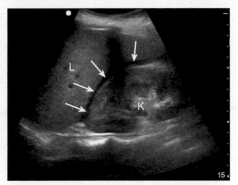

Figure 29.26 Abdominal Free Fluid *(arrows)* **in the Hepatorenal Recess (Morison's Pouch).** *K*, Kidney; *L*, liver.

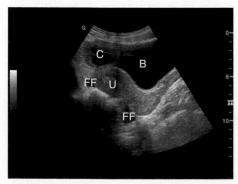

Figure 29.25 Abdominal Free Fluid. A large amount of free fluid *(FF)* is seen tracking up to the uterine fundus. The culprit was a large ruptured hemorrhagic cyst *(C)*, which is seen extending over the uterus *(U)* in this sagittal image. *B*, Bladder.

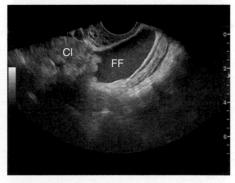

Figure 29.27 Echogenic Free Fluid. Free fluid *(FF)* that contains echogenic, floating particles can be blood that is clotting. *Cl*, Clots.

Free fluid visualized in Morison's pouch is more specific for ectopic pregnancy (Fig. 29.26 and Video 29.24). Echogenic material within intraperitoneal free fluid is often indicative of clotted blood and carries a reported PPV of 90% for ectopic pregnancy (Fig. 29.27 and Video 29.25).[41]

The vast majority of ectopic pregnancies are located within one of the fallopian tubes. Less common locations include the interstitium (2.5%), ovaries (3%), cervix (1%), and abdomen (1.3%).[42] Intramural ectopic pregnancies within the myometrium have been reported but are exceedingly rare.[43] A cervical ectopic pregnancy can be easily confused with a miscarriage in progress, although a closed cervical os and the presence of fetal heart motion suggest cervical implantation. Other criteria exist for the diagnosis of cervical ectopic pregnancy, although this is best confirmed with a comprehensive diagnostic ultrasound exam.[44,45]

The appearance of an interstitial ectopic pregnancy may resemble an IUP, mainly because the pregnancy has implanted at the junction of the uterus and the fallopian tube. Gestational sacs identified on the periphery of the uterus, with little or no myometrial mantle, should raise suspicion for an interstitial ectopic pregnancy (Fig. 29.28; Video 29.26-29.29). A myometrium thicker than 5 mm surrounding the entire gestational sac and the presence of a double decidual sac sign (see Fig. 29.11) are two features that help establish implantation within the endometrium.[46] In general, it should be remembered that when a gestational sac is found, it is important to carefully establish that it is located in a normal position within the uterus to avoid confusion with these rarer forms of ectopic pregnancy.

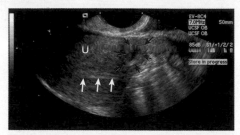

Figure 29.28   Interstitial Ectopic Pregnancy. The red arrows outline a gestational sac within the left cornual region. *U*, Uterus; *white arrows*, endometrial stripe.

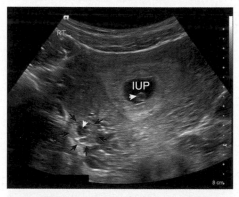

Figure 29.29   Heterotopic Pregnancy. Two separate gestational sacs are present in this image: one within and the other outside of the uterus. Both contain yolk sacs *(white arrows)*. *IUP*, Intrauterine pregnancy; *red arrows*, extrauterine pregnancy.

Finally, the possibility of a heterotopic pregnancy (simultaneous IUP and ectopic) must be considered even when a definite IUP has been identified, particularly in women undergoing treatment for infertility with assisted reproductive techniques (Fig. 29.29; Videos 29.30 and 29.31).[47] Women who are undergoing in vitro fertilization (IVF) in particular are at significantly increased risk of heterotopic pregnancy with an incidence of 1:100 versus 1:30,000 in those with natural conception.[41,47,48]

Gestational Trophoblastic Disease

Gestational trophoblastic disease (GTD) is an uncommon cause of vaginal bleeding and pelvic pain in the first trimester, estimated to occur in 0.1% of pregnancies in the United States. The term encompasses a number of proliferative disorders of the placental trophoblastic epithelium, including partial and complete hydatidiform moles, choriocarcinoma, and other placental tumors.[49] These conditions are often misdiagnosed on ultrasound as incomplete abortion, especially with partial moles, as one study reported only 29% of cases were detected by initial ultrasound.[50] A full understanding of the spectrum of findings in gestational trophoblastic disease is beyond the scope of point-of-care ultrasound, so we will focus on the most common findings of this condition.

Molar pregnancies are nonviable pregnancies by definition. Complete molar pregnancies have more strikingly abnormal ultrasound findings in comparison to partial molar pregnancies and are subsequently diagnosed more frequently on ultrasound.[51] Ultrasound findings in complete molar pregnancies typically include a complex multicystic and often hypervascular intrauterine mass with the absence of fetal tissue. The sonographic appearance of the intrauterine mass has been described as a "snowstorm" or "cluster of grapes" appearance, describing the cystic components corresponding to enlarged chorionic villi in the uterus (Fig. 29.30A). The ovaries may contain multiple theca lutein cysts, a finding that is more common in complete molar pregnancies. Partial molar pregnancies more commonly present with a subtle placental abnormality, in addition to either a live embryo, a spontaneous intrauterine demise, or an empty gestational sac.[51] When choriocarcinoma is present, it may appear as an enlarged uterus containing a hemorrhagic mass (Fig. 29.30B).[52]

The definitive diagnosis of GTD is made by tissue histology. When the suspicion for GTD is raised by a point-of-care ultrasound exam, a comprehensive diagnostic pelvic ultrasound exam and gynecologic consultation are recommended.

Clinical Integration of First-Trimester Pelvic Ultrasound

All symptomatic first-trimester patients should be evaluated with an ultrasound examination along with standard laboratory tests, including a complete blood count, type and screen to determine Rh antigen status, and quantitative serum β-hCG level. After this initial workup, patients will generally fall into one of the following categories:

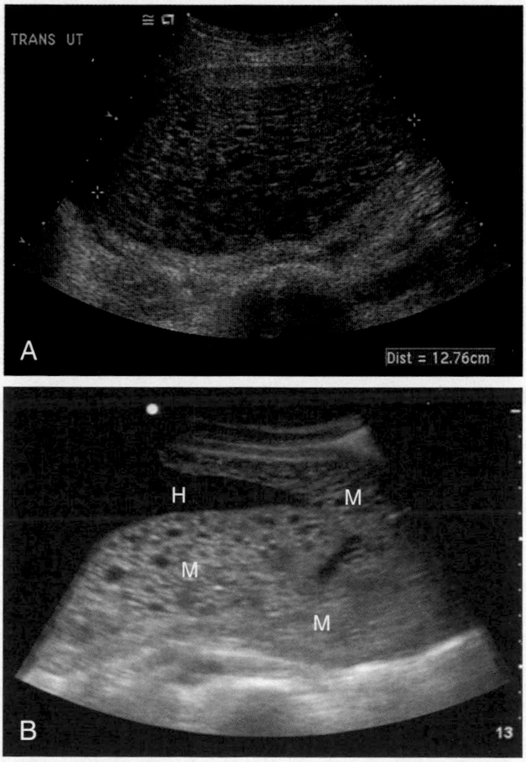

Figure 29.30 Gestational Trophoblastic Disease. (A) Multiple small cystic structures representing enlarged chorionic villi in the uterus of a patient with a molar pregnancy *(M)* are seen from a transabdominal transverse view. The mass measures approximately 13 cm transversely. (B) A mass with multiple cystic components is present within the uterus as seen from a transabdominal transverse view. Intrauterine hemorrhage *(H)* is also present.

(1) **Confirmed IUP.** The presence of an intrauterine gestational sac with a yolk sac, embryo, or both, clearly establishes the diagnosis of IUP (Video 29.32). Care should be taken to ensure that these structures are seen in a normal position inside the uterus to avoid possible confusion with an ectopic pregnancy. As discussed, given the very low risk of heterotopic pregnancy in non-IVF patients, clinicians can generally assume that ectopic pregnancy has been ruled out if an IUP is visualized, but they should be aware of heterotopic pregnancy as a possibility and arrange for follow-up imaging if this is suspected clinically. For routine cases, these patients can be discharged home with outpatient follow-up. Neither a comprehensive ultrasound exam nor consultation with an obstetrician-gynecologist is usually required.

(2) **Pregnancy of Unknown Location, Likely Early IUP of Unknown Viability.** The presence of a round or elliptical intrauterine fluid collection with round edges, even without a decidual reaction, yolk sac, or embryo, is likely to represent an early IUP, regardless of the quantitative β-hCG level or gestational age based on the last menstrual period (LMP) (Video 29.33).[53-55] Although historically there has been considerable concern over the possibility that such a finding may be present in cases of ectopic pregnancy, evidence suggests that the presence of a true pseudogestational sac is far less common that previously thought.[56,57] Unless other findings suggest an ectopic pregnancy (significant intra-abdominal fluid, adnexal mass, etc.), providers should be aware that these patients are highly likely to have an IUP. Nonetheless, a

comprehensive ultrasound exam may be considered during the patient's ED visit or next clinic visit to confirm the findings of the point-of-care ultrasound exam. If an IUP is ultimately identified, the patient can follow up routinely as an outpatient. If no definite evidence of an IUP is noted, these patients need close follow up as an outpatient in 48 hours for a repeat ultrasound examination and serum β-hCG. In this scenario, if pregnancy is desired, methotrexate should *never* be given nor should manual uterine aspiration be performed, regardless of the serum β-hCG level.[53,55,58]

(3) **Confirmed IUP, Nonviable Pregnancy ("Missed Abortion").** In some cases, intrauterine embryonic demise will be identified with point-of-care ultrasound. As mentioned above, current diagnostic criteria for this condition include an intact GS with a mean sac diameter of >25 mm without a yolk sac or embryo, termed an "anembryonic gestation" (see Fig. 29.18 and Video 29.34), or an embryo measuring >7 mm without signs of cardiac activity, often termed "embryonic demise" (Fig. 29.31 and Video 29.35).[4] Any such findings should be confirmed by a diagnostic ultrasound exam before definitive management is undertaken. Because early pregnancy loss is not typically a dangerous or emergent condition, it is normally safe to defer formal imaging and arrange prompt outpatient follow-up based on the patient's preference. If embryonic or fetal demise is confirmed by a diagnostic ultrasound examination, providers should explain the diagnosis to the patient and briefly discuss available treatment options: expectant, medical (misoprostol), or procedural (manual uterine aspiration) therapy. In-person obstetric-gynecology consultation is generally not needed in the ED, but prompt follow-up should be arranged, ideally for the next day.

(4) **Pregnancy of Unknown Location, Likely Miscarriage.** The presence of heavy vaginal bleeding, crampy lower abdominal pain, and passage of tissue strongly suggests a spontaneous abortion. Ultrasound will generally reveal an empty or nearly empty-appearing uterus, in the case of a complete abortion, or areas of mixed echogenicity and debris within the endometrial canal, in the case of an incomplete abortion (Videos 29.36 and 29.37). If the patient is found to have a significant amount of intraperitoneal fluid on ultrasound, concern should be raised for a ruptured ectopic pregnancy. If the patient is having massive vaginal bleeding and is clinically unstable, providers should be concerned for an unstable, incomplete spontaneous abortion. In either case, emergent consultation with an obstetrician-gynecologist should be undertaken. However, if the patient is stable, it should be emphasized that heavy vaginal bleeding with passage of clots and/or tissue is *highly* likely to represent a miscarriage rather than a ruptured ectopic pregnancy.

Providers should perform a thorough exam, including a speculum and bimanual exam to assess the cervix. Any tissue or

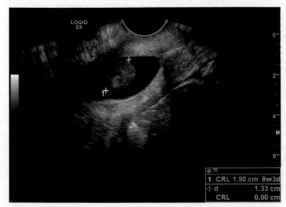

Figure 29.31 Fetal Demise. No identifiable cardiac activity is seen in a fetus with a crown-rump length *(CRL)* of 19 mm corresponding to an estimated gestational age of 8 weeks, 3 days.

products of conception at the cervical os should be removed and sent to pathology to confirm a spontaneous abortion and rule out an ectopic pregnancy. This may also stop the patient's bleeding if present. Patients should be followed to ensure the serum β-hCG is declining in cases where no definitive evidence of an IUP on a prior ultrasound exam was noted.

In cases where the diagnosis of miscarriage is clinically obvious, a comprehensive diagnostic ultrasound exam is not required, but it may be advisable to confirm the diagnosis and detect any residual products of conception in the uterus, which can be helpful when discussing management options.

In most cases, patients who are actively miscarrying but are clinically stable can be treated by acute care providers without in-person consultation of an obstetrician-gynecologist; however, all such patients should have follow-up to ensure adequate resolution. Providers should consider giving misoprostol if confident in the diagnosis. Methotrexate should not be given to women having a miscarriage. Bleeding precautions should be discussed. Generally, if bleeding of >1 pad/hr persists for more than 4 hours or the patient has clinical signs of significant blood loss (dizziness, nausea, fainting, etc.), the patient should follow up promptly for further evaluation.

(5) **Pregnancy of Unknown Location, Concerning for Possible Unruptured Ectopic Pregnancy.** The presence of an empty uterus on TVS in patients who do not appear clinically to be having a miscarriage is concerning for ectopic pregnancy, especially in patients with a serum β-hCG >3000 mIU/mL (see Fig. 29.6 and Video 29.38). However, before a definitive diagnosis of ectopic pregnancy is made, clinicians should realize two important points: (1) In rare instances, viable IUPs will not exhibit a visible gestational sac even above the β-hCG discriminatory zone;[53,58] and (2) a miscarriage is still twice as common in this scenario as an ectopic pregnancy.[4] Thus, the absence of an IUP coupled with a β-hCG above this level does not confirm that an ectopic pregnancy is present. Nonetheless, in this scenario where the uterus appears empty and the serum β-hCG is above

3000 mIU/mL, clinicians should be highly concerned about an ectopic pregnancy.

In cases where the uterus appears empty on point-of-care ultrasound, and the patient does not appear clinically to be having a miscarriage, a diagnostic ultrasound should be obtained as soon as possible, regardless of the serum β-hCG value. If there continues to be high suspicion for ectopic pregnancy after the diagnostic ultrasound, definitive treatment should proceed per recommendations from an obstetrician-gynecologist. This may include performing a manual uterine aspiration to assess for evidence of a failed IUP (chorionic villi, etc) with subsequent administration of methotrexate if no evidence of an IUP is found. If the ultrasound is inconclusive and the patient is stable, a follow-up visit for a repeat ultrasound exam and β-hCG should be arranged within 48 hours.

For women with pregnancy of unknown location (PUL), if the serum β-hCG is very low, an early, normal IUP is still a likely possibility, and the patient should have a 48-hour follow-up before additional management is undertaken. However, as mentioned above, current data suggest that women with a PUL and β-hCG >3000 mIU/mL most likely will have a failed IUP (66%), ectopic pregnancy (33%), or rarely a viable IUP (0.5%).[4] Given these data, if the pregnancy is not desired, sequential treatment with manual uterine aspiration followed by methotrexate should be performed if no chorionic villi/trophoblastic tissue is seen on pathologic examination, or if the β-hCG does not decline. If pregnancy is desired, additional testing at 48 hours should be performed before treating for ectopic pregnancy.[4]

(6) **Likely Ruptured Ectopic Pregnancy.** Any pregnant patient with hemoperitoneum and no clear evidence of an IUP on ultrasound should be assumed to have a ruptured ectopic pregnancy (see Figs. 29.26 and 29.27; Video 29.39). If the patient is unstable, aggressive resuscitation and emergent consultation should be undertaken for immediate operative intervention. In certain cases, if the patient is stable, a comprehensive diagnostic ultrasound exam can be considered since occasionally cases of hemorrhagic corpus luteum cysts may mimic this presentation.

PEARLS AND PITFALLS

- Transabdominal ultrasonography should be performed with a full bladder, as it provides a good acoustic window to the female reproductive system. In contrast, an empty bladder is preferable for transvaginal ultrasonography.
- For transabdominal scanning, ensure sufficient gel is applied between the skin and transducer, and for transvaginal scanning, ensure that no air bubbles are present between the transducer and sterile sheath.
- Scan the uterus and adnexa in multiple planes to better appreciate structures of interest (gestational sac, cysts, adnexal mass) and surrounding anatomy.
- Note the amount and echogenicity of free fluid in the abdomen/pelvis. A small amount of pelvic free fluid can be normal, but moderate to large free fluid is always abnormal, as is increased echogenicity of the fluid.
- Echogenic material within the endometrial cavity does not always represent a miscarriage and can be seen with ectopic pregnancy and gestational trophoblastic disease. When in doubt, a comprehensive diagnostic ultrasound and/or gynecologic consultation is indicated.
- A tubal ring may look like a corpus luteum cyst. Use the criteria described above to differentiate a tubal ring from a corpus luteum cyst.
- Remember to rule out other potential causes of the patient's symptoms, such as a ruptured corpus luteum cyst, ovarian torsion, or other intra-abdominal pathologies.

CHAPTER 30

Second and Third Trimester Pregnancy

Justin R. Lappen ■ Kelly S. Gibson ■ Robert Jones

KEY POINTS

- Point-of-care ultrasound is used in the second and third trimesters of pregnancy when a timely, goal-directed assessment is needed to guide patient care of both critical and noncritical conditions.
- Six fundamental components comprise the point-of-care ultrasound examination during the second and third trimester: determination of fetal lie and presentation, cardiac activity, fetal number, amniotic fluid volume, placental location, and fetal biometry.
- During active labor, determination of fetal presentation, fetal number, placental location, and fetal viability can be assessed with point-of-care ultrasound.

Background

Ultrasonography is integral to the practice of modern obstetrics and is increasingly used at the point-of-care in many countries, especially developing countries.[1] In time-sensitive scenarios, point-of-care ultrasound (POCUS) is used to provide accurate assessment of gestational age, fetal number, presence or absence of cardiac activity, and placental location. POCUS may also aid in the diagnosis of underlying obstetric pathologies, such as fetal demise, premature rupture of membranes (PROM), and antenatal hemorrhage from abnormal placentation, such as placenta previa or accreta. Additionally, POCUS can be used in the assessment of various other conditions that impact pregnant women, including abdominal pain and maternal trauma. As such, POCUS is integral in providing comprehensive care and assessing pregnant women during both routine prenatal visits and during triage in emergency situations.

This chapter provides detailed information on the use of POCUS in the second and third trimesters of pregnancy. A systematic approach to perform a basic ultrasound examination is provided with a focus on the technical aspects. Although ultrasound has a vast array of applications pertaining to fetal anatomy, a goal-directed approach during the second and third trimesters will be the focus of this chapter.

Normal Anatomy

A review of the normal female pelvic anatomy can be found in Chapter 29. Pertaining to the second and third trimesters, it is important to remember that the enlarging uterus will displace the normal position of surrounding structures, and this can affect how the advanced gravid patient presents with intra-abdominal pathology. At approximately 12 to 13 weeks' gestation, the fundus of a gravid uterus will be at the level of the pubic symphysis, and by 20 weeks' gestation, the uterine fundus will be at the level of the umbilicus. After 20 weeks, the distance in centimeters from the pubic symphysis to the fundus of the gravid uterus approximates the gestational age in weeks (Fig. 30.1)

Image Acquisition

The goal of a point-of-care second or third trimester ultrasound examination is to identify key pathologic conditions that will impact the

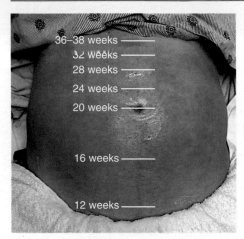

Figure 30.1   Gestational Age. Uterine fundal height from the symphysis pubis can estimate gestational age.

TABLE 30.1   **Second and Third Trimester Point-of-Care Ultrasound Examination**

1. Fetal lie and presentation
2. Fetal cardiac activity
3. Fetal number (singleton, twin, triplet or higher order multiple gestation)
4. Amniotic fluid volume
5. Placental localization and assessment
6. Fetal biometry

---

management of the mother and child. Comprehensive evaluation of the fetal anatomy to identify congenital anomalies requires a much greater degree of training and is beyond the scope of the POCUS examination. The scope of a point-of-care second or third trimester ultrasound examination is summarized in Table 30.1.

The patient should be comfortably positioned supine with the upper body and head slightly inclined and supported by a soft pillow or cushion, unless the patient is in spinal precautions. In the latter part of pregnancy, a pillow may be placed under the patient's right side to provide left lateral tilt and relieve aortocaval compression.

A transabdominal second or third trimester ultrasound examination is best performed with a curvilinear transducer (2–5 MHz) that provides a wide field of view and adequate penetration for pelvic imaging. A phased-array transducer may be used but is less ideal given

its narrow field of view. An obstetric exam preset should be selected to perform some key measurements and calculations. A transvaginal ultrasound examination may be performed when the transabdominal images of placental location at the cervical os are nondiagnostic. However, unlike the assessment of a first trimester patient, transvaginal ultrasound is not part of a routine second or third trimester point-of-care examination and will not be discussed in this chapter.

Image Interpretation

FETAL LIE AND PRESENTATION

Fetal lie and presentation will influence the choice between vaginal or cesarean mode of delivery. Fetal lie is defined as the orientation of the fetal spine relative to the maternal spine. Fetal presentation refers to the anatomical part of the fetus closest to the pelvic inlet. Determination of fetal lie requires obtaining a midsagittal view of the fetal spine. Longitudinal fetal lie occurs when the fetal and maternal spinal columns are parallel, such as a breech or cephalic presentation, and is the most common fetal lie in the second and third trimesters. Transverse lie occurs when the fetal spine is positioned perpendicular to the maternal spine (Fig. 30.2). When the fetal spine is angled between a longitudinal and transverse lie, the fetal lie is described as being oblique.

Fetal presentation may be cephalic or breech. Determination of fetal presentation is technically easier than lie, therefore we recommend assessing fetal presentation first. A fetus in cephalic or breech presentation, by definition, has a longitudinal lie (Fig. 30.3). If the fetal head or sacrum is not visible in the lower uterine segment, then a transverse or oblique lie should be suspected and a midsagittal view of the fetal spine should be obtained to assess the relative angle of the fetal and maternal spines.

To assess fetal presentation, place the transducer over the maternal lower abdomen, just above the pubic symphysis, in a transverse orientation. Tilt the transducer inferiorly toward the cervix to identify the presenting part of the fetus (head, buttocks/sacrum, or other part) (Fig. 30.4 and Video 30.1).

Breech presentation frequently results in cesarean delivery (Fig. 30.5), although attempting vaginal delivery may be appropriate based on clinical factors, experience of the health

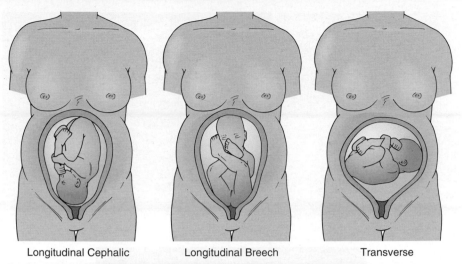

Longitudinal Cephalic   Longitudinal Breech   Transverse

Figure 30.2 Fetal Lie and Presentation. Fetal lie (longitudinal vs. transverse) and fetal presentation (cephalic vs. breech) are shown.

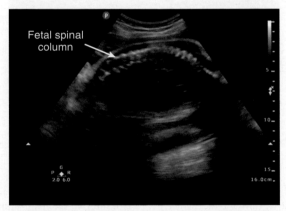

Fetal spinal column

Figure 30.3 Longitudinal Cephalic Presentation. The fetal spine is parallel to the maternal spine and the fetal head is in lower uterus demonstrating a longitudinal cephalic presentation of the fetus as seen from a sagittal transabdominal image.

care provider, and clinical setting.[1] External cephalic version may be recommended to women with oblique lie or breech presentation at term. Persistent transverse lie requires cesarean delivery. However, a classical cesarean delivery is required if the fetal spine is in the lower uterine segment, as the thorax and abdomen obstruct delivery through a hysterotomy in the lower uterine segment.

FETAL CARDIAC ACTIVITY

Determination of fetal cardiac activity is an essential component of any basic obstetric ultrasound examination. Determining the presence or absence of normal fetal cardiac activity in the second and third trimesters has significant management implications. Detection of abnormal cardiac activity may provide an early window to intervene on a maternal or fetal pathological process and can guide management in both hospital and austere settings. Furthermore, the presence of normal cardiac activity (110 to 160 beats/minute) provides an important opportunity for patient reassurance. As such, confirmation of cardiac activity should be performed early in the ultrasound examination. Although a fetal heart rate may

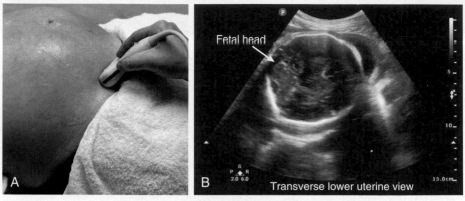

Figure 30.4   Determination of Fetal Lie and Presentation. (A) Transducer position to obtain a transverse view of lower uterine region. (B) Cephalic presentation.

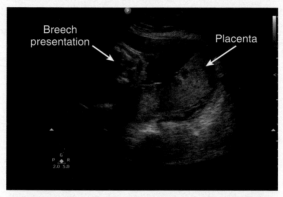

Figure 30.5   Breech Presentation. A transverse lie is seen from a transverse transabdominal image of the lower uterine segment.

be detectable by a Doppler exam alone, assessing fetal cardiac activity during performance of a POCUS examination allows a more timely and comprehensive fetal assessment.

Documentation of fetal cardiac activity can be performed by either obtaining a video loop of cardiac contractions or obtaining a static M-mode or pulsed-wave (PW) Doppler image. Measurement of fetal heart rate is typically done using either PW Doppler or M-mode. Both techniques rely on producing a graphical display of the cardiac cycle (blood flow peaks for PW Doppler and anatomical deflections in M-mode) and measuring the distance between cardiac contractions, analogous to measuring the R-R interval on an electrocardiogram (ECG). For PW Doppler, the first step is to acquire a fetal four-chamber view with the cardiac apex directed toward the transducer. This view is optimal for Doppler interrogation

of flow through the mitral and tricuspid valves. Place the PW Doppler sample gate at the level of the mitral valve, and blood flow throughout the cardiac cycle will be displayed on the screen. Calipers are then placed between consecutive peaks, or every beat ("2 beat" calculation), to calculate the heart rate. (Fig. 30.6 and Video 30.2). It is important to note that spectral Doppler may be used in late pregnancy, whereas it is generally contraindicated in first trimester due to the theoretical risk of heat production in developing organs. M-mode, a function available on most ultrasound machines, is also used to detect fetal cardiac motion and determine the fetal heart rate. This technique is standard for calculating fetal heart rate in the first trimester. Measuring the distance between consecutive deflections, such as ventricular contractions, is used to calculate fetal heart rate (Fig. 30.7 and Video 30.3).

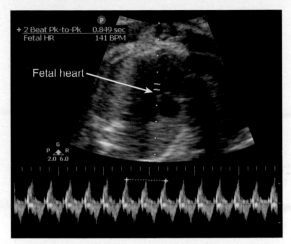

Figure 30.6 Pulsed-Wave Doppler Calculation of Fetal Heart Rate. Calipers are used to measure the distance between 1 or 2 heart beats to calculate the fetal heart rate. The 2-beat method is used in this image and determines the fetal heart rate to be 141 beats/minute.

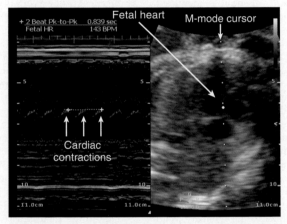

Figure 30.7 M-Mode Calculation of Fetal Heart Rate. M-mode is used to measure the beat-to-beat distance (or 2-beat distance as shown in this image) to calculate the fetal heart rate (143 beats/minute in this fetus).

FETAL NUMBER, CHORIONICITY AND AMNIONICITY

Identifying multiple gestations at the point-of-care is a core skill. Multiple gestations are associated with complications including preterm delivery, preeclampsia, abnormal labor, fetal malpresentation, as well as fetal, neonatal, and infant mortality.[2] Further, fetal risk is influenced by the number of placentae (chorionicity) and amniotic sacs (amnionicity). These numbers should be documented when multiple gestations are present. Twin pregnancies can be dichorionic diamniotic, monochorionic diamniotic, or monochorionic monoamniotic. The assessment of amnionicity and chorionicity is easier to do in the first trimester but sonographic assessment can still be performed in the second- or third-trimester patient who was not scanned during the first trimester. Sonographic findings in the second or third trimester that could help determine chorionicity and amnionicity include fetal gender, placental number, umbilical cord entanglement, membrane insertion, and presence or absence of an intertwin membrane. However, the point-of-care examination focuses on detection of an intertwin membrane and evaluation of the membrane's insertion and thickness.

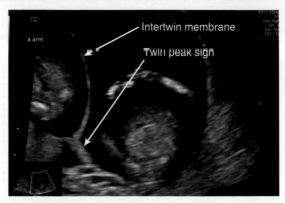

Figure 30.8 **Dichorionic Diamniotic Pregnancy.** An intertwin membrane and twin peak sign are seen.

To assess fetal number, the entire uterine cavity must be assessed in a standardized, systematic manner to identify the number of fetal crania. If more than one head is identified, confirmation of twins should be performed by identifying other body parts. The uterine cavity should be evaluated in both transverse and sagittal planes. In a transverse plane, the entire uterine cavity should be evaluated in sequential parallel planes from superior to inferior, from the uterine fundus to the lower uterine segment. Sequential parallel scanning should then be repeated in a sagittal orientation, from the left to right aspect of the maternal pelvis. Keep the ultrasound transducer perpendicular to the abdominal skin surface to prevent a false diagnosis of twins, which can result from imaging the same head at various angles.

In the early first trimester, the number of gestational sacs is equal to the number of chorions. The presence of two gestational sacs represents a dichorionic pregnancy, but without this finding, monochorionicity is most likely. The number of yolk sacs tends to equal the number of amnions in the early first trimester; however, this is not a reliable diagnostic criterion. Therefore, one gestational sac and two yolk sacs would likely be a monochorionic diamniotic gestation, whereas one gestational sac and one yolk sac would likely represent a monochorionic monoamniotic gestation. Follow-up imaging in the late first-trimester to assess the inter-twin membrane is recommended.

In the second and third trimesters, the yolk sac will no longer be visualized and cannot be used to distinguish amnionicity and chorionicity. The thickness of the intertwin membrane can help in distinguishing between monochorionic diamniotic versus dichorionic diamniotic twin pregnancies. In dichorionic diamniotic pregnancies, the intertwin membrane consists of two layers of chorion and two layers of amnion (Fig. 30.8). Additionally, in a dichorionic diamniotic pregnancy, the placenta extends in between the gestational sacs creating the "twin peak" or "lambda" sign.

In monochorionic diamniotic twin pregnancies, the intertwin membrane will qualitatively appear to be quite thin in appearance, containing only the two layers of amnion. In monochorionic diamniotic pregnancies, the single chorionic membrane surrounds both gestational sacs and prevents the placenta from extending between the two gestational sacs ("T-sign"). Lastly, in a monochorionic monoamniotic pregnancy, the intertwin dividing membrane will be absent (Fig. 30.9).

Due to the increased risk of complications associated with twin pregnancies, these patients require more frequent serial evaluations for early detection of complications. Complications include single fetal demise, intrauterine fetal growth restriction, twin-twin transfusion syndrome, and discordant growth. Considering the elevated complication risk, monochorionic twins should have ultrasound examinations every 2 weeks in the last half of pregnancy, and dichorionic twins should have ultrasound examinations every 4 weeks during the last half of pregnancy.[3]

AMNIOTIC FLUID VOLUME

Amniotic fluid is necessary for normal human development and may protect the fetus against mechanical trauma or intrauterine infection.

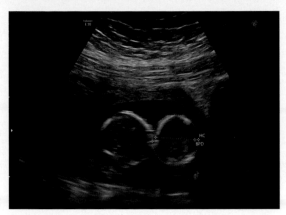

Figure 30.9 Monochorionic Monoamniotic Twin Pregnancy. The absence of an intertwin membrane dividing the two fetal crania is seen.

The primary source of amniotic fluid in the second and third trimesters is fetal urine. Disorders of amniotic fluid volume may suggest underlying maternal or fetal pathology. Oligohydramnios, or decreased amniotic fluid volume for a particular gestational age, can be caused by PROM, uteroplacental insufficiency (hypertension, preeclampsia, and intrauterine growth restriction), post-term pregnancy, or fetal genitourinary abnormalities. Polyhydramnios, or increased amniotic fluid volume for a particular gestational age, can be idiopathic (approximately 50% of cases) or related to gestational/pregestational diabetes, fetal infection, alloimmunization, or fetal structural or chromosomal abnormalities.[4] Most important, both oligohydramnios and polyhydramnios are associated with an increased risk of perinatal morbidity and mortality.[4-8]

Two sonographic techniques are commonly used for assessing amniotic fluid volume: measurement of the maximal vertical pocket (MVP) and the amniotic fluid index (AFI). MVP is the preferred method given the simplicity of the technique and lower false positive rate for the diagnosis of oligohydramnios, which results in fewer obstetric interventions without affecting perinatal outcomes.[9] Furthermore, a recent multidisciplinary, multisociety consensus recommended the MVP technique and therefore will be the only method discussed here.[10]

The MVP technique is defined as measurement of the single largest vertical pocket of amniotic fluid within the uterine cavity that is free of umbilical cord or fetal parts. With the transducer in a sagittal orientation, the uterine cavity should be scanned in its entirety from left to right, and from the fundus to the lower uterine segment, to identify the single largest pocket of amniotic fluid. After identification of the largest pocket, place the calipers in a vertical straight line to measure the depth in centimeters. Normal MVP ranges from 2 to 8 cm. Oligohydramnios and polyhydramnios are defined as an MVP less than 2 cm and MVP greater than 8 cm, respectively (Figs. 30.10 and 30.11).

PLACENTAL LOCALIZATION AND ASSESSMENT

Placental abnormalities can cause significant maternal and fetal morbidity. For nonexperts, POCUS offers an opportunity for early detection of aberrant placental location or structure that can significantly alter patient management. In general, clinicians should use POCUS to rule-in placental abnormalities, as definitively ruling out placental pathology requires greater expertise.

Placental implantation can occur on any uterine surface: anterior, posterior, lateral, fundal, or overlying the internal os of the cervix. The latter situation, called placenta previa, represents one of the most common causes of bleeding during the second and third trimesters of pregnancy. Placenta previa requires a cesarean delivery, making antenatal identification essential to minimize the risk of fetal and maternal morbidity.[11] In addition to bleeding complications, placenta previa and other types of abnormal placentation, such

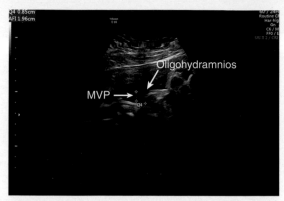

Figure 30.10   Oligohydramnios. Maximal vertical pocket (MVP) less than 2 cm defines oligohydramnios. MVP is 0.85 cm in this patient.

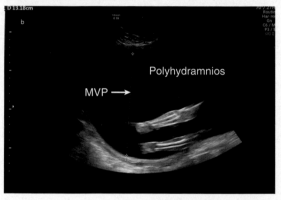

Figure 30.11   Polyhydramnios. Maximal vertical pocket (MVP) greater than 8 cm defines polyhydramnios. MVP is 13.18 cm in this patient.

as placenta accreta, increase the risk of other complications.

With the transducer in a sagittal orientation, scan in parallel, longitudinal paths from superior to inferior, from the uterine fundus to the lower uterine segment, along the maternal abdomen and from the left side to right side (Fig. 30.12) Starting at the uterine fundus will ensure that a fundal placenta is not overlooked. After the placenta is located, the inferior edge must be identified and its relationship to the cervix must be evaluated (Fig. 30.13 and Video 30.4). In patients with a posterior placenta, scanning the lateral abdomen may be helpful to identify the placenta when overlying fetal parts cause shadowing and obscuration of the placental edge.

Placenta previa occurs when the placenta covers the internal os of the cervix and affects approximately 1 in 200 pregnancies at term.[12]

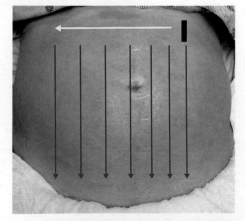

Figure 30.12   Placental Localization Technique. Place the transducer in the left upper quadrant in a sagittal plane *(black bar)*, and slide the transducer in a craniocaudal direction moving sequentially from the patient's left to right side to localize the placenta.

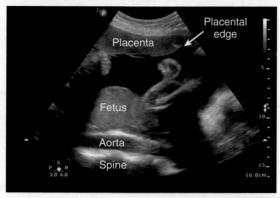

Figure 30.13   Anterior Placenta. An anterior placental edge is seen from a sagittal transabdominal view.

Placenta Previa

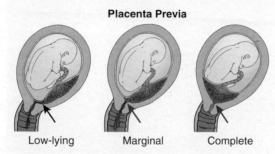

Low-lying   Marginal   Complete

Figure 30.14   Types of Placenta Previa. In low-lying placenta previa, the placental edge is within 2 cm of the internal cervical os *(black arrow)*. In marginal placenta previa, the placental edge abuts the internal cervical os but does not cover it *(blue arrow)*. In complete placenta previa, the placenta covers the internal cervical os *(red arrow)*.

A multispecialty consensus changed the definition of placenta previa to any placenta that overlies the cervical os to any degree.[10] A low-lying placenta occurs when the placental edge is within 2 cm of the internal cervical os but does not touch it (Figs. 30.14 and 30.15). A marginal placenta previa occurs when the placental edge touches the internal cervical os but does not cover it. A complete placenta previa occurs when the placenta covers the internal cervical os (Fig. 30.16).[13] Ideally, the urinary bladder should only be partially full since a full urinary bladder can simulate placenta previa by causing apposition of the anterior and posterior uterine walls. On the contrary, a completely empty urinary bladder can make visualization of the lower uterine segment and cervical os difficult. Further, if the patient was experiencing a contraction during the examination, the examination should be repeated after the contraction has resolved because contractions can distort the placenta and myometrium resulting in a false positive diagnosis of placenta previa. A diagnosis of placenta previa should be confirmed by a transvaginal ultrasound exam only if the transabdominal ultrasound exam is nondiagnostic.[13] Assessment of placenta accreta, increta, and percreta require systematic transabdominal scanning that is beyond the scope of a point-of-care obstetric ultrasound examination.

Vasa previa, a rare but potentially catastrophic complication, occurs when fetal vessels are present in the membranes covering the cervical os. A vasa previa can form in the following two scenarios:

1. Velamentous insertion of the umbilical cord: umbilical vessels course within the fetal membranes (amnion and chorion) before inserting into placental disk
2. Bilobed or succenturiate placenta: a variation of placental morphology with two equally sized lobes (bilobed placenta) or

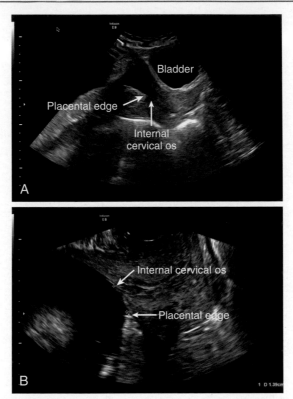

Figure 30.15   Low-Lying Placenta. (A) Sagittal *transabdominal* view of a low-lying placenta previa. Note proximity of the placental edge to the internal cervical os. (B) Sagittal *transvaginal* view of the cervix confirming the presence of a low-lying placenta previa. The placental edge measures 1.39 cm from the internal cervical os.

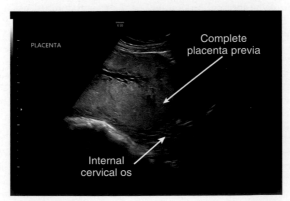

Figure 30.16   Complete Placenta Previa. A sagittal transabdominal view reveals a complete placenta previa with the placenta covering the internal cervical os.

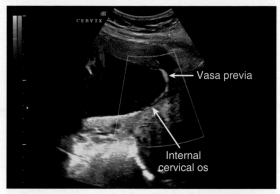

Figure 30.17   Vasa Previa. A sagittal transabdominal image reveals fetal vessels overlying the internal cervical os consistent with vasa previa.

unequally sized lobes with a smaller lobe (succenturiate lobe) that has fetal vessels connecting in the membranes overlying the cervix.

Undiagnosed vasa previa carries a perinatal mortality rate of approximately 60% as a result of fetal and neonatal exsanguination upon spontaneous or artificial rupture of membranes.[14] Prior to the incorporation of ultrasound into prenatal care, the morbidity from vasa previa was thought to be unavoidable. However, in the era of ultrasound, the majority of morbidity from vasa previa is circumvented with prenatal diagnosis and cesarean delivery prior to the onset of labor.

Flow within the vessels overlying the internal cervical os can be seen with transabdominal ultrasound (Fig. 30.17). A diagnosis of vasa previa can be confirmed by transvaginal ultrasound with color flow Doppler documenting the presence of fetal vessels overlying the internal cervical os. PW Doppler should be performed to ensure the vascular flow is fetal in origin and not maternal uterine flow. Consideration should be given to performing the study in a Trendelenburg position or after the patient is repositioned to ensure a funic presentation (umbilical cord pointing towards the internal cervical os or lower uterine segment) is ruled out.

Placental abruption, or premature placental separation with bleeding at the placental-decidual interface, affects approximately 1% of all pregnancies and is associated with an increased risk of maternal and fetal morbidity and mortality.[15,16] Most important, a diagnosis of placental abruption is based on

clinical findings of vaginal bleeding accompanied by pelvic pain because the majority of clinical placental abruption will not be detected by ultrasound. Therefore, the absence of sonographic findings of placental abruption does not rule out the diagnosis.[17] Sonographic findings include presence of a hematoma as a result of the separation. The hematoma will usually be located retroplacental but can also be preplacental (Fig. 30.18). The sonographic appearance of hematomas can vary in appearance from hypoechoic, isoechoic, and hyperechoic relative to surrounding tissue.[17] Visualization of a retroplacental hematoma has a high positive predictive value for placental abruption. Most of these patients typically present with a substantial amount of bleeding and placental separation.

FETAL BIOMETRY

Fetal biometry refers to the anatomic measurements of the fetus that can be used to estimate both fetal age and fetal weight. Some common biometric parameters used for estimation of gestational age and fetal size in the second and third trimesters include: head circumference (HC), biparietal diameter (BPD), abdominal circumference (AC), and femur length (FL). It is important to remember that ultrasound evaluation of an embryo or fetus in the first trimester using crown-rump length through the 13 6/7 week of gestation is the most accurate method to determine gestational age.[18] The gestational age, or estimated due date, of a pregnancy based on first trimester ultrasonography should not be changed based on biometric

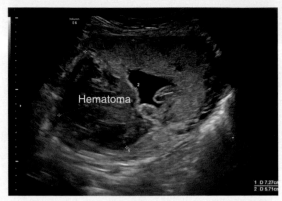

Figure 30.18   Placental Abruption. A large retroplacental hematoma appears hypoechoic and measures 7.27 cm × 5.71 cm in a patient with placental abruption.

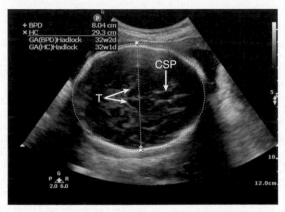

Figure 30.19   Biparietal Diameter (BPD) and Head Circumference (HC). The BPD and HC are obtained at the level of the thalami *(T)* and the cavum septi pellucidi *(CSP)*. Note that the BPD is obtained from the outer edge of the proximal parietal bone to the inner edge of the lower parietal bone. The HC is obtained at the same level with the ellipse over the outer edge of the parietal bone.

assessment in the second or third trimester. Therefore, the earliest ultrasound in pregnancy should be used for gestational dating. When dating a pregnancy, we recommend following the guidelines endorsed by The American College of Obstetricians and Gynecologists (ACOG), Society for Maternal-Fetal Medicine (SMFM), and American Institute of Ultrasound in Medicine (AIUM).[18]

Biparietal Diameter and Head Circumference

The BPD and HC should be measured in a transverse cross-section of the head at the level of the thalami and cavum septi pellucidi. Other landmarks include the midline falx and symmetrical appearance of the bilateral cerebral hemispheres (Fig. 30.19). The cerebellar hemispheres should not be visible. To measure the BPD, activate the biometry software on the ultrasound console. Place the upper caliper on the outer edge of the proximal parietal bone in the near field and the lower caliper on the inner edge of the distal parietal bone in the far field. The line between the calipers should be perpendicular to the midline falx.

The HC can be measured in the same plane as the BPD. Position the calipers on the *outer* edges of the proximal and distal parietal bones in the near and far fields, respectively. The line between the calipers should be perpendicular to the midline falx. Fit the ellipse over the contour of the fetal skull to measure the circumference. The ellipse can be adjusted to fit

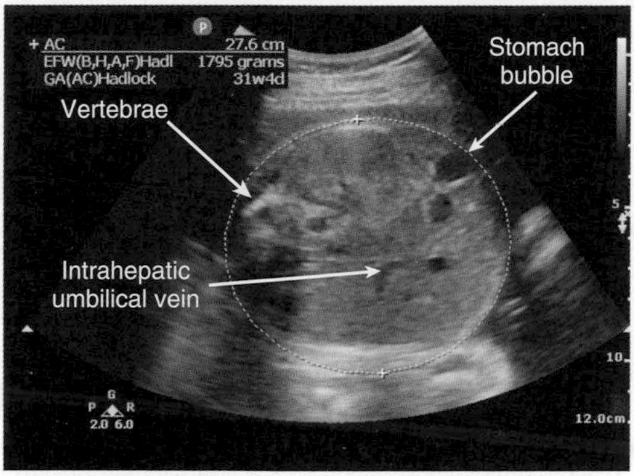

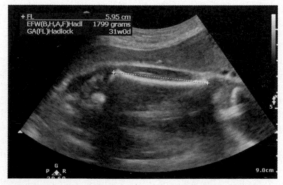

Figure 30.20 Abdominal Circumference. The stomach bubble, vertebrae, and intrahepatic umbilical vein are identified and an ellipse is traced over the contour of the fetal abdomen to calculate the abdominal circumference.

Figure 30.21 Femur Length Measurement. Note that only the metaphysis is being measured. The epiphysis should not be included in the measurement.

over the fetal skull by adjusting the position of the calipers (Video 30.5). The ultrasound machine's biometry software will calculate the estimated gestational age.

Abdominal Circumference

The AC is measured in a symmetrical, circular, transverse cross-section of the fetal abdomen. Anatomic landmarks to identify the proper plane of measurement include: visualization of the vertebrae in cross section along with the stomach bubble and intrahepatic umbilical vein with portal sinus (Fig. 30.20). The fetal kidneys should not be visualized. Measuring the AC with the fetal spine at 3 o'clock or 9 o'clock will minimize shadowing. Similar to measurement of the HC, after selecting AC from the biometry menu, calipers will appear.

Place the calipers on the outer edges of the fetal skin such that the line between them is perpendicular to the midline. Open and fit the ellipse over the contour of the fetal abdomen. The ellipse can be adjusted to improve the fit by adjusting the position of the calipers (Video 30.6).

Femur Length

FL should be measured with the full length of the bone, excluding the epiphysis (Fig. 30.21, Video 30.7). The measurement is obtained by selecting FL from the biometry menu and placing the calipers on the ends of the ossified diaphysis.

Most ultrasound machines include a biometry software package that can estimate fetal weight from biometric measurements. A complete discussion of the methodology to estimate fetal weight is beyond the scope of this chapter. If using an ultrasound machine that does not have biometry software, the calipers can be used to measure BPD and FL, and the ellipse function can be used to measure HC and AC.

PEARLS AND PITFALLS

- If the fetal head or sacrum is not visualized in the lower uterine segment, then a transverse or oblique lie should be suspected. A midsagittal view of the fetal spine should be obtained to assess the relative angle of the fetal and maternal spines.
- Fetal heart rate can be measured using either pulsed-wave Doppler or M-mode. The distance between cardiac contractions is used to calculate fetal heart rate, similar to an ECG.
- The maximal vertical pocket (MVP) technique is the preferred method to determine amniotic fluid volume given its simplicity and lower false positive rate for diagnosing oligohydramnios.
- Monochorionic twins should have an ultrasound examination every 2 weeks, and dichorionic twins should have an ultrasound examination every 4 weeks during the last half of pregnancy.

- Point-of-care ultrasound should be used only to rule-in placental pathology as ruling out the presence of hazardous placental structure or function requires greater expertise.
- When assessing for placenta previa, the urinary bladder should be partially full since a full urinary bladder can simulate placenta previa by causing apposition of the anterior and posterior uterine walls. On the contrary, avoid a completely empty urinary bladder as visualization of the lower uterine segment and internal cervical os can be difficult.
- The majority of cases of clinical placental abruption will not be detected by ultrasound, and the absence of sonographic findings of placental abruption cannot rule out the diagnosis.
- Gestational age or estimated due date of pregnancy based on the first trimester ultrasonography should not be changed based on a biometric assessment in the second or third trimester because late pregnancy ultrasound findings can be impacted by pathologic processes, such as fetal growth restriction.
- Rapid techniques to estimate gestational age include measurement of fundal height above the symphysis pubis and measurement of fetal femur length. It is important to recognize that in critical situations the quickest and easiest measurement of fetal biometry should be obtained.

CHAPTER 31

Testicular Ultrasound

Daniel Lakoff ■ Stephen Alerhand

KEY POINTS

- Acute scrotal pain can be rapidly evaluated using point-of-care ultrasound to diagnose multiple conditions, including testicular torsion, epididymitis, and inguinal hernias.
- A thorough understanding of Doppler ultrasound techniques, including use of color Doppler, improves evaluation of the testicles and epididymis.
- For providers who perform testicular ultrasonography infrequently, a low threshold for consultation with radiology and urology should be maintained.

Background

Ultrasound has emerged as a preferred modality for evaluation of acute scrotal pain. Point-of-care ultrasound (POCUS) can facilitate diagnosis of most testicular pathologies, with particular emphasis on the emergent pathologies that threaten the viability of the testicle. The three most common etiologies of acute scrotal pain are testicular torsion, epididymitis, and inguinal hernia.[1,2] Other common etiologies that may present acutely include varicocele, hydrocele, and trauma.

This chapter provides basic instruction on how to perform a point-of-care testicular ultrasound exam. The imaging techniques described in this chapter can mitigate diagnostic dilemmas that arise in acute care settings and can be used to rule in certain pathologies. When POCUS findings are indeterminate, a comprehensive diagnostic testicular ultrasound exam should be obtained.

Normal Anatomy

Normal male testicular anatomy is illustrated in Fig. 31.1.

Image Acquisition

Image acquisition begins with patient comfort and proper positioning. After ensuring patient

privacy and administering adequate analgesia, place the patient in a supine, frog-legged position. The penis should be positioned upward onto the abdomen and covered with towels, leaving only the testicles exposed. The scrotum should be elevated with towels for comfort and to facilitate ultrasound imaging. An ultrasound machine with a high-frequency transducer should be brought to the patient's bedside and cleaned with antiseptic wipes before use. A transparent dressing or ultrasound probe cover can be placed over the probe.

Providers should always take advantage of anatomic symmetry by initially imaging the unaffected testicle to first gain familiarity with the patient's normal findings, as well as adjust the ultrasound machine settings (depth, gain, and Doppler). The same settings should be used when imaging the symptomatic testicle. A testicular ultrasound examination should be approached systematically to evaluate all elements during the exam (Fig. 31.2).

Image Interpretation

TESTICLES

The testicles lie in the scrotum and can easily be identified with ultrasound (Fig. 31.3). A normal two-dimensional (2D) image of the testicle in a longitudinal plane demonstrates an oval structure with homogeneous

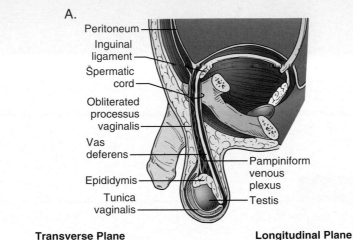

A.

Peritoneum

Inguinal ligament

Spermatic cord

Obliterated processus vaginalis

Vas deferens

Epididymis

Tunica vaginalis

Pampiniform venous plexus

Testis

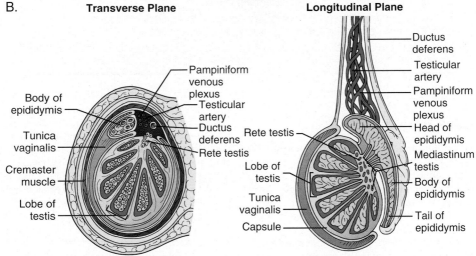

B.

Transverse Plane

Pampiniform venous plexus

Body of epididymis

Testicular artery

Tunica vaginalis

Ductus deferens

Cremaster muscle

Rete testis

Lobe of testis

Longitudinal Plane

Ductus deferens

Testicular artery

Pampiniform venous plexus

Rete testis

Head of epididymis

Lobe of testis

Mediastinum testis

Tunica vaginalis

Body of epididymis

Capsule

Tail of epididymis

Figure 31.1   Normal Testicular Anatomy. (A) Gross anatomy of the testicle. (B) Cross-sectional anatomy of the testicle in transverse and longitudinal planes.

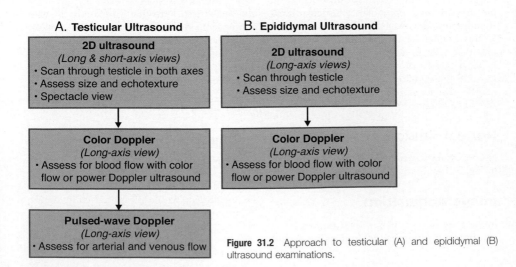

A. Testicular Ultrasound

2D ultrasound
(Long & short-axis views)
• Scan through testicle in both axes
• Assess size and echotexture
• Spectacle view

↓

Color Doppler
(Long-axis view)
• Assess for blood flow with color flow or power Doppler ultrasound

↓

Pulsed-wave Doppler
(Long-axis view)
• Assess for arterial and venous flow

B. Epididymal Ultrasound

2D ultrasound
(Long-axis views)
• Scan through testicle
• Assess size and echotexture

↓

Color Doppler
(Long-axis view)
• Assess for blood flow with color flow or power Doppler ultrasound

Figure 31.2   Approach to testicular (A) and epididymal (B) ultrasound examinations.

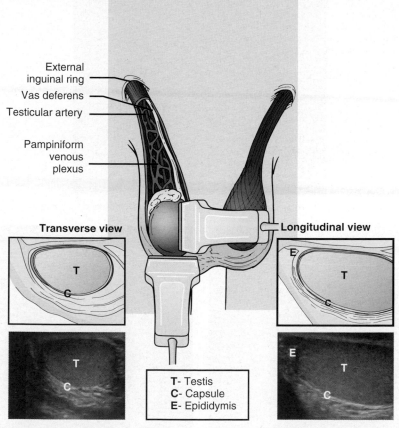

External inguinal ring
Vas deferens
Testicular artery
Pampiniform venous plexus

Transverse view

T
C

Longitudinal view

E
T
C

T
C

E
T
C

T- Testis
C- Capsule
E- Epididymis

Figure 31.3 **Transducer Position.** Acquisition of transverse *(short-axis)* and longitudinal *(long-axis)* views.

echotexture and smooth rounded edges measuring on average 4 cm × 3 cm × 3 cm (Fig. 31.4 and Video 31.1). In a transverse plane, the short-axis view shows a circular structure (Fig. 31.5). A spectacle view (Fig. 31.6) is obtained by centering the transducer over the midline to partially visualize both testicles in short axis, allowing side-by-side comparison of both testicles. The mediastinum testis is the confluence of septa and appears as a hyperechoic linear structure in a long-axis view. The rete testis can be identified adjacent to the mediastinum, and it appears as small anechoic areas. The testicular appendage is a remnant of the müllerian duct and can occasionally be seen at the superior pole of the testicle.

In a normal testicle, color flow Doppler shows blood flow throughout the testicle. Color power Doppler (CPD) is more sensitive for low-flow areas and is often preferred

for testicles (Fig. 31.7 and Video 31.2). When assessing either arterial or venous flow of a testicle, pulsed-wave Doppler (PWD) must be used to differentiate arteries from veins. Arterial waveforms have a high-velocity, pulsatile pattern (Fig. 31.8), whereas veins have a low-velocity, nonpulsatile pattern (Fig. 31.9).

EPIDIDYMIS

The epididymis lies posterior and lateral to the testicle. The head of the epididymis is superior to the testicle, the body is posterior, and tail is at the inferior pole. The tail tapers into the ductus deferens, which becomes part of the spermatic cord, and ultimately ascends into the abdominal cavity via the inguinal canal. The epididymal head appears wrinkled with a heterogeneous echotexture that is either isoechoic or slightly hyperechoic relative to the

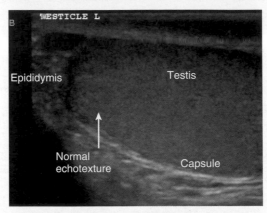

Figure 31.4   Normal Testicle. A normal testicle in long axis (longitudinal plane).

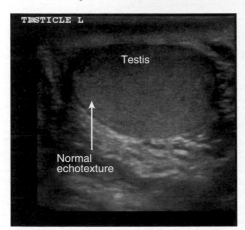

Figure 31.5   Normal Testicle. A normal testicle in short axis (transverse plane).

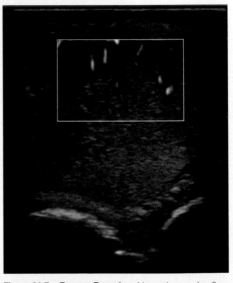

Figure 31.7   Power Doppler. Normal vascular flow of the testicle by power Doppler ultrasound.

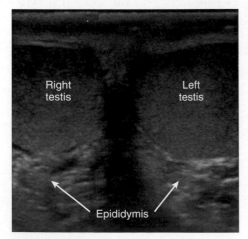

Figure 31.6   Spectacle View. Both testicles are visualized simultaneously in side-by-side short-axis views.

testicle. These findings are more exaggerated when using zoom. The epididymal head has a pyramidal shape, measures approximately 5 to 12 mm, and is located at the superior pole of the testicle (Fig. 31.10). A normal and healthy epididymal body and the tail are challenging to visualize. The epididymal appendage is a remnant structure at the epididymal head that is usually not visible in the absence of pathology. Color flow or power Doppler should be used to demonstrate intraepididymal flow (Fig. 31.11).

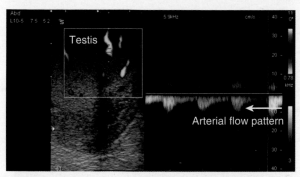

Figure 31.8 Arterial Flow. Pulsatile, relatively high-velocity arterial flow of the testicle is seen with pulsed-wave Doppler.

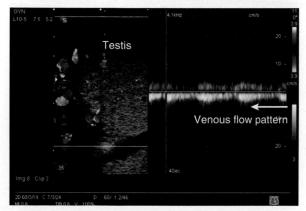

Figure 31.9 Venous Flow. Nonpulsatile, low-velocity venous flow of the testicle is seen by pulsed-wave Doppler.

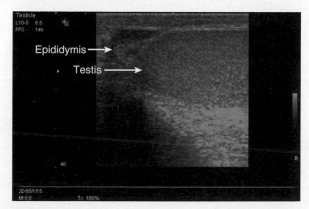

Figure 31.10 Normal Epididymis. Normal epididymal head is seen at the superior pole of the testicle.

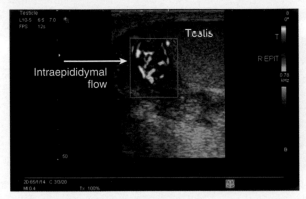

Figure 31.11 **Epididymal Flow.** Color flow Doppler pattern of a normal epididymis.

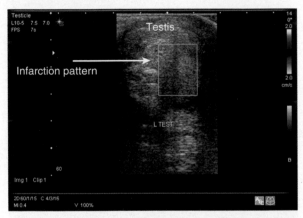

Figure 31.12 **Testicular Torsion.** Testicular torsion demonstrates heterogeneous echotexture, infarction pattern (hypoechoic lesion), and absence of flow by color Doppler.

Pathologic Findings

TESTICULAR TORSION

A variety of ultrasound findings can be seen in torsion. Based on studies by radiologists, ultrasound has high sensitivity and specificity to diagnose testicular torsion.[3] In studies performed by emergency medicine physicians, similar results have been obtained with a sensitivity of 90% to 100% and specificity nearing 100%.[4]

The testicle is affected primarily and the epididymis secondarily in torsion. 2D findings of testicular torsion include an enlarged testicle secondary to venous congestion or inflammation, heterogeneous testicular echotexture, reactive hydrocele, edema of the scrotal wall,

infarction pattern, and enlargement of the epididymis with diminished flow (Fig. 31.12).

Color Doppler generally shows a decrease or absence of blood flow in torsion, although an increase in flow can be seen in the torsion/detorsion phenomenon (Fig. 31.13). Vascular occlusion starts with loss of the low-pressure venous flow at the onset of testicular torsion. Venous obstruction is followed by the loss of high-pressure arterial flow. As the testicle twists on its vascular supply and the arterial flow is crimped, the pulsatile arterial flow is diminished or lost (Videos 31.3–31.5). Decreased or absent blood flow of the testicle is seen with PWD, including absence of arterial and venous flow waveforms compared to the contralateral side.[5,6] It is imperative to obtain PWD waveforms of both arteries and veins to avoid

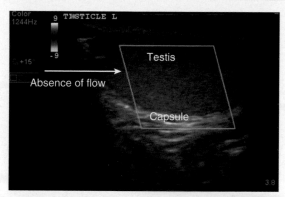

Figure 31.13   Testicular Torsion by Color flow Doppler. Absence of blood flow by color flow Doppler is seen in testicular torsion.

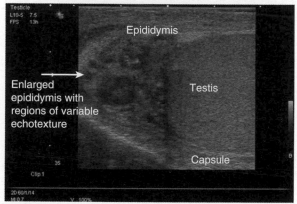

Figure 31.14   Epididymitis. An enlarged epididymis with variable echotexture (hypoechoic areas) is seen in epididymitis.

mistaking low flow as venous when it is actually dampened arterial flow.

In cases of potential detorsion, ultrasound may show isolated hyperemia, which may sway a provider to diagnose orchitis or epididymo-orchitis, given the testicular enlargement. Interpretation of this finding should be done in conjunction with a careful history and complete testicular physical exam. Providers are advised to consult with urology, ensure expedited follow-up, and provide strict return precautions.

EPIDIDYMITIS

Most patients with epididymitis exhibit a constellation of ultrasound findings that confirm the diagnosis. False-negative or false-positive findings occur in few patients. Therefore,

ultrasound examination for epididymitis should be integrated with the history (i.e., post-pubertal male with a painful tender scrotum, dysuria, and fever), physical examination, and lab and urine results. An enlarged epididymis (>17 mm) with areas of variable echotexture, most often hypoechoic areas due to edema, are seen on 2D ultrasound imaging with the epididymal head being most commonly affected (Fig. 31.14). Hyperechoic areas may be seen due to hemorrhage. Nonspecific secondary findings that may be seen include reactive hydrocele or pyocele and scrotal wall thickening (normal range 2–8 mm) (Fig. 31.15). Abscess formation may appear as an avascular, hypoechoic pocket within the epididymis. Using color flow Doppler, the affected epididymis will demonstrate increased vascularity and flow compared with the unaffected side (Fig. 31.16; Videos 31.6

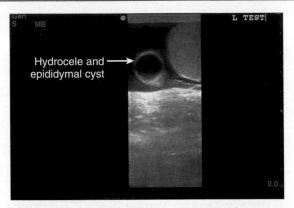

Figure 31.15 Hydrocele. Epididymitis with a reactive hydrocele.

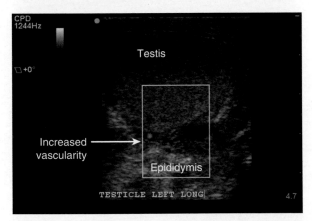

Figure 31.16 Epididymitis. Increased vascularity by color power Doppler is seen with epididymitis.

and 31.7).[6-8] Sensitivity of color Doppler for detecting scrotal inflammation is nearly 100%.[9]

EPIDIDYMO-ORCHITIS

Epididymo-orchitis occurs in about 20% to 40% of epididymitis cases due to direct spread of the infection from the epididymis to the testicle,[10] with multiple sonographic findings to assist in the diagnosis. Epididymal hyperemia will continue to be present on color Doppler as seen in epididymitis.[11] The testicle will appear enlarged and hyperemic with loss of its homogeneous echotexture (Figs. 31.17 and 31.18; Video 31.8). A reactive hydrocele may also be present.[12] In severe cases, swelling can obstruct blood flow and lead to an infarction pattern, similar to testicular torsion; however, the clinical history, persistent hyperemia, and scrotal warmth will point toward a diagnosis of epididymo-orchitis rather than torsion.

SCROTAL CELLULITIS

Cellulitis of the scrotum occurs most often in patients who are obese, diabetic, or otherwise immunocompromised.[13,14] On ultrasound, the scrotal wall will appear thickened with increased echogenicity, showing increased vascular flow on color Doppler. If the cellulitis is severe, it may exhibit the classic cobblestoning pattern.[7] An abscess may develop and appear as septated lobules interspersed within loculated, anechoic fluid collections.[14] These loculations may contain low-level internal echoes.

INGUINAL HERNIA

Ultrasound offers excellent diagnostic performance for detecting inguinal hernias with a sensitivity of 97%, specificity of 75%, and positive predictive value of 93% when performed by experienced providers.[15] Different

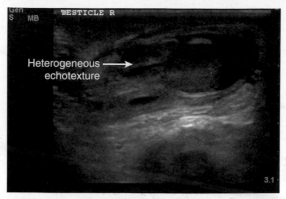

Figure 31.17 Epididymo-Orchitis. Epididymo-orchitis with heterogeneous echotexture of the testicle is seen in a long-axis view.

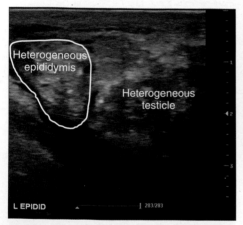

Figure 31.18 Epididymo-Orchitis. Note the heterogeneous echotexture of both the epididymis and testicle.

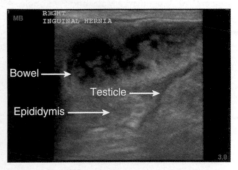

Figure 31.19 Inguinal Hernia. An inguinal hernia is seen with small bowel adjacent to the testicle and epididymis.

approaches have been described to evaluate for an inguinal hernia. The first approach is to use a linear transducer to scan the hemiscrotum for any bowel contents, which can rapidly diagnose an inguinal hernia when moderate to high pretest probability exists (Fig. 31.19 and Video 31.9).

A more systematic approach can be used to diagnose subtle hernias. The first step is to identify the inferior epigastric artery (IEA) using a linear transducer in a transverse plane. The IEA is traced inferolaterally on the anterior abdominal wall to the external iliac artery, and the inguinal ring is identified between the root of the IEA and external iliac artery. Over the inguinal ring, the transducer is rotated to align the ultrasound beam parallel to the inguinal ligament, acquiring a long-axis view of the inguinal canal. With the transducer placed longitudinally along the inguinal ligament, either a hernia sac (blind-ending tubular structure) or preperitoneal fat can be identified. Once a hernia sac is identified, compression can be performed to differentiate clinically significant, painful hernias from clinically insignificant hernias. Experienced providers may be able to assess hernia neck size to predict reducibility, as well as identify the spermatic cord to categorize the hernia as direct or indirect.

If a hernia sac cannot be found with the above techniques, then provocative, dynamic imaging may be performed if the clinical suspicion remains high. The transducer is positioned over the inguinal canal and the patient is asked to increase his/her intraabdominal pressure by standing or performing a Valsalva

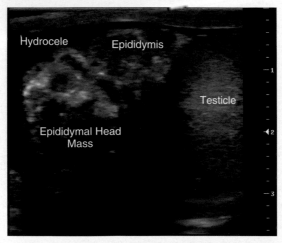

Figure 31.20   Epididymal Mass and Hydrocele. A reactive hydrocele due to an epididymal head mass is seen in a zoomed view.

maneuver. If a hernia is present, the preperitoneal fat or bowel will descend into the inguinal canal.

HYDROCELE

Hydroceles are fluid collections between the parietal and visceral layers of tunica vaginalis and can develop for a variety of reasons. In children, hydroceles develop due to a patent processus vaginalis, resulting in a communicating track that allows fluid to shift from the abdominal cavity to the scrotum. This can result in the development of unilateral or bilateral hydroceles, as well as hernias. Generally, the hydrocele and track resolve within 1 year in newborns.

As men age, hydroceles most often develop due to infection, inflammation, trauma, or malignancy.[16] Although the presentation of painless scrotal swelling may seem benign, malignant hydroceles are present in about 10% of testicular tumors (Fig. 31.20).[17] Most hydroceles are not true emergencies. However, if the hydrocele volume is large enough, it can compromise perfusion of the testicle. In most circumstances, scrotal ultrasound can initiate the evaluation and determine the urgency with which a patient should seek follow-up (Fig. 31.21 and Video 31.10). Infectious hydroceles can also demonstrate septations (Fig. 31.22 and Video 31.11).

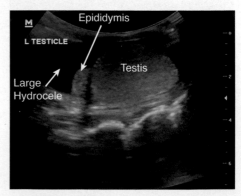

Figure 31.21   Hydrocele. A large hydrocele is seen surrounding the testicle.

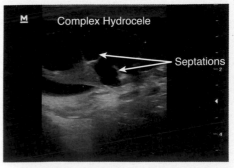

Figure 31.22   Hydrocele With Septations.

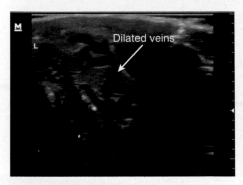

Figure 31.23 Varicocele. Note the dilated veins that appear as anechoic tubular structures.

VARICOCELE

Varicocele formation may arise from defective valves or venous compression by a nearby structure, the most common latter etiology being renal cell carcinoma. The dilated veins of the pampiniform plexus appear as multiple hypoechoic or anechoic dilated tubular structures. Their diameter will be greater than 2 to 3 mm,[7,14] as opposed to their normal range of 0.5 to 1.5 mm.[7] Varicoceles occur more frequently on the left side due to the abrupt 90-degree angle of the left gonadal vein's drainage into the left renal vein. Upon standing or performing the Valsalva maneuver, a varicocele will enlarge and demonstrate increased blood flow on color Doppler and flow reversal on spectral Doppler.[7] If blood flow does not increase on the right side or flow reversal does not occur when supine, further workup should be pursued to rule out a retroperitoneal malignancy that is compressing the inferior vena cava.[18] A common technical pitfall is applying excessive pressure to the skin of the scrotum with the ultrasound transducer, reducing venous diameter while increasing the Doppler flow rate (Fig. 31.23 and Video 31.12).[19]

ACUTE SCROTAL TRAUMA

Blunt testicular trauma may occur from sports injuries, motor vehicle accidents, assaults, or straddle injuries. Using ultrasound, visualization of a normal testicle virtually excludes significant injury. Testicular trauma may appear in the form of a fluid collection (hematocele, hydrocele, hematoma), testicular disruption (fracture, rupture), or vascular injury.

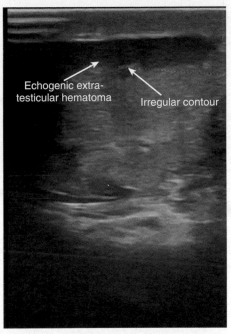

Figure 31.24 Hematocele. A hematocele is seen adjacent to a testicle with traumatic disruption of its tunica albuginea.

Acute hematoceles (blood collections within the tunica vaginalis) are the most common scrotal complication from blunt trauma.[8] These echogenic extratesticular hematomas may compress the surrounding vasculature and thus reduce blood flow, necessitating surgery in order to salvage the testis (Fig. 31.24 and Video 31.13).[20] Acute hematomas will appear as focal areas of heterogeneous echogenicity.[21] Of note, 10% to 15% of testicular tumors first manifest as hematomas after trauma, even if the trauma is minimal.[22] In contrast to hematomas, these masses show flow on color Doppler.[4]

A testicular fracture appears as a linear hypoechoic, avascular area within the parenchyma with or without tunica albuginea disruption. A discrete fracture plane is reported to be seen in only 17% of cases.[23] Normally, the tunica albuginea is seen as an echogenic line outlining the testis. In testicular rupture, there is discontinuity of the contour of the tunica albuginea and heterogeneous parenchymal extrusion.[20] The sensitivity and specificity of ultrasound for testicular fracture is 50% and

75%, respectively.[21] Disruption of the arteries associated with the tunica albuginea may also occur,[24] manifesting as regions of avascularity.[13] For disruption of the tunica albuginea, surgery is indicated to prevent pressure necrosis, atrophy, and orchiectomy.[26] The salvage rate is 80% if surgery occurs in the first 72 hours.[27] Conversely, small hematomas without rupture can be managed conservatively.[25]

Testicular torsion is also associated with trauma or physical exertion in up to 20% of cases.[28] This may result from forceful contraction of the cremaster muscle.[20] Ultrasound findings will be similar to those described previously for torsion.

PEARLS AND PITFALLS

- Providers should be proficient in color and pulsed-wave Doppler ultrasound to perform testicular ultrasound examinations. If available, color power Doppler is preferred to assess the low-velocity blood flow of testicles.
- Start by evaluating the unaffected testicle first to have a baseline for comparison with the affected side.
- The three most common etiologies of acute scrotal pain are testicular torsion, epididymitis, and inguinal hernia. Venous followed by arterial blood flow is generally decreased or absent with torsion, whereas increased flow is seen with epididymitis.
- A focused ultrasound examination to detect bowel or preperitoneal fat in the inguinal canal or scrotum can rapidly detect an incarcerated inguinal hernia. Nonincarcerated hernias can be detected by using dynamic evaluation methods (standing, Valsalva).
- Though not often an emergency, hydroceles should be evaluated thoroughly because malignant hydroceles are present in about 10% of testicular tumors. Similarly, 10% to 15% of testicular tumors first manifest as hematomas after trauma, even if the trauma is minimal.
- Recognize normal findings and remember that normal findings do not always equate with the absence of pathology; if the pain persists or diagnosis is uncertain, a low threshold for consultation with radiology and urology should be maintained.

Abdominal Pain

John Eicken ■ Patricia C. Henwood

- Point-of-care ultrasound assessment of *unstable* patients with abdominal pain should begin with an evaluation for hemorrhage, followed by an evaluation for infectious sources.
- Point-of-care ultrasound assessment of *stable* patients with abdominal pain should focus on etiologies based on the patient's history, examination, and demographics with an emphasis on detecting time-sensitive emergencies.
- Ultrasound is the initial diagnostic imaging modality of choice for children with abdominal pain because most etiologies can be diagnosed in this population without exposure to ionizing radiation.

Background

Point-of-care ultrasound (POCUS) has become an essential component in the evaluation of acute abdominal pain. Providers can integrate the clinical history and physical exam findings with a focused bedside ultrasound examination to guide diagnostic and therapeutic decisions. POCUS results are immediately available, saving both time and personnel resources, and avoiding the use of ionizing radiation or intravenous contrast agents.[1]

A wide range of acute abdominal pathologies can be diagnosed or supported with a focused abdominal ultrasound exam, including but not limited to the following: abdominal aortic aneurysm (AAA) or dissection, intraperitoneal fluid, appendicitis, renal or biliary calculi, acute cholecystitis, bowel obstruction, tubo-ovarian abscess, ectopic pregnancy, ovarian torsion, ruptured ovarian cyst, abdominal wall abscess, intussusception, and bowel perforation (Fig. 32.1).

Previous chapters have addressed image acquisition and interpretation of the focused abdominal ultrasound exams highlighted in Fig. 32.1. This chapter presents a framework to conceptualize integration of the various POCUS techniques into the initial evaluation of urgent or emergent abdominal complaints. Providers may perform a focused evaluation of one organ or a combination of abdominal organs. We review the most important applications in the evaluation of unstable and stable patients with abdominal pain.

Unstable Patients

Initial evaluation of unstable patients with abdominal pain should focus on a limited number of conditions for which point-of-care abdominal ultrasound results will dramatically change acute management decisions. Ultrasound is used in these patients to broadly search for two things: evidence of intraperitoneal hemorrhage or an infectious source within the abdomen (Fig. 32.2).

HEMORRHAGE

Evaluation of unstable patients with abdominal pain begins with a search for hemoperitoneum, best performed with the abdominal views of the Focused Assessment with Sonography in Trauma (FAST) exam.[2] Whereas many providers are aware that unstable trauma patients with

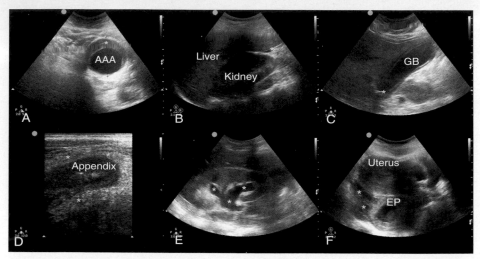

Figure 32.1   Abdominal Pain Pathologies Diagnosed by Point-of-Care Ultrasound. (A) Abdominal aortic aneurysm. A 5-cm abdominal aortic aneurysm (AAA) containing a mural thrombus *(asterisk)*. (B) Hemoperitoneum. Trace amount of intraperitoneal free fluid *(asterisk)* in Morison's pouch after liver laceration. (C) Acute cholecystitis. Note the gallbladder *(GB)* with a thickened wall, pericholecystic fluid, and gallstone lodged in the gallbladder neck *(asterisk)*. (D) Acute appendicitis. The appendiceal tip is surrounded by hyperechoic periappendiceal fat stranding *(asterisks)*. (E) Obstructive uropathy. Dilated calyces in the renal pelvis *(asterisks)* consistent with mild to moderate hydronephrosis in a patient with an obstructing ureteral stone. (F) Ruptured ectopic pregnancy *(EP)* with extrauterine gestation visualized posterior to the uterus. Complex free fluid *(asterisks)* is seen due to hemoperitoneum.

positive FAST exams should undergo immediate operative exploration, it is also important to remember that hemoperitoneum can result from nontraumatic etiologies, including ruptured ectopic pregnancy or ovarian cysts, aneurysmal disease of the aorta or visceral vessels, anticoagulant use, blood dyscrasias, or tumor-associated hemorrhage.[3] Detection of free fluid in Morison's pouch (Video 32.1), the perisplenic space (left subdiaphragmatic space) (Video 32.2), or pelvis (Video 32.3) is critical to promptly identify patients in whom aggressive resuscitation with blood products is indicated while arranging for definitive care.

Conversely, it is vital to recognize the limited sensitivity of the FAST exam; an initial negative FAST exam should not be used by providers to definitively "rule out" a traumatic intra-abdominal injury.[4] Ultrasound has limited utility in evaluating the retroperitoneal space. Computed tomography (CT) imaging should be invoked when serial FAST exams are negative but an intra-abdominal source of hemorrhage is suspected. Performance of a repeat FAST exam within 24 hours of hospital admission has been shown to increase sensitivity for intra-abdominal injury, which may be useful for providers practicing in resource-limited settings without access to immediate CT scans.[5]

Evaluation for AAA is included in the bedside abdominal ultrasound exam for hemorrhage and multiple studies have supported the use of ultrasound by emergency physicians to assess for AAA in symptomatic patients (Video 32.4).[6] Given that the majority of ruptured AAAs cause retroperitoneal hemorrhage, the role of POCUS is more to detect the presence of an AAA that is large or dissecting (Video 32.5), rather than to detect intraperitoneal hemorrhage. Rapid identification of an AAA with suspected or impending rupture can dramatically expedite definitive management for patients who might otherwise have a broad differential diagnosis.[7,8] The abdominal aorta must be visualized from the diaphragm through its bifurcation into common iliac arteries in both long and short axes. Although an abdominal aortic diameter >3 cm is considered aneurysmal, it is unusual for aneurysms <4.5 cm to rupture, and clinicians must consider the entire clinical presentation when incorporating ultrasound findings into decision making.

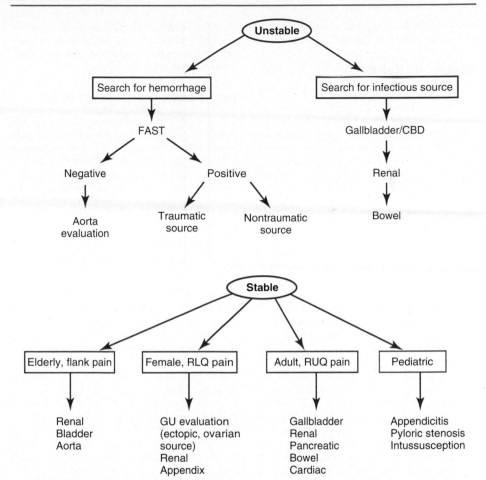

Figure 32.2 Approach to Acute Abdominal Pain Using Point-of-Care Ultrasound in Unstable and Stable Patients. *CBD*, Common bile duct; *FAST*, Focused Assessment with Sonography in Trauma; *GU*, genitourinary; *RLQ*, right lower quadrant; *RUQ*, right upper quadrant.

Patient demographics play an important role in evaluation of unstable patients. For example, a young female is far more likely to have a ruptured ectopic pregnancy than an AAA, whereas the opposite is true for an elderly patient. Thus, clinicians should individualize their diagnostic approach accordingly.

INFECTION

Point-of-care abdominal ultrasound can play an important role in identifying an infectious source in unstable patients with septic shock.[9] The gallbladder should be assessed for signs of acute cholecystitis, including wall thickening (Video 32.6), pericholecystic fluid, gallstones (Video 32.7 and Video 32.8), and a positive sonographic Murphy sign. Assessment of the common bile duct for dilation can confirm suspected acute cholangitis, most often due to a lodged gallstone. Unilateral hydronephrosis with or without a visualized ureteral stone indicates obstructive uropathy which is often associated with infection due to an infected renal stone or pyelonephritis (Video 32.9). Intra-abdominal abscess, perforated appendicitis, small bowel obstruction, and pneumoperitoneum may be detected but cannot be ruled out with POCUS. However, detection of any of these conditions can guide acute management, including prompt initiation of appropriate antibiotics, ordering of comprehensive or confirmatory imaging, and consultation with surgical services, if indicated.[10-14]

Stable Patients

Point-of-care abdominal ultrasound can help narrow the broad differential diagnosis and expedite care in stable patients with abdominal pain.[15] Four classic patient scenarios in which POCUS can be most useful will be reviewed: an adult patient with right upper quadrant, right lower quadrant, or flank pain; and a pediatric patient with generalized abdominal pain (see Fig. 32.2).

FLANK PAIN

The differential diagnosis for an adult patient with flank pain includes benign etiologies, such as muscle strain; urgent etiologies, such as renal colic; and life-threatening etiologies, such as aortic dissection or ruptured AAA.

In patients with acute unilateral flank pain, ultrasound can identify hydronephrosis due to an obstructing ureteral stone (Video 32.9). It is important to remember that unilateral hydronephrosis with or without hematuria may result from external compression of the ureter by an AAA, lymphadenopathy, or a retroperitoneal mass. A low threshold to image the abdominal aorta in patients at risk for AAA should be maintained. For certain patient populations in whom there is high clinical suspicion for renal colic, studies have shown that ultrasound is a reasonable first line imaging modality. For patients who are nonobese, nonpregnant, and who do not have a history of kidney transplant or dialysis, the use of ultrasound as the initial imaging modality has been shown to significantly decrease cumulative radiation exposure and emergency department length of stay without significant differences in adverse events, pain scores, return visits, or hospital admissions compared to patients who underwent CT imaging.[16,17]

In patients with urinary retention, providers may visualize bilateral hydronephrosis secondary to bladder outlet obstruction due to prostatic hypertrophy or medication side effects (Video 32.10). In patients with pyuria and flank pain, evaluation of kidneys for evidence of obstruction, stones, or abscess is critical to determine the need for further intervention or imaging. In patients with abdominal or back pain and acutely decreased urine output, bladder ultrasound to assess postvoid residual volume can help differentiate between decreased urine production versus acute urinary retention.

RIGHT LOWER QUADRANT PAIN

Ultrasound can rapidly evaluate for several possible etiologies of acute abdominal pain in the right lower quadrant.[18] In young female patients with acute onset of severe pain isolated to the lower abdomen, ruptured ectopic pregnancy and ovarian torsion are high-priority diagnoses to exclude (Video 32.11). Ultrasound is the imaging modality of choice to assess for both conditions and may also reveal other, often less emergent, causes of these symptoms, such as a ruptured hemorrhagic ovarian cyst or ovarian mass.[19]

In patients with acute onset of right lower quadrant pain that radiates from the flank to the groin, renal ultrasound should be used to evaluate for hydronephrosis due to an obstructing ureteral stone. Keep in mind that patients with ovarian torsion may also present with colicky pain. Although ovarian torsion is associated with large ovarian cysts and presents with decreased blood flow to the ovaries, the presence of normal blood flow and absence of ovarian cysts do not rule out ovarian torsion. Therefore further gynecologic evaluation for intermittent or persistent ovarian torsion should be pursued if there is high clinical suspicion.

A gradual onset of progressively worsening abdominal pain localizing to the right lower quadrant, calls for an evaluation of appendicitis (Video 32.12). Although evaluation may be limited by obesity and bowel gas, bedside ultrasound should be attempted as an initial imaging modality to avoid ionizing radiation associated with CT imaging, decrease imaging resource utilization, and expedite care if a grossly inflamed appendix is identified.[20,21]

RIGHT UPPER QUADRANT PAIN

Right upper quadrant or epigastric abdominal pain carries a broad differential diagnosis. The gallbladder remains a sensible starting point for stable patients and is easily evaluated with point-of-care ultrasound. As reviewed in chapter 27, the point-of-care exam may, include an assessment for gallstones, gallbladder wall thickening, pericholecystic fluid, common bile duct dimensions, and a sonographic Murphy sign. Ultrasound at the bedside can rapidly and effectively augment the diagnosis of biliary colic, acute cholecystitis, choledocholithiasis, and acute cholangitis.[22,23] Renal ultrasound may reveal evidence of stones or infection as a possible source of pain. Pancreatic ultrasound may also be attempted and can be useful to support a diagnosis of pancreatitis. Although the pancreas is often obscured by bowel gas, large pancreatic cysts or pseudocysts may be seen (Videos 32.13 and 32.14).[24]

PEDIATRIC ABDOMINAL PAIN

Due to safety concerns related to ionizing radiation, abdominal ultrasound is especially valuable as an initial diagnostic imaging modality in pediatric patients.[25] Ultrasound should be considered as the initial diagnostic test in children presenting with abdominal pain suspected to be acute appendicitis.[26-28] Integration of a clinical assessment or score, such as the Pediatric Appendicitis Score, can help guide patient care when ultrasound results are negative or equivocal.[29] POCUS can expedite diagnosis, surgical consultation, and disposition to the operating room.

Ultrasound is also useful for other gastrointestinal conditions in children, especially infants with vomiting. In infants less than 6 months old with vomiting in whom pyloric stenosis is a consideration, an ultrasound examination to evaluate for a hypertrophic pylorus is the test of choice.[30] Similarly, for those children in whom intussusception is a consideration, ultrasound is preferred to plain radiography as the initial imaging modality[31] and can be performed effectively by frontline physicians at the bedside.[32-34] Although more prevalent in the pediatric population, intussusception can also present in adults and be diagnosed by POCUS.[35] See also chapters 47 and 48 for pediatric and neonatal point-of-care ultrasound applications.

Conclusion

POCUS can be extremely informative in the evaluation of both stable and unstable patients with acute abdominal pain. In addition to evaluating for hemorrhage, infection, and obstruction, POCUS can be used to diagnose pneumoperitoneum,[12] bowel obstruction,[36] abdominal wall pathologies,[37] and aortic dissection,[38] as well as guide performance of diagnostic or therapeutic paracentesis.[39] Early integration of POCUS in the care of patients with acute abdominal pain can improve diagnostic efficiency while limiting exposure to ionizing radiation.

PEARLS AND PITFALLS

- Bring the ultrasound machine to the bedside during your initial evaluation of patients who present with abdominal pain. A focused abdominal ultrasound exam can be performed simultaneously while collecting the medical history.
- Unstable patients benefit from immediate evaluation with point-of-care ultrasound as transport to imaging departments may be hazardous and introduces delays in management.
- POCUS exams are best utilized when integrated with other clinical data to either rule in or rule out a specific pathology. The clinical utility of decreasing the likelihood of certain diagnoses can be equally as useful as increasing the likelihood of other diagnoses.
- POCUS is a goal-directed approach to imaging the abdomen. The broad differential diagnosis of abdominal pain often means that POCUS is used in conjunction with other imaging modalities to effectively address the full scope of possible diagnostic considerations.

CHAPTER 33

Trauma Ultrasound

Patrick Murphy ■ W. Robert Leeper

KEY POINTS

- The EFAST (extended focused assessment with sonography in trauma) exam is an essential component of the primary survey in blunt and penetrating trauma, and in both stable and unstable patients.
- The EFAST exam includes rapid assessment for intra-abdominal hemorrhage (right upper quadrant, left upper quadrant, and pelvic windows), hemopericardium (subxiphoid window), and hemopneumothorax (thoracic and pleural ultrasound).
- Only five anatomic locations are capable of accumulating sufficient blood in blunt trauma to produce instability: *chest*, *belly*, *pelvis*, *femurs*, and *floor* (external hemorrhage). Hemorrhage into the pelvis can be more challenging to diagnose, and EFAST has a low sensitivity for retroperitoneal hemorrhage.

Background

Many studies have demonstrated the utility of ultrasound in thoracoabdominal trauma.[1-3] Evidence and techniques for the individual components of the EFAST (Extended Focused Assessment with Sonography in Trauma) exam, including thoracic, cardiac, and abdominal ultrasound examinations, have been covered in previous chapters. This chapter will focus on clinical cases to synthesize the previously described techniques into comprehensive algorithms for the four principle scenarios encountered in trauma:

1. Unstable penetrating trauma
2. Unstable blunt trauma
3. Stable penetrating trauma
4. Stable blunt trauma

In addition to these four principal types of trauma, this chapter will present special circumstances where unique indications, findings, pitfalls, and applications of point-of-care ultrasound (POCUS) exist. These special cases will be used to highlight individual considerations for each circumstance.

General Principles

The principles taught in the Advanced Trauma Life Support (ATLS) course remain the guiding and unifying language of trauma care. In the 10th edition of ATLS, ultrasound retains its designation as an "adjunct" to the primary survey.[4] Given the superiority of ultrasound to traditional primary survey techniques (e.g., auscultation), many trauma providers argue that ultrasound should be considered as an integrated component of the primary survey, reflecting how most ultrasound-trained providers actually practice. To this end, we present cases and approaches in this chapter that assume ultrasound is fully integrated into the ABCs of the primary survey.

Differentiation of "stable" versus "unstable" patients is both a critical and contentious determination. For the purposes of this chapter, "unstable" refers to life-threatening symptomatology (stridor, severe dyspnea, dense coma, significant external hemorrhage), or unresponsive states of hemodynamic compromise, including only transient responsiveness

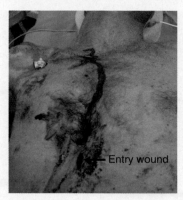

Figure 33.1 Penetrating Epigastric Wound.

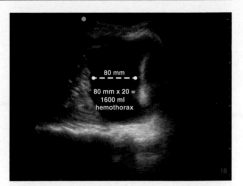

Figure 33.2 Pleural Fluid Volume. Pleural fluid volume (hemothorax in this case) is estimated using this formula: Distance between the diaphragm and base of the lung (mm) × 20 = volume (mL).

to resuscitation. The benefits of ultrasound in trauma have shown to be different between the stable and unstable populations. In unstable patients, ultrasound guides immediate decision-making, directs interventions, and can potentially save lives, whereas in stable patients, ultrasound expedites care, reduces or replaces ancillary testing, and educates providers.

The FAST (Focused Assessment with Sonography in Trauma) exam was originally designed to assess for both intra-abdominal hemorrhage (RUQ, LUQ, and pelvic windows), as well as hemopericardium (subxiphoid window).[4] Over time, the examination was expanded to include assessment of the thorax for pneumothorax (PTX) and hemothorax (HTX). This composite examination comprises the extended FAST or EFAST exam and assesses for life-threatening traumatic conditions of the pleural, pericardial, and peritoneal spaces. The following four cases highlight the integration of the EFAST exam into the care of critically injured patients.

CASE SCENARIO 1: UNSTABLE PENETRATING TRAUMA

A 23-year-old man presents to the emergency department (ED) after being stabbed in the epigastrium by an unknown assailant. His blood pressure on presentation is 90/40 and heart rate is 115. He is alert and oriented, speaking in full sentences, and has an open epigastric wound (Fig. 33.1).

A (Airway) is addressed immediately. Delayed airway management is preferred given the hemodynamic consequences of induction medications. Ultrasound has a role only in confirming endotracheal tube (ETT) placement or in the rare assessment of tracheal anatomy as part of a surgical airway.

B (Breathing) is addressed next. Critical information can be gained within seconds of patient arrival with ultrasound and without the attendant delay of portable chest radiography. Ultrasound is more sensitive than an upright chest x-ray (CXR) for PTX which can be **ruled in** by the presence of lung point (Video 33.1) and **ruled out** by the presence of normal lung sliding (Video 33.2), B-lines (Video 33.3), or any non-A pattern of the lungs. Although false-positive findings do exist for the absence of lung sliding (apnea, bullae, adhesions), this finding should lead directly to tube thoracostomy (TT) in unstable patients where delays in definitive diagnosis can increase morbidity and mortality.[5] Additionally, a HTX can be detected, and the volume can be estimated based on the distance from the diaphragm to the inferior aspect of the lung (Fig. 33.2). Multiplying this distance in millimeters by 20 estimates the volume of HTX in milliliters.[6] Detection of HTX permits providers to begin administering blood and plasma, as well as prepare for operative intervention, even prior to placement of a TT. If more than 1500 mL of blood is estimated on ultrasound, then the operating room should be prepared, and if more than 1500 mL is drained upon TT placement, an exploratory thoracotomy should be performed as soon as possible.

C (Circulation) is then addressed through evaluation for occult hemorrhage. Epigastric wounds, such as the one pictured (Fig. 33.1), are equally prone to lacerate the liver or myocardium. Differentiating these two sources of bleeding can be performed quickly with cardiac and abdominal ultrasound. In penetrating

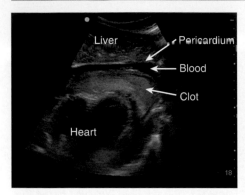

Figure 33.3 **Hemopericardium.** A large hemopericardium is seen from the subxiphoid window after penetrating cardiac injury. Note the large amount of clotted blood in the pericardial sac.

trauma, the subxiphoid cardiac view should be obtained first. The presence of pericardial fluid is an indication for immediate thoracotomy or sternotomy (Fig. 33.3 and Video 33.4). False-negative findings for cardiac injury may occur when a hemopericardium is draining into a left HTX. Specifically, a wound to the cardiac box and a large left HTX must be further investigated to rule out cardiac injury, even in the presence of a negative subxiphoid cardiac view. The most appropriate approach is to perform a diagnostic pericardial window in the operating room with the ability to rapidly convert to sternotomy if significant cardiac injury is detected.[7]

Positive findings on any of the three abdominal views mandate immediate laparotomy in an unstable patient (Fig. 33.4). Given the high stakes involved in an unstable patient after penetrating injury, equivocal findings from either the pericardial or abdominal ultrasound exams should lead directly to invasive testing with a subxiphoid pericardial window or diagnostic peritoneal aspiration/lavage (DPA/DPL), respectively. Negative findings on both the pericardial and abdominal ultrasound exams should lead to a reassessment of patient stability and consideration of retroperitoneal hemorrhage or nonhemorrhagic causes of shock (see algorithm, Fig. 33.5).

CASE SCENARIO 2: UNSTABLE BLUNT TRAUMA

A 39-year-old man is referred to the trauma service from a rural ED following a high-velocity all-terrain

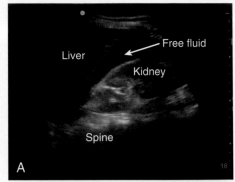

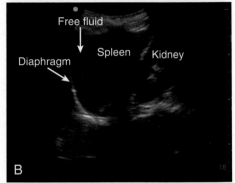

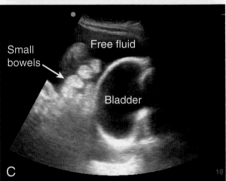

Figure 33.4 **Abdominal Free Fluid.** (A) Right upper quadrant view showing anechoic free fluid in the hepatorenal interface (Morison's pouch). (B) Left upper quadrant view showing anechoic free fluid between the spleen and diaphragm. (C) Pelvic free fluid seen from a sagittal view in a male patient with free-floating loops of bowel and bladder.

vehicle (ATV) rollover injury. Air paramedics report the patient became unstable en route. Despite intubation and mechanical ventilation his arterial oxygen saturation remains 88% to 90%. His heart rate is 90. His blood pressure is 85/40. Bolused intravenous fluids produce only a transient rise in

Unstable penetrating trauma

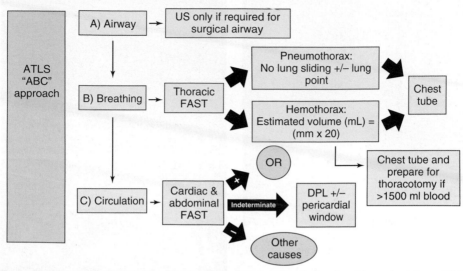

Figure 33.5 Unstable Penetrating Trauma Algorithm. *ABC,* Airway, breathing, circulation; *ATLS,* Advanced Trauma Life Support; *DPL,* diagnostic peritoneal lavage; *FAST,* Focused Assessment with Sonography in Trauma; *OR,* operating room; *US,* ultrasound.

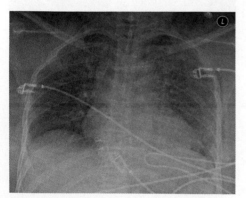

Figure 33.6 Flail Chest. A portable chest x-ray demonstrates multiple left-sided rib fractures and a flail chest.

blood pressure. The chest radiograph supplied by the rural ED is shown in Fig. 33.6.

A (Airway) has been previously addressed. Ultrasound has a role to confirm ETT placement.[8]

B (Breathing) is an urgent concern. Flail chest is evident on radiography; however, superimposed PTX and HTX are suboptimally demonstrated on this portable, supine plain film. Ultrasound allows prompt identification and intervention for PTX and HTX in a fashion identical to the thoracic portion of the *"unstable penetrating"* algorithm (see Fig. 33.5). Special consideration in unstable blunt trauma should be given to the possibility of diaphragmatic rupture. Misleading studies in the left chest can be produced by diaphragmatic rupture and careful attention to any intestinal or gastric viscera on pleural ultrasound should lead to prompt laparotomy, rather than TT in this setting. The ultrasound images seen in Videos 33.5 and 33.6 demonstrate a diaphragmatic rupture, along with the CXR image which is shown in Fig. 33.7. Note a TT was carefully inserted superior to the observed diaphragmatic herniation in order to avoid visceral injury.

C (Circulation) can now be approached. The principle mission for trauma providers dealing with unstable blunt trauma is to **find** the bleeding and **stop** the bleeding. Practically speaking, there are only five anatomic locations capable of accumulating sufficient blood in blunt trauma to produce instability: chest, belly, pelvis, femurs, floor (external hemorrhage). Combining the cardiac component of the EFAST exam with a pleural study rules in or out the chest as the source. Positive findings on the cardiac exam should lead to thoracotomy or sternotomy, whereas indeterminate studies

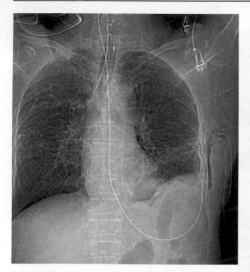

Figure 33.7   Traumatic Diaphragmatic Hernia. Chest x-ray of a traumatic left-sided diaphragmatic hernia.

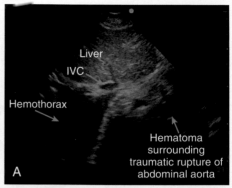

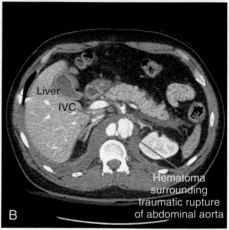

Figure 33.8   Ruptured Aorta. (A) A hematoma is seen surrounding the aorta at the supraceliac level from a transverse upper abdominal view. (B) Computed tomography scan confirmed a hematoma at the supraceliac level. *IVC,* Inferior vena cava.

may require a subxiphoid window. Bleeding in the "belly" or peritoneal space is well demonstrated on the abdominal components of the EFAST exam (see Fig. 33.4), and positive results lead to laparotomy, whereas indeterminate results may require DPL. External hemorrhage ("floor") and femur fractures associated with thigh hematomas are obvious on cursory physical exam. However, hemorrhage into the pelvis and retroperitoneum ("pelvis") can be considerably more challenging to diagnose. Rarely, trauma ultrasound can identify a retroperitoneal source of hemorrhage (Fig. 33.8). More commonly, retroperitoneal hemorrhage is a diagnosis of exclusion supported by clinical findings of an unstable pelvis or flank hematoma, and radiographic evidence of a pelvic fracture. In the unstable blunt trauma algorithm (Fig. 33.9), this pathway leads to a difficult management decision. The patient may either undergo laparotomy with extraperitoneal packing or external pelvic stabilization in the operating room, or angioembolization of bleeding retroperitoneal vasculature in the angiography suite. The evolution of hybrid operating rooms plus angiography suites may alleviate this dilemma.[9]

Use of the resuscitative endovascular balloon occlusion of the aorta (REBOA) device has had a significant impact on controlling hemorrhage in trauma patients. REBOA is a percutaneously inserted, intra-arterial device

that is inflated in the aorta above the level of hemorrhage. The device provides temporary proximal control of bleeding, enhances afterload immediately, and augments mean arterial pressure in the upper body circulation.[10] Use of REBOA has proliferated across the globe, and prospective data are being gathered to assess the impact of its use in trauma patients. See below for additional discussion of REBOA.

CASE SCENARIO 3: STABLE PENETRATING TRAUMA

A 19-year-old man is stabbed by his neighbor during an altercation. There is a single wound, 1.5 cm in size, just inferior to his left nipple. He is hemodynamically stable. His cardiorespiratory status appears satisfactory. He is agitated and wishes to leave the ED.

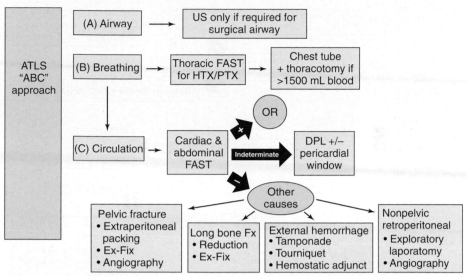

Figure 33.9 Unstable Blunt Trauma Algorithm. *ABC,* Airway, breathing, circulation; *ATLS,* Advanced Trauma Life Support; *DPL,* diagnostic peritoneal lavage; *Ex-Fix,* external fixation; *FAST,* Focused Assessment with Sonography in Trauma; *Fx,* fracture; *HTX,* hemothorax; *OR,* operating room; *PTX,* pneumothorax; *US,* ultrasound.

A (Airway) is seldom a concern in stable patients. If so, their stability should be reassessed.

B (Breathing) is a key concern for this patient. His injury pattern is highly likely to result in PTX, even though none is obvious initially. Clinical exam is essential to determine the depth and trajectory of penetration. In the absence of concerning exam findings or of significant HTX or PTX on CXR, controversy exists as to best practice guidelines. Some providers would recommend a 6- to 8-hour observation period with serial CXRs. Providers proficient in POCUS may perform serial pleural ultrasound exams and consider an early discharge strategy for this otherwise resource-intensive population. Positive findings for PTX or HTX, regardless of stability, should trigger immediate TT, as well as admission to the trauma service.

Additional consideration should be given to the *level of injury.* Traditional teaching dictates that all penetrating wounds to the left thoraco-abdominal region should be considered for laparoscopic exploration to rule out injury of the left hemidiaphragm.[11] A focused ultrasound exam at the level of injury during maximal expiratory effort may provide valuable

information about the likelihood of diaphragmatic injury. If the diaphragm is visible on ultrasound at the level of injury, then it should be considered definitively reachable by the offending weapon, and all such injuries should undergo laparoscopic exploration owing to an otherwise high rate of missed injury.[11]

C (Circulation) is of paramount concern with injuries to the cardiac box, such as the one described in this case. In this setting, bleeding in the pericardial space must be ruled out (Video 33.7). Demonstration of pericardial fluid on any cardiac views in patients with penetrating trauma is presumed to be hemopericardium until proven otherwise and requires operative exploration. Given the stable status of this patient, a diagnostic subxiphoid window was performed in the operating room with the sternal saw on standby. Hemopericardium in a stable patient is initially explored with a subxiphoid pericardial window because up to 50% result from minor, superficial cardiac injuries. If blood is cleared with irrigation and aspiration, then the patient can be spared the morbidity of a sternotomy.[7]

Positive findings on the abdominal ultrasound exam should lead to prompt laparotomy in noncirrhotic patients with penetrating

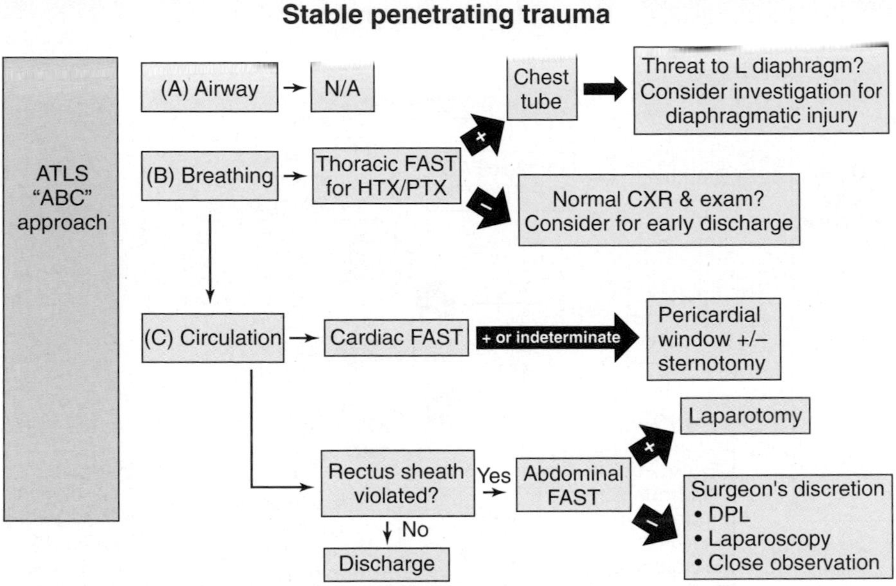

Stable penetrating trauma

Figure 33.10   Stable Penetrating Trauma Algorithm. *ABC,* Airway, breathing, circulation; *ATLS,* Advanced Trauma Life Support; *CXR,* chest x-ray; *DPL,* diagnostic peritoneal lavage; *FAST,* Focused Assessment with Sonography in Trauma; *HTX,* hemothorax; *PTX,* pneumothorax.

thoracoabdominal trauma. Blood, urine, and intestinal contents are the most common causes of abdominal free fluid and all generally require operative management. Although evidence exists supporting the safety of observation for stable penetrating trauma,[12] operative management is favored for two reasons. First, most medium- to low-volume trauma centers are unlikely to have the observation capability and diagnostic accuracy of CT imaging found at large urban trauma centers, and second, no study has specifically investigated the subpopulation of stable trauma patients with abdominal free fluid. Negative or indeterminate results are more troublesome. Ultrasound is not capable of ruling out peritoneal penetration. If peritoneal penetration can be excluded by close inspection of the superficial wound on physical exam, then further evaluation is likely not indicated. However, if the physical exam is suspicious for penetration into the rectus sheath and the abdominal EFAST scan is negative, then a number of management strategies exist: serial observation (even in abdominal gunshot wounds),[11] laparoscopic exploration to exclude peritoneal penetration, or mandatory laparotomy. Currently, the preferred management strategy for this scenario depends on the surgeon and institutional protocols (Fig. 33.10).

CASE SCENARIO 4: STABLE BLUNT TRAUMA

A 32-year-old woman is transported to the ED by paramedics following a T-bone mechanism motor vehicle collision at city speeds. She was the belted front seat passenger in the vehicle T-boned on her passenger side door. The paramedics describe modest passenger space intrusion. She is wearing a C-spine collar and is asymptomatic. Her pulse is 62 and blood pressure is 118/69. She reports currently undergoing infertility investigations.

A (Airway) is seldom a concern in stable patients. If so, their stability should be reassessed.

B (Breathing) is not an immediate concern for this patient. However, an EFAST exam should be performed, but positive findings carry some special considerations in a stable patient. Positive findings of PTX in this setting may *not* lead to immediate TT placement, in contrast to all previous algorithms (see Figs. 33.5, 33.9, and 33.10). Clinical equipoise exists regarding the treatment of occult PTX in blunt trauma.[13] If portable CXR is normal (that is, the PTX remains small enough to be "occult" on CXR), then one may consider omitting TT in stable blunt trauma. This question remains controversial, and a study (OPTICC trial) is under way to better understand this topic.[14]

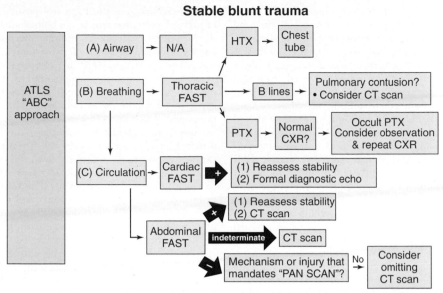

Figure 33.11 Stable Blunt Trauma Algorithm. *ABC,* Airway, breathing, circulation; *ATLS,* Advanced Trauma Life Support; *CT,* computed tomography; *CXR,* chest x-ray; *FAST,* Focused Assessment with Sonography in Trauma; *HTX,* hemothorax; *PTX,* pneumothorax.

Despite a normal physical exam and CXR, lung ultrasound may show early patterns of interstitial lung injury consistent with pulmonary contusion (Video 33.8). This finding may expedite decisions about early admission or transfer to higher level of care.

C (**Circulation**) assessment in the stable blunt trauma patients represents an opportunity for ultrasound to educate providers performing the study, expedite discharge of patients, and avoid unnecessary ancillary testing. In this stable patient, an ample amount of time exists for providers new to POCUS to practice acquiring EFAST windows on a "control" patient. The benefit for the patient is that a negative study in this low-risk setting might expedite discharge by providing reassurance that a major abdominal injury does not exist. Young patients with fertility concerns are particularly averse to radiographic imaging with ionizing radiation, and a negative EFAST exam is a key component in clinical decision-making to omit further testing, such as CT scans. On the contrary, if the abdominal component of the EFAST exam shows abdominal free fluid, the patient's stability should be reassessed and an expeditious CT scan should be obtained to characterize any intra-abdominal injury. Detection of pericardial fluid on the cardiac component of an EFAST exam in a stable blunt trauma patient should similarly trigger a reassessment of the patient's stability, additional diagnostic imaging (CT scan or echocardiogram), and possibly additional workup for nontraumatic causes of pericardial effusion (Fig. 33.11).

Special Circumstances

Whereas the four previous cases represent models to categorize trauma patients with a systematic approach, the following cases highlight unique circumstances where POCUS has an indication, application, or pitfall that exists outside of the standard approach. These scenarios serve to highlight nuances of POCUS for experienced trauma providers.

SPECIAL CIRCUMSTANCE #1: WITNESSED TRAUMA ARREST

A 45-year-old man is brought to the ED after a head-on motor vehicle collision. His vital signs on arrival are a pulse of 120, blood pressure of 90/50, and a Glasgow Coma Scale (GCS) of 12. During the primary survey, the patient becomes comatose and pulseless. Cardiopulmonary resuscitation (CPR) is initiated.

A (Airway) is addressed by the ED physician, and the patient is intubated. Ultrasound has a role in confirmation of ETT placement.

B (Breathing) is an urgent concern. A number of possible reasons exist to explain why this blunt trauma patient arrested. Although ultrasound may be used to identify PTX or HTX, immediate tube-thoracostomy is diagnostic and therapeutic, and this patient should receive immediate bilateral TTs without prior ultrasound imaging. In fact, there is expert opinion and animal data that suggest CPR may be briefly deferred in order to rapidly perform TT and other emergent resuscitative procedures.[15-17]

C (Circulation) is assumed to be compromised due to hypovolemia in an arrested trauma patient. Immediate goals are to stop any hemorrhage and volume resuscitate the patient. In an arrested patient, performance of a resuscitative thoracotomy (RT) or placement of a REBOA device must be considered depending on local resources and practice patterns. In blunt trauma, an indication for ED thoracotomy with cross-clamping of the aorta in the trauma bay is cardiac arrest. Ultrasound can be used to determine which patients may benefit from RT versus placement of a REBOA device. Transthoracic subxiphoid views or transesophageal echocardiography (TEE) guide the critical decision matrix as follows:

1. Cardiac activity present with hemopericardium or massive HTX = **RT**
2. Cardiac activity present without hemopericardium or massive HTX = **REBOA device placement** (Zone 1 Deployment)[a]
3. No cardiac activity present = **termination of resuscitation**

To better understand this decision matrix, let us consider the rationale for each branch point of the matrix and the supporting evidence. First, the use of TEE in cardiac arrest has been demonstrated to be a safe and effective tool in the ED.[18] While high-quality transthoracic subxiphoid views can provide useful clinical data, they are often not obtainable during CPR. In this setting, TEE is a more reliable option (see Chapter 20).

The first scenario of trauma arrest and cardiac activity with hemopericardium or massive HTX demands an immediate ED RT. Evidence-based practice management

guidelines indicate a small but real possibility of survival, even after arrest from blunt trauma. In the setting of hemopericardium, one must assume a full thickness, blunt cardiac injury. In the setting of a large HTX, one must assume exsanguinating thoracic hemorrhage as the cause of arrest. In either scenario, thoracotomy is the only hope for the simultaneous relief of tamponade and control of hemorrhage.

Special note should be made that "cardiac activity" in this setting refers to organized cardiac contractions that are not able to produce an appreciable pulse—a common state of classic pulseless electrical activity (PEA) arrest from a combination of hypovolemia and tamponade. For providers who doubt the absence of a pulse, a more reliable and quantifiable measure is the end-tidal CO_2 ($EtCO_2$) for reassurance that RT is indicated. In this setting, an $EtCO_2$ less than 20 mm Hg is pathognomonic for cardiac arrest and should be managed with immediate thoracotomy.

In the second scenario of cardiac activity without hemopericardium or HTX (Video 33.9), it is likely most advisable to proceed with the percutaneous deployment of a Zone 1 REBOA device to occlude the thoracic aorta for a presumed infradiaphragmatic source of hemorrhage (intra-peritoneal or retroperitoneal hemorrhage) (Fig. 33.12). This approach avoids the attendant risks of thoracotomy for both the patient and provider. In an arrested patient, the abdominal portion of the EFAST may be

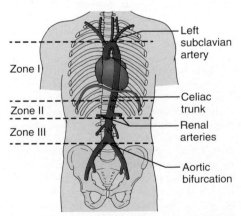

Figure 33.12. REBOA Aortic Landing Zones. Zone I extends from the origin of the left subclavian artery to the celiac artery, zone II extends from the celiac artery to the renal artery, and zone III extends from the lowest renal artery to the bifurcation of the aorta.

[a]If REBOA is not available, perform RT with aortic cross-clamping

deferred until REBOA deployment or thoracotomy performance, and return of spontaneous circulation has been obtained.

In the third scenario, regardless of the circumstances, it is most appropriate to terminate resuscitation when absence of cardiac activity is seen on POCUS (Video 33.10). In a retrospective review of all resuscitative thoracotomies over a 4-year period, the absence of cardiac activity on initial ultrasound was associated with a 100% rate of death. However, the small group of patients (5%) that either survived or achieved stabilization for organ procurement had initial cardiac activity on ultrasound.[19] Given the resources consumed, risks to providers, and low probability of meaningful survival, the absence of cardiac activity should herald the end of any trauma resuscitation.

SPECIAL CIRCUMSTANCE #2: EQUIVOCAL FAST IN AN UNSTABLE TRAUMA

A 65-year-old man is transported from an outside hospital for ongoing instability after a motor vehicle collision. Upon arrival, his pulse is 110, he is confused, and his oxygen saturation is 95% on face mask. Blood pressure on arrival is 100/70 but drops to 80/40 after 5 minutes. Massive blood transfusion is initiated. He is morbidly obese and his EFAST is indeterminate. Adequate views on the abdominal and cardiac EFAST exams were not obtained and intra-abdominal hemorrhage and cardiac tamponade cannot be ruled out.

A (Airway) shows acute decompensation requiring intubation given patient's aspiration risk. Ultrasound is used to confirm ETT placement.

B (Breathing) Given the acute decline in the patient's status, intrathoracic hemorrhage and PTX need to be ruled out. Although ultrasound can rapidly assess for hemorrhage or PTX, when a patient acutely declines, the provider must consider proceeding directly with bilateral TT, as was advocated in the setting of witnessed traumatic arrest. Bilateral TT is both diagnostic and therapeutic.

C (Circulation) In a stable trauma patient, time is less of a concern and a nondiagnostic EFAST exam is followed by CT scans to assess for intra-abdominal and retroperitoneal sources of hemorrhage. In an unstable patient, providers must quickly determine the source of hypotension. This patient may have an abdominal source of hypotension or a less common cause of shock, such as high spinal cord injury (neurogenic shock), pulmonary embolism, aortic dissection, or myocardial infarction. In this setting it is critical to consider both of these options:

1. Perform serial multi-system ultrasound examinations as resuscitation progresses
2. Proceed with more invasive diagnostic testing:
   a. DPL/DPA to rule out abdominal hemorrhage
   b. TEE to rule out cardiac tamponade

The value of serial ultrasound examinations in this setting cannot be overstated. In this case of a highly unstable blunt trauma patient, both the initial abdominal and pericardial EFAST images were read as negative (Videos 33.11 and 33.12), although a trained eye can now clearly see that both of these images were positive. After 30 minutes and administration of several units of blood, the repeat abdominal ultrasound exam revealed gross intra-abdominal hemorrhage (Video 33.13). The patient underwent both laparotomy and sternotomy for intra-abdominal hemorrhage and full thickness blunt cardiac injury. Exsanguination and low central venous pressure can make major cardiac injury and intra-abdominal hemorrhage occult, and therefore serial ultrasound exams after resuscitation are vitally important.

Trauma scenarios such as this one remind us that invasive diagnostic testing still has a role in modern trauma care. Providers must consider DPL/DPA to rule out intraperitoneal hemorrhage and consider TEE for a more detailed assessment of the pericardium. These tests can be life-saving, despite their invasiveness. Consider the patient in Fig. 33.13 who spent 120 minutes in the trauma bay, received 18 units of blood for an occult source of hemorrhage, and had a negative EFAST exam. A CT scan revealed massive hemoperitoneum (Fig. 33.13). Perhaps the laminated thrombus around the liver was misinterpreted as liver parenchyma on ultrasound.

SPECIAL CIRCUMSTANCE #3: EXSANGUINATING PELVIC HEMORRHAGE

A 25-year-old man sustains a crush injury to his pelvis and lower abdomen when a piece of heavy machinery malfunctions at a local construction site. Upon arrival to the ED, his pulse is 130 and blood pressure is 70 systolic by palpation. His airway is

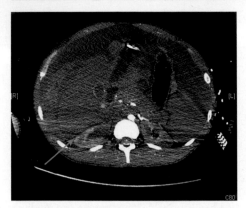

Figure 33.13 False-Negative Abdominal FAST Exam. An isoechoic, small thrombus *(green arrow)* that blends in with the liver parenchyma was missed by ultrasound. A computed tomography scan of abdomen revealed massive hemoperitoneum with only scant blood in Morison's pouch.

clear. He is somnolent but arouses to voice. Primary survey is completed and the EFAST is negative for pleural, pericardial, or intra-abdominal blood. The patient has a grossly unstable pelvis on exam and a pelvic binder is placed. Massive transfusion is initiated, but after 4 units of blood, his blood pressure remains 75/40.

A (**Airway**) is tenuous given his somnolent state, and a judicious approach may be to withhold invasive airway management, as induction medications and positive end expiratory pressure are likely to trigger cardiac arrest in this state of hypotension.

B (**Breathing**) appears stable given the absence of chest trauma and reassuring based on this point-of-care pleural or parenchymal lung ultrasound exams.

C (**Circulation**) needs to be addressed immediately due to suspected rapid exsanguination from a catastrophic pelvic hemorrhage.

Although a variety of options exist for interventional therapy (angiography, preperitoneal pelvic packing, external fixation, etc.), this patient is likely to arrest without more urgent intervention. REBOA of the aorta must be considered.

Although mentioned earlier in this chapter, a more complete discussion of REBOA is presented here. Life-threatening pelvic hemorrhage is perhaps the most attractive disease state to treat with REBOA. As a temporary means of obtaining inflow control to the pelvic vessels, REBOA can be employed to rapidly halt pelvic bleeding and transiently increase mean arterial pressure to vital organs while targeted interventions to control hemorrhage are undertaken.

The REBOA device is a percutaneous balloon that is inflated either in the lower thoracic aorta (zone 1) or lower abdominal aorta (zone 3) to control abdominal or pelvic hemorrhage, respectively (see Fig. 33.12). Indications for REBOA are relatively straightforward and an example of a REBOA activation algorithm is provided (Fig. 33.14). If a REBOA is being considered, it is of paramount importance to ensure mandatory placement of a carefully targeted femoral arterial line. This represents a paradigm shift from traditional trauma teaching that invasive arterial access is unnecessary and wastes time in an otherwise busy trauma bay. However, obtaining arterial access specifically in the common femoral artery allows upsizing to an appropriately sized sheath and rapid deployment of a REBOA once a decision has been made to proceed. Therefore, all trauma providers should be familiar with the sonographic anatomy of the common femoral artery and vein in the groin (Fig. 33.15). Accessing the superficial femoral artery or the external iliac will unnecessarily complicate REBOA placement and should be avoided.

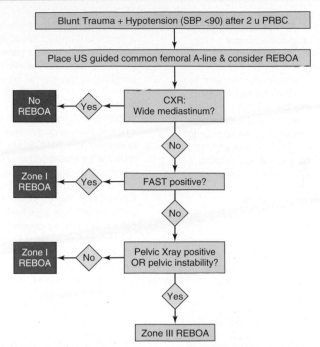

Figure 33.14 Example of One Trauma Center's Resuscitative Endovascular Balloon Occlusion of the Aorta *(REBOA)* **Activation Algorithm.** *A-line*, arterial line; *CXR*, Chest x-ray; *FAST*, Focused Assessment with Sonography in Trauma; *OR*, operating room; *PRBC*, packed red blood cells; *SBP*, systolic blood pressure; *u*, unit; *US*, ultrasound.

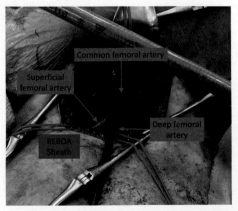

Figure 33.15 Resuscitative Endovascular Balloon Occlusion of the Aorta *(REBOA)* **Landmarks.** The ideal location for insertion of a REBOA sheath is in the common femoral artery, caudal to the inguinal ligament but cephalad to the bifurcation into the superficial and deep femoral arteries.

PEARLS AND PITFALLS

Extended Focused Assessment With Sonography in Trauma & the Primary Survey

- The Extended Focused Assessment with Sonography in Trauma (EFAST) exam is simultaneously carried out with the assessment of airway and breathing but is generally thought of as an adjunct to circulation (the "C" of the ABCs)
- Serial EFAST exams can be valuable if the patient's condition changes or the initial exam is negative or indeterminate.

Unstable Trauma Patients

- Positive findings on any of the three abdominal views mandate immediate laparotomy and, if any of the cardiac views show pericardial fluid, then a subxiphoid window or sternotomy should also be performed.
- False-negative findings for cardiac injury may occur when a hemopericardium is draining into a left hemothorax (HTX), particularly with penetrating wounds to the cardiac box.
- A negative EFAST exam in an unstable patient should raise suspicion of retroperitoneal hemorrhage, pelvic hemorrhage, or external hemorrhage. Further diagnostic assessment (e.g., diagnostic peritoneal aspiration [DPA]/ diagnostic peritoneal lavage [DPL]) or empiric treatment (e.g., laparotomy or resuscitative endovascular balloon occlusion of the aorta [REBOA] deployment) should be performed.
- In unstable blunt trauma patients, the goal is to find and stop the bleeding that can be in five anatomic locations capable of accumulating sufficient blood to produce instability: chest, belly, pelvis, femurs, floor (external hemorrhage).

- Use of the REBOA device has had a significant impact on controlling hemorrhage in trauma patients by providing temporary aortic occlusion proximal to the area of bleeding.

Stable Trauma Patients

- Absence of lung sliding on EFAST exam is both sensitive and specific for pneumothorax (PTX) in trauma; however, multiple rib levels (≥2) should be assessed to ensure accuracy. Negative or indeterminate lung sliding should be followed by a 6- to 8-hour observation period with serial chest x-rays (CXRs) or pleural ultrasound exams.
- Demonstration of pericardial fluid on any cardiac views in patients with penetrating trauma is presumed to be hemopericardium until proven otherwise and requires operative exploration with a diagnostic subxiphoid window or sternotomy.
- Positive findings on the abdominal ultrasound exam should lead to prompt laparotomy in noncirrhotic patients with penetrating thoracoabdominal trauma.
- In penetrating stable trauma, if peritoneal penetration cannot be excluded by close inspection of the superficial wound, then serial observation, laparoscopic exploration, or mandatory laparotomy are all reasonable options.
- Detection of an occult PTX in stable blunt trauma may not require tube thoracostomy (TT) and can be observed with serial imaging.
- If the abdominal or pericardial free fluid is detected on the EFAST exam of a stable blunt trauma patient, the patient's stability should be reassessed and a computed tomography (CT) scan and/ or echocardiogram should be obtained expeditiously.

SECTION 5

Vascular System

CHAPTER 34

Lower Extremity Deep Venous Thrombosis

Ariel L. Shiloh

KEY POINTS

- Providers can accurately detect lower extremity deep venous thrombosis with point-of-care ultrasound after limited training.
- Compression ultrasound exams are as accurate as traditional duplex and triplex vascular ultrasound exams.
- Compression ultrasound exam at only two sites, the common femoral vein and popliteal vein, permits rapid and accurate assessment of deep venous thrombosis.

Background

Venous thromboembolic disease (VTE) is a common cause of morbidity and mortality in hospitalized patients and is especially prevalent in critically ill patients.[1-3] Approximately 70% to 90% of patients *with an identified source* of pulmonary embolism (PE) have a proximal lower extremity deep venous thrombosis (DVT). Conversely, 40% to 50% of patients with a proximal DVT have a concurrent pulmonary embolism at presentation, and similarly, in only 50% of patients presenting with a PE can a DVT be found.[4-6]

Point-of-care ultrasound is readily available as a diagnostic tool for VTE. Both emergency medicine and critical care medicine literature have demonstrated that after brief, focused training sessions, physicians and other health

care providers can perform lower extremity compression ultrasonography exams rapidly and with high diagnostic accuracy to detect DVT.[7-13] A meta-analysis of 16 studies showed that point-of-care ultrasound can accurately diagnose lower extremity DVTs with a pooled sensitivity of 96% and specificity of 97%.[14]

Traditional vascular studies, the duplex and triplex exams, use a combination of two-dimensional (2D) imaging with compression along with the use of color and/or spectral Doppler ultrasound. More recent studies have demonstrated that 2D compression ultrasound exams alone yield similar accuracy as traditional duplex or triplex vascular studies.[9,11,15-17] Furthermore, reporting of duplex or triplex exams is often delayed due to limitations in the availability of radiology services. Delays in obtaining such test results can compromise the

323

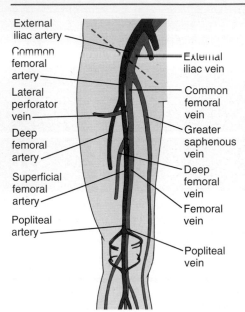

External
iliac artery

Common
femoral
artery

Lateral
perforator
vein

Deep
femoral
artery

Superficial
femoral
artery

Popliteal
artery

External
iliac vein

Common
femoral
vein

Greater
saphenous
vein

Deep
femoral
vein

Femoral
vein

Popliteal
vein

Figure 34.1 Vascular Anatomy of the Right Lower Extremity.

care of acutely ill patients.[9] Thus, the importance of avoiding such delays, along with the minimal training needed to accurately perform the exam, has made point-of-care lower extremity compression ultrasonography an essential skill for health care providers.

This chapter focuses on 2D ultrasonography to detect proximal lower extremity DVT. Distal lower extremity DVTs are not discussed because of their low embolic potential and the lower accuracy of compression ultrasound to detect DVTs below the knee, even by expert sonographers.[18-20]

Anatomy

The proximal lower extremity deep venous system consists of the external iliac, common femoral, deep femoral, femoral, and popliteal veins (Fig. 34.1). Deep veins are accompanied by an adjacent artery. The external iliac vessels are named common femoral vessels distal to the inguinal ligament. Arteries are typically lateral to veins in the thigh. The greater saphenous vein (GSV) is the first venous branch of the common femoral vein (CFV) located anteromedially in the upper thigh. Next, the adjacent common femoral artery (CFA) divides into the deep and superficial femoral arteries.

Lateral perforator veins are usually seen just distal to the division of the CFA. Distal to the lateral perforator veins, the CFV divides into a deep femoral vein (DFV) posteriorly and femoral vein (FV) anteriorly. The FV, traditionally referred to as the femoral vein, is actually a deep vein. Thus, current guidelines recommend calling it the femoral vein to avoid confusion. The FV is visualized with ultrasound until it dives deep into the adductor canal (Hunter's canal) in the distal thigh. In the popliteal fossa, the popliteal vein (PV) overlies the popliteal artery until the vein trifurcates in the distal fossa into the anterior and posterior tibial and peroneal veins.

Image Acquisition

A high-frequency (5–12 MHz) linear transducer is best suited for the evaluation of lower extremity vasculature because it provides high resolution of superficial structures. Vessels typically appear as well-defined, circular, anechoic structures that are contiguous when tracked proximally and distally. A key step in compression ultrasonography is differentiating veins from arteries. Even though no single feature is entirely specific, arteries are generally rounder, thicker walled, pulsatile, and smaller than accompanying veins. Most important, veins are normally fully compressible under light pressure, whereas arteries require substantial pressure to compress. Color flow Doppler can help differentiate arteries from veins when the above features are equivocal, when vessels are deeper in the leg, or when evaluating obese or edematous patients. When utilizing color flow Doppler, one should preferentially tilt the transducer face towards the heart. Using the default Doppler settings, venous blood flow will appear blue as the direction of flow is away from transducer. Normally, color fills the entire venous lumen, and manual compression of the distal leg will cause a transient increase in flow (augmentation) seen as a burst of color within the vein.

A compression ultrasound exam is ideally performed with the patient supine and the leg externally rotated with the knee slightly flexed. The ultrasound machine should be placed ipsilateral, distal to the site of examination with the screen directly facing the provider. The transducer is placed in a transverse orientation at the most proximal point above the inguinal ligament where the external iliac vessels can

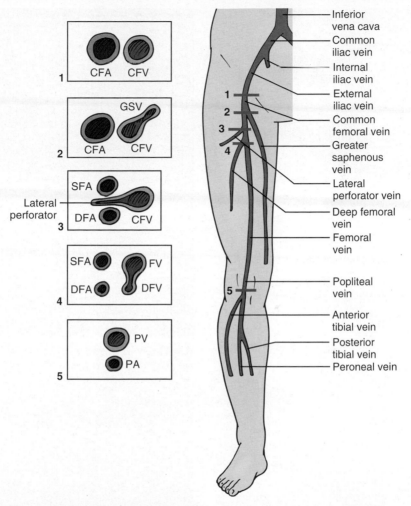

Figure 34.2 Cross-Sectional Anatomy of Lower Extremity Vasculature. Compressions should be performed at each of the following ultrasound exam points: (1) common femoral artery *(CFV)*, (2) CFV–greater saphenous vein *(GSV)*, (3) CFV–lateral perforators, (4) deep femoral vein *(DFV)*–femoral vein *(FV)*, and (5) popliteal vein *(PV)*. *DFA,* Deep femoral artery; *PA,* popliteal artery; *SFA,* superficial femoral artery.

still be identified without obscuration from overlying bowel gas.

Compressions should be applied every 1 to 2 cm along the lower extremity veins. While sliding the transducer distally along the CFV, identify and compress each of the main branch points (Figs. 34.2 and 34.3). Start by compressing the CFV proximal to the GSV branch (Video 34.1) and then the CFV-GSV anastomosis (Video 34.2). The proximal portion of the GSV should be examined as thrombus here has high risk of extending into the CFV

(Videos 34.3 and 34.4). Continuing distally, the CFA branches into superficial and deep branches before the CFV braches into the femoral vein (FV) and the deep femoral vein (DFV). Along the CFV, lateral perforator veins are usually seen coursing laterally between the superficial and deep femoral arteries (Video 34.5). Distal to the lateral perforators, the CFV divides into the DFV and FV (Video 34.6).

Data have shown high diagnostic utility of a limited two- or three-point compression ultrasound exam in patients who have physical

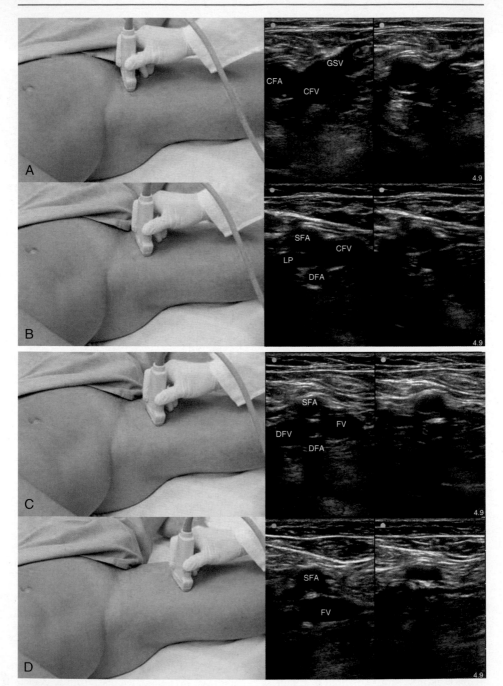

Figure 34.3 Lower Extremity Compression Ultrasound Exam. Transducer position and corresponding precompression *(left)* and postcompression *(right)* ultrasound images are shown at different levels. (A) Common femoral vein–greater saphenous vein *(CFV–GSV)* level. (B) CFV–lateral perforator *(LP)* vein level, distal to the bifurcation of the common femoral artery *(CFA)* into superficial femoral artery *(SFA)* and deep femoral artery *(DFA)*. (C) Bifurcation of the common femoral vein into femoral (FV) and deep femoral veins *(DFV)*. (D) The femoral vein is deep to the SFA from the mid- to distal thigh.

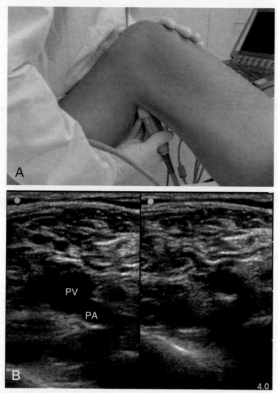

Figure 34.4 Transducer position in popliteal fossa (A) with corresponding precompression and postcompression ultrasound images (B). *PA*, Popliteal artery; *PV*, popliteal vein.

exam findings or symptoms of a DVT (calf pain, tenderness, edema, or redness). A limited compression ultrasound exam must evaluate at a minimum: the CFV-GSV level, the bifurcation of the CFV into DFV and FV, and the PV level. The distal course of the FV is not examined in a limited two- or three-point exam. However, given the relative ease and rapidity of performing compression ultrasonography, we recommend performing compressions distally from the CFV along the FV in select patients with high suspicion for lower extremity DVT. Studies have shown that thrombi can be isolated to the FV and not involve a branch point.[21-24] Compressions are continued every 1 to 2 cm along the proximal (Video 34.7), middle (Video 34.8), and distal FV (Video 34.9) until the vein dives deep into the adductor canal (Hunter's canal) in the distal thigh.

Next, the examiner should examine the PV by placing the transducer within the popliteal fossa with the transducer in a transverse orientation (Fig. 34.4). The transducer should be held gently to avoid inadvertently collapsing the PV. If an adequate seal between the transducer and skin cannot be attained in the popliteal fossa without applying excessive pressure, consider using a narrower linear transducer or applying copious gel. The PV is typically superficial or lateral to the artery in the center of the popliteal fossa (Video 34.10). If only small veins are visualized, the transducer is positioned too distal and should be slid proximally toward the posterior thigh. Compressions are performed sequentially to the trifurcation of the PV into anterior and posterior tibial and peroneal veins.

Normal and Pathologic Findings

Normal veins should fully compress; opposing walls should touch with application of

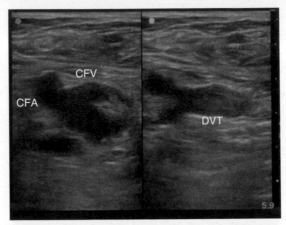

Figure 34.5   Common Femoral Vein Deep Venous Thrombosis. Noncompression of the common femoral vein *(CFV)* is revealed by the precompression *(left)* and postcompression *(right)* images demonstrating a deep venous thrombosis *(DVT)*. *CFA*, Common femoral artery.

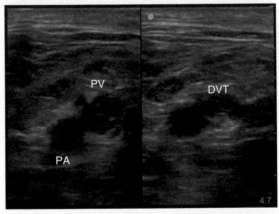

Figure 34.6   Popliteal Vein Deep Venous Thrombosis. Noncompression of the popliteal vein *(PV)* is revealed by the precompression *(left)* and postcompression *(right)* images demonstrating a deep venous thrombosis *(DVT)*. *PA*, Popliteal artery.

less pressure than is required to compress the adjacent artery. Most deep venous thrombi usually develop around valve sinuses, especially at bifurcations, where decreased blood flow exists.[25] Inability to completely compress the venous lumen is the main criterion for diagnosis of DVT using compression ultrasonography, even if thrombus is not visualized in the vein (Figs. 34.5 and 34.6). Lower extremity DVTs can be detected at any of the examination points: CFV (Video 34.11), CFV-GSV anastomosis (Video 34.12), CFV-lateral perforator vein anastomosis (Video 34.13), FV (Video 34.14), and PV (Video 34.15).

Providers should keep in mind that thrombosis is a spectrum. Early thrombus formation begins with venous stasis, usually seen as spontaneous echo contrast or "smoke" around valve leaflets, and fibrin deposition (Video 34.16). The sonographic appearance of venous thrombi varies based on age, extent, and location. Acute thrombi are gelatinous in consistency, appear anechoic or hypoechoic, and cause greater venous distention than chronic thrombi. Subacute and chronic thrombi are more echogenic due to fibrin deposition and can often be visualized without compression (Video 34.17). Chronic thrombi recanalize, retract to the vessel wall, and can cause thickening of the vessel wall. Partial compressibility can be seen with chronic thrombi that have retracted to the vessel wall (Video 34.18) or acute, gelatinous thrombi that are adherent to a vessel wall.

Due to their similar appearance and noncompressibility, inguinal lymph nodes can be mistaken for DVTs. It is important to recognize that lymph nodes are discrete, ovoid structures with a hypoechoic cortex and hyperechoic hilum (Video 34.19; see Chapter 41). Additionally, lymph nodes are generally more superficial, not paired, and cannot be tracked proximally or distally along the extremity.

PEARLS AND PITFALLS

- Providers should have a thorough understanding of lower extremity venous anatomy, including the main segments and branch points, before performing venous compression ultrasound exams.
- Lower extremity compressions should begin at the most proximal visualizable vein segment above the inguinal ligament (external iliac vein).
- Compression ultrasound should always be performed in a transverse orientation because compressions in a longitudinal orientation are prone to the operator sliding to one side of the vessel resulting in erroneous exam findings.
- Firm, rapid, downward compressions of veins should be used to reduce false-positive results. Conversely, forceful compressions should be avoided to reduce false-negative results. Adequate force is being applied if the adjacent artery is slightly compressed.
- After diagnosing a lower extremity deep venous thrombosis (DVT), serial compressions should be avoided in cases of acute, free-floating thrombus.
- Besides DVT, some veins may not compress due to operator error, depth of the vein, obesity, or edema. The depth of some lower extremity deep veins, such as the distal femoral vein, often precludes adequate compression. Compressing the vein at an angle, rather than perpendicularly, can also result in false positives.

CHAPTER 35

Upper Extremity Deep Venous Thrombosis

Lewis Satterwhite ■ Maykol Postigo Jasahui

KEY POINTS

- Upper extremity deep venous thrombosis (DVT) is underdiagnosed. The incidence is increasing, mostly due to the increasing use of central venous catheters. Although the risk of pulmonary embolism is less than lower extremity DVTs, the risk is substantial.
- The cardinal feature of a DVT is noncompressibility of the vein. The deep veins should be visualized in a transverse plane to evaluate for DVT, with the exception of the subclavian vein.
- Acute thrombi appear hypoechoic or anechoic and are loosely attached to vein walls, whereas chronic thrombi are hyperechoic and adherent to the walls.

Background

Ultrasonography of the upper extremity veins has a wide array of applications, including evaluation for thrombosis, guidance of venous catheter insertion, preoperative mapping for hemodialysis access, and postoperative assessment of venous patency.[1] This chapter focuses on use of point-of-care ultrasound (POCUS) to diagnose upper extremity deep venous thrombosis (DVT), including examination techniques, imaging protocols, and common pitfalls.

Primary upper extremity DVTs are uncommon and are typically associated with strenuous and repetitive activity of the upper extremities in individuals with anatomical abnormalities of the veins at the thoracic outlet.[2] Effort-related thrombosis of the upper extremities is also called Paget-Schroetter syndrome. Repetitive microtrauma to the subclavian vein's intima leads to fibrosis and activation of the coagulation cascade, leading to effort-related thrombosis.[3]

Secondary upper extremity DVTs are far more common and associated with unique risk factors. These cases account for approximately 10% of all DVTs with an incidence of 0.4 to 1 case per 10,000.[3,4] The incidence has been increasing due to the increasing use of central venous catheters. The use of central venous catheters and malignancies are the strongest risk factors for upper extremity venous thrombosis, increasing the risk by more than 1100-fold in one study.[5] Risk factors for catheter-related upper extremity DVT include use of a peripherally inserted central catheter (PICC), history of DVT, subclavian venipuncture site, and improper positioning of the catheter tip (tip not in the superior vena cava or at the cavo-atrial junction).[6,7] The number of lumens and catheter gauge relative to the vein size have also been associated with PICC-related thrombosis.[8-10]

The misconception that upper extremities have a lower rate of pulmonary embolism (PE) may lead to fewer diagnostic workups of the upper extremities compared to the lower extremities. Although upper extremity DVT poses one-third of the risk of PE compared to lower extremity DVT, the risk is not trivial with an incidence ranging from 1% to 11%.[3,11-13]

One study reported symptomatic PE in 9% versus 29% of patients with upper versus lower extremity DVT, respectively.[14] The risk of PE by site has been reported to be highest with brachial vein DVTs (11%), followed by axillary (6%) and subclavian vein (5%) DVTs.[13]

Whereas validated algorithms for diagnosis of lower extremity DVT have been published, few algorithms for evaluation of upper extremity DVT have been developed, although a few risk prediction tools have been proposed.[15,16] One of these tools provides a scoring system from 0 to 3 based on individual patient risk factors. However, while this tool may be useful, 13% of patients with a score of 0 were diagnosed with upper extremity DVT in the validation study.[15] The use of D-dimer has not been recommended in patients with suspected upper extremity DVT because it is common to have an elevated D-dimer secondary to comorbidities such as cancer, recent procedures, or an indwelling central venous catheter.

Venography is the gold standard test for diagnosing an upper extremity DVT, but ultrasonography has replaced venograms in most clinical practices.[17-19] Although different ultrasound modalities can be combined to diagnose upper extremity DVTs (i.e., two-dimensional [2D], color flow Doppler, and spectral Doppler), a systematic review showed that 2D compression ultrasound (CUS) has the highest sensitivity (97%) and specificity (96%) for diagnosing upper extremity DVTs.[20]

Once an upper extremity DVT has been accurately diagnosed, there are three main goals of treatment: (1) alleviate symptoms, (2) prevent progression of the thrombus, and (3) decrease the risk of PE.[2] The American College of Chest Physicians created consensus guidelines for the treatment of upper extremity DVTs in 2016. These guidelines suggest anticoagulant therapy alone over thrombolysis for upper extremity DVTs involving the axillary or more proximal veins.[21]

Anatomy

Veins of the upper extremity are divided into deep and superficial veins (Fig. 35.1). Deep veins of the upper extremity are paired with arteries and both are named similarly. The ulnar and radial veins ascend medially and

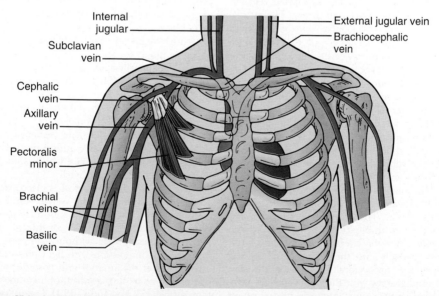

Figure 35.1 Anatomy of the Upper Extremity Veins. From proximal to distal, the superior vena cava branches into the right and left brachiocephalic (innominate) veins, which divide into the internal jugular and subclavian veins posterior to the sternoclavicular joint. The subclavian vein becomes the axillary vein at the lateral border of the first rib. The axillary vein branches into the brachial and basilic veins in the upper arm. The brachial veins become the ulnar and radial veins in the forearm. The superficial veins are the cephalic, basilic, and median cubital veins (see also Fig. 35.5).

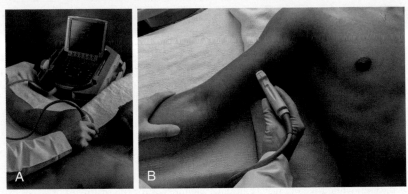

Figure 35.2 Patient Positioning. (A) Position the patient and ultrasound machine in the operator's direct line of sight. (B) Abduct the arm 90 degrees, and orient the transducer with the marker pointed toward the patient's right side.

laterally, respectively, along the forearm to form the brachial veins in the area of the antecubital fossa. The brachial veins anastomose with the basilic vein in the upper arm to become the single axillary vein at the inferior margin of the teres major muscle. The axillary vein becomes the subclavian vein at the lateral aspect of the first rib. The subclavian vein lies anterior to the subclavian artery. The subclavian and internal jugular veins anastomose behind the medial aspect of the clavicle to form the innominate, or brachiocephalic, vein that drains into the superior vena cava.

An ultrasound examination of the upper extremity veins is not complete without assessing the internal jugular vein, even though it is located in the neck. The internal jugular vein travels from the jugular foramen in the base of the skull to behind the clavicle, where it fuses with the subclavian vein to form the brachiocephalic vein.

The main superficial veins of the upper extremities are the cephalic, basilic, and median cubital veins. The superficial veins do not have accompanying arteries. The cephalic vein ascends along the lateral aspect of the biceps, turns medially into the deltopectoral groove, pierces the clavipectoral fascia below the clavicle, and merges with the upper axillary vein. The basilic vein runs along the medial aspect of the upper arm, pierces the deep fascia in the mid-upper arm, and joins the brachial vein to become the axillary vein. The median cubital vein runs in the antecubital fossa between the cephalic and basilic veins.

Image Acquisition

The patient should be supine with the arm externally rotated and abducted 90 degrees from the chest, resting comfortably (Fig. 35.2). The patient's head is turned to the contralateral side and kept elevated above the extremity being examined to avoid external compression of the distal subclavian vein between first rib and clavicle.

A high-frequency (5–12 MHz) linear transducer is used to scan all upper extremity vessels. For superficial veins, the frequency can be increased to 10 MHz for better resolution of smaller vessels.

With the operator facing the patient, the transducer orientation marker is pointed toward the operator's left side (patient's right side) to image veins in a transverse plane, except for the subclavian vein, which is imaged longitudinally below the clavicle.

In 2D mode, the transducer is placed transversely over a vein, and the vein is tested for compressibility. The lumen of a normal, patent vein appears anechoic. CUS consists of visualizing the vessel first without compression, followed by compression with light pressure to assess whether the anterior and posterior walls of the vein come into contact, obliterating the lumen (Fig. 35.3 and Video 35.1). Lack of complete, wall-to-wall compressibility is diagnostic of intraluminal thrombus, even if echogenic thrombus is not visualized in the lumen (Fig. 35.4 and Video 35.2). Compressions are performed every 1 to 2 cm along the course of

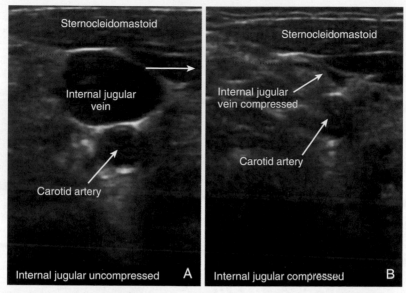

Figure 35.3 Normal Internal Jugular Vein. (A) A patent internal jugular vein is seen superficial to the common carotid artery. (B) Compression with light pressure completely obliterates the entire lumen of the vein.

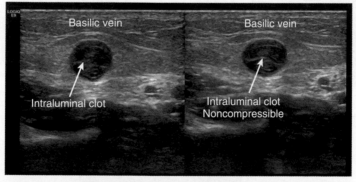

Figure 35.4 Basilic Vein Deep Venous Thrombosis (DVT). Uncompressed *(left)* and compressed *(right)* transverse views of the basilic vein demonstrate noncompressibility consistent with DVT.

the vein, requiring a detailed understanding of venous anatomy. An upper extremity DVT ultrasound examination includes evaluation of the following veins (Fig. 35.5):

- Internal jugular vein (Video 35.3)
- Subclavian vein
- Axillary vein (Video 35.4)
- Brachial veins (Video 35.5)
- Basilic vein (Video 35.6)
- Cephalic vein (Video 35.7)

Although the basilic and cephalic are superficial veins, they are included in the upper extremity DVT compression ultrasound exam. If a thrombus in identified in the proximal segments of these superficial veins, then anticoagulation may be considered to prevent extension into the deep veins. Because thrombosis often occurs at venous junctions, providers must carefully examine the three major upper extremity venous junctions: (1) cephalic-axillary, (2) basilic-axillary, and (3) internal jugular–subclavian vein junctions. Evaluate the internal jugular vein starting at the most cranial segment. Normal venous valves are often seen in the internal jugular and subclavian veins and should not be

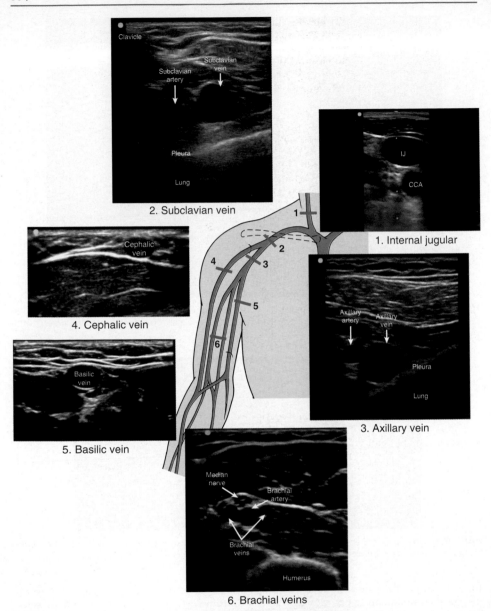

Figure 35.5 Upper Extremity Compression Ultrasound Examination. An upper extremity compression ultrasound exam evaluates the following veins: *(1)* internal jugular vein, *(2)* subclavian vein, *(3)* axillary vein, *(4)* cephalic vein, *(5)* basilic vein, and *(6)* brachial veins. *CCA,* Common carotid artery; *IJ,* internal jugular vein.

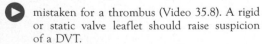

mistaken for a thrombus (Video 35.8). A rigid or static valve leaflet should raise suspicion of a DVT.

Forearm veins are not usually assessed unless focal findings are suspicious for thrombosis.

Image Interpretation

Acute thrombi are typically hypoechoic or anechoic and are loosely attached to the wall of a vein. An acute thrombus fills the central portion of the venous lumen, and as the thrombus expands, the vein becomes distended and rounder compared to normal (Fig. 35.6 and Video 35.9). Nonocclusive thrombi usually do not cause rounding and enlargement of the vein (Fig. 35.7; Videos 35.10 and 35.11). Thrombosis is often seen around central venous catheters (Videos 35.12 and 35.13). Chronic thrombi differ in appearance from acute thrombi; chronic thrombi appear more echogenic and eccentric (retracted to the wall) and are easily recognizable by ultrasound

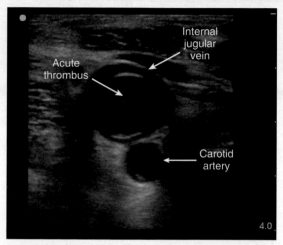

Figure 35.6 Acute Thrombus. An acute, nearly occlusive deep venous thrombus in the left internal jugular vein.

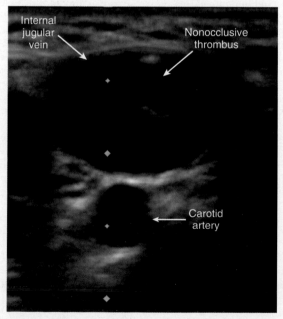

Figure 35.7 Nonocclusive Thrombus. A nonocclusive deep venous thrombus is seen in the internal jugular vein.

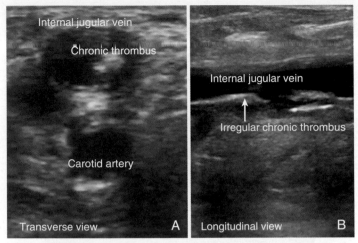

Figure 35.8 Chronic Thrombus. A hyperechoic thrombus adherent to the internal jugular vein wall suggestive of a chronic deep venous thrombosis is seen in transverse (A) and longitudinal views (B).

(Fig. 35.8 and Video 35.14). The smooth walls of normal veins become irregular, thickened, calcified, and hyperechoic after recanalization of thrombus. Visualization of collateral veins should raise suspicion for the presence of chronic thrombosis. Superficial vein DVT can be of concern when extension into a deep vein is likely (Video 35.15)

POCUS is being used more often to assess arteriovenous fistulas in patients receiving chronic hemodialysis. Although a comprehensive evaluation of arteriovenous flow is beyond the scope of POCUS, most providers can rapidly detect large, occlusive thrombi (Video 35.16).

COLOR DOPPLER INTERROGATION

Color flow Doppler can be used to help distinguish vessels from surrounding structures and complement a compression ultrasound exam of the deep veins. This technique can be considered an adjunct in the diagnosis of upper extremity DVT, but should not be used alone to determine the presence or absence of a thrombus. Both the symptomatic and asymptomatic extremities should be examined and compared. Normally, the entire vessel lumen fills with color, especially with squeezing of the distal extremity (augmentation) (Fig. 35.9 and Video 35.17). When a thrombus is present, a "filling defect" is seen with lack of color in the

portion of lumen with thrombus (Videos 35.18 and 35.19).

SPECTRAL DOPPLER

Spectral Doppler can be useful in evaluating veins that are not accessible to direct compression during an upper extremity DVT ultrasound examination: medial subclavian and brachiocephalic veins, and the superior vena cava. Variation or collapse of the venous lumen during respirations, or with techniques such as the "sniff maneuver" that decrease intrathoracic pressure, can help rule out an occlusive thrombus in these inaccessible proximal veins. Complete collapse of the internal jugular or subclavian veins in response to sniffing is associated with absence of a proximal DVT or obstruction.[22]

Spectral Doppler interrogation requires positioning the pulsed-wave Doppler box over the vein in a longitudinal plane with an angle of insonation <60 degrees. Normally, large veins demonstrate spontaneous flow (spontaneity), respiratory variation (phasicity), and cardiac pulsations (pulsatility) (Fig. 35.10). It is important to compare the spectral Doppler findings on both sides. Unilateral loss of spontaneity, phasicity, or pulsatility suggests proximal obstruction, most often due to intraluminal thrombosis (Fig. 35.11).

Similar to color Doppler, spectral Doppler can be useful in the diagnosis of upper

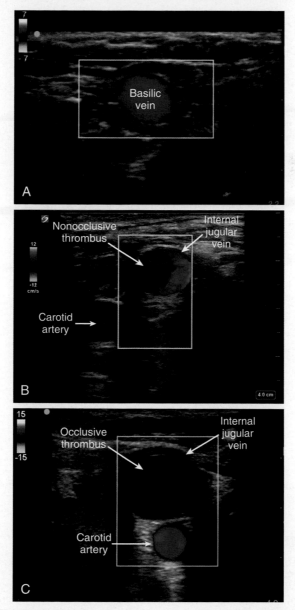

Figure 35.9 Color Flow Doppler Ultrasound. Normally, the entire venous lumen fills with color (A). A filling defect is seen in a partially occluded vein (B). Absence of flow is seen in a completely occluded vein (C).

extremity DVT; however, it does not provide definitive proof of thrombosis and should not be the only diagnostic modality used due to its low sensitivity and specificity.[22,23]

Ultrasound evaluation of the upper extremity venous system is considered to be more challenging than evaluation of the lower extremities. Even though the minimum amount of training needed to perform upper extremity DVT ultrasound exams has not been established, providers can gain competence and confidence through repeated practice.

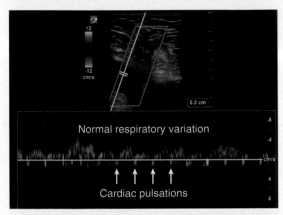

Figure 35.10 Normal Spectral Doppler Ultrasound. Normally, spontaneous venous flow with respiratory variation (phasicity) and cardiac pulsations (pulsatility) is seen.

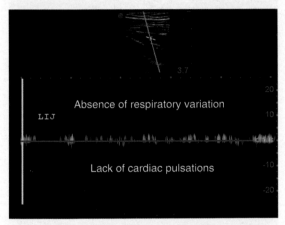

Figure 35.11 Abnormal Spectral Doppler Ultrasound. Proximal obstruction from a deep venous thrombosis causes diminished flow with loss of respiratory variation and cardiac pulsations.

PEARLS AND PITFALLS

- Compression ultrasonography: When evaluating patients for deep venous thrombosis (DVT), compression ultrasonography is considered the standard examination, and use of color and spectral Doppler ultrasound is supplementary.
- Inadequate acoustic windows: The presence of venous catheters, pacemakers, infusion ports, and dressings limits the ability to perform a compression ultrasound (CUS) exam of the target veins. However, because intravascular lines pose a higher risk

for venous thrombosis, providers should carefully assess these patients with multiple views and use color and spectral Doppler ultrasound when uncertainty exists.
- Low venous flow: Faint, mobile echoes may be visualized in the lumen of compressible proximal veins (internal jugular, subclavian, axillary), especially in critically ill patients with low-flow states. These echoes are produced by aggregates of red cells and should not be confused with true thrombosis.

CHAPTER 36

Central Venous Access

Ricardo A. Franco-Sadud ■ Nilam J. Soni

KEY POINTS

- Ultrasound guidance for central line placement reduces mechanical complications, including pneumothorax, hematoma, and arterial punctures, and is now the standard of care for placement of central venous catheters in the internal jugular vein.
- Complication rates associated with central venous catheterization correlate with the number of needle passes, and use of ultrasound guidance reduces the number of needle passes during central vein catheterization.
- Tracking the needle tip in real time using a transverse or longitudinal approach is the primary skill that must be mastered to insert both central and peripheral venous catheters with ultrasound guidance.

Background

Use of ultrasound to guide central venous access was first described in 1984.[1] Initially, ultrasound was used only to help locate the target vein when using the traditional landmark, or "blind," technique. Although the potential to reduce complication rates was recognized, early studies did not definitively conclude that use of ultrasound guidance was beneficial, and use of ultrasound was felt to be too cumbersome, and potentially too expensive, for widespread implementation.[2]

Over the past 25 years, ultrasound guidance for vascular access has evolved from use of Doppler alone to detect the location of vessels to use of high-resolution, two-dimensional ultrasound to track the needle tip in real time. High-frequency, linear-array transducers on modern ultrasound machines allow detailed visualization of vascular anatomy and adjacent structures. In the neck, the internal jugular vein (IJV) and common carotid artery (CCA) are easily recognized with two-dimensional ultrasound and can be confirmed with Doppler ultrasound. Adjacent structures in the neck, such as the thyroid gland, trachea, and pleura, can also be readily visualized.

Several studies have demonstrated that use of real-time ultrasound guidance for central venous catheter (CVC) insertion can increase success rates and decrease mechanical complications, primarily arterial puncture and pneumothorax.[3-15] Use of real-time ultrasound guidance for insertion of CVCs has evolved to become the standard of care and is recommended by the Agency for Healthcare Research and Quality (AHRQ), Institute of Medicine (IOM), National Institute for Health and Clinical Excellence (NICE), Centers for Disease Control (CDC), and several professional societies.[10,16-21] Benefits of real-time ultrasound guidance for CVC insertion have expanded to include cost-effectiveness and reduction of catheter-related bloodstream infections. Currently, providers are expected to have very low complication rates when inserting CVCs.[18,20] Use of real-time ultrasound guidance for CVC insertion is now recommended for both elective and emergency IJV catheterization.[17]

As providers' confidence with use of ultrasound guidance for venous access has increased, the spectrum of large and small vessels that can be accessed with ultrasound has also increased. Following use of ultrasound guidance for IJV cannulation, its use became routine for insertion of peripherally inserted central catheters (PICCs).[22-24] More recently, providers have recognized the benefits of ultrasound guidance for subclavian/axillary vein access.[25-28] Despite a meta-analysis of randomized trials demonstrating the benefits of ultrasound guidance for insertion of CVCs since the mid-1990s,[3] use of ultrasound guidance for CVC insertion has not been universally adopted.[29-34] Two evidence-based consensus statements include recommendations for training because lack of training is a known barrier to use of ultrasound guidance for CVC insertion.[20,23]

This chapter reviews the techniques for CVC insertion in the IJV and subclavian vein (SCV), or proximal axillary vein, using real-time ultrasound guidance.

Internal Jugular Vein Catheterization

ANATOMY

The IJV runs vertically on the anterolateral side of the neck, lateral to the CCA. The IJV joins the SCV to form the brachiocephalic, or innominate, vein that drains into the superior vena cava (Fig. 36.1). In the neck, CVCs are generally inserted into the IJV between the clavicular and sternal heads of the sternocleidomastoid muscle (SCM).

TECHNIQUE

High-frequency, linear-array transducers, often called vascular probes, are used for vascular access procedures. The high-frequency waves give a high-resolution image to a maximum depth of 6 to 10 cm, and the IJV and the axillary/SCV are typically only a few centimeters below the skin.

Images are generated from sound waves reflected from each tissue interface, which determines the tissue echogenicity, or "brightness," displayed on the screen. Dense tissue, such as needles, bones, and pleura, appear bright or hyperechoic. Fluid-filled structures, including arteries and veins, transmit and do not reflect sound waves, and therefore appear black or anechoic.

The ability to distinguish arteries from veins is essential. Veins are oval or triangular shaped, thin-walled, fully compressible, and change size with breathing (respiratory variation) or Valsalva. Arteries are round, thick-walled, partially compressible, and pulsatile.

Preprocedural scanning of the left and right neck should be performed to determine the best CVC insertion site. A linear transducer is placed transversely on the anterolateral neck and the IJV is assessed from the angle of jaw to the inferior anastomosis with the SCV (Fig. 36.2 and Video 36.1). Turn the patient's head slightly,

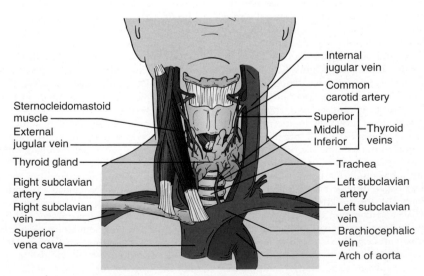

Figure 36.1 Normal Neck Vascular Anatomy.

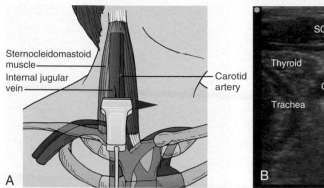
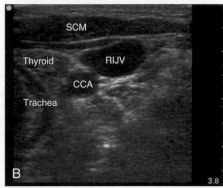

Figure 36.2 Cross-Sectional Anatomy of the Neck. (A) The transducer is placed on the anterolateral neck in a transverse orientation. (B) The internal jugular vein is anterior and lateral to the common carotid artery *(CCA)*. The thyroid gland and trachea are medial to both vessels. *RIJV*, Right internal jugular vein; *SCM*, sternocleidomastoid muscle.

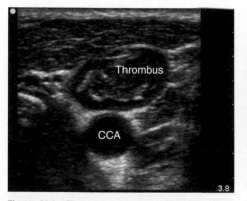
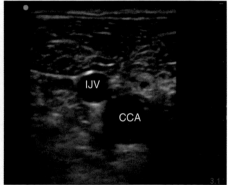

Figure 36.3 Thrombus in the Internal Jugular Vein. A large, echogenic thrombus is visualized in the lumen of the internal jugular vein. *CCA*, Common carotid artery; *IJV*, internal jugular vein. It should be noted that even without thrombus present, this would not be a safe needle trajectory given the CCA lying immediately deep to the IJV.

Figure 36.4 Stenotic Internal Jugular Vein. *CCA*, common carotid artery; *IJV*, Internal jugular vein.

no more than 30 degrees, to the contralateral side with the neck extended. Evaluate the IJV's size, shape, depth, compressibility, proximity to CCA, and distal anastomosis with SCV. Respirophasic variation of the size of the IJV can be noted (Video 36.2). Center the IJV on the screen, then slide the ultrasound transducer slowly toward the clavicle. Once the transducer cannot be advanced distally, tilt the transducer aiming the ultrasound beam toward the feet to visualize the subclavian and brachiocephalic veins. It is important to assess for complete compressibility of the IJV (Video 36.3). Asymptomatic thrombosis in the IJV is

not uncommon in hospitalized and critically ill patients, and lack of compressibility is diagnostic for deep venous thrombosis. Both complete and partially occluding thrombi manifest with lack of compression (Fig. 36.3 and Videos 36.4-36.6). Color and spectral Doppler can supplement the compression ultrasound exam when evaluating for deep venous thrombosis (Video 36.7) (see Chapter 35). Avoid serial compressions after diagnosing IJV thrombosis given the potential risk of dislodging the thrombus. Patients who have had multiple prior IJV cannulations, especially large-caliber temporary hemodialysis catheters, may have a stenotic IJV (Fig. 36.4 and Video 36.8).

Select the safest needle insertion site based on the following characteristics: 1) absence of thrombus, 2) widest diameter, 3) shallowest depth, and 4) relationship to the CCA (preferably not overlying the CCA). If the IJV directly overlies the CCA, the transducer should be rocked to assess whether the needle trajectory would avoid the CCA if the posterior wall were punctured.

After the best insertion site has been determined, the ultrasound machine should be prepared. Position the ultrasound machine in the operator's direct line of sight to avoid head turning to view the screen. Cover the transducer with a sterile sheath prior to placing it on the sterile field. Hold the transducer in the nondominant hand while holding the needle in the dominant hand. Orient the transducer in the nondominant hand such that the left side of the transducer corresponds with the left side of the screen. Two approaches to real-time needle guidance are described: transverse (short-axis) and longitudinal (long-axis) (see Chapter 4, Figs. 4.8).

TRANSVERSE APPROACH

In a transverse or short-axis approach, the introducer needle crosses the plane of the ultrasound beam, and only a portion of the needle shaft is visualized, rather than the actual tip of the needle, unless care is taken to first identify the needle tip. First, center the IJV in a transverse view on the screen and assess the depth to the vessel (Fig. 36.5). Tilt the transducer pointing the ultrasound beam toward the operator. Insert the needle at a 45- to 60-degree angle relative to skin in the center of the transducer (Fig. 36.6). Identify the needle tip on the screen by very subtly tilting the transducer to and from the needle insertion site. The first appearance of the hyperechoic needle with shadow is assumed to be the tip of the needle. It is imperative to identify and track the needle tip. Advance the needle only 1 to 2 mm at a time while continuously tracking the needle tip by tilting the transducer back and forth. Redirect the needle as needed if its trajectory is off target. As the skin is traversed as described above, the needle tip will be visualized denting the IJV (Video 36.9), followed by puncturing and entering the vessel (Fig. 36.7 and Video 36.10). The needle tip should be confirmed to be in the IJV (Video 36.11).

After the needle enters the IJV, a guidewire is inserted to maintain the track. After placing the guidewire, the operator should confirm proper placement of the guidewire in the IJV

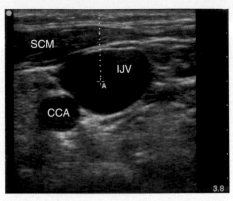

Figure 36.5 Depth of Internal Jugular Vein. Measure the distance from skin surface to center of the vessel lumen. In this example, this distance is 1.5 cm. *CCA*, Common carotid artery; *IJV*, internal jugular vein; *SCM*, sternocleidomastoid muscle. Note also that an orientation of the IJV and CCA is achieved whereby the CCA is not immediately deep to the IJV.

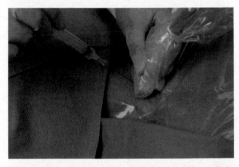

Figure 36.6 Transverse Approach (Short-Axis Technique). The transducer is held tilted toward the needle. The needle insertion angle is 45 to 60 degrees to the skin surface and approximately 90 degrees relative to the ultrasound beam to maximize visualization of the needle tip.

and not the CCA (Fig. 36.8 and Video 36.12). Emerging literature supports visualization of the guidewire in the brachiocephalic vein to confirm proper placement prior to dilation of the vein.[35] Compression and Doppler ultrasound (color flow, power, pulsed-wave) may also be used to confirm placement of the guidewire in the vein. If any doubt exists about placement of the guidewire in the IJV versus the CCA, the guidewire should be removed promptly with minimal risk of harm to the patient; however, if the IJV is dilated and a CVC is inadvertently inserted in the CCA, major complications can

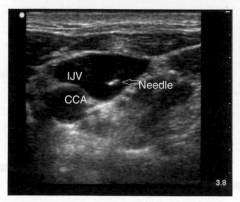

Figure 36.7 Needle Tip in the Internal Jugular Vein. The needle tip is seen in the center of the venous lumen before inserting the guidewire. *CCA*, Common carotid artery; *IJV*, internal jugular vein.

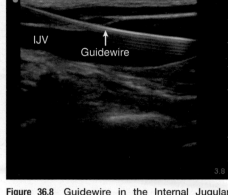

Figure 36.8 Guidewire in the Internal Jugular Vein. Visualization of the guidewire within the internal jugular vein to confirm proper placement without traversing the posterior wall of the vessel is a critical step.

occur, including stroke. After the guidewire has been confirmed in the IJV, proceed using standard technique: make a skin nick, dilate, and insert the catheter over the guidewire.

LONGITUDINAL APPROACH

In a longitudinal or long-axis approach, the plane of the ultrasound beam is parallel to the course of the target vessel. Insertion of CVCs in the IJV using a longitudinal approach is an advanced skill that should be attempted by providers experienced in performing real-time ultrasound-guided procedures. First, the IJV should be centered in a transverse view on the screen and then the transducer is rotated 90 degrees with the transducer orientation marker pointed toward the operator. Once the transducer is centered over the IJV in a longitudinal plane, the operator must focus on ensuring the transducer remains in the same plane without sliding medially or laterally. Care must be taken to prevent the transducer from sliding medially over the arterial lumen, and mistaking the CCA for the IJV. The pulsatility and thick walls distinguish the CCA from IJV in a longitudinal view. Insert the needle at a 45- to 60-degree angle relative to skin in the center of the short side of the transducer (Fig. 36.9). The needle insertion angle and distance from the transducer should be appropriate for the depth of the target vessel. Shallow needle insertion angles are used for superficial vessels, whereas steep angles are used for deep vessels (Fig. 36.10). The needle tip and shaft have to remain

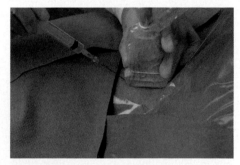

Figure 36.9 Longitudinal Approach (Long-Axis Technique). The transducer is positioned longitudinally over the course of the internal jugular vein. The needle insertion angle is steep (45–60 degrees) relative to the skin surface.

in the plane of the ultrasound beam to ensure visualization throughout needle advancement. Adjust the needle trajectory to aim the tip toward the target vessel at its widest diameter in a longitudinal view. Track the needle tip in real time as it traverses the soft tissues and enters the IJV.

Transverse Versus Longitudinal Approach

Limited data exists comparing the longitudinal versus transverse approach to CVC insertion at the IJV site, and most experts of ultrasound-guided procedures recommend learning the transverse approach first.[36] A

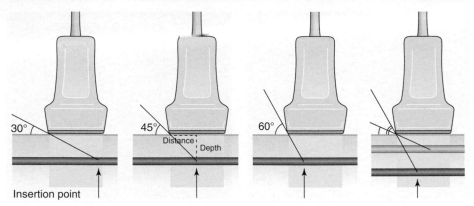

Figure 36.10   Needle Insertion Angle and Vessel Depth. The needle insertion angle is normally 30–60° and should be adjusted for the depth of the target vessel.

randomized controlled trial comparing the short-, long-, and oblique-axis approaches found that both short- and oblique-axis approaches had higher first-attempt success rates and lower complication rates compared to a long-axis approach.[37]

The hand–eye coordination needed to use the transverse approach is generally learned easier than the longitudinal approach. Visualization of the IJV in long axis is limited by the jaw and clavicle, and stabilizing the transducer longitudinally on the curvature of the neck can be challenging. Additionally, most studies demonstrating reduced complications with real-time ultrasound guidance utilized the transverse approach at the IJV site. Regardless of the approach utilized, it is most important for providers to track the needle tip in real time and confirm placement of the guidewire in the lumen of the IJV.

Subclavian and Axillary Vein Catheterization

BACKGROUND

Early studies concluded that ultrasound could not be used for SCV access due to the presence of overlying bony structures. Subsequently, widespread adoption of ultrasound-guided IJV access overshadowed the potential use of ultrasound at the SCV site. Recent research has turned its attention to using real-time ultrasound guidance for placement of subclavian central lines and has shown a significant decrease in complication rates, including

inadvertent arterial punctures, pneumothorax, and hematoma formation, and a reduction in number of puncture attempts.[27,38,39] Most of these studies describe using real-time ultrasound to insert CVCs in the axillary vein.[25,40]

When comparing complication rates of sites for central venous access, one study that reviewed data from over 2600 tunneled CVCs inserted by anesthesiologists found low complication rates for both ultrasound-guided distal axillary vein versus ultrasound-guided IJV cannulation (0.7% vs. 1.2%). The study concluded that ultrasound-guided axillary vein access is technically more difficult than the IJV because the axillary vein is deeper and surrounded by the axillary artery, brachial plexus, chest wall, and pleura. However, once the technique is mastered, ultrasound-guided axillary vein access is safe and reliable.[40] A meta-analysis of 10 randomized controlled studies with 2168 patients concluded that use of real-time ultrasound guidance for SCV cannulation reduced the risk of complications and incidence of failed attempts compared to landmark-based techniques.[38]

This section will focus on ultrasound-guided axillary vein catheterization. In clinical practice, the term ultrasound-guided SCV access is commonly used, although providers are technically referring to the axillary vein access because the needle insertion site is lateral to the first rib.

ANATOMY

The axillary vein is formed by the anastomosis of the brachial and basilic veins. The axillary

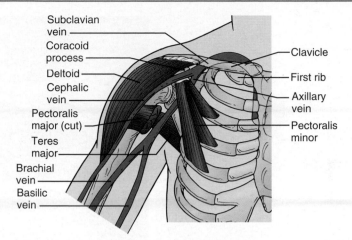

Figure 36.11 Anatomy of the Axillary and Subclavian Veins. The basilic and brachial veins anastomose to form the axillary vein, and the cephalic and axillary vein anastomose to form the subclavian vein. The axillary vein extends from the lateral border of teres major to the lateral border of the first rib.

vein extends from the lateral border of the teres major to the lateral border of the first rib where it joins the cephalic vein to form the SCV (Fig. 36.11). Start by scanning along the inferior margin of the mid-clavicle with the transducer in a longitudinal plane, and slide the transducer laterally. Select the site where the axillary vein is most superficial and can be clearly distinguished from the axillary artery. Avoid selecting a site too distal because of increased risk of brachial plexus or long thoracic nerve injury. We recommend selecting a site no more than 4 cm from the mid-clavicle.

TECHNIQUE

In a transverse or oblique plane, scan the axillary vein from glenohumeral joint to the point where the vein passes between the clavicle and first rib. Identify the axillary vein, axillary artery, cephalic vein, distal SCV, and first rib (Fig. 36.12 and Video 36.13). Once all of these structures have been identified, scan 1 to 2 cm proximally toward the first rib. The distal SCV can be identified where the cephalic vein joins the axillary vein (Video 36.14). Afterward, scan laterally and identify the distal axillary vein before it dives deep and divides into the basilic and brachial veins (Video 36.15).

Choose the most proximal and superficial needle insertion site on the axillary vein where vital structures surrounding the vein, specifically the axillary artery and pleura, can be well

visualized. We recommend the use of color flow and pulsed-wave Doppler ultrasound to confirm correct differentiation of the axillary artery and vein (Fig. 36.13 and Video 36.16). If thrombus is visualized in the subclavian or axillary vein, an alternative insertion site should be selected (Video 36.17).

With the transducer in a longitudinal or oblique plane, inject local anesthesia under real-time ultrasound visualization using a steep 60–80 degree insertion angle. The needle trajectory should be toward the center of the anterior wall of the axillary vein or distal SCV. Once the anticipated needle tract has been anesthetized, use the same technique to insert the introducer needle in a longitudinal approach as described above for the IJV. Choosing an angle whereby the 1st or 2nd rib is just deep to the vein and on the anticipated the needle trajectory can help prevent pneumothorax in case of posterior venous wall puncture. Follow the needle tip using real-time ultrasound visualization until the needle tip punctures the vein and is seen in the center of the venous lumen (Fig. 36.14 and Videos 36.18). Once the needle is in the vein, consider reducing the needle insertion angle to less than 60 degrees to facilitate insertion of the guidewire. After the guidewire is confirmed to be in the axillary or subclavian vein, proceed using the standard insertion technique: make a skin nick, dilate the tract, and insert the catheter over the guidewire.

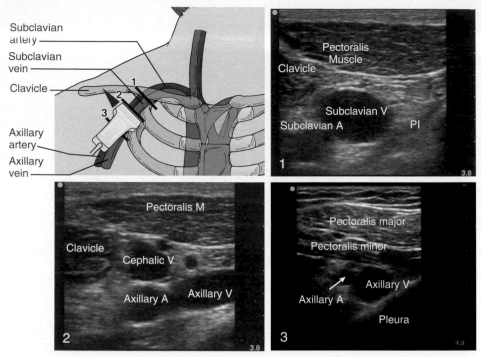

Figure 36.12   Cross-Sectional Anatomy of the Subclavian and Axillary Vessels. The cross-sectional anatomy is shown in the infraclavicular space in a longitudinal orientation at three levels. (1) The subclavian vein is seen anterior and superior to the subclavian artery. (2) The cephalic and axillary veins anastomose to form the distal subclavian vein. (3) The distal axillary vein and artery are seen deep to the pectoralis major and minor muscles. Note the pleural line and lung are seen deep to both vessels. A, Artery; M, muscle; V, vein.

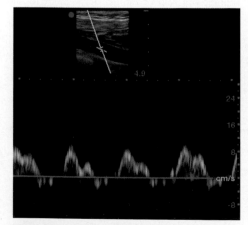

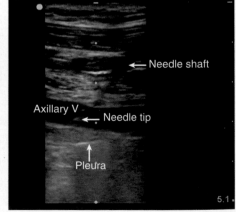

Figure 36.13   Pulsed-Wave Doppler of Subclavian Vein. Normally, the spectral Doppler waveform of the subclavian vein demonstrates respirophasic variation.

Figure 36.14   Ultrasound-Guided Axillary Vein Cannulation. The needle tip is tracked in real time and is seen inside the lumen of the axillary vein.

PEARLS AND PITFALLS

- When prescanning the patient to determine the best CVC insertion site, evaluate for distal stenosis, thrombus in the vein, and anatomic anomalies increasing the risk of arterial puncture. Also, ensure the diameter of the venous lumen is sufficiently wide to allow insertion of the venous catheter.
- Avoid sites that may increase the difficulty of the procedure: scars in neck, sites of previous tunneled catheters, tracheostomy, cellulitis.
- Novice operators should only move one hand at a time. When advancing or changing the direction of the needle, hold the ultrasound transducer still. When adjusting or moving the transducer to improve ultrasound visualization, stop advancing the needle until the needle tip is clearly identified.
- Measure the depth of the anterior vein wall in relation to the skin surface. If the needle has been advanced to the expected depth and a flash of venous blood has not been seen, confirm the location of the needle tip. If the needle tip is not visualized, withdraw the needle to a shallow depth and resume tracking the tip toward the anterior wall of the target vessel.
- Most central venous catheter (CVC) kits contain an introducer needle that is 4 to 6 cm long, whereas the depth of most internal jugular or axillary veins is less than 3 cm. When supervising novice operators, it is imperative to recognize that less than half of the introducer needle needs to be inserted before venous blood is obtained in most patients.
- To maintain a firm grip on the transducer and syringe, do not place an excessive amount of sterile ultrasound gel in your immediate work area. Drop a small amount directly on your probe and an additional amount within reach on the sterile drape.
- Visualizing the needle tip within the target vessel is important, but the most critical step is ensuring the guidewire is within the vein. Inadvertent placement of the guidewire through the vein and into the artery will result in dangerous placement of the CVC in the adjacent artery.
- Ultrasound-guided placement of CVCs should be mastered at the internal jugular and femoral vein sites using a transverse approach before attempting the axillary vein site. Practicing a longitudinal approach for placement of arterial lines and peripheral venous catheters can improve an operator's skills and comfort prior to attempting an ultrasound-guided axillary CVC insertion.

CHAPTER 37

Peripheral Venous Access

Felipe Teran ■ Bret P. Nelson

KEY POINTS

- Use of ultrasound guidance to insert peripheral intravenous catheters increases procedure success rates compared to traditional techniques, and reduces the need for placement of central venous catheters.
- Preprocedural ultrasound evaluation allows selection of a peripheral vein with the high likelihood of successful placement of an intravenous catheter.
- Both transverse and longitudinal approaches can be used to insert peripheral intravenous catheters, although the transverse approach may be faster and easier to learn.

Background

Even though insertion of peripheral intravenous (PIV) catheters is the most common procedure performed in emergency departments (EDs) in the United States,[1] clinicians often encounter difficulty in obtaining peripheral venous access with first- and second-attempt failure rates reported to be as high as 39% and 22%, respectively.[2] Another study in an ED showed that 12% of patients had difficult PIV access, defined as requiring more than three attempts or physician intervention to obtain venous access.[3]

Several factors have been associated with difficult peripheral venous access: body habitus (obesity, underweight), anatomical variations (small, nonvisible, nonpalpable veins), subcutaneous edema, multiple failed attempts, intravenous drug abuse, volume depletion, and certain chronic medical conditions (diabetes, sickle cell disease).[3-5]

Multiple studies have demonstrated benefits of placing PIV catheters using ultrasound guidance.[6-16] In general, these studies have demonstrated a reduction in number of attempts, reduction in time to cannulation, and an increase in overall success rates; however, these studies are limited by small sample sizes,

different patient populations, and variable training of providers. Two meta-analyses that pooled data from these studies concluded that use of ultrasound guidance to insert PIVs can improve overall success rates when compared with traditional techniques, although there was no significant difference in number of attempts or time to cannulation.[17,18]

One advantage of ultrasound-guided PIV catheter placement is the avoidance of central venous catheters. In an ED, ultrasound-guided placement of PIVs reduced the need for central venous access in 85% of patients.[19] Additionally, placement of PIVs with ultrasound guidance is more likely to be successful than blind placement of external jugular IVs.[20]

Ultrasound-guided placement of PIVs can be used in any patient, but the technique is particularly useful in patients with nonpalpable or nonvisible peripheral veins. Nurses, physicians, and other health care providers have successfully learned ultrasound-guided PIV placement through focused training courses.[6,21-23]

Currently, there are no guidelines recommending specific indications for use of ultrasound guidance to insert PIV catheters. Performance of ultrasound-guided PIV insertion should be considered by trained providers in any patient with known difficult venous

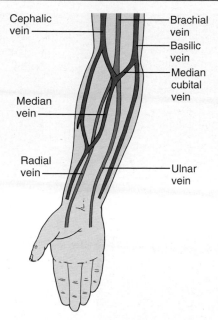

Figure 37.1 Normal Vein Anatomy of the Arm and Forearm. The median cubital, basilic, cephalic, and brachial veins are most commonly accessed.

access or after failed attempts using traditional techniques.

Anatomy

The anterior forearm, antecubital fossa, and medial upper arm are the most common sites for performing ultrasound-guided PIV placement (Fig. 37.1). The brachial (Video 37.1), cephalic (Video 37.2), and basilic (Video 37.3) veins are the largest upper extremity veins and most commonly accessed for placement of PIVs with ultrasound guidance (Fig. 37.2).

When selecting a vein for ultrasound-guided PIV insertion, an important consideration is the depth of the target vessel, with greatest success seen with a depth between 0.3 cm and 1.5 cm and lower success rates reported when depth from the skin is greater than 1.6 cm.[24,25] Furthermore, successful PIV insertion is more likely when veins with a diameter ≥0.4 cm are targeted.[24] Lastly, veins travelling a straight path are preferred, as they are easier to cannulate than tortuous vessels.

Arteries can be differentiated from veins based on pulsatility, compressibility, wall thickness, and Doppler appearance. Whereas arterial walls are thicker, more echogenic, and

less compressible, peripheral venous walls are thinner, less echogenic, and fully compressible with minimal pressure (Video 37.4). Color or spectral Doppler may be used when uncertainty exists between arteries and veins (Video 37.5). When paired arteries and veins are visualized together, small amounts of pressure will collapse the vein, whereas much greater pressure is required to compress the artery (Table 37.1).

Technique

A high-frequency linear-array transducer (5–12 MHz) is used for this procedure because it provides high resolution of superficial structures. If available, a narrow linear, or "hockey stick", transducer is advantageous because of the ease of tracking fine movements.

Position the patient either sitting or supine, but most important is to maximize both operator and patient comfort. The ultrasound machine should be positioned within the operator's direct line of sight to provide an unobstructed and easily achievable view of the screen. The patient's arm should be fully extended and externally rotated with the palm facing upward.

Scan the arm in a transverse plane to identify potential PIV insertion sites. Imaging depth should be set to 2 to 2.5 cm to avoid vessels more than 2.5 cm deep, which have a lower likelihood of successful cannulation. Evaluate the vein's size, depth, proximity to arteries/nerves, and compressibility to rule out thrombosis (Fig. 37.3 and Video 37.6). Select the most accessible vein that is superficial and distal.

After an insertion site has been chosen, all supplies should be gathered. Most standard IV catheters are too short to reach deep peripheral veins. Long IV catheters have less risk of premature failure due to dislodgement compared to short IV catheters, especially in obese and edematous patients.[26] Catheters that are 48 mm (1.88 inches) in length are generally preferred, but a good rule of thumb is to leave twice as much catheter within the vessel as it takes to reach the vessel. An arterial line catheter may be considered as an alternative.

After a target vein has been selected, place a tourniquet proximal to the insertion site to increase the diameter of the vessel. We recommend placing the tourniquet as high as possible, ideally next to the axilla.

Sterilization of the skin and preparation of the sterile field must be performed per local

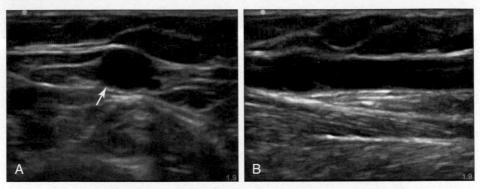

Figure 37.2 Transverse (A) and longitudinal (B) views of the basilic vein *(arrow)*.

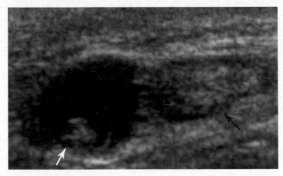

Figure 37.3 **Peripheral Vein Thrombosis.** A peripheral vein with a partially occluding thrombus *(white arrow)* and adjacent lymph node *(red arrow)* are seen in a transverse view.

TABLE 37.1 Characteristics of Arteries and Veins by Ultrasound

Arteries	Veins
Noncompressible with light pressure	Compress easily with light pressure
Thick, echogenic walls	Thin, nearly imperceptible walls
Round shape	Variable shape
Pulsatile	Nonpulsatile (may appear pulsatile due to transmission of pulses from an adjacent artery)
Color flow unchanged with distal compression	Color flow augmented by distal compression

protocol. We recommend sterilizing the skin with chlorhexidine and cleaning the transducer face and sides with antiseptic wipes. A sterile transducer cover and sterile gel may be used. We recommend performing the procedure under strict sterile conditions, and at minimum, a sterile transparent waterproof film should be placed over the transducer. If available, we recommend use of a local anesthetic for cannulation of deep veins to minimize patient discomfort and facilitate performance of the procedure.

TRANSVERSE VERSUS LONGITUDINAL APPROACH

Peripheral veins, similar to central veins, can be cannulated using either a transverse or a longitudinal approach. One small study found no difference in success rates using a transverse versus longitudinal approach, yet a transverse approach was found to be faster.[27]

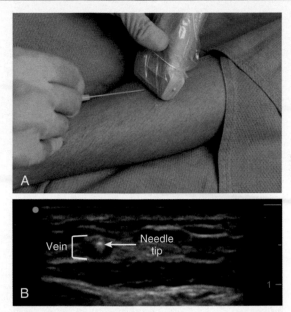

Figure 37.4   Transverse Approach. (A) Transducer and needle position. (B) Needle tip in the target vein in a transverse view.

We recommend that novice operators initially learn a transverse approach. More experienced operators that are skilled in performing real-time, ultrasound-guided procedures may prefer to use a longitudinal approach.

Transverse Approach

With the transducer held in the nondominant hand and transducer marker pointed toward the operator's left side, the target vein is centered on the screen (Fig. 37.4). The operator should insert the needle at the center of the transducer with an angle of approximately 45 degrees. Slowly advance the needle and subtly tilt the transducer to maintain the needle tip in sight. Once the needle reaches the vein, tenting of the anterior vein wall will be seen. At this point, a brisk acceleration of the needle is needed to puncture the wall. Once a flash of blood is observed, the needle tip should be seen in the lumen as a bright hyperechoic dot. Next, reduce the angle of the needle to 20 to 30 degrees, align the needle trajectory with the course of the vessel, and advance the catheter into the vein. For long catheters in deep veins, we recommend to further advance the needle into the vein a few millimeters, visualizing the needle tip at all times, before advancing the catheter. This allows penetration past venous

valves that may cause kinking of the catheter and ensures enough catheter is inside the lumen to avoid extravasation (Video 37.7).

Longitudinal Approach

Start by centering the transducer over the target vessel as described for a transverse approach. Rotate the transducer 90 degrees to visualize the vessel in a longitudinal plane (Fig. 37.5). The probe marker should be pointed toward the operator. If the vessel walls are not seen, the transducer is not directly over the vein or is completely compressing the vein. With a longitudinal approach, the needle should be inserted just under the center of the short end of the transducer. In contrast to the transverse approach in which the operator tracks only the needle tip as it advances to the target vessel, the longitudinal approach allows the operator to visualize the entire needle as it advances to the target vessel. If there are adjacent structures to avoid, such as arteries or nerves, the needle may be initially inserted using a transverse approach, and then rotated 90 degrees to switch to a longitudinal approach to visualize the needle approaching the target vessel. Both the needle advancement and threading of the catheter should be performed under real-time, direct visualization (Video 37.8). The ability to

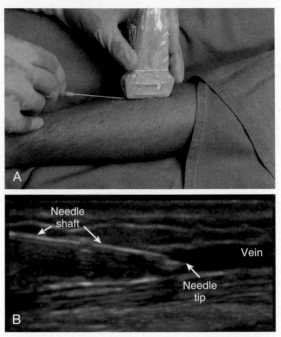

Figure 37.5   Longitudinal Approach. (A) Transducer and needle position. (B) Needle tip entering the target vein in a longitudinal plane.

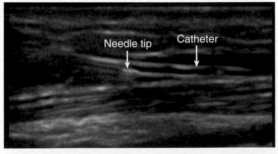

Figure 37.6   Catheter in Vein. The catheter is being advanced off the needle into the peripheral vein shown in a longitudinal view.

follow the course of the IV catheter throughout the procedure and assess the length of catheter inserted into vessel is the main advantage of using a longitudinal approach (Fig. 37.6 and Video 37.9).

Complications

Potential complications include arterial puncture, nerve injury, extravasation, hematoma, infection, and thrombophlebitis (Video 37.10). Few studies have reported complication rates with or without the use of ultrasound guidance for PIV insertion. One study reported 1 arterial puncture (4%) during ultrasound-guided PIV cannulation, which is similar to previously reported brachial artery puncture rates of 2%.[8,13] In comparison, brachial artery puncture rates have been reported to be 25% without the use of ultrasound.[28]

PEARLS AND PITFALLS

- Ensure comfort of the operator and patient before beginning the procedure and ensure the screen is in the operator's direct line of sight. To minimize the patient's discomfort, use a local anesthetic for cannulation of any deep veins.
- Ensure that at least two-thirds of the length of catheter is inside the vein lumen. A minimum length of 48 mm (1.88 inches) is recommended for most peripheral veins identified by ultrasound. Avoid using shallow insertion angles that can result in insufficient catheter length to thread into the vein.
- The needle tip must coincide with the ultrasound beam to be visualized on the screen and subtly tilting or sliding the transducer will maintain the needle tip in sight.
- Maintaining control of the needle during cannulation is key to avoid complications. If the needle tip cannot be visualized during insertion, avoid further advancement until either the needle tip, or its "ring down" artifact, can be seen.
- Complications such as arterial puncture, nerve injury, and hematoma formation are infrequent with use of ultrasound and can be prevented by continuous visualization of the needle tip during peripheral intravenous catheter insertion.

CHAPTER 38

Arterial Access

Anita Cave

KEY POINTS

- Use of ultrasound to guide arterial line placement increases the success rate of cannulation and reduces the risk of periprocedural complications.
- Nontraditional arterial cannulation sites with few landmarks can be accessed using ultrasound guidance.
- Arteries can be differentiated from veins using ultrasound based on compressibility, pulsatility, and Doppler appearance.

Background

Arterial cannulation is performed to facilitate hemodynamic monitoring, measure cardiac output, and sample arterial blood. Historically, this procedure was performed using landmark-based techniques, and success depended on knowledge of vascular anatomy and clinical experience. A major limitation of landmark-based techniques is variance in patient anatomy due to obesity, edema, hypotension, vessel thrombosis, and congenital anomalies. Repeated attempts at arterial cannulation may become progressively more difficult secondary to arterial vasospasm, hematoma formation, and intimal dissection.

Ultrasound guidance for arterial cannulation has been shown to increase the success rate of cannulation while reducing the number of attempts, time to cannulation, and complications.[1] In a meta-analysis of randomized controlled trials comparing radial artery cannulation with and without ultrasound guidance, ultrasound guidance improved first-attempt success rates from 34% to 57%. First-attempt success rates were as high as 95%.[2,3] Ultrasound guidance has also been shown to facilitate arterial access in patients with low perfusion and after multiple failed attempts using a landmark-based technique.[4,5] In the pediatric population, which has a greater proportion of subcutaneous fat and smaller arterial diameter,

ultrasound guidance has significantly improved first-attempt success rates and reduced the number of attempts.[2] Ultrasound can guide arterial access at traditional insertion sites (radial, femoral, brachial, and dorsalis pedis arteries) and nontraditional insertion sites, such as the axillary, ulnar, and temporal arteries, where landmarks are not useful.[5]

Anatomy

RADIAL ARTERY

The radial artery is the most common site for arterial cannulation. The artery's superficial location, ease of access, and low rate of complications make it a favorable site.[6] Also, the dual blood supply to the hand provided by the radial and ulnar arteries minimizes the risk of distal ischemia if a complication arises resulting in a loss of radial artery blood flow.[7] The necessity and optimal method to assess adequacy of collateral blood flow to the hand before radial artery cannulation are controversial.[7,8] The modified Allen test is most commonly used, although a number of studies refute its predictive value.[8,9]

At the level of the wrist, the radial artery is superficial and lies medial to the brachioradialis tendon and lateral to the flexor carpi radialis tendon (Fig. 38.1 and Video 38.1). Cannulation proximal to the wrist is more challenging because the artery runs deep through the

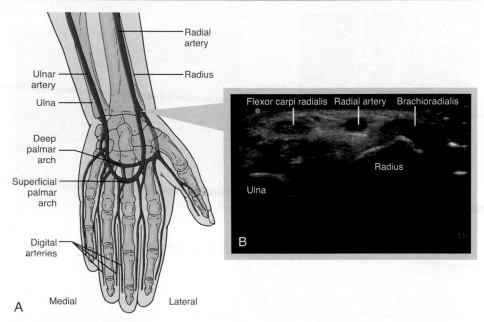

Figure 38.1 Radial Artery Anatomy. (A) Radial artery lies superficial to the radius on the lateral, volar aspect of the wrist. (B) Cross-sectional anatomy of the radial artery in between the brachioradialis and flexor carpi radialis tendons.

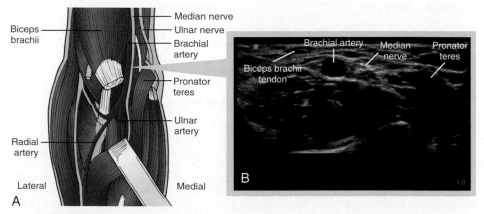

Figure 38.2 Brachial Artery Anatomy. (A) Brachial artery lies in the antecubital fossa medial to the biceps brachii and lateral to the pronator teres. (B) Cross-sectional anatomy of the brachial artery.

brachioradialis muscle.[10] Anatomical variants of the origin or course of the radial artery occur in up to 30% of the population.[11]

BRACHIAL ARTERY

The brachial artery is a continuation of the axillary artery and can be palpated on the medial side of the antecubital fossa. The brachial artery lies along the medial border of the biceps brachii muscle and the lateral border of the pronator teres muscle (Fig. 38.2 and Video 38.2).[12] This location is the most accessible site for brachial artery cannulation. Some prefer a more proximal insertion site where there is less chance of kinking or occluding the catheter.

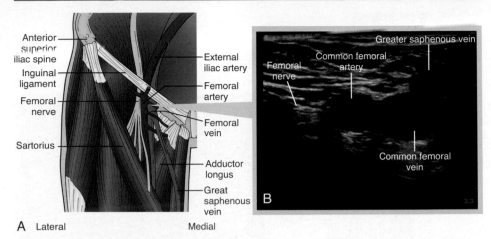

Figure 38.3 Femoral Artery Anatomy. (A) Femoral artery lies in the femoral triangle (inguinal ligament, sartorius, adductor longus) in between the femoral vein and nerve. (B) Cross-sectional anatomy of the femoral artery.

The brachial artery is a less favored site for cannulation because it lacks the benefit of collateral circulation, and obstruction may lead to compromise of radial and ulnar perfusion, resulting in distal ischemia.

FEMORAL ARTERY

After the external iliac artery crosses beneath the inguinal ligament, it is called the femoral artery. The femoral artery is contained within a neurovascular bundle between the femoral vein and nerve (Fig. 38.3 and Video 38.3) in the femoral triangle. The superior border of the femoral triangle is the inguinal ligament, the medial border is the adductor longus muscle, and the lateral border is the sartorius muscle. The femoral artery is palpated midway between the anterior superior iliac spine and the symphysis pubis.[12] In 65% of patients, a portion of the common femoral artery overlaps the common femoral vein.[13] The large vessel diameter and abundant collateral circulation make the femoral artery a favorable site for cannulation.

DORSALIS PEDIS

The dorsalis pedis artery runs from the level of the ankle along the medial side of the dorsal foot to the great toe (Fig. 38.4 and Video 38.4).[12] The dorsalis pedis artery can be palpated between the tendons of the extensor hallucis longus medially and the extensor

digitorum longus laterally. The dorsalis pedis artery is a less favored site for cannulation because it is distant from the central circulation and difficult to cannulate in patients with hypotension or peripheral vascular disease.[14]

Technique

The technique for ultrasound-guided arterial cannulation is similar at all sites. A general description of the procedure is provided below followed by site-specific details.

PREPARATION

A high-frequency (≥7 MHz) linear-array transducer is required. High-frequency transducers provide better resolution of superficial structures close to the skin surface.[5] The ultrasound screen should be in the direct line of sight of the operator. Aligning the operator, transducer, target vessel, and screen minimizes head turning during needle insertion. The entire procedure should be performed using sterile technique. Skin overlying the insertion site should be sterilized using a chlorhexidine-based solution per local protocol. Procedure supplies should be placed on a sterile field within the operator's close reach; specifically, the guidewire, scalpel, and catheter should be within reach. A sterile transducer sheath should be placed over the transducer, using sterile gel both inside and outside of the sterile sheath.

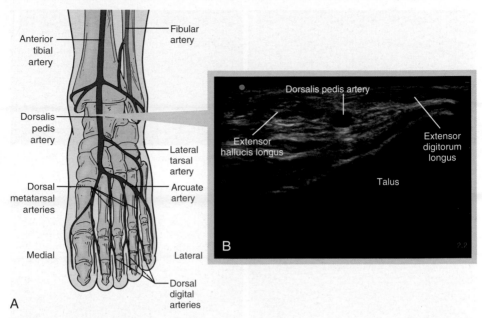

Figure 38.4   Dorsalis Pedis Artery Anatomy. (A) Dorsalis pedis artery lies superficial to the talus bone in between the tendons of the extensor hallucis longus medially and the extensor digitorum longus laterally. (B) Cross-sectional anatomy of the dorsalis pedis artery.

Percutaneous cannulation may be performed using a modified Seldinger technique or a catheter over-the-needle technique.[15] In a modified Seldinger technique, a guidewire is advanced through the needle into the vessel lumen before catheter advancement. A 20-gauge, 3- to 5-cm Teflon catheter is most commonly used for radial, brachial, or dorsalis pedis artery cannulation. For the femoral artery, a longer catheter length is required, usually 12 to 15 cm.

Imaging depth varies depending on the insertion site and patient's body habitus. The transducer should be held in the operator's nondominant hand. The artery is identified in a transverse (short-axis) view (Fig. 38.5A), and then the transducer is rotated 90 degrees to visualize the artery in a longitudinal (long-axis) view (see Fig. 38.5B and Video 38.5). Several characteristics differentiate arteries from veins by ultrasound. Arteries are pulsatile with lumens that cannot be fully collapsed by external compression from the transducer.[5] Arterial walls are thicker and more echogenic. Color-flow Doppler of arteries shows pulsatile flow that is detected predominantly during systole (Fig. 38.6; Videos 38.6 and 38.7),[5] and the color cannot be completely obliterated with

external compression of the vessel (Video 38.8). Flow may appear turbulent due to high velocities within the artery. Pulsed-wave Doppler of arteries shows a systolic-diastolic pattern with high velocities.[5]

TRANSVERSE VERSUS LONGITUDINAL APPROACH

Needle insertion can be performed using either a transverse (short-axis) or a longitudinal (long-axis) approach. Choice of approach depends on the artery's location, operator preference, and anatomic relationships.[16] In a transverse approach (Video 38.9), it can be challenging to distinguish the true needle tip from the needle shaft. The evidence comparing the two approaches is inconclusive. One study showed that a transverse approach was faster than a longitudinal approach to obtain vascular access for novices.[17] Another study showed experienced ultrasound users favored a longitudinal approach, with higher success rates at first attempt and lower complication rates.[18] We focus on a transverse approach, which is most commonly used (see Chapters 4 (Fig 4.8), 36 (Fig 36.10), and 37 for a description of the longitudinal approach).

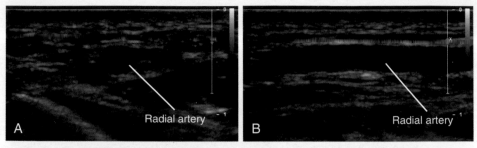

Figure 38.5   Radial Artery. (A) Transverse view. (B) Longitudinal view.

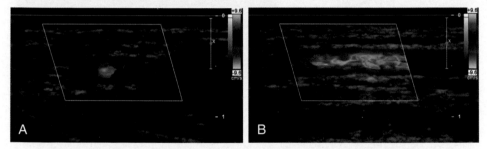

Figure 38.6   Color Flow Doppler of Radial Artery. (A) Transverse view. (B) Longitudinal view.

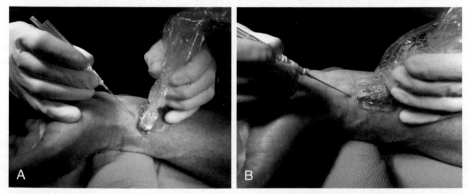

Figure 38.7   Radial Artery Cannulation. (A) Transverse approach. (B) Longitudinal approach.

In a transverse view, center the target vessel on the ultrasound screen (see Fig. 38.5A). Insert the needle in line with the center of the transducer at a 45-degree angle to the skin (Fig. 38.7).[5] Generally, the closer the artery is to the skin surface, the shallower the angle of the needle should be. With more acute angles, the needle tip is more likely to inadvertently advance past the posterior wall of the vessel. Slowly advance the needle while maintaining visualization of the tip at all times.[5] As described by Fujii et al., this can be accomplished by

tilting the transducer away from the operator until the needle tip disappears from the screen. When the needle tip disappears, the needle is advanced until the tip reappears but at a slightly deeper location.[19] This same maneuver of tilting the transducer and following the needle tip is repeated in small increments until the tip is visualized entering the vessel. Success is improved by ensuring that the center of the vessel is penetrated. Puncturing the artery off center will often lead to a flash of blood with inability to advance the wire or the catheter.

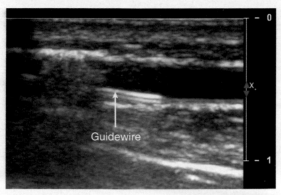

Figure 38.8 **Guidewire Confirmation.** The guidewire is seen within the radial artery in a longitudinal view.

In a longitudinal approach, the entire needle should be visualized as it is advanced toward the target vessel.

When the needle is observed entering the vessel, a flash of blood is obtained, and the guidewire should then be advanced into the artery. A second operator can assist with advancing the guidewire and catheter. If alone, the operator has to put the transducer down before advancing the guidewire and catheter. Confirm placement of the guidewire in the lumen of the artery by visualizing it within the vessel in transverse and longitudinal views, before advancing the catheter (Fig. 38.8). If using an arterial catheter without a guidewire, the catheter is advanced over the needle.

RADIAL ARTERY

Position the patient supine with the arm fully extended onto an arm board. A small towel may be rolled under the wrist to maintain mild dorsiflexion, but avoid overextending the wrist, which can compress the vessel. Tape may be used to secure the hand in position with the palm facing upward. Scan the lateral volar surface of the wrist to locate the radial artery in a transverse plane.

BRACHIAL ARTERY

Position the patient supine with the arm fully extended. Scan the medial side of the antecubital fossa to locate the brachial artery in a transverse view. If a more proximal insertion site is desired, trace the brachial artery proximally by sliding the transducer superiorly and medially toward the upper arm.

FEMORAL ARTERY

Position the patient supine with the leg slightly abducted and externally rotated.[5] The femoral artery should be accessed more than 1 to 2 cm below the inguinal ligament to reduce the risk of retroperitoneal hemorrhage and allow adequate compression of the femoral artery in case of local bleeding.

DORSALIS PEDIS ARTERY

Position the patient supine with the foot slightly plantar flexed for ease of access. Because the artery is superficial and curves with the dorsum of the foot, a shallow needle insertion angle of ≤30 degrees to the skin should be used (Fig. 38.9).

Complications

The most common complications of arterial cannulation include hematoma and temporary occlusion of the artery. Less common complications include pseudoaneurysm, hemorrhage (retroperitoneal hemorrhage with femoral artery cannulation), thrombosis, arteriovenous fistula, limb ischemia, peripheral neuropathy, and local or systemic infection.

OCCLUSION

Occlusion is a common occurrence after arterial cannulation. Temporary radial artery occlusion has a reported incidence of 19.7%.[6] Thrombotic occlusion may occur as early as 2 hours after radial artery catheter insertion and up to a week after catheter removal.[20]

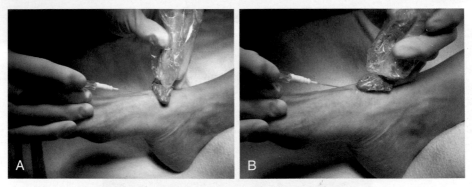

Figure 38.9   Dorsalis Pedis Artery Cannulation. (A) Transverse approach. (B) Longitudinal approach.

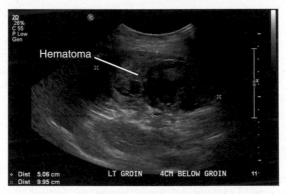

Figure 38.10   Hematoma. A large hematoma is seen after femoral artery cannulation.

Generally, temporary occlusion of the artery has no serious sequelae. The incidence of permanent occlusion of a radial artery is reported as 0.09%.[6] Rarely, this can lead to distal limb ischemia, nerve damage, or necrosis. Risk factors associated with arterial occlusion include duration of cannulation, ratio of outer catheter diameter to vessel lumen diameter, non-Teflon catheter, low cardiac output, and presence of hematoma.[6] Evaluation of flow using Doppler ultrasound distal to the insertion site is the most reliable technique to diagnose occlusion.

HEMATOMA

Hematoma has been reported as a complication in 14.4% of radial and 6.1% of femoral artery cannulations.[6] Rates have not been reported in the literature for brachial or dorsalis pedis artery cannulation. Clinically, patients present with pain, bruising, and nonpulsatile swelling at the insertion site. Ultrasound shows a soft

tissue mass with heterogeneous echogenicity adjacent to the wall of the vessel or within the muscle bed (Fig. 38.10).[21] It is important to use color and pulsed-wave Doppler to demonstrate absence of internal blood flow to differentiate a hematoma from a pseudoaneurysm.[21]

PSEUDOANEURYSM

A pseudoaneurysm develops when at least one layer of the arterial wall is disrupted and persistent blood flow causes an outpouching of the residual arterial wall.[22] It presents as a pulsatile or palpable mass with a palpable thrill at the puncture site. Pseudoaneurysm has been reported as a complication in 0.09% of radial and 0.3% of femoral artery cannulations.[6] Pseudoaneurysms appear as soft tissue masses with heterogeneous echogenicity by ultrasound (Fig. 38.11). Blood flow within the neck or lumen of the pseudoaneurysm must be seen using color or pulsed-wave Doppler to distinguish it from a hematoma.[21]

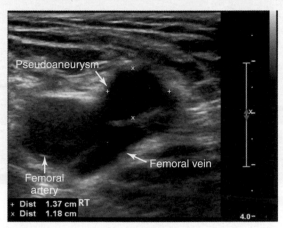

Figure 38.11 Pseudoaneurysm. A pseudoaneurysm after femoral artery cannulation is seen compressing the adjacent common femoral vein.

PEARLS AND PITFALLS

- Position the ultrasound screen in the direct line of sight of the operator to avoid head turning, and place the procedure supplies within arm's reach before beginning the procedure.
- The target vessel should be centered on the screen, and the insertion point of the needle should be exactly in the center of the ultrasound transducer.
- Penetrating the target vessel in the center helps ensure successful cannulation. Puncturing off-center will often lead to a flash of blood with inability to advance the wire or catheter.
- Sterile gel should be used both inside and outside of the sterile sheath in case the sterile sheath is punctured during the procedure.
- Because complications from brachial artery cannulation can compromise blood flow of the hand, the brachial artery is a less preferred site and should be considered a secondary choice when selecting a site.

SECTION 6

Head and Neck

CHAPTER 39

Ocular Ultrasound

Gregg L. Chesney ■ Marsia Vermeulen

KEY POINTS

- Measurement of optic nerve sheath diameter by ocular ultrasound provides a rapid, noninvasive method to assess for elevated intracranial pressure at the bedside, with a measurement of more than 5 mm considered elevated.
- Ocular ultrasound is a valuable tool in the evaluation of ocular trauma and can be used to assess for foreign bodies, globe rupture, traumatic detachments, lens dislocation, and vitreous hemorrhage.
- In patients with painless vision loss, ocular ultrasound can be used to evaluate for posterior vitreous detachment or retinal detachment and assess blood flow of the central retinal artery and vein.

Background

The eye's superficial location and fluid-filled constitution are ideal for a point-of-care ultrasound evaluation. The well-defined borders of the globe and deeper ocular structures, including the optic nerve, retinal artery, and retinal vein, can be easily imaged with ultrasound. Although ocular ultrasonography has appeared in the ophthalmology literature since the late 1950s, we have only begun to appreciate its diagnostic potential since the late 1990s.[1] Minimal training is required to acquire the skills to perform an accurate point-of-care ocular ultrasound examination for specific findings.[2-4]

A point-of-care ocular ultrasound is particularly useful when physical examination is limited by bright lighting, facial swelling, or pain due to trauma. Ocular ultrasound allows rapid assessment for potentially vision-threatening conditions when evaluation by an ophthalmologist or imaging by computed tomography (CT) or magnetic resonance imaging (MRI) may be unavailable or delayed. Furthermore, ocular ultrasound enables providers to evaluate the posterior chamber of the eye when direct visualization through the lens is limited by hyphema, hypopyon, or cataracts. A noninvasive assessment for elevated intracranial pressure (ICP) can also be performed using ocular ultrasound.

The five primary indications to perform an ocular ultrasound examination are:
- Acute loss of vision (partial or complete)
- Ocular trauma
- Atraumatic eye pain
- Intraocular foreign body (IOFB)
- Elevated ICP

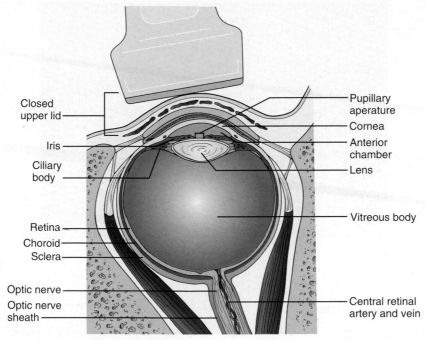

Closed upper lid

Iris

Ciliary body

Retina

Choroid

Sclera

Optic nerve

Optic nerve sheath

Pupillary aperature

Cornea

Anterior chamber

Lens

Vitreous body

Central retinal artery and vein

Figure 39.1 Normal Ocular Anatomy.

Normal Anatomy

The eye normally appears as a circular, well-circumscribed, anechoic structure on ultrasound (Figs. 39.1 and 39.2). The human eye is 24 to 25 mm in anteroposterior diameter, with minimal variation from person to person.[5] The cornea appears as a thin, arch-shaped, hyperechoic layer parallel to the overlying eyelid and is contiguous with the sclera. The anterior chamber lies beneath the cornea and is filled with aqueous humor, thus appearing anechoic by ultrasound. The iris and anterior reflection of the lens constitute the posterior wall of the anterior chamber and appear as a hyperechoic line that abuts the pupillary aperture. The lens appears as a biconvex structure with distinct anterior and posterior borders and an anechoic center.

Posterior to the lens is a large, anechoic space that is the vitreous body. In younger patients, the vitreous body appears black (anechoic), but in older patients, small, low-intensity echoes are scattered in the vitreous body ("floaters") due to vitreous syneresis, or liquefaction of

vitreous gel. The retina, choroid, and sclera form the posterior border of the globe, and these layers cannot be differentiated by ultrasound, except when pathologic findings, such as retinal detachment (RD), are present.

Posterior to the globe, the optic nerve and surrounding echogenic retro-orbital fat can be visualized. The optic nerve extends posteriorly and appears as an echogenic, linear structure perpendicular to the retina. A hyperechoic sheath surrounds the optic nerve. The optic nerve enters the eye slightly inferior and medial to the posterior pole of the globe. With subtle adjustment of the transducer angle, the optic nerve can be visualized longitudinally in the center of the screen. The central retinal artery and vein are within the center of the optic nerve and can be identified using color flow Doppler over the distal optic nerve. The central retinal artery and vein can be distinguished from one another by evaluating the waveforms using pulsed-wave Doppler. In both transverse and sagittal imaging planes, dense orbital bones create acoustic shadows that form the lateral borders of the globe.

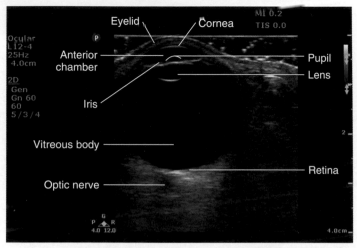

Figure 39.2   Normal Ocular Ultrasound Image.

Image Acquisition

Because the eye is superficial and requires high-resolution images to be evaluated, a high-frequency linear-array transducer (7.5 MHz or greater) is used. Ophthalmologists often use transducers with higher frequencies (20–50 MHz) to maximize resolution. A two-dimensional (B-mode) ultrasound mode and an "ocular" exam preset should be selected.

The patient should be positioned lying supine. The head of the bed may be elevated if the patient cannot tolerate lying completely flat. The exam is performed with the patient's eyelids closed. A copious amount of ultrasound gel should cover the entire eyelid to allow placing the transducer on the gel without applying any pressure to the eye. Chilling the ultrasound gel increases its viscosity and allows the gel to stack easily. Ultrasound gel is safe if it comes into contact with the eye, but we recommend use of sterile gel or placing a transparent film dressing, such as a Tegaderm (3M, St. Paul, MN), over the eyelid to prevent contamination of the conjunctiva. Also, a transparent film may improve patient comfort and should be carefully removed without pulling eyebrow hairs or eyelashes.[6]

While standing to the patient's side, scan the unaffected eye first and compare the appearance of the normal eye to the abnormal eye. Begin scanning in a transverse plane by placing the transducer across the eyelid with

the transducer marker pointing to the patient's right (Fig. 39.3). The provider's wrist can be stabilized against the patient's zygomatic arch or nose bridge to steady the image. Instruct the patient to look straight ahead, and identify the cornea, iris, lens, vitreous body, retina, and optic nerve. The transducer may need to be positioned slightly laterally and angled infero-medially to capture a true longitudinal view of the eye, including the optic nerve. Adjust the depth of the image to visualize 1 to 2 cm of the optic nerve posterior to the globe. Tilt or fan the transducer systematically to thoroughly visualize the entire eye throughout the globe. While holding the transducer centered over the eye, ask the patient to slowly look in all four directions and evaluate the eye for any abnormalities. Objects that disappear as the eye is moved are most likely artifacts, rather than true pathology.

After imaging in a transverse plane, turn the transducer 90 degrees clockwise to a sagittal plane with the transducer marker pointing toward the patient's head. Obtain a mid-eye view of the cornea, iris, lens, vitreous body, retina, and optic nerve. Repeat the process of tilting or fanning the transducer while having the patient maintain a static gaze. Scan the entire orbit from its medial to lateral edge, noting any abnormalities and correlating findings with those seen on transverse images. After returning to the initial mid-eye view, hold the transducer steady and have the patient slowly

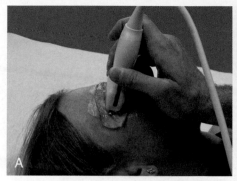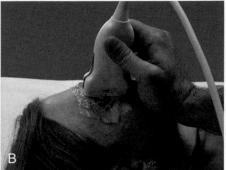

Figure 39.3 Transducer Position. The transducer is held like a pen with the hand resting on the zygomatic arch or nose bridge to obtain transverse (A) and sagittal (B) views.

look in all four directions to assess the extraocular muscles.

After imaging the entire globe, the optic nerve sheath diameter should be evaluated. Measure the optic nerve sheath diameter from mid-eye transverse and sagittal views and then evaluate the central retinal artery and vein with color flow and pulsed-wave Doppler.

Even though animal studies suggest that prolonged high-frequency ocular ultrasound is safe, these studies are limited.[7] The eye is considered a particularly sensitive organ to the potential mechanical and thermal effects of ultrasound energy. Using an ocular ultrasound preset limits the mechanical and thermal output of the transducer to relatively safer levels; however, ocular ultrasound should still be performed in concordance with the ALARA (As Low As Reasonably Achievable) principle. Limiting the duration of an ocular ultrasound exam (especially the amount of time spent with the transducer in a single position) and minimizing the use of color flow and spectral Doppler ultrasound (modes with higher thermal output than standard two-dimensional imaging) can lessen the potential risk for damage to the sensitive tissues of the eye.[8]

Image Interpretation

EXTRAOCULAR MOVEMENTS AND PUPILLARY REFLEX

Significant periorbital edema can preclude evaluation of extraocular muscles and the pupillary light reflex, and ocular ultrasound can be a valuable adjunct in these patients.

From a transverse or sagittal view, identify the anterior chamber, iris, lens, and globe and then ask the patient to look in all four directions to assess ocular movements by ultrasound (Video 39.1). To evaluate the pupillary reflex, place the patient in a dark room and position the transducer in a transverse plane along the inferior eyelid just above the infraorbital ridge. Tilt the transducer superiorly until the pupil is visualized obliquely (Fig. 39.4 and Video 39.2). Shine a light over the closed eyelid of the contralateral eye and look for pupillary constriction on the screen.[9] The pre- and post-contraction diameters of the pupil can be measured and trended in patients at risk of cerebral herniation, but the measurements may overestimate or underestimate the actual diameter when imaging in an oblique plane.

LENS DISLOCATION

Lens dislocation is a cause of acute vision loss in the setting of blunt trauma. Normally, the lens lies immediately posterior to the iris and is tethered to the ciliary body by suspensory ligaments. If these ligaments are traumatically disrupted, the lens can be displaced.[5] Complete lens dislocation is seen on ultrasound with the lens in a remote location.[10] Most often the lens is dislocated posteriorly and seen floating in the vitreous body (Fig. 39.5; Videos 39.3 and 39.4), although it can be displaced anteriorly or laterally.[11] Lens subluxation is often more subtle and difficult to diagnose (Video 39.5). If lens subluxation is suspected, evaluate the lens position with eye movements. The lens will normally remain fixed in position with ocular

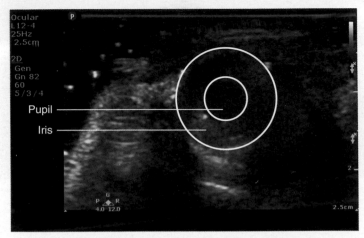

Figure 39.4 Pupillary Aperture. To test the pupillary light reflex, a coronal view of the pupil and iris is obtained by placing the transducer under the inferior eyelid and tilting superiorly.

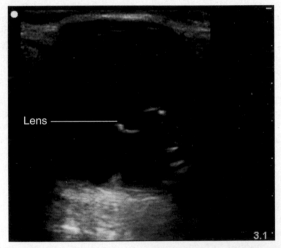

Figure 39.5 Lens Dislocation. A displaced lens is seen as a biconvex structure with hyperechoic borders floating in the vitreous body.

movements, but if the lens is subluxed, it may slip behind the iris with ocular movements.[12]

VITREOUS HEMORRHAGE

Vitreous hemorrhage can cause symptoms of seeing floaters, photopsia, and impaired vision. Vitreous hemorrhage may occur either spontaneously with diabetic retinopathy or in conjunction with trauma, RD, or posterior vitreous detachment (PVD). The ultrasound appearance of vitreous hemorrhage (Fig. 39.6 and Video 39.6) is heterogeneous, echogenic

layers in the posterior chamber that may appear to tumble with ocular movement, similar to clothes in a washing machine.[2]

RETINAL DETACHMENT AND POSTERIOR VITREOUS DETACHMENT

RD and PVD have characteristic findings that can be difficult to detect with an ophthalmoscope. However, both of these conditions can be readily diagnosed with ocular ultrasound. PVDs occur most often in older and myopic patients. PVD is due to separation of the

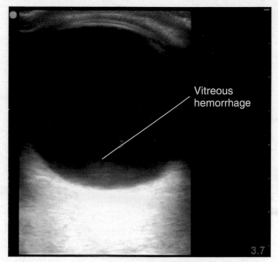

Figure 39.6 Vitreous Hemorrhage. An acute vitreous hemorrhage is seen as murky, heterogeneously echogenic material layering posteriorly. Note the image is overgained to accentuate the vitreous hemorrhage.

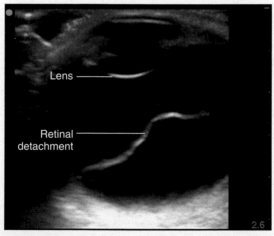

Figure 39.7 Retinal Detachment. The thick, hyperechoic, folded retina is separated from the posterior wall of the globe, consistent with a large retinal detachment.

vitreous body from the posterior portion of the retina, and patients complain of seeing "floaters" or brief flashes (photopsia). RD is due to separation of the sensory retina from the retinal pigment epithelium. There are several causes of RDs, but acute PVD with retinal tear is the most common cause. RDs may be preceded clinically by increased visualization of floaters or flashers followed by perception of a curtain coming down and visual field loss. If RD involves the macula, there may be a loss of central vision and impaired acuity.[13]

RDs appear on ultrasound as thick, hyperechoic, membrane-like structures with multiple folds that appear to be lifted off the posterior surface of the globe and move in conjunction with ocular movements (Fig. 39.7 and Video 39.7). Vitreous detachments appear similarly as linear structures lifted off the posterior surface of the globe (Fig. 39.8 and Video 39.8), but they are thinner and smoother than RDs and have a more mobile, undulating appearance.[2,14] The retina is firmly tethered to the choroid posteriorly at the optic nerve and anterolaterally

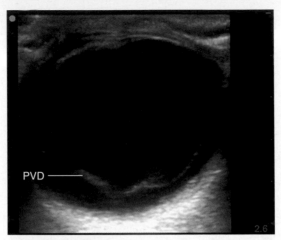

Figure 39.8 Posterior Vitreous Detachment. A posterior vitreous detachment *(PVD)* is seen as a smooth hyperechoic structure off the posterior wall of the globe.

at the ora serrata in the ciliary body. Therefore, RDs do not cross over the optic nerve or extend to the ciliary body, but a PVD may do so. The macula can be seen just lateral (temporal) to the optic nerve on transverse views, and it may be possible to distinguish macular involvement by ultrasound. A choroid detachment, where the choroid separates from the underlying sclera, may also appear similar to a PVD or RD, but a choroid detachment can be distinguished by its smooth, bulging convex shape that does not move with eye movements and possibly extends anteriorly to include the ciliary body.[15]

INTRAOCULAR FOREIGN BODY

Patients with an IOFB usually present with a complaint of acute eye pain or visual changes. IOFBs may be occult or traumatic and can lead to cataract formation, infection, retinal tears, RDs, and retinal degeneration. In almost all cases, IOFBs need to be surgically removed. Although CT scan remains the gold standard, point-of-care ultrasound is sensitive (87%-96%) and specific (92%-96%) for diagnosing IOFBs, regardless of the object's radiopacity.[16,17] Metallic, glass, and plastic IOFBs have irregular edges, are highly reflective, and produce predictable artifacts, such as reverberation, ring-down artifact, and acoustic shadowing (Fig. 39.9 and Video 39.9). Wood or vegetable matter is less echogenic and more difficult to detect, especially when lodged next to the highly echogenic iris or retina. Intraocular air

bubbles are highly reflective and can be mistaken for an IOFB; however, air bubbles do not change in appearance or echogenicity with changes in transducer angle. Air bubbles often shift with eye movements, whereas IOFBs remain in a static position.[18,19]

GLOBE RUPTURE

Globe rupture is an ophthalmologic surgical emergency. In the setting of blunt or penetrating trauma, globe rupture is generally considered to be a contraindication to performing ocular ultrasound because applied pressure from the transducer may increase intraocular pressure and worsen extrusion of vitreous. However, globe rupture can be difficult to diagnose by physical exam. There are numerous reports of globe rupture diagnosed by ultrasound,[1,20] and animal studies suggest that only minimal increases in intraocular pressure occur with ocular ultrasound exams.[21] An ocular ultrasound exam should be performed as described previously with an overlying transparent film dressing and with the transducer suspended in a large bed of ultrasound gel (1-2 inches thick) to minimize pressure on the globe. Ultrasound appearance of globe rupture includes buckling of the sclera, asymmetric loss of the normal spherical shape of the globe, and flattening or compression of the anterior chamber (Fig. 39.10 and Video 39.10).[22] If a globe rupture is detected on ultrasound, the exam should be stopped and an ophthalmologist consulted immediately.

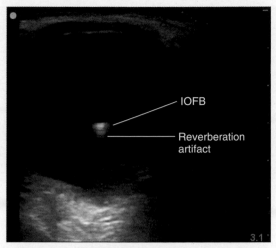

Figure 39.9 Intraocular Foreign Body *(IOFB).* A metallic IOFB is seen as a hyperechoic structure within the vitreous body with associated reverberation artifact.

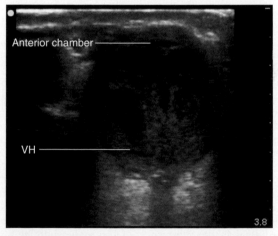

Figure 39.10 Globe Rupture. A ruptured globe with loss of the smooth spherical shape of the globe and collapse of the anterior chamber is seen, in addition to a large vitreous hemorrhage *(VH).*

OPTIC NERVE SHEATH DIAMETER

The optic nerve is considered to be part of the central nervous system, as opposed to the peripheral nervous system, because it is an extension of the brain. The optic nerve sheath encircles the optic nerve and is composed of three layers of meninges. The subarachnoid space surrounding the optic nerve sheath is contiguous with that of the brain and spinal cord, and the same cerebrospinal fluid (CSF) circulates in the subarachnoid space around the brain, spinal cord, and optic nerve. Increases in ICP are transmitted to the CSF in the optic nerve sheath and result in dilation of the optic nerve sheath. The optic nerve sheath diameter (ONSD) can be measured with ocular ultrasound, and a growing body of literature has demonstrated a correlation between increased ONSD and increased ICP when compared to intraventricular pressure monitoring or evidence of increased ICP on CT scan.[23,24]

To measure the ONSD accurately, an on-axis, longitudinal cross-sectional view of the optic nerve sheath must be obtained. The borders of the sheath appear sharply

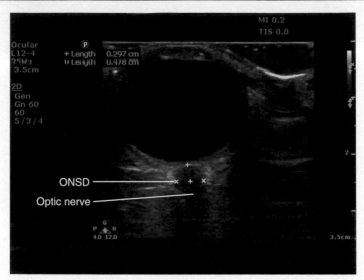

Figure 39.11   Optic Nerve Sheath Diameter *(ONSD)*. The optic nerve appears as a hypoechoic, tubular structure extending posteriorly from the retina. The diameter of the optic nerve sheath is measured 3 mm posterior to the retina and is measured as 4.78 mm in this patient (normal <5 mm).

demarcated and are parallel to one another. Because the optic nerve enters the globe slightly inferior and medial to the posterior pole, the ideal view of the optic nerve will show an off-axis view of the anterior chamber, iris, and lens. It is imperative to acquire a true on-axis, longitudinal cross-section of the optic nerve sheath because off-axis images result in erroneous measurement of the ONSD. The ONSD should be measured 3 mm posterior to where the optic nerve sheath engages the retina. The subarachnoid space in the optic nerve sheath does not dilate uniformly, and the greatest variability and most pronounced response to increased fluid in the subarachnoid space occurs 3 mm posterior to the optic nerve–retina junction.[25] Starting in a transverse plane, measure the width of the optic nerve sheath 3 mm posterior to the retina and then rotate the transducer 90 degrees to measure the ONSD in a sagittal plane, perpendicular to the first measurement (Fig. 39.11). Repeat these steps in the contralateral eye to obtain transverse and sagittal measurements of the ONSD. The ONSD is reported as the average of these four values. Any intracranial process causing elevated ICP should affect ONSD of both eyes equally. The presence of unilateral increased ONSD suggests a lateralizing process, such as optic neuritis or compressive optic neuropathy. Papilledema may also be noted as optic disc bulging into the retina and protruding into the vitreous body (Fig. 39.12).[22]

The cutoff value for increased ONSD correlating with increased ICP is debatable. Based on the initial study of ultrasound measurement of ONSD,[26] many authors cite a diameter greater than 5 mm as elevated in patients older than 4 years. Two recent meta-analyses of six studies evaluated the correlation between ONSD and ICP greater than 20 mm Hg and calculated a pooled sensitivity and specificity of 87% to 90% and 79% to 85%, respectively; however, the cutoff for abnormal ONSD varied from 5.0 to 5.9 mm in these studies, with half of the studies utilizing a cutoff ≥5.7 mm.[24,27] As the cutoff for abnormal ONSD increases from 5.0 mm to 5.9 mm, the sensitivity for elevated ICP decreases, whereas the specificity increases. Based on the current body of literature, ONSD may be better utilized as an initial test to rule out rather than rule in elevated ICP. Therefore, we recommend using an ONSD greater than 5 mm as abnormal in patients with clinical concern for elevated ICP. Particularly in resource-limited situations or in an effort to reduce unnecessary head imaging, ONSD may be utilized as a screening exam for diseases associated with elevated ICP, such as tuberculous meningitis, acute mountain sickness, or idiopathic intracranial hypertension.[28-30]

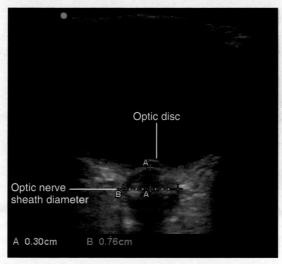

Figure 39.12 Dilated Optic Nerve Sheath and Papilledema. The optic nerve sheath diameter is markedly dilated at 7.6 mm due to elevated intracranial pressure. Papilledema is seen as the optic disc bulges into the retina.

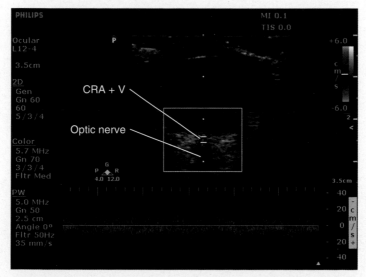

Figure 39.13 Central Retinal Artery and Vein. Color flow Doppler with arterial and venous waveforms using pulsed-wave Doppler can assess blood flow in the central retinal artery and vein (*CRA + V*)

CENTRAL RETINAL ARTERY AND VEIN OCCLUSION

Central retinal artery or vein occlusion presents with acute, painless loss of vision. The retinal artery and vein are enveloped in the center of the optic nerve and can be visualized by applying color flow Doppler at the entry site of the optic nerve in the posterior globe (Video 39.11). The presence of bidirectional blood flow indicates patency of both vessels, and pulsed-wave Doppler can be used to confirm arterial and venous waveforms (Fig. 39.13). Absence of color flow or loss of waveforms suggests vascular occlusion or ischemia (Video 39.12).[31]

PEARLS AND PITFALLS

- Small foreign bodies and subtle retinal detachments can be difficult to distinguish. Increasing the gain to high levels and then slowly reducing the gain can improve detection of these pathologic findings.
- Insufficient amounts of gel is a common cause of blurry images and unwanted artifacts. The eyelid is curved, and copious amounts of gel are needed to maintain contact between the transducer and eyelid. Using large quantities of gel improves visualization of the eye and minimizes pressure applied to the eye.
- Artifacts of ocular ultrasound may be mistaken for pathology. Reverberation artifact through the lens is common in the posterior chamber. Adjusting the transducer's angle of interrogation and decreasing the gain can facilitate differentiation of artifacts from true pathologies. If a suspected abnormal finding persists in multiple views with different angles and levels of gain, then it is most likely a pathologic finding.
- When measuring optic nerve sheath diameter, small increments separate normal from abnormal. An optic nerve sheath diameter less than 5 mm is a safe cut-off to rule out elevated intracranial pressure in adults. An optic nerve sheath diameter greater than 5 mm should be considered abnormal, and additional testing should be considered depending on the clinical scenario.

CHAPTER 40

Thyroid Gland

Sara Ahmadi ■ Stephanie Fish

KEY POINTS

- Thyroid ultrasound is the preferred modality to evaluate thyroid nodules. Nodules detected incidentally on cross-sectional imaging (computed tomography [CT]), magnetic resonance imaging (MRI), or positron emission tomography (PET) should be further evaluated by thyroid ultrasound.
- Thyroid nodules with suspicious findings by ultrasound, such as hypoechogenicity, irregular or infiltrative margins, microcalcifications, "taller than wide" shape, or evidence of extra-thyroidal extension have an increased risk of malignancy.
- Ultrasound-guided fine-needle aspiration is a safe procedure with minimal complications and is the method of choice for definitive evaluation of thyroid nodules.

Background

A thyroid nodule is a discrete lesion within the normal thyroid parenchyma. Widespread use of neck ultrasound and other imaging modalities has led to an increase in the diagnosis of thyroid nodules.

Thyroid nodules are common but few are malignant. In iodine-sufficient countries, the prevalence of a palpable thyroid nodule is 5% in women and 1% in men.[1] However, high-resolution thyroid ultrasound is able to detect thyroid nodules in 19% to 67% of randomly selected individuals.[1]

Ultrasound-guided fine-needle aspiration (FNA) is widely accepted as the method of choice for the evaluation of thyroid nodules that meet the criteria for biopsy. Using ultrasound guidance for FNA improves the rate of obtaining an adequate biopsy specimen and lowers the rate of false-negative results when compared to palpation-guided FNA.[2-5]

Several factors should be considered in determining which nodules should undergo FNA, including nodule size, ultrasound appearance, and high-risk history. High-resolution thyroid ultrasound is the method of choice to evaluate thyroid nodules, and the American Thyroid Association (ATA) recommends that thyroid ultrasonography be performed in all patients with a thyroid nodule.[1] Ultrasound features of thyroid nodules that need to be evaluated include echogenicity, structure, vascularity, calcifications, margins, shape, and presence or absence of suspicious cervical lymph nodes.

Normal Anatomy

The thyroid gland is an encapsulated organ located in the anterior mid-portion of the neck, inferior to the cricoid cartilage. The thyroid gland is composed of two lobes that are connected by an isthmus. The sternocleidomastoid muscle and carotid sheath are located lateral to the thyroid gland. Three of the strap muscles (sternohyoid, sternothyroid, and omohyoid) are located anterior to the thyroid gland. The trachea is normally located posterior to the thyroid isthmus in the midline, and the right and left thyroid lobes wrap around the trachea. The longus colli muscles are located posterior to each thyroid lobe. The esophagus can be seen adjacent to the trachea, posterior to the left lobe of the thyroid. Peristalsis can be seen

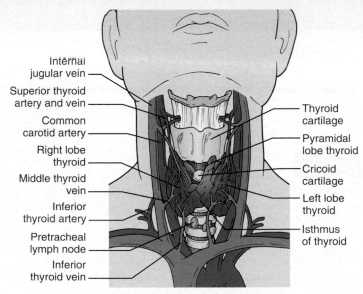

Internal jugular vein

Superior thyroid artery and vein

Common carotid artery

Right lobe thyroid

Middle thyroid vein

Inferior thyroid artery

Pretracheal lymph node

Inferior thyroid vein

Thyroid cartilage

Pyramidal lobe thyroid

Cricoid cartilage

Left lobe thyroid

Isthmus of thyroid

Figure 40.1 Thyroid Gland Anatomy.

when the patient swallows, which helps differentiate the esophagus from a thyroid nodule (Fig. 40.1).

Image Acquisition

A high-frequency linear transducer is used to image the thyroid gland. Images should be obtained in both transverse and sagittal planes (Fig. 40.2). A high-frequency linear transducer provides excellent axial and lateral resolution of the superficial neck structures, including the thyroid gland, lymph nodes, and blood vessels. However, a low-frequency transducer may be necessary when these structures are deep in the neck in morbidly obese patients or in the setting of a large multinodular goiter. Thyroid lobes and nodules should be measured in three dimensions: depth (anterior-posterior), width (transverse), and length (superior-inferior). In the transverse imaging plane, depth is measured at the maximal anterior-posterior distance, and width is measured from the medial to the lateral border of the thyroid lobe. A normal thyroid gland is 2 cm or less in both anterior-posterior (depth) and transverse (width) dimensions. Length is measured in a sagittal imaging plane from the cranial to caudal border of the thyroid lobe and is normally 4.5 to 5.5 cm (Fig. 40.3).[6]

Image Interpretation

THYROIDITIS

Normal thyroid gland parenchyma is homogeneous and hyperechoic when compared to the surrounding strap muscles (Fig. 40.4).

The ultrasound appearance of thyroid tissue changes in diffuse autoimmune thyroid disorders, such as Hashimoto's thyroiditis.[6] The thyroid parenchyma in Hashimoto's thyroiditis appears heterogeneous with patchy hypoechoic and hyperechoic areas.[7] Thyroid size may be normal, enlarged, or small, with variable vascularity depending on the duration of disease. Ultrasound findings manifest the underlying histologic changes, primarily diffuse infiltration of the gland with lymphocytes and fibrosis (Fig. 40.4).

THYROID NODULES

The following characteristics should be described in the evaluation of a thyroid nodule: nodule size in three dimensions, location of the nodule, echogenicity (isoechoic, hypoechoic, or hyperechoic), structure (solid, mixed, cystic, spongiform), margins (well-defined, irregular, or infiltrative), presence and type of calcification (microcalcification, macrocalcification, or eggshell calcification), vascularity (absent,

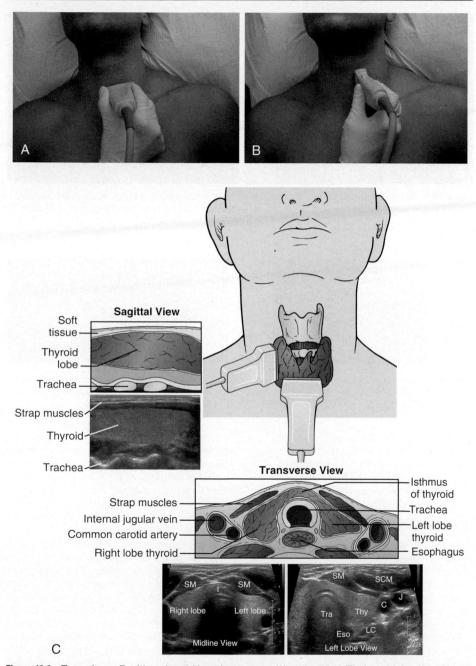

Figure 40.2 Transducer Position. Acquisition of transverse (A) and sagittal (B) views of the thyroid gland and the cross-sectional anatomy (C) of the thyroid gland. *C*, Common carotid artery; *Eso*, esophagus; *I*, isthmus; *J*, internal jugular vein; *LC*, longus colli; *SCM*, sternocleidomastoid; *SM*, strap muscle; *Thy*, thyroid; *Tra*, trachea.

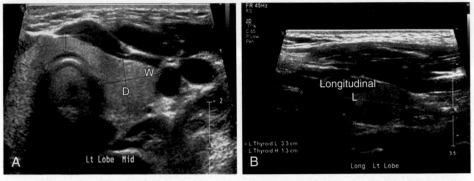

Figure 40.3 Normal Thyroid Gland. (A) Transverse view measuring a thyroid lobe's depth (anterior-posterior) and width (transverse) and (B) sagittal view measuring the length (superior-inferior). *D*, Depth; *L*, length; *W*, width.

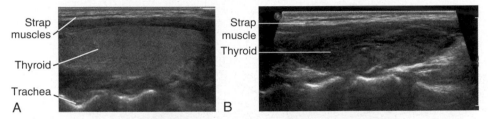

Figure 40.4 Hashimoto's Thyroiditis. The normal thyroid gland has a homogeneous, ground-glass echogenicity (A). Hashimoto's thyroiditis has a heterogeneous echogenicity with patchy hypoechoic and hyperechoic areas. Infiltration by lymphocytes causes the tissue to appear more hypoechoic (B).

peripheral, or intranodular), and shape (round, tall). As described below, the ultrasound characteristics with the highest specificity for thyroid cancer are microcalcifications, irregular margins, and tall shape.

Echogenicity

Echogenicity is the brightness of a thyroid nodule in comparison to normal thyroid parenchyma. Nodules are described as isoechoic (same echogenicity as surrounding thyroid tissue), hypoechoic (darker than surrounding thyroid tissue), or hyperechoic (brighter than surrounding thyroid tissue) (Fig. 40.5). Hypoechogenicity is associated with an increased risk of malignancy.[8,9] However, 50% of benign nodules are hypoechoic, so this feature is less specific for malignancy.[10]

Structure

The structure of nodules is important to note during an ultrasound evaluation. A simple cyst is anechoic with a bright signal posterior to the

cyst (posterior acoustic enhancement). A simple cyst is always benign and does not require further evaluation with FNA.[11] A colloid cyst often contains comet-tail artifact, which is an echogenic focus with reverberation (Fig. 40.6). This can be mistaken for microcalcification by less experienced sonographers.

A spongiform nodule is defined as one with multiple microcystic components in more than 50% of the nodule's volume. This appearance is highly specific for a benign nodule.[10-12] Some nodules are partially cystic with an eccentric solid component (Fig. 40.7). When a nodule is predominantly cystic, there is an increased rate of nondiagnostic FNA specimens because samples contain avascular debris and fibrosis rather than follicular cells. When performing FNA, providers must focus on sampling solid areas that contain follicular cells.[12]

The vast majority of thyroid cancers are solid. In a study of 360 malignant thyroid nodules which were surgically removed, Henrichsen et al. found that 88.3% were solid to

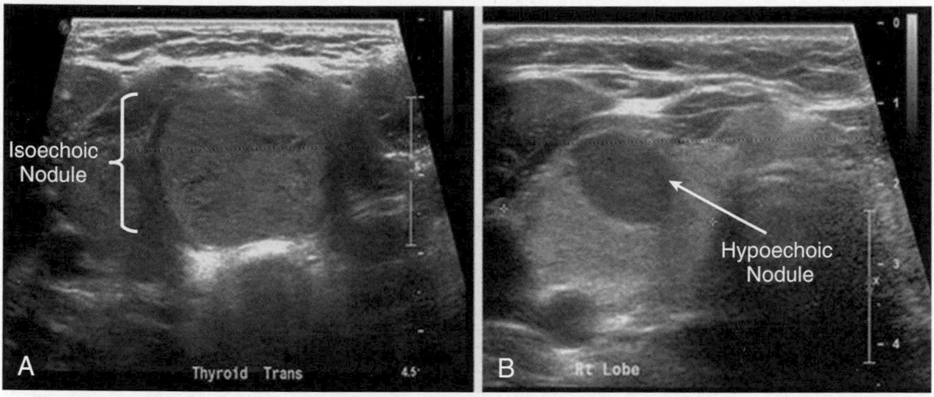

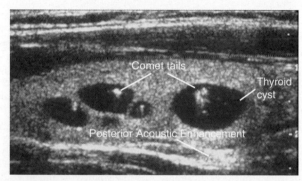

Figure 40.5 Echogenicity of Thyroid Nodules. (A) An isoechoic nodule. (B) A hypoechoic nodule.

Figure 40.6 Comet-Tail Artifacts. The benign colloid cysts display comet-tail artifacts and posterior acoustic enhancement in the far field.

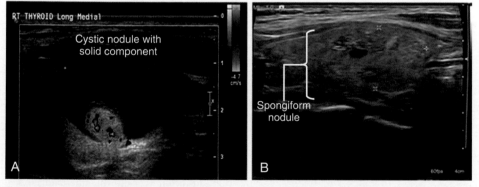

Figure 40.7 Cystic Nodules. A predominantly cystic thyroid nodule with a solid component (A) and a spongiform thyroid nodule (B) are shown.

minimally cystic (<5% cystic change), 9.2% were partially cystic (6%–50% of nodule had cystic change), and 2.5% were mostly cystic (>50% of nodule had cystic change). Of the 2.5% of malignancies with >50% cystic change (n=9), all of the nodules had other suspicious ultrasound findings including mural nodules, microcalcifications, increased vascularity, or a thick irregular wall around the cystic portion.[13]

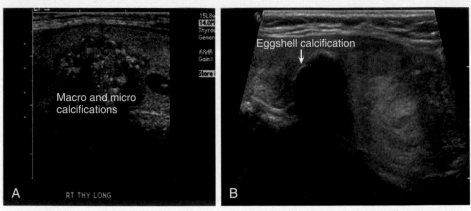

Figure 40.8   Calcification of Thyroid Nodules. (A) Macrocalcifications and microcalcifications. (B) Eggshell calcification with acoustic shadowing.

Margins

Margins of a nodule should be carefully evaluated with ultrasound. The margins may be smooth and well-defined or irregular. Spiculated or irregular margins are associated with an increased risk of malignancy.[10]

Calcifications

Calcifications are seen in almost one-third of thyroid nodules. Calcifications in thyroid nodules can appear as microcalcifications (<1 mm) without acoustic shadowing, rim (eggshell) calcifications, or macrocalcifications (>2 mm) with acoustic shadowing (Fig. 40.8). Microcalcifications are associated with an increased risk of malignancy because they often represent the psammoma bodies that are frequently seen in papillary thyroid carcinoma. Macrocalcifications are often the result of degeneration and necrosis within a thyroid nodule and can be seen in both benign and malignant nodules. Eggshell calcifications can also be seen in both malignant and benign nodules.[14] However, interrupted eggshell calcifications associated with a rim of soft tissue outside the calcification is a worrisome ultrasound finding for malignancy.[15]

Vascularity

Vascular flow within a nodule can be determined using color flow or power Doppler. Three grades are used to describe vascularity of thyroid nodules: type 0 (absence of flow), type 1 (peripheral flow), and type 2 (intranodular flow) (Fig. 40.9). Two studies with a large number of follicular thyroid carcinomas showed that intranodular vascularity is correlated with malignancy.[16,17] However, in a study where 98% of cancers were papillary thyroid carcinoma, intranodular vascularity was not reported as an independent predictor for malignancy.[18]

Shape

The shape of thyroid nodules can be assessed with ultrasound. One study suggested that spherical shape is associated with increased risk of malignancy.[19] Cappelli et al. reported that a ratio of anterior-posterior diameter to transverse diameter of greater than 1 is associated with increased risk of malignancy.[20] In general, experts agree that "taller than wide" thyroid nodules have higher risk of malignancy.

In summary, thyroid nodules are best characterized with ultrasound, and certain ultrasound findings are associated with an increased risk of malignancy. Characterizing thyroid nodules by ultrasound is important to determine which nodules require further evaluation with FNA.

The 2015 ATA guidelines classify thyroid nodules into five different categories according to their sonographic appearance[21] (Table 40.1): high suspicion (Fig. 40.10), intermediate suspicion (Fig. 40.11), low suspicion (Fig. 40.12), very low suspicion (Fig. 40.13), and benign (Fig. 40.14).

In the absence of suspicious cervical lymphadenopathy, the ATA recommends FNA for high and intermediate suspicion nodules ≥1 cm, low suspicion nodules ≥1.5 cm, and very low suspicion nodule ≥2 cm. The

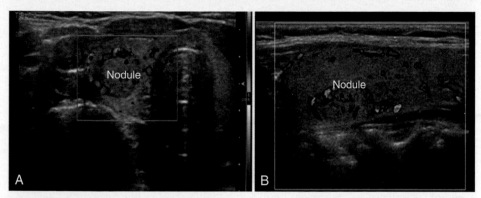

Figure 40.9 **Vascularity of Thyroid Nodules.** (A) Peripheral vascularity (transverse view). (B) Intranodular vascularity (sagittal view).

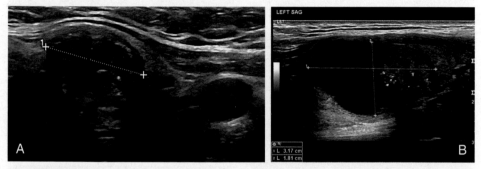

Figure 40.10 **High Suspicion Thyroid Nodule.** (A) A solid hypoechoic nodule with irregular margins and microcalcifications and (B) a solid hypoechoic component of a partially cystic nodule with microcalcifications are both considered high suspicion nodules.

TABLE 40.1   **Sonographic Classification of Thyroid Nodules**

Sonographic Pattern	Ultrasound Features	Risk of Malignancy	FNA Size Cutoff
High suspicion	Solid hypoechoic nodule or solid hypoechoic component of a partially cystic nodule with one or more other suspicious ultrasound features: irregular margin, taller than wide shape, interrupted eggshell calcification with extrusive soft tissue component, or extra-thyroidal extension	>70%–90%	≥1 cm
Intermediate suspicion	Hypoechoic solid nodule with smooth margin and no other suspicious ultrasound features	10%–20%	≥1 cm
Low suspicion	Isoechoic or hyperechoic solid nodule or partially cystic nodule with eccentric solid areas without other suspicious ultrasound features	5%–10%	≥1.5 cm
Very low suspicion	Spongiform or partially cystic nodule with no other suspicious ultrasound features	<3%	≥2 cm versus observation
Benign	Purely cystic nodule	<1%	No biopsy

FNA, Fine-needle aspiration.

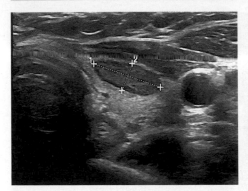

Figure 40.11 Intermediate Suspicion Thyroid Nodule. A hypoechoic solid nodule with smooth margins and no other suspicious ultrasound features is seen.

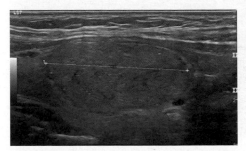

Figure 40.12 Low Suspicion Thyroid Nodule. An isoechoic solid nodule or cystic nodule with an eccentric solid component (see Fig 40.7A) without other suspicious ultrasound features is considered a low suspicion nodule.

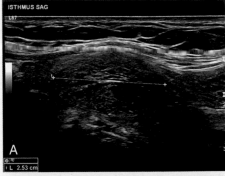

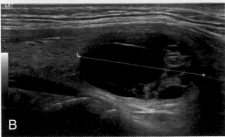

Figure 40.13 Very Low Suspicion Thyroid Nodule. A spongiform (A) or partially cystic (B) nodule without any other suspicious ultrasound features is considered a very low suspicion nodule.

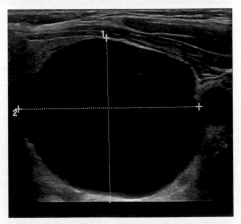

Figure 40.14 Benign Thyroid Nodule. A purely cystic nodule without solid components is considered benign.

suspicious sonographic findings described in Table 40.1 are typically seen in papillary thyroid cancers, which represent 70% of thyroid malignancies (Fig. 40.15).

A follicular neoplasm is less common and usually does not exhibit classic malignant sonographic features. Jeh et al. reported that 65.2% of follicular neoplasms are isoechoic and 72.7% have an oval shape.[22] Hurthle cell neoplasm and follicular variant of papillary thyroid cancer may have a sonographic appearance similar to a follicular neoplasm.[23,24]

Thyroid Fine-Needle Aspiration

Although ultrasound features are useful in determining which thyroid nodule requires additional evaluation, ultrasound-guided FNA is the method of choice for definitive evaluation of thyroid nodules. FNA is a safe procedure with minimal complications. In general, ultrasound-guided FNA is not recommended in patients with high bleeding risk, though it can be safely performed in most patients. The overall incidence of hematoma formation associated with ultrasound-guided FNA has been reported to be as low as 1%, and an increased incidence of hematoma formation in patients receiving anticoagulation was not seen. However, caution is recommended in patients on anticoagulation undergoing ultrasound-guided FNA.[25]

After obtaining written consent, place the patient in a supine position with a rolled towel or pillow behind the shoulders to extend the neck. Position the ultrasound machine in the operator's direct line of sight. Using a high-frequency 10 to 14 MHz linear transducer, perform a pre-procedural scan of the thyroid gland, central neck, and lateral neck to identify any abnormalities, particularly lymphadenopathy.

The overlying skin must be cleaned with alcohol, iodine, or chlorhexidine. The transducer should be cleaned thoroughly with antiseptic wipes pre-procedurally. Only sterile

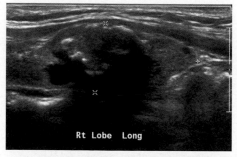

Figure 40.15 Papillary Thyroid Cancer. Macrocalcification with acoustic shadowing is seen in this solid hypoechoic nodule with irregular margins that was biopsy-proven to be papillary thyroid cancer.

ultrasound gel should be used during the procedure. Sterile gel is applied to the transducer face before covering it with a sterile transducer sheath. Local anesthesia with lidocaine spray and 1% lidocaine injection is recommended. A small (25-27 gauge) needle is recommended for FNA. Risk of bleeding is higher with larger gauge needles. The ultrasound probe is maneuvered with the non-dominant hand while the needle is held in the dominant hand.

There are two approaches to perform thyroid FNA: parallel (in-plane) and perpendicular (out-of-plane) (Fig. 40.16).

PARALLEL APPROACH

The needle is inserted at the center of the short edge of the transducer. While holding the transducer steady, the needle tip should be tracked from the point of insertion at the skin to the nodule by maintaining the transducer and needle in the same plane. The nodule should be positioned close to the lateral edge of the screen, on the side where the needle is being inserted (Fig. 40.17).

PERPENDICULAR APPROACH

Using this approach, the nodule is positioned in the center of the screen, and the needle is inserted at the center of the long edge of the transducer. The entire needle shaft is not seen in this approach, but the needle tip is tracked as it is advanced to penetrate the nodule.

SAMPLING TECHNIQUE

There are two sampling techniques to obtain cellular material: fine-needle capillary sampling and FNA.

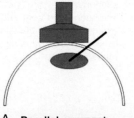 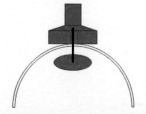

A **Parallel approach**   B **Perpendicular approach**

Figure 40.16 Fine-Needle Aspiration Technique. Parallel (in-plane) approach (A), and perpendicular (out-of-plane) approach (B).

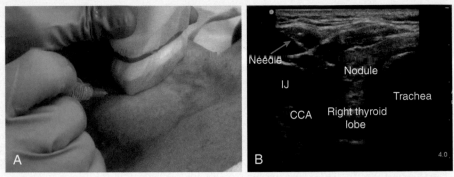

Figure 40.17   Parallel (In-Plane) Approach. The needle is inserted in the center of the short edge of the sterilely sheathed ultrasound transducer (A). The needle is seen as a hyperechoic line traversing the soft tissues as it approaches the nodule to perform fine-needle aspiration (B). *CCA,* Common carotid artery; *IJ,* internal jugular vein.

For fine-needle capillary sampling, the needle is observed entering the nodule and is then moved up and down multiple times within the nodule for 3 to 10 seconds. The thyroid follicular cells travel into the needle through capillary action. With this technique, the needle can be placed on a 10 mL syringe with 1 to 3 mL of air in the syringe, or the needle can be used alone. In the needle-only technique, the needle is grasped at the hub by the thumb and middle finger, and the index fingertip is placed over the hub as the needle is withdrawn. The needle is then attached to a syringe to expel the tissue sample onto a slide.

With the FNA technique, the needle is attached to a 10 mL syringe. After the needle penetrates the nodule, negative pressure is applied to the syringe to obtain a sample. Negative pressure is released before withdrawing the needle.

Both fine-needle capillary sampling and FNA sampling have almost identical rates of obtaining an adequate sample.[26]

PEARLS AND PITFALLS

- Thyroid nodules should be visualized by ultrasound in both longitudinal and transverse planes to confirm findings. Nodules that are seen in only one plane are most likely pseudo-nodules.
- Appropriate adjustment of depth and frequency of the ultrasound machine is required to obtain clear images of deep structures in the neck, especially in morbidly obese patients.
- The esophagus is posterior to the left lobe of the thyroid and should not be mistaken for a thyroid nodule.
- The ultrasound characteristics with the highest specificity for thyroid cancer are microcalcifications, irregular margins, and tall shape.
- Obtaining accurate measurements of thyroid nodules extending into the mediastinum is challenging and requires application of pressure over the clavicle while aiming the ultrasound beam inferiorly.
- The lateral and central neck should be examined to identify suspicious cervical lymphadenopathy in all patients with a thyroid nodule.

CHAPTER 41

Lymph Nodes

Ricardo Franco-Sadud

KEY POINTS

- Evaluation of enlarged lymph nodes with ultrasound includes assessment of size, shape, echogenicity, borders, and vascularity. In general, normal-sized lymph nodes are less than 1 cm, but normal size varies by location in the body from 0.5 to 2 cm.
- Abnormal lymph nodes are markedly hypoechoic, especially the hilum, and may have irregular borders, increased cortical thickness, and increased peripheral vascularity.
- In patients with enlarged cervical lymph nodes, a core-needle biopsy can be safely performed at the bedside using ultrasound guidance. Biopsy of lymph nodes less than 1 cm is not recommended because the procedure has low diagnostic yield and poses unnecessary risk to the patient.

Background

Increased availability of portable ultrasound machines has allowed providers to safely perform procedures at the bedside, including percutaneous needle biopsies of head, neck, axillary, and inguinal lymph nodes. Differentiation of pathologic versus reactive lymph nodes is important for diagnosis and when deciding to perform a biopsy. This chapter focuses on the evaluation of superficial lymph nodes of the neck. The basic principles described in this chapter can be applied to superficial lymph nodes in the supraclavicular, axillary, and inguinal lymph nodes.

Normal Anatomy

Lymph nodes are solitary structures composed of lymphoid tissue and are distributed along the course of lymphatic vessels. A lymph node is divided anatomically into an outer cortex and inner medulla and is surrounded by a fibrous capsule. The afferent lymphatic vessels bring lymph to the node through the cortex, whereas the efferent lymphatic vessel carries lymph away from the node exiting at the hilum. Lymph nodes are permeated by blood

vessels, and both the artery and vein enter and exit the lymph node at the hilum (Fig. 41.1).

In general, normal lymph nodes are not larger than 0.7 to 1 cm, but the normal size of lymph nodes varies greatly from 0.5 to 2.0 cm depending on the location in the body.[1,2] The normal distribution of lymph nodes of the head and neck is illustrated in Fig. 41.2. In the cervical chains, at least six nodes can be routinely identified. The normal size of cervical nodes ranges from 0.3 to 0.8 cm. Lymph nodes in the upper neck, specifically submandibular and upper cervical nodes, tend to be larger.[3,4]

Superficial lymph nodes less than 12 mm in diameter are often missed by physical examination, whereas nodes greater than 15 mm are nearly always detected by palpation. Disadvantages of computed tomography (CT) in the evaluation of neck lymph nodes include the inability of CT to depict the longitudinal diameter of enlarged nodes and differentiate the margins of nodes from adjacent vessels.[5] Evaluation of superficial lymph nodes with ultrasound is well established. Two-dimensional (2D) ultrasound allows accurate assessment of lymph node site, size, shape, border, internal architecture, matting and adjacent soft tissue edema, and color Doppler allows characterization of the vascular flow pattern.[6]

Image Acquisition

A high-frequency, linear-array ultrasound transducer (5–15 MHz) provides maximal resolution of soft tissues while giving an adequate

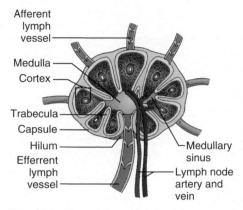

Afferent lymph vessel
Medulla
Cortex
Trabecula
Capsule
Hilum
Efferent lymph vessel
Medullary sinus
Lymph node artery and vein

Figure 41.1   Normal Cross-Sectional Anatomy of a Lymph Node.

penetration of 6 to 10 cm to visualize lymph nodes, vessels, and soft tissues.

For optimal imaging of neck lymph nodes, place the patient in a supine position with a pillow between the scapulae. Rotate the head to the contralateral side, with the neck extended. Start by scanning the neck in a transverse plane in the submental area. Next, slide the transducer toward the submandibular area with the transducer parallel to the lower edge of the mandible, and aim the ultrasound beam superiorly toward the head. Slide the transducer laterally toward the angle of the mandible. To image the parotid lymph nodes, slide the transducer superiorly from the angle of mandible over the parotid gland. To image the cervical lymph nodes, start at the angle of the mandible with the transducer in a transverse orientation. Slide the transducer inferiorly to sequentially evaluate the upper, middle, and lower cervical nodes along the path of the internal jugular vein and common carotid artery from the angle of the mandible to the junction of the internal jugular and subclavian veins.

Lymph nodes are evaluated using 2D and color Doppler ultrasound. 2D ultrasound is used to assess the lymph node's size, shape,

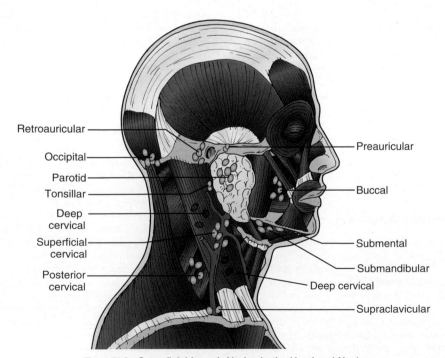

Retroauricular
Occipital
Parotid
Tonsillar
Deep cervical
Superficial cervical
Posterior cervical

Preauricular
Buccal
Submental
Submandibular
Deep cervical
Supraclavicular

Figure 41.2   Superficial Lymph Nodes in the Head and Neck.

borders, and echogenicity; measure the long- and short-axis diameters; assess for intranodal necrosis and calcification; and detect matting and soft tissue edema. Color flow or power Doppler ultrasound is used to assess a lymph node's vascularity.

Image Interpretation

The normal size of head and neck lymph nodes is generally less than 0.8 cm. Diagnostic yield of biopsy will increase with lymph node size, and specificity might decrease if biopsy is performed of nodes less than 1 cm in size. Normal lymph nodes are oval and have a homogeneous echotexture. The normal appearance of the outer cortex is hypoechoic due to lymphoid follicles, whereas the central medulla is hyperechoic due to a dense network of lymphatic cords and sinuses (Fig. 41.3 and Video 41.1). The center of lymph nodes may have some distinctly echogenic foci. Lymph node atrophy with cortical thinning, and fatty replacement of the hilum is seen with aging.[1]

Abnormal lymph nodes have distinct characteristics. A thin, hypoechoic hilum is suspicious of a pathologic lymph node that is infiltrated, inflamed, or malignant. Metastatic nodes are markedly hypoechoic with heterogeneous echotexture and often change shape from oval to round with a long-to-short axis ratio of less than 2 (Fig. 41.4; Videos 41.2 and 41.3). Asymmetric cortical thickening is seen with subcapsular and sinusoidal metastatic invasion. Cortical thickness more than half the transverse diameter of the hilum is abnormal.

Metastatic lymph nodes tend to have sharp nodal borders due to intranodal tumor infiltration. However, with extracapsular invasion in advanced tumors, the borders are ill-defined and surrounding soft tissue edema with nodal matting may be seen (Fig. 41.5 and Video 41.4).

When color flow or power Doppler is applied to normal or reactive lymph nodes, vascularity is primarily seen in the hilar and perihilar areas (Video 41.5). In contrast, malignant lymph nodes tend to show increased peripheral vascularity (Fig. 41.6 and Video 41.6). Abnormal lymph nodes with necrotic centers have a heterogeneous appearance with little to no vascularity detected (Fig. 41.7 and Video 41.7).[6]

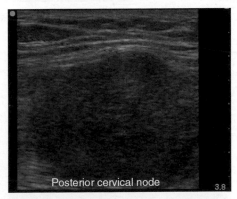

Figure 41.4 Pathologic Cervical Lymph Node. The heterogeneous appearance, sharp borders, enlarged size (approximately 3 × 3 cm), asymmetric cortex, and central hypoechogenicity are all signs of a pathologic lymph node.

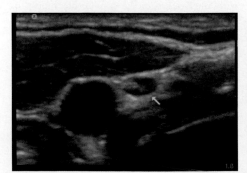

Figure 41.3 Normal Cervical Lymph Node. A normal lymph node *(arrow)* that is oval shaped with a homogeneous echotexture with central hyperechogenicity is seen adjacent to the common carotid artery.

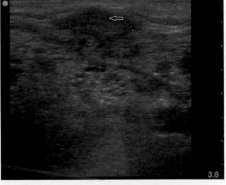

Figure 41.5 Extracapsular Invasion. An abnormal supraclavicular lymph node is shown with infiltration into the deep tissues and apical pleura.

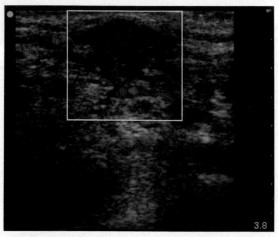

Figure 41.6 Peripheral Vascularity. Color flow Doppler of a malignant supraclavicular lymph node shows increased peripheral vascularity.

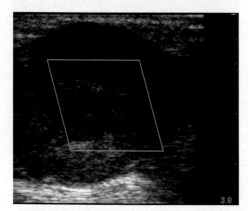

Figure 41.7 Necrotic Lymph Node. A pathologic lymph node shows no blood flow by color flow Doppler in the hypoechoic hilum, suggesting a necrotic center.

Lymph Node Biopsy

Evaluation of head and neck lymph nodes for suspected lymphoma has traditionally been made by excisional biopsy. Ultrasound-guided core-needle biopsy of enlarged lymph nodes has distinct advantages over excisional biopsy (reduced exposure to ionizing radiation and reduced morbidity) and is currently preferred over fine-needle aspiration (FNA).[7-12] A recent study found ultrasound-guided core-needle biopsy to have a higher sensitivity (92% vs. 50%) and diagnostic accuracy (99% vs. 90%) compared to fine-needle

aspiration in differentiating malignant from benign lymphadenopathy.[13] Most important, ultrasound-guided core-needle biopsy can be performed safely at the bedside using local anesthesia in patients with high operative risk.

In general, ultrasound-guided core-needle biopsy of neck lymph nodes is preferred to FNA, especially if clinical suspicion for lymphoma is high.[11,12,14-17] A definitive diagnosis can be made by core-needle biopsy because cellular architecture is preserved in core biopsy samples. Sensitivity and specificity of ultrasound-guided core-needle biopsy to diagnose lymphoma have been reported as 89% to 97% and 97% to 99%, respectively.[18] One study reported that a histologic diagnosis was made with ultrasound-guided core-needle biopsy in 146 of 155 (94%) patients studied, achieving a sensitivity, specificity, and diagnostic accuracy of 97.9%, 99.1%, and 97.9%, respectively, with no procedure-related complications.[19]

Ultrasound-guided FNA is the standard modality to work up thyroid nodules (see Chapter 40) and is commonly used to evaluate lesions in other head and neck tissues, such as salivary glands. The goal of FNA is to obtain cellular material among the aspirate and use analytic methods, such as immunocytochemistry, flow cytometry, cytogenetics, and molecular genetics, to make a diagnosis. Ultrasound-guided core biopsy can also be used to evaluate salivary gland lesions of the head and neck with high diagnostic accuracy.[20] For neck lymph nodes, ultrasound-guided core-needle biopsy is preferred to FNA in general.[21] Table 41.1 lists indications for an ultrasound-guided biopsy of the neck.

ULTRASOUND-GUIDED FINE-NEEDLE ASPIRATION

Insert a 21G needle into the target lymph node, preferably with a butterfly needle. Apply constant negative pressure on the syringe. Perform several forward and backward passes of the needle through the node. Make subtle changes in direction, depth, and orientation with each

pass. Release the negative pressure while the needle is still in the lymph node. Withdraw the needle and use positive pressure from the syringe to release the contents from the needle hub or butterfly onto the slides (Video 41.8).

ULTRASOUND-GUIDED CORE-NEEDLE BIOPSY

Although any suspicious lymph node can be biopsied, it is imperative to evaluate the surrounding anatomy before attempting a core-needle biopsy to avoid injury to nerves and vessels. Pre-procedural ultrasound scanning allows identification of adjacent nerves and vessels (Video 41.9), and direct visualization of the needle tip during the procedure avoids puncturing adjacent structures. Place the ultrasound transducer directly above the node, and reconfirm the position, echogenicity, and vascularity of the node (Fig. 41.8).

Once the target node has been reconfirmed, sterilize the skin surface, drape the procedure site, and place a sterile probe cover on the transducer. Core biopsy devices have a hollow advancing needle that houses a biopsy needle. The advancing needle is inserted into the lymph node, and the spring-loaded biopsy needle is released to capture a tissue sample. Center the lymph node on the screen, and insert the advancing needle under direct visualization at a steep 60- to 90-degree angle relative to the skin (Fig. 41.9 and Video 41.10).

TABLE 41.1 Indications for Ultrasound-Guided Biopsy of the Neck

- Suspected squamous cell carcinoma of any primary origin
- Persistently enlarged (>4 weeks) or rapidly enlarging lymph node
- Thyroid gland nodules (fine-needle aspiration is standard)
- Differentiation of benign from malignant tumors
- Confirmation of suspected malignancy
- Salivary gland pathology[a]
- Obtain sample for tissue culture[b]

[a]Ultrasound-guided core-needle biopsy has higher accuracy than fine-needle aspiration.
[b]Ultrasound-guided core-needle biopsy and fine-needle aspiration are equivalent.

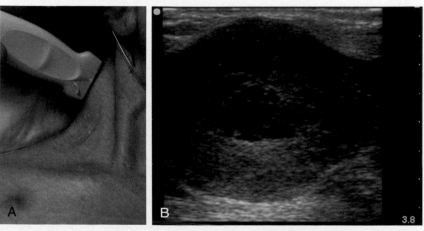

Figure 41.8 Evaluation of an Enlarged Posterior Cervical Lymph Node. (A) Transducer position along the long axis of an enlarged posterior cervical lymph node. (B) An abnormal lymph node is seen that measures approximately 3 × 3 cm. Note the markedly heterogeneous appearance, central hypoechogenicity, enlarged size, and effaced borders due to capsular invasion.

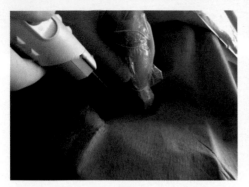

Figure 41.9 Core-Needle Biopsy Technique. Insert the needle at a steep angle (60–90 degrees) relative to the skin under direct visualization with ultrasound.

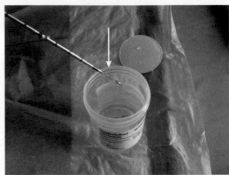

Figure 41.11 Core Tissue Sample. Adequacy of the core tissue sample *(arrow)* can be assessed before placing it in a container with fixating solution.

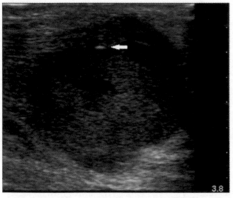

Figure 41.10 Tip of the Advancing Needle. Position the advancing needle tip on the superficial edge of an abnormal lymph node *(arrow)*. Optimal needle positioning is as superficial as possible, which allows the biopsy needle to be fired 2 cm deep.

Position the advancing needle tip on the superficial edge of the lymph node; this is especially important when the node is less than 2 cm in diameter (Fig. 41.10 and Video 41.11). The biopsy needle deploys 2 cm beyond the advancing needle tip, and it is critical to avoid puncturing any adjacent vessels. If a lymph node is superficial, a large-gauge biopsy needle (14G) is preferred, and risk of complications from superficial biopsies is low. If significant risk of injury to adjacent structures exists, an 18G core biopsy needle may be used safely. Once you confirm the location of the advancing needle tip, deploy the biopsy needle. Evaluate

the adequacy of the core sample in the needle (Fig. 41.11), and then flush the tissue core sample into a container with fixating solution.

PEARLS AND PITFALLS

- Lymph nodes can be differentiated from deep venous thrombi by tilting the transducer to identify the node margins.
- Key characteristics that distinguish malignant lymph nodes are their round shape and hypoechoic hilum.
- Evaluate several superficial lymph nodes, if possible, before selecting a superficial node to biopsy.
- Ultrasound evaluation is essential to identify adjacent blood vessels and nerves to avoid and confirm proper positioning of the advancing needle tip before deploying the biopsy needle when performing a core biopsy.
- Providers should acquire experience performing ultrasound-guided biopsies of large lymph nodes before attempting to biopsy lymph nodes less than 2 cm in diameter.
- Identify the lymph node hilum, and avoid biopsy of the hilum when possible, due to the presence of hilar vessels. Control any bleeding with direct digital pressure for 5 to 10 minutes.
- Review institutional policies for minor surgical procedures in patients with bleeding diathesis or anticoagulation when deciding whether or not to perform a lymph node biopsy.

CHAPTER 42

Peripheral Nerve Blocks

Arun Nagdev ■ Shankar LeVine ■ Daniel Mantuani

KEY POINTS

- An ultrasound-guided single-injection nerve block can be a primary or adjunctive tool to reduce pain from acute injuries or procedures.
- Targeted deposition of local anesthetic near specific nerves has been shown to be effective outside of the operating room and is an ideal technique in a multimodal approach to pain management.
- An ultrasound-guided femoral nerve block can effectively reduce pain from acute hip fractures.

Background

Alleviating pain is one of the basic tenets of medical care. Ultrasound-guided peripheral nerve blocks are a newer technique that can be part of a multimodal approach to pain management. A recent Cochrane review of peripheral nerve blocks revealed that ultrasound guidance in the hands of anesthesiologists is an efficacious technique for surgical anesthesia. Ultrasound guidance reduces time to onset of a nerve block and volume of anesthetic required compared to classic nerve stimulation and landmark-based techniques.[1,2] Ultrasound-guided nerve blocks allow providers to reduce the amount of adjunctive analgesic therapy needed for pain relief, in particular, use of intravenous opioids, thereby reducing undesired dose-related side effects such as respiratory depression. This chapter focuses on three commonly performed nerve blocks that can be incorporated into clinical practice: femoral, distal sciatic, and brachial plexus nerve blocks.

Indications

Single-injection ultrasound-guided nerve blocks are ideal to relieve pain from acute injuries and painful procedures. Common indications include wound debridement and irrigation, laceration repair, incision and drainage, fracture reduction, and joint relocation. Depending on the effectiveness of a nerve block, adjunctive therapies can be added to maximize patient comfort.

389

PATIENT SELECTION

Single-injection ultrasound-guided nerve blocks should be performed only in patients who are awake, alert, and able to cooperate with a neurologic exam. Patients with preexisting neurologic deficits in the distribution of the nerve being blocked are not candidates because these deficits obscure the ability to screen for postprocedural peripheral nerve injury (PNI). Caution is recommended in injuries that are at high risk for compartment syndrome (e.g., distal tibia fractures, crush injuries). Since ultrasound-guided nerve blocks may mask an evolving compartment syndrome, we recommend consulting the primary surgical service (e.g., trauma surgery, orthopedics) to assess the potential risks and benefits before performing a nerve block in a patient at risk for compartment syndrome.

PERIPHERAL NERVE INJURY

PNI is an uncommon event defined as a persistent motor or sensory deficit or pain after a nerve block. Its incidence ranges from 0% to 2.2%.[3] The mechanism of injury is not well understood; direct needle trauma from the needle, increased intrafascicular pressures from the anesthetic, direct cytotoxic effects of the anesthetic, and nerve ischemia secondary to the metabolic stress of the anesthetic have been proposed as possible mechanisms. For these reasons, we recommend three intuitive steps to reduce the risk of PNI. First, place the needle tip close to, but not in, the nerve fascicle. Second, slow low-pressure injections should be performed, and the procedure should be stopped if the patient experiences any new pain or paresthesias. Finally, we recommend not performing an ultrasound-guided nerve block in patients with underlying peripheral neuropathy.

POSITIONING

The ultrasound system is generally positioned in front of the provider, on the opposite side of the body (Fig. 42.1). To improve ergonomics, the ultrasound screen should be positioned in the provider's direct line of sight, allowing visualization of both the needle and ultrasound screen without significant head turning. All nerve blocks should be performed with the patient on a cardiac monitor with continuous pulse oximetry.

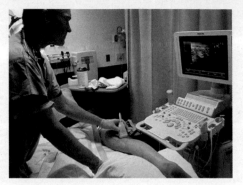

Figure 42.1 Positioning of the Patient, Operator, and Ultrasound Machine. The procedure site is between the provider and ultrasound machine with the screen in the operator's direct line of sight.

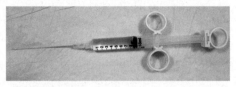

Figure 42.2 Control Syringe. A control syringe is filled with anesthetic and preferably attached to a 20G, 3.5-inch spinal needle.

SUPPLIES

The skin overlying the injection site should be cleaned with chlorhexidine or an equivalent solution. A small-gauge needle (25–30G) is used to anesthetize the skin at the site of injection. The ultrasound transducer should be covered with a transparent adhesive dressing or a sterile transducer sheath. Selection of a needle gauge and length depends on the specific block. A control syringe is preferred (Fig. 42.2). Block-specific needles with blunt tips can be used but are not necessary to perform peripheral nerve blocks.[4]

ANESTHETIC AGENTS

Consider both the duration and safety profile when choosing an anesthetic agent. In general, 2-chloroprocaine and lidocaine are preferred for novice providers over the longer acting agents due to their favorable safety profile. These agents are ideal for short procedures such as joint reductions, simple incision and drainage, and laceration repairs. The concentration of

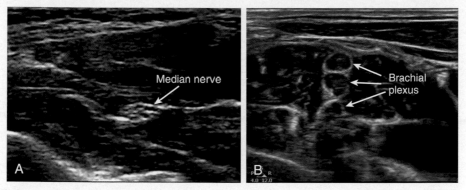

Figure 42.3 Appearance of Nerves. (A) The median nerve is covered in connective tissue and has the classic "honeycomb" appearance by ultrasound. (B) The brachial plexus nerve in the interscalene groove appears as anechoic bundles that can be mistaken for vasculature.

the anesthetic agent determines the rate of diffusion to the nerves and the onset of action; therefore, 3% 2-chloroprocaine and 2% lidocaine would have a more rapid onset when needed.

When a longer duration of anesthesia is required for pain control, such as with femoral or humeral fractures, bupivacaine and ropivacaine are preferred. These agents can be toxic to the heart and central nervous system, and novice providers who are less facile with real-time needle tip visualization should only use the shorter acting agents. Local anesthetic systemic toxicity (LAST) can occur with administration of an excessive dose, rapid absorption, or accidental intravenous injection, even when meticulous injection techniques are used. The addition of a vasoconstrictor, most commonly epinephrine, to shorter acting anesthetic agents can delay vascular absorption and increase the duration of action, which is a reasonable alternative to using a longer acting anesthetic.

Regardless of which agent is used, providers should be familiar with the signs and symptoms of LAST. Classically, the patient complains of tongue numbness and lightheadedness, which then progresses to muscle twitching, unconsciousness, seizures, and cardiovascular depression. Signs and symptoms can occur in any order. In cases where bupivacaine has been inadvertently injected into the vascular system, the use of a hyperlipophilic solution (20% Intralipid; 1.5 mL/kg bolus with a continued infusion of 0.25 mL/kg/min) should be infused. Providers who perform ultrasound-guided nerve blocks should have ready access to 20%

Intralipid (Baxter, Deerfield, IL). Standard safety precautions mandate that providers never inject without visualizing the needle tip and always aspirate to confirm lack of vascular puncture before injecting anesthetic.[5,6]

Anesthetic	Approximate Duration (hours)	Maximum Dose (mg/kg)
2-Chloroprocaine	0.5–1	12
Lidocaine	1.5–2	4
Bupivacaine	4–8	3
Ropivacaine	4–8	3

IDENTIFICATION OF NERVES

Locating peripheral nerves with ultrasound requires knowledge of adjacent anatomy. Nerves are best visualized, and targeted for blocks when oriented in cross-section. Distal peripheral nerves appear as bundles of hyperechoic circles or as a "cluster of grapes" (Fig. 42.3A). However, proximal peripheral nerves, such as the roots of the brachial plexus, appear as individual anechoic circles that can be mistaken for blood vessels (see Fig. 42.3B). Subtle tilting of the transducer may be necessary to obtain the highest quality images and minimize effects of anisotropy. Ultrasound image quality of nerves is more sensitive than other structures to the angle of insonation. Novice providers should verify that the intended target is not a vessel using color flow Doppler (Fig. 42.4). For single-injection ultrasound-guided nerve blocks discussed in this chapter, a high-frequency linear transducer (6–13 MHz)

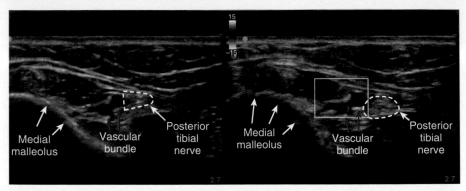

Figure 42.4   Color Flow Doppler. Color flow Doppler demonstrates a vascular bundle next to the posterior tibial nerve.

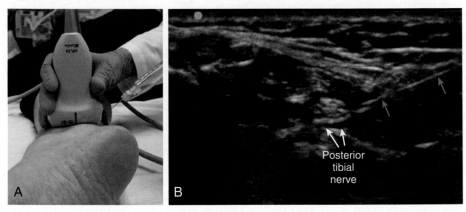

Figure 42.5   Longitudinal Approach. (A) A longitudinal or in-plane approach is shown for an ultrasound-guided posterior tibial nerve block. The needle *(red arrows)* is inserted parallel to the long axis of the transducer (B). Anechoic anesthetic agent is seen surrounding the needle tip on the ultrasound image.

is needed. Providers must maintain image orientation during ultrasound-guided peripheral nerve blocks by aligning the transducer marker ("notch") and screen marker, depending on the approach (transverse vs. longitudinal) and type of nerve block.

Needle Orientation

LONGITUDINAL APPROACH

The longitudinal approach is also called an in-plane or long-axis approach. The needle is inserted parallel to the long axis of the transducer (Fig. 42.5A). As the needle passes under the transducer, the entire length of the needle is visualized (see Fig. 42.5B). The needle must be kept exactly in the center of

the long axis of the transducer in order to visualize the needle in its entirety. A longitudinal approach for needle tip visualization is recommended for novice providers performing nerve blocks.

TRANSVERSE APPROACH

The transverse approach is also called an out-of-plane or short-axis approach. The needle is inserted in the center of and perpendicular to the long axis of the transducer at a steep angle (>60–80 degrees) to the skin (Fig. 42.6). The needle tip is visualized only as a hyperechoic dot as it passes through the ultrasound beam (Fig. 42.7). Safe and successful execution of this technique relies on confident visualization of the needle tip, which requires proficient

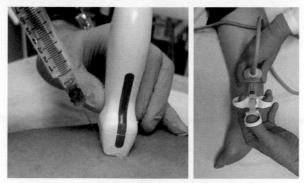

Figure 42.6 **Transverse Approach.** In a transverse or out-of-plane approach to ultrasound-guided nerve blocks, the needle is inserted in the center of and perpendicular to the long axis of the transducer at a steep angle.

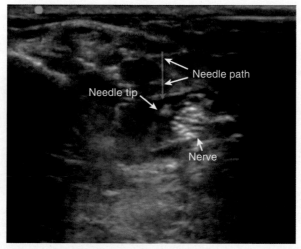

Figure 42.7 **Transverse Approach.** An ultrasound image of a transverse approach shows only the needle tip and anechoic anesthetic spread above the nerve.

spatial-motor skills to manipulate both the transducer and needle. For this reason, a transverse approach may be considered more suitable for experienced providers.

Femoral Nerve Block

INDICATIONS

An ultrasound-guided femoral nerve block is an excellent method to decrease pain from proximal lower extremity injuries. In particular, the femoral nerve block is ideal for pain reduction in patients with hip fractures (intertrochanteric

and subtrochanteric), femur fractures, and patellar injuries. In patients with a hip fracture, the femoral nerve block gives moderate pain reduction but does not provide complete analgesia because the obturator nerve, one of the three nerves that innervate the hip, is not blocked by this approach.[7] However, this method can significantly decrease the need for intravenous opioid medications, reducing the risk of adverse events such as respiratory depression, confusion, and hypotension, especially in elderly patients.

A well-performed femoral nerve block with anesthetic tracking laterally under the fascia

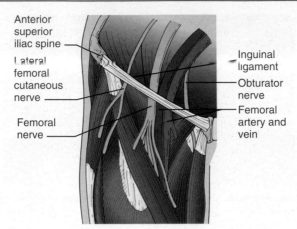

Figure 42.8 Anatomy of the Femoral Triangle. The femoral nerve and the lateral femoral cutaneous nerve are lateral to the femoral artery.

iliaca can also anesthetize the lateral cutaneous nerve. Both nerves innervate the anterior and lateral thigh and this approach can be used for lacerations or abscesses of the thigh. Even though the risk of developing compartment syndrome of the thigh is very rare, we recommend consulting with the primary surgical service before performing a femoral nerve block.

ANATOMY

The femoral nerve is one of the branches of the lumbar plexus arising from the L1 to L4 ventral rami before descending toward the lower extremity. At the level of the inguinal canal, the femoral nerve is located just lateral to the femoral artery, beneath the fascia iliaca and superficial to the iliopsoas muscle; together these structures constitute important landmarks for this nerve block (Fig. 42.8).

TECHNIQUE

With the patient in a supine position, place the linear high-frequency transducer parallel to and just below the inguinal canal (Fig. 42.9). The transducer marker should be pointing to the patient's right side. After locating the femoral artery and vein in cross-section, slide the transducer laterally to locate the femoral nerve. The femoral nerve appears as a hyperechoic triangular region immediately below the fascia iliaca and above the iliopsoas muscle (Fig. 42.10 and Video 42.1). Fanning the transducer superiorly

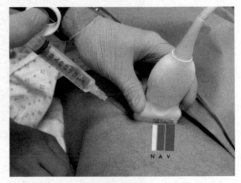

Figure 42.9 Femoral Block Transducer Position. The ultrasound transducer is placed just below the inguinal crease for a longitudinal (in-plane) approach for a femoral nerve block. Note the needle entering the skin lateral and underneath the probe with the orientation of structures superimposed: (N) femoral nerve, (A) femoral artery, (V) femoral vein.

and inferiorly can improve identification of the triangular femoral nerve and its characteristic "honeycomb" appearance.

We recommend using a longitudinal (in-plane) approach from lateral to medial for femoral nerve blocks and depositing the anesthetic agent lateral to the femoral nerve, far from the femoral artery. After making a small skin wheal with local anesthetic, draw 20 mL of 2% lidocaine with epinephrine using a 3.5-inch (9 cm) 20G spinal needle. With the syringe in your dominant hand and the ultrasound transducer in your nondominant

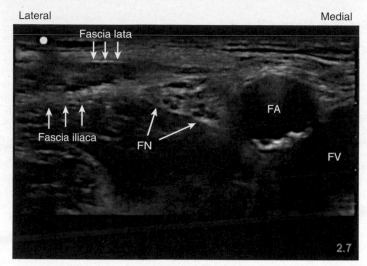

Figure 42.10 Femoral Nerve. The femoral nerve *(FN)* is a triangular structure lateral to the femoral artery *(FA)* and femoral vein *(FV)* and deep to the fascia iliaca, a key landmark.

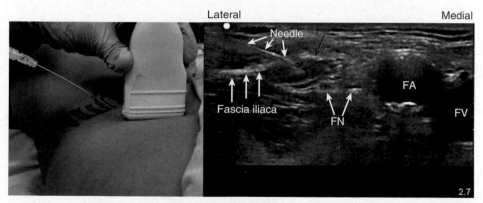

Figure 42.11 Femoral Nerve Block. A lateral to medial longitudinal (in-plane) approach for ultrasound-guided femoral nerve block. The needle tip is deep to the fascia iliaca, and an anechoic pocket of fluid is stretching the tissues with injection of anesthetic *(red arrow)*. *FA,* Femoral artery; *FN,* femoral nerve; *FV,* femoral vein.

hand, enter the skin approximately 0.5 to 1 cm lateral to the transducer using a longitudinal (in-plane) approach. Needle insertion angle depends on the target depth of the fascia iliaca (Fig. 42.11).

Advance the needle toward the junction of the hyperechoic fascia iliaca and lateral corner of the femoral nerve. Once beneath the fascia iliaca, aspirate to confirm the needle tip has not entered a vessel and then slowly inject 1 to 2 mL of local anesthetic. Placing anesthetic just below the hyperechoic fascia iliaca is key to obtaining an effective femoral nerve block.

During injection of the anesthetic, an anechoic fluid pocket appears and can be seen stretching the fascia iliaca (see Fig. 42.11 and Video 42.2). After confirming an optimal needle tip location, proceed to inject a total of 10 to 20 mL of local anesthetic in 3 to 5 mL aliquots. If at any point the spread of local anesthetic is not visualized, then intravascular injection should be suspected and the procedure should be halted. Targeting your needle tip 1 cm lateral to the femoral nerve and vessels, yet deep to the fascia iliaca, reduces the risk of vascular puncture and intraneural injection.[7]

Distal Sciatic Nerve Block

INDICATIONS

The distal sciatic nerve innervates the lower extremity, making it an ideal block for fractures of the ankle, distal tibia, and fibula, and for injuries of the foot. A distal sciatic nerve block does not anesthetize the medial aspect of the lower leg, which is innervated by the saphenous nerve, a distal branch of the femoral nerve. Tibial fractures are high-energy fractures commonly associated with compartment syndrome. Since a distal sciatic block obscures many clinical findings of compartment syndrome (pain, most notably), this block should only be performed after consulting with the primary surgical service.

ANATOMY

The distal sciatic nerve originates from the L4 to S3 nerve roots. The popliteal fossa is bound by the semimembranosus and semitendinosus tendons medially and the biceps femoris tendon laterally. At the most proximal point in the popliteal fossa, the large sciatic nerve bifurcates into the tibial nerve (medially) and the common peroneal nerve (laterally) (Fig. 42.12). The sciatic nerve can be blocked at any location from the proximal deep gluteal region to the distal superficial popliteal fossa. The proximal region is technically more difficult and a

distal location is ideal because many providers are already familiar with the popliteal fossa anatomy.

TECHNIQUE

If possible, the patient should be in a prone position, allowing easy access to the popliteal fossa and posterior aspect of the patient's lower extremity. In patients who are unable to lay prone, the affected extremity must be elevated and supported with mild flexion of the knee to fit the transducer between the popliteal fossa and bed.

Using a high-frequency linear transducer, locate the popliteal artery and vein. The tibial nerve is usually located superficial to the popliteal vein and appears as a hyperechoic "honeycomb" (Fig. 42.13). If you are unable to locate the neural bundle, a more perpendicular view of the nerve may improve visualization due to anisotropy. Once the tibial nerve is visualized, slowly slide the transducer proximally and follow the tibial nerve approximately 5 to 10 cm until the common peroneal nerve is seen joining the tibial nerve laterally to form the distal sciatic nerve (Fig. 42.14 and Video 42.3). The operator should mark this location and note the depth of the nerve.

In contrast to a femoral nerve block in which the needle is inserted immediately adjacent to the transducer, for a distal sciatic

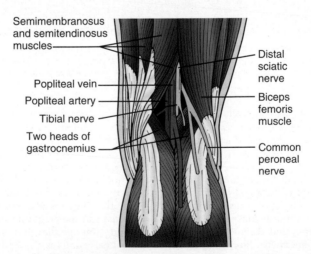

Figure 42.12 Anatomy of Distal Sciatic Nerve. The distal sciatic nerve bifurcates into the tibial and common peroneal nerves in the popliteal fossa.

Labels:
Semimembranosus and semitendinosus muscles
Popliteal vein
Popliteal artery
Tibial nerve
Two heads of gastrocnemius
Distal sciatic nerve
Biceps femoris muscle
Common peroneal nerve

Medial Lateral

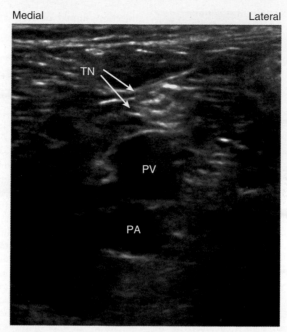

Figure 42.13 Tibial Nerve Anatomy. The tibial nerve *(TN)* in the popliteal fossa. Note the popliteal artery *(PA)* and vein *(PV)* just deep to the nerve.

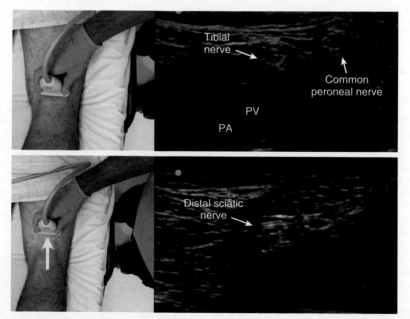

Figure 42.14 Distal Sciatic Nerve. Identify the tibial nerve in the popliteal fossa and slide the transducer proximally to identify the common peroneal nerve *(top)*. The tibial and common peroneal nerves merge to form the distal sciatic nerve *(bottom)*.

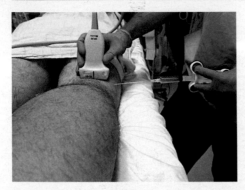

Figure 42.15 Distal Sciatic Nerve Block Transducer Position. The needle is inserted at a flat angle to the skin on the lateral leg and not adjacent to the transducer.

nerve block, we recommend inserting the needle farther away from the transducer on the lateral aspect of the leg (Fig. 42.15). The distal sciatic nerve is often 2 to 4 cm deep to the skin surface, and a steep needle angle would prevent visualization of the needle tip on the ultrasound screen. We recommend measuring the nerve depth and entering the lateral leg at a similar depth with a fairly flat angle, a technique that improves needle visualization. After placing a small skin wheal, fill 20 mL of local anesthetic in a syringe attached to a 20G, 3.5-inch (9 cm) spinal needle.

Advance the needle slowly underneath the transducer, using a longitudinal (in-plane) approach and maintain the needle shaft and tip in view at all times. We recommend performing the distal sciatic nerve block just before it bifurcates into the common peroneal nerve and tibial nerve. Target the honeycomb appearing sciatic nerve without placing the needle directly into the nerve. Place the needle tip just superficial to the nerve to reduce intraneural injection risk. Aspirate to confirm that there has been no vascular puncture and then slowly inject 3 to 5 mL of local anesthetic. With the needle tip in view, the spread of anechoic anesthetic should be visualized in real time (Fig. 42.16 and Video 42.4). We recommend not attempting to inject on the inferior aspect of the nerve, which is close to the popliteal vasculature, because the risk of inadvertent intravascular injection at this location may be higher. If at any point the spread of local anesthetic is not visualized, intravascular

injection should be suspected and the procedure halted.[7]

Brachial Plexus Nerve Block: Interscalene Approach

INDICATIONS

An ultrasound-guided interscalene brachial plexus block provides anesthesia to the proximal upper extremity including the shoulder. In the acute care setting, an interscalene brachial plexus block is primarily indicated for pain control of upper extremity fractures (distal clavicle and humerus) and as an alternative to procedural sedation for the reduction of a shoulder dislocation. Other indications include large abscess drainage, burns, deep wound exploration, and complex laceration repair.

The risk of phrenic nerve–related transient diaphragmatic hemiparesis exists with an interscalene block. With the use of ultrasound guidance, the rate of this event has decreased due to lower volume of anesthetic administration and increased precision of anesthetic delivery.[8,9] Even though the clinical significance of transient unilateral phrenic nerve paralysis is debated, we recommend caution when performing an interscalene block in patients with poor pulmonary reserve (e.g., severe chronic obstructive pulmonary disease, sleep apnea).

ANATOMY

Interscalene blocks target the brachial plexus at the level of the roots or trunks as they pass through the interscalene groove. Just deep to the clavicular head of the sternocleidomastoid muscle and at the level of the cricoid cartilage, the interscalene groove is bordered medially by the anterior scalene muscle and laterally by the middle scalene muscle (Fig. 42.17 and Video 42.5). The targeted C5 to C7 nerve roots are positioned vertically within the interscalene groove. Anesthetic placed in this fascial plane commonly does not track around the inferiorly located C8 to T1 nerve roots and therefore, does not reliably provide anesthesia for injuries distal to the elbow. Important landmarks include the carotid artery and internal jugular vein that lie medial to the anterior scalene muscle. The dome of the pleura is located caudally and the risk of pleural puncture is low if

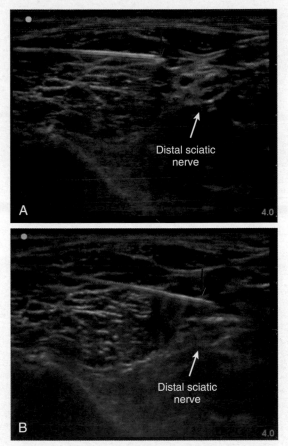

Figure 42.16 Distal Sciatic Nerve Block. (A) The needle *(red arrow)* is advanced toward the distal sciatic nerve using a longitudinal approach. (B) Note the spread of anechoic anesthetic fluid above the distal sciatic nerve.

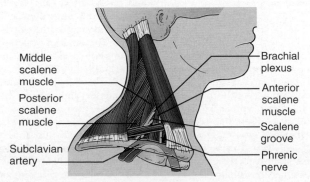

Figure 42.17 Anatomy of the Interscalene Brachial Plexus. Roots of the brachial plexus are in the scalene groove, the space between the anterior and middle scalene muscles.

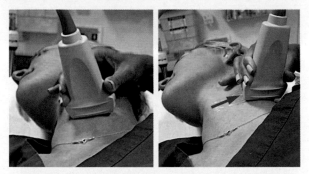

Figure 42.18 **Interscalene Block Transducer Position.** Place the ultrasound transducer at the level of the cricoid cartilage, locate the internal jugular vein and common carotid artery, and then slide the ultrasound transducer laterally to identify the sternocleidomastoid muscle and brachial plexus roots deep to the sternocleidomastoid muscle.

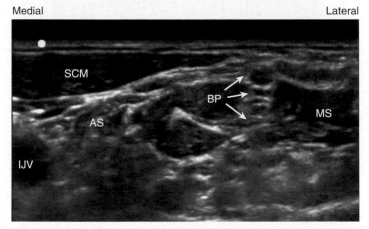

Figure 42.19 **Brachial Plexus Roots.** The brachial plexus *(BP)* roots are seen in the interscalene groove. Borders of the interscalene groove are the middle *(MS)* and anterior scalene *(AS)* muscles. Note the more superficial sternocleidomastoid muscle *(SCM)*. *IJV*, Internal jugular vein.

the block is performed correctly with real-time ultrasound guidance.

TECHNIQUE

The patient is positioned in an upright or semirecumbent position with the head turned partially toward the contralateral side. An interscalene block should be performed using a longitudinal (in-plane) approach. Patient positioning is critical to insert the needle tip safely in the interscalene groove. The ipsilateral shoulder may be elevated using towels or a pillow under the scapula to flatten the skin surface and increase needle visibility.

Using a high-frequency linear transducer in a transverse orientation at the level of the cricoid cartilage, locate the internal jugular vein and carotid artery (Fig. 42.18). Slide the transducer laterally until the clavicular head of the sternocleidomastoid muscle is centered on the screen. The anterior scalene muscle lies deep to the sternocleidomastoid muscle. The roots of the brachial plexus originate from the spinal cord and run in the scalene groove between the anterior and middle scalene muscles as they make their way to innervate the upper extremity. At this level, the C5 to C7 roots of the brachial plexus appear as hypoechoic round or ovoid structures vertically aligned, referred to as the "traffic light" sign (Fig. 42.19). Color flow Doppler can differentiate the hypoechoic cords of the brachial plexus from vessels in the anterior neck.

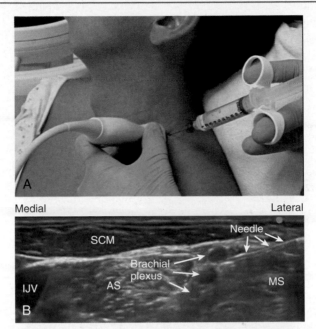

Medial

Lateral

Figure 42.20 Interscalene Block. (A) Transducer position for a longitudinal (in-plane) approach. (B) The needle is inserted from lateral to medial into the interscalene groove to perform an ultrasound-guided interscalene nerve block. *AS,* Anterior scalene; *IJV,* internal jugular vein; *MS,* Middle scalene; *SCM,* sternocleidomastoid muscle.

After prepping the neck and injecting a skin wheal, a 21 to 23G, 1.5-inch needle is inserted using a longitudinal (in-plane) approach. The needle tip is advanced through the middle scalene muscle to the lateral border of the deepest nerve root. Approximately 10 to 20 mL of local anesthetic is then injected into the potential space between the middle scalene muscle and brachial plexus sheath (Fig. 42.20 and Video 42.6). With a successful block, local anesthetic tracks in the fascial plane between the middle scalene muscle and the nerve roots.

Supraclavicular Brachial Plexus Nerve Block

INDICATIONS

A supraclavicular brachial plexus nerve block (SCB) provides anesthesia to injuries of the upper extremity from the mid-humerus, elbow, forearm, and hand. An SCB provides anesthesia for the reduction of elbow dislocations and distal radius fractures, as well as management of complex wounds of the forearm. The suprascapular nerve branches proximal to the brachial plexus in the supraclavicular fossa; and in contrast to an interscalene block, an SCB does not provide pain relief for injuries of the distal clavicle and shoulder.

An SCB targets the brachial plexus distal to the interscalene nerve block. The risk of inadvertent paralysis of the phrenic nerve and hemidiaphragm or an iatrogenic Horner's syndrome exists but is less frequent.[10] The brachial plexus in the supraclavicular fossa lies both adjacent to the subclavian artery and superficial to the dome of the pleura, necessitating the mastery of needle tip visualization prior to incorporating this procedure into practice.

ANATOMY

Distal to the interscalene groove in the supraclavicular fossa, the trunks and divisions of the brachial plexus are compactly arranged within a fascial sheath that runs superficial to the middle scalene muscle and lies lateral to the subclavian artery. At the midpoint of the clavicle, the subclavian artery is readily visualized

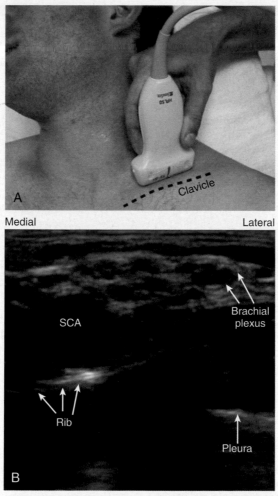

Figure 42.21   Supraclavicular Brachial Plexus. (A) Transducer position for a supraclavicular brachial plexus block. (B) The subclavian artery *(SCA)* and adjacent brachial plexus are superficial to the first rib and pleura when the transducer is placed parallel to the rib and pointed caudally.

in cross-section just superficial to the first rib. The brachial plexus at this level appears as an ovoid or triangular-shaped hypoechoic bundle that looks like a honeycomb. Deep and lateral to the first rib is the hyperechoic pleura which slides back and forth during the respiratory cycle. (Fig. 42.21 and Video 42.7)

TECHNIQUE

Similar to the setup for an interscalene brachial plexus block, the patient is positioned upright or semirecumbent with their head turned toward the contralateral side. The ultrasound machine is placed opposite the patient in direct line of sight of the operator. The SCB is always performed using a longitudinal (in-plane) approach with a lateral to the medial trajectory.

A high-frequency linear transducer is placed in the supraclavicular fossa just posterior and parallel to the mid-portion of the clavicle. As the transducer is tilted or fanned anteriorly, the subclavian artery will be seen in a transverse cross-section as a pulsatile, hypoechoic circular structure that lies just superficial to the first rib. Lateral to the subclavian artery lies the hyperechoic, honeycomb-like brachial plexus as it runs superficial to the middle

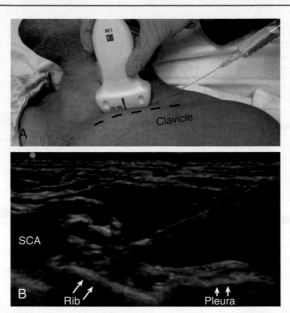

Figure 42.22 Supraclavicular Brachial Plexus Block. (A) The transducer is placed above the clavicle and the needle is inserted longitudinally underneath the transducer. (B) The brachial plexus is visualized lateral to the anechoic subclavian artery *(SCA)*. Note the rib and sliding pleura. Injection of the local anesthetic hydrodissects the tissues around the brachial plexus.

scalene muscle. Identify the shimmering and sliding pleura which lies deep and lateral to the first rib.

After prepping the area and anesthetizing the skin, use a longitudinal (in-plane) approach to insert a 21 to 23G, 1.5-inch (3.8 cm) needle lateral to the transducer. A 3.5-inch (9 cm) needle may be needed in obese patients. The needle is then advanced longitudinally underneath the superficial fascial plane to the lateral border of the brachial plexus. With the needle tip in view, low-pressure injections using small aliquots of 3 to 5 mL of local anesthetic are used to hydrodissect above and below the brachial plexus (Fig. 42.22 and Video 42.8). A total of 20 to 30 mL of local anesthetic may be used to achieve dense anesthesia distal to the mid-humerus.

PEARLS AND PITFALLS

- Peripheral nerves can look like vasculature on ultrasound. Use color flow Doppler over the area of interest to confirm that the anechoic proximal nerve roots are not vasculature. Reduce the Doppler pulse repetition frequency (PRF) to a low-flow setting to detect small vessels.
- Ultrasound-guided femoral nerve blocks do not offer complete anesthesia for hip fractures but rather deliver significant pain relief. This block in conjunction with standard intravenous analgesics should reduce rates of opioid-related adverse events.
- The femoral nerve innervates only the anterior aspect of the thigh and a small portion of the medial leg (via the saphenous nerve). A femoral nerve block will not anesthetize the entire thigh.
- The goal of a femoral nerve block is to place anesthetic under the fascia iliaca while staying away from the nerve. Inject small aliquots of anesthetic to spread the soft tissues and then reposition the needle tip for better visualization.
- For ultrasound-guided distal sciatic nerve blocks, patients should be

placed in a prone position if possible. This position facilitates identification of relevant anatomy and improves the success of the procedure.

- An ultrasound-guided interscalene nerve block usually spares the C8 and T1 nerve roots, making this block less effective for injuries of the hand and wrist.

- An ultrasound-guided interscalene nerve block is ideal for anesthesia of the distal clavicle and shoulder, whereas a supraclavicular nerve block is ideal for injuries of the distal upper extremity below the elbow. A supraclavicular nerve block may provide anesthesia above the elbow to the mid-humerus if a large volume of anesthetic is deposited.

CHAPTER 43

Lumbar Puncture

Paul G. McHardy ■ Daniel J. Schnobrich ■ David M. Tierney ■
Nilam J. Soni

KEY POINTS

- Ultrasound increases the success rate of lumbar puncture by improving identification of the lumbar spine's midline and interspaces by visualizing the bony processes in transverse and longitudinal planes, respectively.
- The greatest improvement in success rate of lumbar puncture with ultrasound guidance has been shown in morbidly obese patients and those with difficult to palpate landmarks.
- For experienced operators, real-time ultrasound guidance may provide additional benefit beyond static guidance.

Background

Ultrasound was first described as a useful bedside tool to identify lumbar spine anatomy in 1971.[1] The most common technique for using ultrasound to guide lumbar puncture is preprocedural mapping of the lumbar spine to choose a needle insertion site. Ultrasound can identify the lumbar spine level more accurately than physical examination.[2-7] A meta-analysis of 14 randomized trials showed that selecting a needle insertion site with ultrasound prior to lumbar puncture or epidural catheterization reduced the number of attempts, needle redirections, failed procedures, and traumatic taps.[8] Similar benefits have been demonstrated in a meta-analysis that included only randomized trials of lumbar puncture.[9] Although lumbar spine mapping has shown greatest benefit in obese patients in whom the palpation of landmarks is difficult,[10-13] benefits have also been demonstrated in obstetric, orthopedic, and emergency department patients.[14-21] A reduction in postprocedure back pain after lumbar puncture and headache after spinal anesthesia has been demonstrated with the use of ultrasound.[10,21-25] Studies have shown that mapping can be accomplished by nonradiologists after brief training,[26,27] and that high-quality images can usually be obtained in under a minute.[28]

Training requirements to obtain consistently high-quality images in one study included review of ultrasound images and 10 practice scans.[28]

Spinal ultrasound can additionally be used to accurately measure the distance between the skin and ligamentum flavum. Because the ligamentum flavum is adjacent to the dura mater, this measurement can guide selection of the most appropriate length spinal needle and anticipation of how deep the needle should be inserted to obtain cerebrospinal fluid.[11,12,14,29-31] Patients with a body mass index (BMI) <25 had an average difference of 2 cm of depth when compared to morbidly obese patients with BMI >30 (4.4 cm vs. 6.4 cm).[3] This measurement is best performed using a longitudinal paramedian view.[11,12,14,30-33]

Lumbar puncture using real-time ultrasound guidance, a technically advanced skill, has been described using a paramedian approach.[17,34-40] However, static ultrasound guidance to map the lumbar spine and mark a needle insertion site has greater supporting evidence and is the more common technique in clinical practice.

Anatomy

The spine consists of 24 vertebral bodies (7 cervical, 12 thoracic, and 5 lumbar), intervertebral

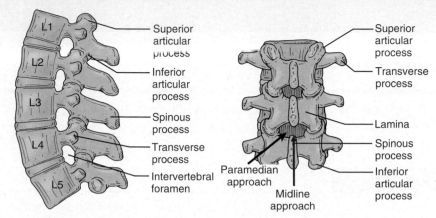

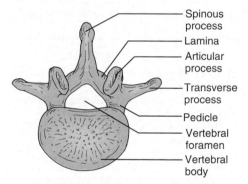

Figure 43.1 Anatomy of Lumbar Spine. The lumbar spinous processes are rectangular, or tombstone-shaped. The L2–L3 and L3–L4 midline interspinous spaces are often the widest and preferred for lumbar puncture. The foramina for the two approaches to lumbar puncture are shown: midline *(red arrow)* and paramedian *(blue arrow)*.

Figure 43.2 Anatomy of Lumbar Vertebra.

cartilaginous discs, sacrum, and coccyx. The five lumbar vertebrae are relatively larger than those of the cervical or thoracic spine (Fig. 43.1). Each vertebra has a vertebral body, the weight-bearing and largest part, connected to pedicles, laminae, and transverse and spinous processes (Fig. 43.2). The spinous processes extend posteriorly and are the most superficial component of vertebrae that are palpable in the midline. Connecting the transverse processes to the spinous process are the superior and inferior articular processes, or facet joints, and laminae. The spinous processes are connected at the tips by the supraspinous ligament and at the shafts by the interspinous ligament. Ligamentum flavum lines the vertebral foramina and connects the laminae. The posterior longitudinal ligament runs along the posterior aspect of the vertebral bodies (Fig. 43.3).

Technique

PATIENT POSITION

Lumbar puncture can be performed with patients in an upright seated position or lateral decubitus position. In the upright seated position, the patient leans forward with arms folded on a table, and the feet are supported with a chair or stool. In a lateral decubitus position, the patient lies on his left or right side with the knees flexed to the chest. Lumbar puncture success rates tend to be lower in the lateral decubitus position than in the upright seated position because the vertebral column bows or twists on the soft bed surface and the interspinous spaces open less in a lateral decubitus position.[2,41,42] However, in a hospital setting, some patients may not tolerate sitting upright for the duration of the procedure, and for these patients, the lateral decubitus position should be used.

If the patient is in a lateral decubitus position, it is important to square the shoulders and hips perpendicular to the bed surface. If the hips and shoulders are not perfectly vertical in a lateral decubitus position, the spine will twist, which often leads to failed attempts. The lateral decubitus position allows measurement of the opening pressure using manometry because the patient's head is at the same level as the spinal needle entry site. Manometry is not performed when the patient is in an upright seated position.

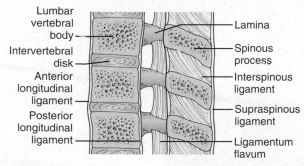

Figure 43.3 Ligaments of Lumbar Spine. In a midline approach, the spinal needle passes through the supraspinous and interspinous ligaments before piercing the ligamentum flavum to enter the epidural space.

ULTRASOUND EXAM

For patients with a low or normal BMI, a high-frequency, linear array transducer may be used to provide high resolution of superficial bony structures. For obese patients with a high BMI, a low frequency, curvilinear transducer is used because deeper penetration is needed to visualize the spinal structures.[43]

In adults, the spinal cord terminates at L1, and therefore lumbar puncture can be safely performed below L2. The level of the posterior superior iliac crests is approximately L4. In patients with palpable landmarks, the L4 lumbar spine level may be approximated by drawing an imaginary line between the posterior superior iliac crests. One interspace above or below the level of the posterior superior iliac crests is ideal for lumbar puncture because the spinal needle enters in the L3–L4 or L4–L5 interspinous space. In general, the L3–L4 interspinous space is preferred for lumbar puncture because it is wider and has less soft tissue overlying the spinous processes compared to the L4–L5 interspinous space (Fig. 43.4).

IDENTIFICATION OF THE LUMBAR SPINE

In morbidly obese patients or those with few palpable bone landmarks, all five lumbar spinous processes can be identified with ultrasound. Starting in a transverse plane, place the transducer over the sacrum, just above the intergluteal cleft, with the transducer orientation marker pointed to the operator's left. The sacrum is distinguished by its ragged, superficial surface and hyperechoic, fused bones. Slide the transducer superiorly until the first

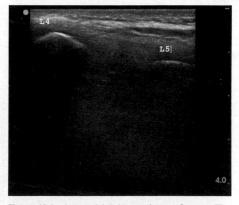

Figure 43.4 L4 and L5 Interspinous Space. The L4 and L5 spinous processes are shown in a longitudinal plane. In general, the L2–L3 or L3–L4 interspinous spaces are preferred for lumbar puncture because the L4–L5 interspinous space is deeper due to overlying soft tissue.

lumbar spinous process (L5) is seen. The L5 spinous process is relatively small and deep in soft tissue, even in thin patients (see Fig. 43.4 and Video 43.1). Sliding the transducer superiorly can identify the L4, L3, L2, and L1 lumbar spinous processes (Fig. 43.5). Marking the lumbar spine in transverse and longitudinal views is described below.

TRANSVERSE VIEW: MIDLINE IDENTIFICATION

With the transducer oriented in a transverse plane to the spine, the tips of the spinous processes are seen as hyperechoic, pointed structures in the near field of the screen. Each spinous process casts a vertical shadow that extends to the far field of the screen (Fig. 43.6A, B; Video 43.2). The spinous process appears much thinner in a transverse versus longitudinal view. Several centimeters deep and lateral to the superficial midline spinous

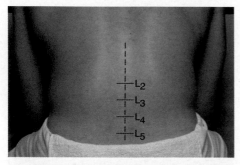

Figure 43.5 Lumbar Spine Mapping of the L2–L5 Spinous Processes.

processes, the transverse processes can be seen as two horizontal white lines and can confirm identification of the midline (Fig. 43.7 and Video 43.3). Center the transducer exactly on the spinal midline and make a mark perpendicular to the transducer along the spinous processes (see Fig. 43.6C). The midline should be marked at a minimum of two or three levels.

LONGITUDINAL VIEW: INTERSPINOUS SPACE IDENTIFICATION

After identifying the L3 and L4 vertebrae, rotate the transducer 90 degrees clockwise to align the transducer in a longitudinal plane over the midline. Identify the L3–L4 interspinous space in a longitudinal orientation (Fig. 43.8A, B; Video 43.4). Adjust the depth to visualize the spinous processes, and the ligamentum flavum may be seen deep in the

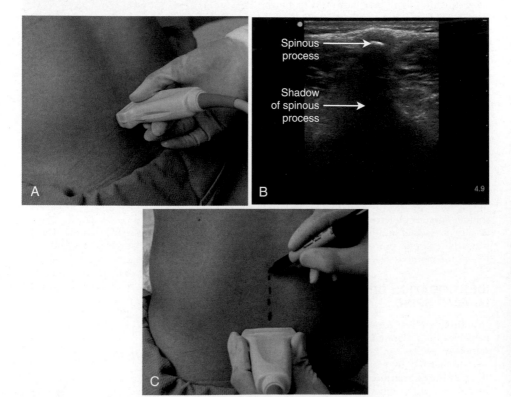

Figure 43.6 Marking the Midline of the Lumbar Spine. (A) The transducer is centered over a lumbar spinous process in a transverse plane. (B) The spinous process appears as a hyperechoic, pointed structure in the center of the screen. (C) To mark the midline of the spine, a mark is made perpendicular to the transducer.

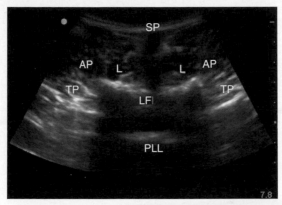

Figure 43.7 Transverse Midline View of the Lumbar Spine. A curvilinear transducer allows visualization of the deep structures of the spine. *AP*, Articular process; *L*, lamina; *LF*, ligamentum flavum; *PLL*, posterior longitudinal ligament; *SP*, spinous process; *TP*, transverse process.

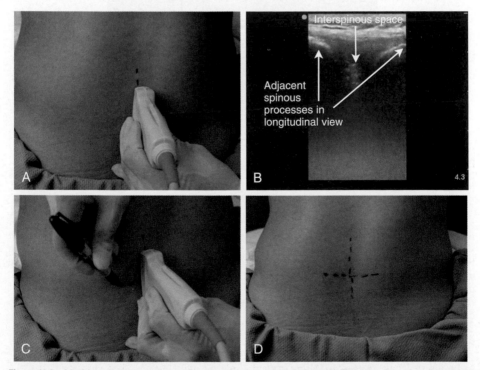

Figure 43.8 Marking the Interspinous Space of the Lumbar Spine. (A) The transducer is oriented longitudinally and centered over two spinous processes. (B) The interspace between two lumbar spinous processes is shown in a longitudinal plane. (C) A mark is made perpendicular to the center of the transducer to denote the interspinous space. (D) The vertical line identifying the midline crosses the horizontal line identifying the interspinous space, and an "X" marks the site for spinal needle insertion.

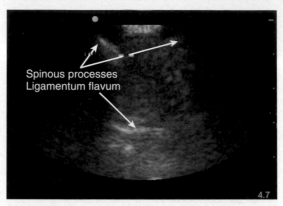

Figure 43.9 Ligamentum Flavum. A longitudinal, midline view of the spine using a curvilinear transducer allows visualization of the ligamentum flavum deep to the spinous processes.

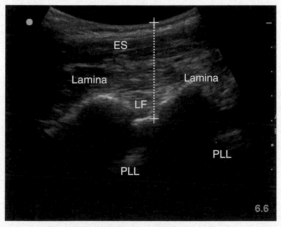

Figure 43.10 Measurement of Depth of Ligamentum Flavum. The ligamentum flavum *(LF)* is best visualized in between laminae from a longitudinal paramedian view and the skin-ligamentum flavum depth can be measured *(vertical line)*. *ES*, Erector spinae muscles; *PLL*, posterior longitudinal ligament.

interspinous space (Fig. 43.9). The depth of the ligamentum flavum and distance from skin surface to ligamentum flavum are more reliably visualized from a longitudinal paramedian view (Fig. 43.10). The posterior dura is only a few millimeters deep to the ligamentum flavum. Measuring the depth of the ligamentum flavum helps providers select an appropriate length spinal needle and anticipate when the subarachnoid space will be entered; for example, a typical 8–9 cm spinal needle needs to be inserted only halfway in a thin patient with a ligamentum flavum depth of 4 cm, whereas the same needle will not suffice in an obese patient with a ligamentum flavum depth of 10 cm.

It is critical to recognize that a longitudinal paramedian view can be mistaken for a midline view. The laminae in a paramedian view can be misinterpreted for spinous processes. Sweeping the transducer from left to right in a longitudinal plane and visualizing both the laminae and spinous processes is a technique to confirm the spinous processes are being visualized. Additionally, only skin and subcutaneous tissues are seen superficial to the spinous processes in the midline, whereas muscle fibers of the erector spinae muscles are seen superficial to the laminae when in a longitudinal paramedian plane (Videos 43.5 and 43.6).

The ultrasound appearance of lumbar spinous processes in this orientation is rectangular, like "tombstones," and shadowing is seen deep to the spinous processes. The transducer is centered over two adjacent spinous processes, and the interspinous space is marked with a line perpendicular to the transducer (see Fig. 43.8C). The intersection of the markings of the spinal midline and interspinous space is the entry point for the spinal needle (see Fig. 43.8D).

REAL-TIME ULTRASOUND GUIDANCE

Most of this chapter focuses on the use of static ultrasound guidance for lumbar puncture site marking, but there are at least three different real-time, ultrasound-guided approaches to lumbar puncture—all of which use a paramedian approach to the spinal canal.[17,34-40] An advantage of the paramedian approach is the needle is advanced through the interlaminar space, which is wider than the midline interspinous space. The disadvantage is the spinal needle is inserted at an oblique angle which requires practice to master.

Real-time ultrasound guidance requires use of the nondominant hand to maneuver the transducer while the dominant hand manipulates the needle. The procedure can be performed in an upright seated or lateral decubitus position. A curvilinear transducer is preferred and must be placed in a sterile plastic sheath with sterile gel. The skin surface must be sterilely prepped and draped. There is no data regarding the safety of sterile gel that may be carried by the spinal needle into the epidural and subarachnoid space. Thus, the operator should either use sterile gauze to wipe off the gel from the needle insertion site, or use sterile saline between the transducer and skin.

When using real-time ultrasound guidance, the clinician should first identify the widest interlaminar space of the lumbar spine, or space with the greatest visibility of spinal ligaments, using a longitudinal paramedian view. Center the transducer over the widest interlaminar space, rotate the transducer 45 degrees with the transducer notch pointing toward the midline in an oblique paramedian plane, and align the ultrasound beam in a plane from the spinous process of the superior vertebra to the lamina of the inferior vertebra (Fig. 43.11). The lamina, ligamentum flavum, and posterior longitudinal ligament are visualized. A critical step is to slide the transducer 1 to 2 cm craniomedially towards the midline to ease insertion

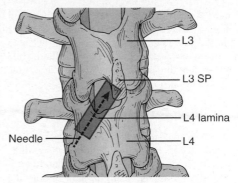

Figure 43.11 Transducer Orientation for Real-Time Ultrasound Guidance. An oblique paramedian view is used to perform real-time ultrasound-guided lumbar puncture. The ultrasound transducer (blue rectangle) is oriented obliquely from the superior vertebra's spinous process to the inferior vertebra's lamina. The needle (red arrow) is inserted under the transducer aiming toward the ligamentum flavum at the base of the superior spinous process. SP, Spinous process.

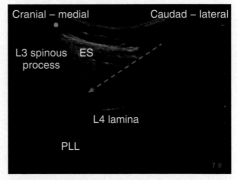

Figure 43.12 Real-Time Ultrasound-Guided Lumbar Puncture. This oblique paramedian view shows the trajectory of the spinal needle (dotted arrow) toward the base of the L3 spinous process just medial to the L4 lamina. ES, Erector spinae; PLL, posterior longitudinal ligament.

of the needle underneath the transducer. After optimizing the image, the provider should wipe away any excess gel. The spinal needle is inserted in the plane of the ultrasound beam and visualized as it is passes through the interlaminar space. The needle is aimed toward the ligamentum flavum at the base of the superior spinal process (Fig. 43.12), but visualization of the needle tip penetrating the ligamentum flavum is usually obscured by shadowing from the spinous process. Resistance increases as the needle traverses the ligamentum flavum, and after a loss of resistance is felt, the provider should put down the transducer and begin to sequentially check for cerebrospinal fluid while advancing the needle 1 to 2 mm at a time (Video 43.7).

Lumbar Puncture

When using static ultrasound to mark the spinal needle insertion site, the patient must remain in the same position in the interim between ultrasound mapping and performing lumbar puncture because small changes in position can offset the markings. Once the skin insertion site has been sterilely prepped, draped, and anesthetized, the spinal needle is inserted at the marked site with the bevel parallel to the longitudinal ligaments of the spine. Multiple studies have demonstrated a reduction of post-lumbar puncture headaches if a smaller-gauge (20–22 gauge) atraumatic spinal needle is used.[44-50] Atraumatic needles are not included in most standard lumbar puncture kits but are available in most hospitals. When removing the stylet to check for fluid return, a longer pause is needed when using a 22 gauge atraumatic needles compared to traditional 18–20 gauge cutting (Quincke) needles. The stylet should always be in place when advancing or withdrawing the spinal needle.[51] After the spinal needle passes through the skin and subcutaneous tissue, it encounters resistance from the dense supraspinous and interspinous ligaments, and firm pressure is required to traverse these ligaments. If bone is encountered superficially (<2 cm in depth), the spinal needle is likely hitting a spinous process, and the needle should be redirected, usually cephalad. The first "pop," or release of resistance, is felt as the needle passes through the ligamentum flavum and enters the epidural space. The second "pop" is felt a few millimeters deeper as the needle punctures the dura mater and enters the subarachnoid space where cerebrospinal fluid is obtained. A manometer can be attached to the spinal needle to obtain an opening pressure. Cerebrospinal fluid is collected in sterile tubes and the stylet is replaced before needle withdrawal.

PEARLS AND PITFALLS

- Visualization of the spinous processes in transverse and longitudinal planes is the key element when using ultrasound to map the lumbar spine.
- If a spinous process cannot be definitively identified in a transverse view, slowly slide the transducer cephalad or caudad in the midline until a shadow of a spinous process is visualized. Trace the shadow superficially until you can identify the hyperechoic tip of the spinous process.
- The length of spinal needle required can be determined by measuring the distance from the skin surface to the ligamentum flavum, which is best measured from a longitudinal paramedian view. An additional 5 mm should be added to this distance to account for skin compression and bowing of the dura prior to puncture.
- In a longitudinal plane, laminae must be differentiated from spinous processes. Slide the transducer in a longitudinal orientation from left to right and definitively identify both laminae and spinous processes. Laminae will have erector spinae muscles superficial to the bone, whereas spinous processes will not have any muscle but only a relatively thin layer of subcutaneous tissue superficial to the bone.
- When inserting a spinal needle using a midline approach, a substantial amount of resistance should be encountered as the supraspinous and interspinous ligaments are traversed. If resistance is not encountered, the needle trajectory is most likely off-center, and the needle is passing through erector spinae muscle.
- Novice providers are recommended to practice lumbar spine mapping on thin patients using a linear transducer to become familiar with the normal sonographic appearance of the lumbar spine.

CHAPTER 44

Transcranial Ultrasound

Vincent I. Lau ■ Robert Arntfield

KEY POINTS

- Gross anatomical abnormalities of the brain, including mass effect and midline shift, can be detected using two-dimensional ultrasound through the transcranial windows.
- Point-of-care transcranial Doppler ultrasound can be used at the bedside to evaluate blood flow changes due to increased intracranial pressure.
- Midline shift can be assessed by measuring the distance between the external temporal bone and third ventricle bilaterally.

Background

Neurological evaluation of obtunded patients is often limited to an assessment of the pupils, brainstem reflexes, gross motor function, and verbal responses. Additional investigations often require transportation of patients for computed tomography (CT) or magnetic resonance imaging (MRI) scans, or performance of invasive procedures, such as insertion of an intracranial pressure (ICP) monitor, which are costly, potentially harmful, and often infeasible in critically ill patients. Due to these limitations, many providers have begun to use point-of-care transcranial Doppler (TCD) ultrasound to evaluate patients at the bedside.

TCD has been used in clinical practice since 1982. The thin temporal bone provides an acoustic window to noninvasively evaluate intracranial blood flow velocity using color flow and pulsed-wave Doppler (PWD) ultrasound.[1-3] TCD has also been used to serially monitor the progression of cerebral circulatory arrest and brain death,[4] and to measure midline shift[5] and ICP.[6]

The most common applications of point-of-care TCD ultrasound are detection of midline shift, elevated ICP, and cerebral circulatory arrest. A comprehensive list of TCD applications is listed in Table 44.1.[7]

MIDLINE SHIFT

Midline shift, usually secondary to mass effect, is frequently life-threatening and requires prompt diagnosis to avoid irreparable damage.[8] Use of ultrasound to measure midline shift was first described in 1996.[5] Ultrasound measurements of midline shift correlate well with CT measurements,[5,8] and have been predictive of poor outcomes from midline shift due to ischemic stroke, hemorrhage (subdural, epidural, subarachnoid), and traumatic brain injury (TBI).[2,3,5,8,9]

ELEVATED INTRACRANIAL PRESSURE AND CEREBRAL CIRCULATORY ARREST

As ICP increases and cerebral perfusion pressure (CPP) decreases, intracranial blood flow is compromised. A correlation between elevated ICP and decreased intracranial diastolic blood flow has been described: diastolic flow is initially blunted, and with increasing ICP, flow is reversed.[6] Prolonged elevations in ICP lead to brain ischemia, cerebral circulatory arrest, and eventually brain death.[4] TCD can be used to identify high ICP and guide decision-making about continuous invasive ICP monitoring.[10]

TABLE 44.1 Indications for Transcranial Doppler Ultrasound

Midline shift
Elevated intracranial pressure
Cerebral circulatory arrest (brain death)
Vasospasm (post-subarachnoid hemorrhage)
Arterial stenosis
Arterial occlusion/stroke
Transient ischemic attack (micro-emboli)
Right-to-left shunts
Sickle cell hyperemia
Intracranial hemorrhage monitoring

ADVANCED APPLICATIONS

Advanced point-of-care TCD ultrasound applications include evaluation for vasospasm and intracranial stenosis, but these applications require significant additional training.[3] Ischemic strokes generally show occlusion of a specific vessel with maintenance of flow elsewhere.[3-5,8] Microemboli from transient ischemic attacks (TIAs) show transient increases in vessel velocity that return to baseline, but the utility of TCD is limited in patients with TIAs because continuous monitoring is required.[4,5,8]

Anatomy

Point-of-care TCD utilizes the thin temporal bone as a window to evaluate intracranial structures. The third ventricle is visualized between the two cerebral hemispheres and marks the midline. The circle of Willis is composed of the bilateral anterior cerebral arteries (ACAs), posterior cerebral arteries (PCAs), posterior communicating (PComm) arteries, and the anterior communicating (AComm) artery (Fig. 44.1). Although not part of the circle of Willis, the bilateral middle cerebral arteries (MCAs) supply the majority of the blood to the brain's hemispheres,[11] and will be the focus of this chapter.

Image Acquisition

Patients are placed in a supine position with head of the bed elevated at 30 degrees. A phased-array transducer (1–5 MHz) is used and a TCD exam preset is selected. A cardiac exam preset may be used but the screen orientation marker will be on the right, and essential calculations, such as pulsatility index (PI), will not be available.

Three transcranial windows may be utilized for transcranial Doppler ultrasound: transorbital, transtemporal, and transforaminal (Fig. 44.2). Point-of-care TCD exams rely primarily on the transtemporal window.

To find the transtemporal window, place the transducer on the temporal bone at the level of the eye, just anterior to the ear. The transducer orientation marker should be pointed anteriorly when scanning either the right or left transtemporal window. This orientation will maintain the left side of the screen as being anterior (Fig. 44.3). The first sonographic landmarks seen are the hypoechoic, heart-shaped bilateral thalami or cerebral peduncles (Fig. 44.4A and Video 44.1), or the third ventricle (see Fig. 44.4B and Video 44.2). The third ventricle is distinguished by its echogenic walls and anechoic, fluid-filled center. These structures are typically visualized at a depth of 6 to 8 cm.

To identify the cerebral vasculature, color-flow Doppler is used. A large color flow sampling box should be positioned over most of the near field of the image. A low-flow setting (approximately 20 cm/sec) will detect the MCA in the near field, and the red color signifies blood flow toward the transducer (Fig. 44.5 and Video 44.3).

After identifying the MCA, PWD is used to measure the blood flow velocity within the MCA. The PWD sampling gate is centered over the MCA's red color flow signal (Video 44.4). By convention, spectral Doppler signals found above the baseline are flowing toward the transducer, and signals below the baseline are flowing away from the transducer. The ultrasound beam should be aligned as parallel as possible to the direction of flow for the most accurate measurement of blood flow velocities and angle correction can be used to improve accuracy of velocity measurements.

Image Interpretation

MIDLINE SHIFT

The presence or absence of midline shift can be determined using a two-dimensional, transtemporal image of the third ventricle. The most common technique is to measure the distance from the external temporal bone to the ipsilateral lateral wall of the third ventricle (distance A), then perform the same measurement on the contralateral side (distance B). Normally, distance A equals distance B, but with midline

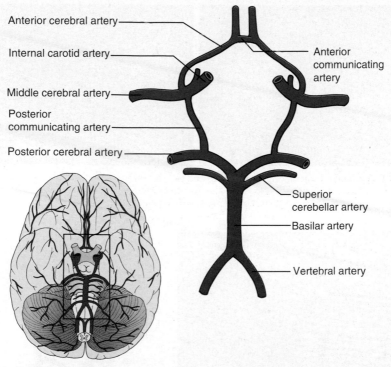

Figure 44.1   Cerebral Circulation. The circle of Willis is shown at the base of the brain. The middle cerebral artery is a key artery in transcranial Doppler imaging, although it is not part of the circle of Willis.

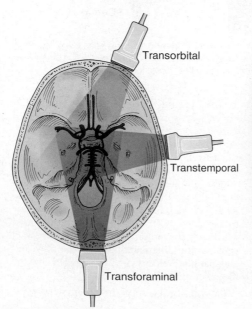

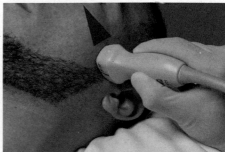

Figure 44.3 Transtemporal Transducer Orientation. Transducer is placed on the pterion of the temporal bone with the transducer orientation marker pointing anteriorly.

Figure 44.2   Transcranial Windows. The three transcranial windows (transorbital, transtemporal, and transforaminal) are shown.

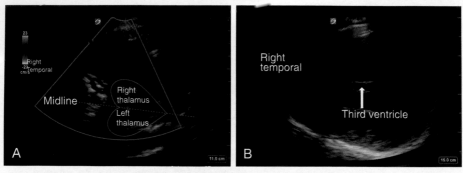

Figure 44.4 Normal Transtemporal Ultrasound image. The midline structures are seen: (A) bilateral thalami that surround the midline and together make a heart shape and (B) third ventricle shown as a thin, midline anechoic stripe flanked by hyperechoic white walls on each side.

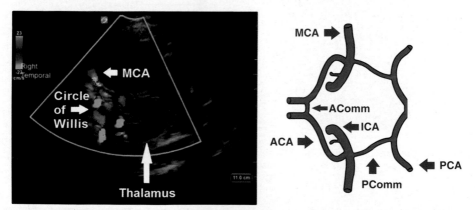

Figure 44.5 Circle of Willis. The circle of Willis and middle cerebral artery *(MCA)*, are seen using color flow Doppler in a transtemporal view. *ACA,* Anterior cerebral artery; *AComm,* anterior communicating artery; *ICA,* internal carotid artery; *PComm,* posterior communicating artery; *PCA,* posterior cerebral artery.

shift, one side will measure greater than the other (Fig. 44.6). The following equation is used to calculate the midline shift deviation:

$$\text{Midline shift} = (\text{distance A} - \text{distance B}) / 2$$

INTRACRANIAL PRESSURE AND CEREBRAL CIRCULATORY ARREST

TCD detects changes in blood flow velocity due to changes in vascular resistance associated with increased ICP. Normally, MCA blood flow velocity shows a steep systolic upstroke with a stepwise deceleration during diastole (Fig. 44.7). Elevated ICP causes external compression of the cerebral vessels resulting in increased resistance to flow. The increased resistance to flow causes a characteristic change

in the spectral Doppler tracing: the MCA velocity has a steep upstroke and is increased during systole and decreased, or blunted, during diastole. When ICP is severely elevated, the diastolic flow may be zero or reversed (Fig. 44.8 and Video 44.5).[6]

Various methods exist to quantify the difference between the increased peak systolic velocity (PSV) and blunted diastolic velocity due to increased ICP. The most commonly used method is the pulsatility index (PI), which is equal to the difference between the PSV and end-diastolic velocity (EDV), divided by the mean velocity (MV)[6]:

$$\text{Pulsatility index (PI)} = [\text{PSV} - \text{EDV}]/\text{MV}$$

The spectral Doppler waveform is used to calculate the PI, and some machines may calculate PI as part of the TCD preset (see Video

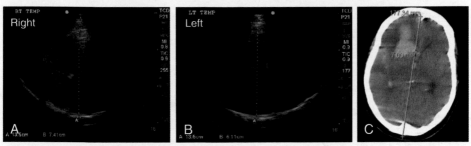

Figure 44.6   Midline Shift Measurement. Using the calipers, the distances between the external temporal bones and right (A) and left (B) lateral walls of the third ventricle are measured. The midline shift is half of the difference in distances, which is 6.5 mm in this patient [(7.41-6.11)/2=0.65 cm]. Computed tomography head confirmed a midline shift of 7 mm toward the left (C).

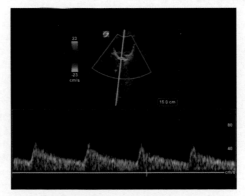

Figure 44.7   Normal Middle Cerebral Artery *(MCA)* Blood Flow. A normal pulsed-wave Doppler tracing of MCA blood flow shows a sharp systolic upstroke with a step-wise diastolic deceleration.

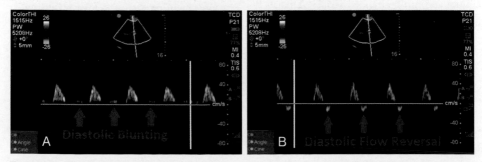

Figure 44.8   Elevated Intracranial Pressure (ICP) and Middle Cerebral Artery Blood Flow. Elevated ICP causes decreased diastolic flow relative to systolic flow with initial diastolic blunting (A) followed by diastolic flow reversal (B) with severely elevated ICP.

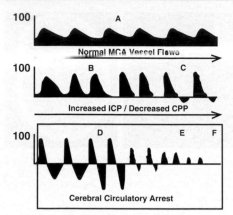

Figure 44.9 Progressive Changes of Increasing Intracranial Pressure *(ICP).* A step-wise progression of increased ICP leads to eventual intracranial cerebral circulatory arrest. (A) Normal systolic upstroke with normal step down of diastolic flow. (B) Increased peak systolic flow with decreasing diastolic flow and eventual blunting of diastolic flow. (C) Peaked systolic flow with diastolic flow reversal. (D) Biphasic or oscillating flow with peaked systolic flow and diastolic flow reversal that approaches equal velocity as systolic flow. (E) Isolated systolic spike flows of <50 cm/s in velocity and <200 msec in duration. (F) Zero flow—where there was previously documented transcranial Doppler flow. The *red* box (D, E, and F) denotes states in which cerebral circulatory arrest can be diagnosed. *CPP,* Cerebral perfusion pressure; *MCA*; middle cerebral artery.

44.4). As the difference between the PSV and the EDV increases, so will the PI. Thus, higher PI values can be associated with higher ICP values and can be trended serially. Though PI values do not correlate exactly with ICP values, in general, a PI value greater than 2 is pathologic, corresponding to an ICP greater than 20 mm Hg.[6]

Serial measurements of TCD are required to diagnose cerebral circulatory arrest and brain death. The progressive stages of cerebral circulatory arrest are illustrated in Fig. 44.9.[4] Because the absence of flow could be due to poor or inappropriate Doppler interrogation, one must be cautious when diagnosing complete cerebral circulatory arrest, unless serial images have shown progressive worsening and the clinical context is appropriate.[12]

PEARLS AND PITFALLS

- The angle of insonation between the ultrasound beam and direction of flow can affect the measurement of blood flow velocity using spectral Doppler ultrasound. An angle of insonation <15 degrees is ideal to avoid underestimating velocities. Most machines include an angle correction feature that should be utilized to maximize accuracy of velocity measurements, though some ultrasound societies advise against using the angle correction feature.
- A goal-directed, point-of-care transcranial Doppler (TCD) exam through the transtemporal window can rule in certain diagnoses, such as midline shift or elevated intracranial pressure (ICP). However, to rule out pathologies, a comprehensive TCD examination with evaluation of all cerebral vessels (anterior cerebral artery, posterior cerebral artery, vertebral, and basilar arteries) using all three TCD windows (transtemporal, transorbital, and transforaminal) is required.
- Diastolic blunting, zero diastolic flow, and diastolic flow reversal using pulsed-wave Doppler are indicative of elevated ICP.
- The pulsatility index (PI) quantifies the difference between increased peak systolic velocity and blunted diastolic velocity using the pulsed-wave Doppler tracing of patients with elevated ICP.
- Although higher PI values correspond to higher ICP values, the exact precision of PI as a surrogate for ICP has shown wide confidence intervals and insertion of an invasive ICP monitor remains the gold standard for patients with elevated ICP.

CHAPTER 45

Skin and Soft Tissues

Michael Y. Woo ■ Elizabeth Lalande

KEY POINTS

- Point-of-care ultrasound can aid in the diagnosis of cellulitis and identify patients with an underlying abscess or necrotizing fasciitis.
- Diagnosis and removal of retained foreign bodies can be guided by use of bedside ultrasound.
- Tendonitis and fracture are two common conditions that can be accurately diagnosed using point-of-care ultrasound.

Background

Ultrasonography of the skin and soft tissues offers providers of all specialties a powerful bedside diagnostic tool for a wide variety of conditions. Interrogation of the skin and soft tissues can diagnose the presence of a broad array of ailments including cellulitis, abscess, foreign bodies, fractures, and tendonitis.[1]

INFECTION

Distinguishing between cellulitis and abscess is a fundamental application of point-of-care ultrasound (POCUS).[2,3] With the high prevalence of methicillin-resistant *Staphylococcus aureus* (MRSA) in the community, presentation of patients with abscesses requiring incision and drainage in emergency departments is increasing.[4] In many circumstances, physical examination is limited in differentiating cellulitis from

abscess, and for those with an abscess, incision and drainage may be delayed. Ultrasound expedites initiation of appropriate management in both adult and pediatric patients with cellulitis with or without abscess by increasing diagnostic accuracy over clinical evaluation.[5-7] If ultrasound confirms nonpurulent cellulitis, a randomized study demonstrated that antibiotic treatment with a single agent without MRSA coverage is adequate.[8,9] When clinical concern for necrotizing fasciitis is present, ultrasonography can be performed rapidly at the bedside to expedite confirmation of diagnosis and initiation of emergent therapy.[10,11]

TENDONITIS AND FRACTURE

Use of bedside ultrasonography to diagnose tendonitis and fractures has increased rapidly due to the availability of less expensive, portable devices that generate high-quality images.[12]

419

A focused ultrasound exam following physical examination has been used to diagnose various tendon pathologies, including tendonitis and tendon rupture or tear.[12,13]

Ultrasound offers a simple and accurate technique to diagnose fractures at the bedside in time-sensitive situations.[14,15] Additionally, it has high diagnostic accuracy for frequently occult fractures, such as rib and sternal fractures.[14,16] When assessing the adequacy of reduction of long bone fractures, a meta-analysis found that POCUS has a sensitivity of 94%–100% and specificity of 56%–100%.[17] Providers seeking to reduce fractures without parenteral sedation may use ultrasound to identify the most appropriate location for the administration of a hematoma block.[18]

FOREIGN BODIES

Retained foreign bodies are common and can be nidi for soft tissue infection. Physical examination is insensitive for detecting foreign bodies, and retained foreign bodies are associated with high medical-legal risk.[19,20] Along with the identification of retained foreign bodies such as wood, metal, or glass,[21] ultrasound can delineate the borders of a foreign body to guide removal.[22]

NEOPLASM

Providers can use ultrasonography to differentiate soft tissue tumors from fluid collections (cysts, abscesses) in patients presenting with a soft tissue nodule. Abnormal findings seen on ultrasound must be considered in clinical context, and additional workup, including imaging or biopsy of the lesion, should be obtained if a neoplasm is suspected.[23] Most importantly, providers can avoid attempting an incision and drainage of a solid soft tissue nodule, or vascular lesion, that was mistaken for an abscess or cyst based on physical examination.

Image Acquisition

A high-frequency linear-array transducer (5 to 12 MHz) should be used to provide the best resolution when imaging the skin and soft tissues. When visualizing structures deeper than 4 cm, a high-frequency transducer may not provide adequate penetration, and a low-frequency curvilinear transducer may be preferred. For example, a low-frequency transducer is often required to visualize a deep abscess over the femur in an obese adult patient.

When imaging an open wound with suspected infection, it is recommended to cover the transducer with a barrier, such as a disposable plastic sheath, to minimize contamination of the transducer with potentially resistant bacteria. Gel should be placed inside the barrier. A copious amount of gel minimizes the amount of pressure required to maintain contact between the transducer and skin, thereby decreasing patient discomfort during the examination. After every ultrasound examination, the transducer must be cleaned with approved antiseptic wipes per local protocol.

The area of interest should be evaluated with ultrasound methodically and systematically. Orthogonal views (i.e., longitudinal and transverse views) should be obtained of the area of interest to elucidate the surrounding tissue anatomy. Important surrounding structures, such as blood vessels, nerves, and lymph nodes, should be identified. Dimensions of fluid collections should be measured in two planes, along with depth of collections. Compressibility may help differentiate fluid collections from solid lesions. Color flow Doppler and power Doppler can be used to evaluate the vascularity of the area of interest and identify surrounding vessels to avoid if incision and drainage is planned.

In adult and pediatric patients, a water-bath method may be used for sonographic evaluation of superficial structures of the extremities, such as fingers. A water bath provides an acoustic standoff to place the area of interest within the focal zone of the ultrasound beam and improve image resolution.[24,25] Further, a water bath (Videos 45.1–45.3) decreases discomfort by avoiding direct contact of the transducer with the skin, provides a large field of view that is unaffected by the contour of the extremity, and allows real-time dynamic evaluation of the affected tendons or joints with visualization of the entire region during a dynamic maneuver.

Pathologic Findings

CELLULITIS, SUBCUTANEOUS ABSCESS, AND NECROTIZING FASCIITIS

Normal areas should be compared to abnormal areas with suspected pathology (Fig. 45.1 and

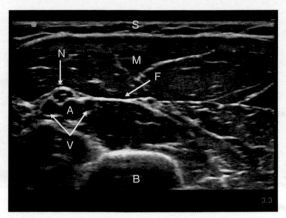

Figure 45.1   Normal Skin and Soft Tissues. Normal soft tissues and bone of the upper arm are shown: subcutaneous tissue *(S)*, biceps muscle *(M)*, fascia *(F)*, median nerve *(N)*, brachial artery *(A)*, brachial veins *(V)*, and humerus bone *(B)*.

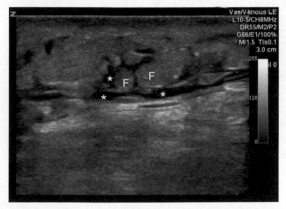

Figure 45.2   Cobblestoning. Cellulitis has a "cobblestone" pattern due to subcutaneous edema. *asterisks*, areas of edema; *F*, subcutaneous fat.

Video 45.4). Initially, cellulitis will result in thickening of the subcutaneous layer. As cellulitis progresses, subcutaneous edema increases and appears as a "cobblestone" pattern (Fig. 45.2 and Video 45.5). This is a result of edema forming around subcutaneous fat globules and connective tissue. Color flow Doppler may highlight areas of hyperemia due to inflammation (Fig. 45.3). It is important to recognize that cobblestoning is a nonspecific sign of subcutaneous edema, and diagnosing cellulitis requires other clinical signs, such as erythema, tenderness, or leukocytosis.

Ultrasound appearance of abscess contents can vary from anechoic to hyperechoic, but all abscesses typically exhibit posterior acoustic enhancement (see Chapter 6: Artifacts) (Fig. 45.4

and Video 45.6). A hyperechoic rim often surrounds abscesses with some hyperemia demonstrated by color flow Doppler. Absence of flow centrally within a suspected abscess ensures that the anechoic area is not a vascular structure, such as a pseudoaneurysm. Compression of an abscess may cause swirling of pus to be visualized sonographically (Videos 45.7 and 45.8).

In clinically suspected cases of necrotizing fasciitis, availability of bedside ultrasound can confirm the diagnosis and expedite care. The presence of air within soft tissues is pathognomonic for necrotizing fasciitis. Air creates multiple comet-tail artifacts that create dirty shadows and obscure visualization of deep structures (Fig. 45.5 and Video 45.9). In addition, fluid along the deep fascia greater than 5 mm in

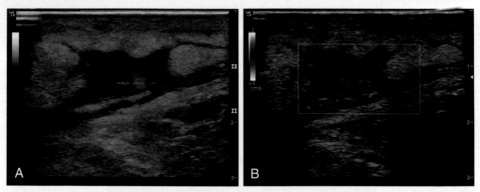

Figure 45.3 (A) Abscess. (B) Color flow Doppler demonstrating hyperemia surrounding the abscess cavity.

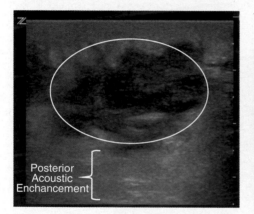

Figure 45.4 Skin Abscess. The abscess cavity *(oval)* is filled with pus and posterior acoustic enhancement is seen in the far field.

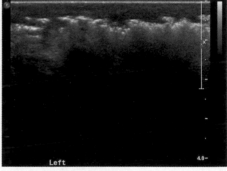

Figure 45.5 Necrotizing Fasciitis. Hyperechoic areas in the near field represent trapped air within the soft tissue that creates dirty shadows.

thickness may be an early sonographic sign of necrotizing fasciitis. The STAFF (Subcutaneous Thickening, Air, and Fascial Fluid) mnemonic can be used to help remember the characteristics of necrotizing fasciitis on ultrasound.[26]

TENDONITIS

Normal tendons appear as discrete fibrillar structures (Video 45.10). Tendonitis is seen on ultrasound as thickened, hypoechoic areas as a result of edema within the tendon (Fig. 45.6, Video 45.11). It is important to recognize that a hypoechoic area of tendon may result from anisotropy rather than actual pathology, particularly at tendon insertion points. Anisotropy occurs when tendons are visualized at an oblique angle.[12] Hypoechoic areas created by anisotropy disappear by tilting the transducer

and changing the angle of insonation. Therefore, tendons should be visualized in orthogonal planes, especially when pathology is suspected (Fig. 45.7 and Video 45.12).

FRACTURE

The outer cortex of bone appears as a hyperechoic line and casts a shadow (Fig. 45.8 and Video 45.13). Disruption of the hyperechoic cortical line represents a fracture and is best visualized in a longitudinal plane (Figs. 45.9 and 45.10; Video 45.14). Reverberation artifact can sometimes appear in a longitudinal plane, and determining which hyperechoic line is bone versus artifact may be difficult. Turning the probe to a transverse plane and noting the depth of the cortex helps determine which hyperechoic line represents bone.

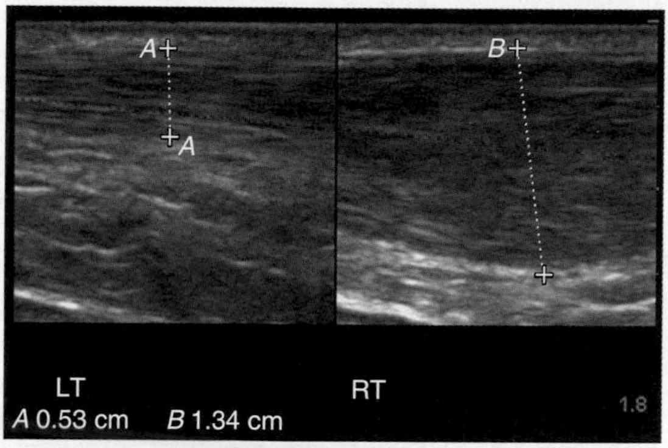

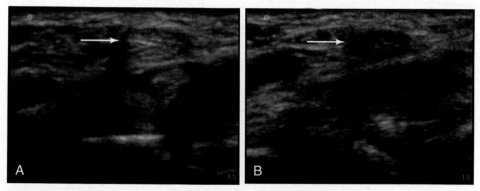

Figure 45.6 Tendonitis. Comparison of a normal Achilles tendon *(left)* with Achilles tendonitis *(right)* in a longitudinal view. Note the hypoechoic areas within the Achilles tendon *(right)* demonstrating edema, as well as increased overall thickness, when compared with the normal Achilles tendon *(left)*.

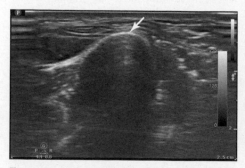
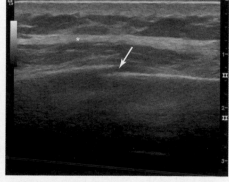

Figure 45.7 Anisotropy. The echogenicity of a superficial wrist tendon *(arrow)* changes from hyperechoic (A) to hypoechoic (B) by tilting the transducer and changing the angle of insonation.

Figure 45.8 Normal Bone. The hyperechoic cortical line *(arrow)* of a bone and its shadow are seen.

Figure 45.9 Rib Fracture. An abrupt disruption of the smooth cortical line of a rib denotes a fracture. *asterisk*, fascia; *arrow*, fracture.

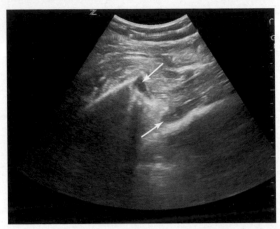

Figure 45.10   Femur Fracture. Comminuted femur fracture is demonstrated using a low-frequency curvilinear transducer. *arrows*, fracture.

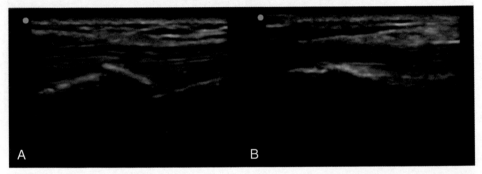

Figure 45.11   Fracture Reduction. A distal radius fracture is seen prereduction (A), and postreduction (B).

For ultrasound-guided reduction of long bone fractures, the fracture should be visualized in two planes prior to attempting a reduction. Postreduction ultrasound images can be compared to pre-reduction ultrasound images (Fig. 45.11) until a satisfactory angulation and step-off reduction is obtained.[17] Ultrasound may be used to identify the appropriate location for the administration of a hematoma block prior to fracture reduction (Video 45.15).

FOREIGN BODY

Ultrasound can often detect foreign bodies within soft tissues missed by physical examination. Radiopaque foreign bodies, such as metal, are relatively easy to identify because they appear hyperechoic and create shadowing and reverberation artifact (Video 45.16).

Radiolucent foreign bodies, such as wood, and small foreign bodies (<5 mm) are more challenging to identify due to size and lack of artifacts to assist with identification. It is important to visualize any suspected foreign body in both transverse and longitudinal planes.

When foreign bodies are very superficial, they may be located too close to the transducer to be visualized. To minimize this effect, a standoff pad can be used (Fig. 45.12). For extremities, a water bath has been shown to increase the accuracy of ultrasonography to detect foreign bodies.[27] An extremity is placed in a pool of water and the transducer is suspended in the water without direct contact with the skin (Video 45.17).

If uncertainty exists regarding whether a foreign body is present, local anesthetic can be injected around the suspected foreign

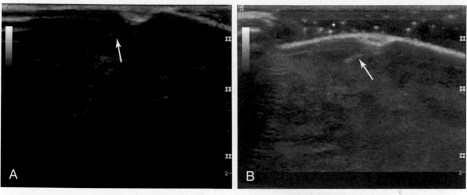

Figure 45.12 Foreign Body. (A) A retained piece of wood *(arrow)* is seen without a gel standoff pad. (B) Using a gel standoff pad *(asterisk)*, visualization of the retained wood *(arrow)* is improved.

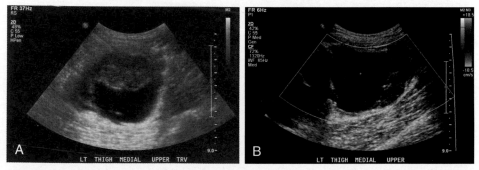

Figure 45.13 Soft Tissue Thigh Mass. (A) A palpable soft tissue mass of the left thigh in a transverse plane. Note the mixed echogenicity. Biopsy confirmed a myxoma. (B) Color flow Doppler of the soft tissue mass demonstrates absence of flow within the mass.

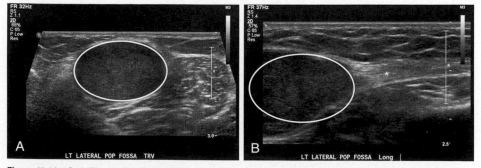

Figure 45.14 Soft Tissue Popliteal Mass. Soft tissue mass arising from the nerves in the popliteal fossa is seen in transverse (A) and longitudinal (B) planes. *asterisk*, peroneal nerve.

body, which enhances its appearance. Care must be taken not to inject any air, since this will obscure visualization of the area. Various normal and pathological structures, such as sesamoid bones and calcified scar tissue, can also be mistaken for foreign bodies, resulting in false positives.[28]

SOFT TISSUE MASS

Ultrasound findings must always be interpreted while considering the clinical presentation. Occasionally, atypical ultrasound findings, such as mixed echogenicity or irregular-shaped masses arising from nerves or muscle, may be encountered (Figs. 45.13 and 45.14). If ultrasound findings are suspicious for a soft tissue mass, then additional imaging should be obtained with either comprehensive ultrasonography, computed tomography (CT) or magnetic resonance imaging (MRI), before performing any invasive procedure at the bedside.

PEARLS AND PITFALLS

- High-frequency transducers are preferred for imaging skin and soft tissues, but low-frequency transducers may be needed to evaluate obese patients or deep structures.
- Cobblestoning is seen with any condition that causes subcutaneous edema and is not specific for cellulitis. Diagnosing cellulitis requires other supporting clinical signs (erythema, tenderness, leukocytosis) in addition to cobblestoning.
- Using color flow Doppler can highlight the hyperemia that typically surrounds an abscess and differentiates an abscess from surrounding vessels. Swirling of pus may be seen with compression of an abscess.
- Anisotropy of tendons can be mistaken for edema, leading to a misdiagnosis of tendonitis. Imaging tendons in multiple planes and tilting the transducer can help differentiate anisotropy from tendonitis.
- Use a gel standoff pad or water bath to improve resolution of superficial tissues when evaluating for retained foreign bodies.

CHAPTER 46

Joints

Sahar Janjua ■ Chan Kim ■ Eugene Kissin

KEY POINTS

- Understanding joint anatomy is key to efficient and accurate ultrasound imaging. Bone landmarks are critical to guide transducer placement and identification of soft tissue structures by ultrasound.
- Diagnostically, musculoskeletal ultrasound has advanced beyond demonstration of fluid collections in or around joints and is now used for identification of subclinical joint inflammation and erosion, as well as prediction of joint damage progression.
- Therapeutically, substantial evidence supports the use of ultrasound guidance for joint and soft tissue aspiration and injection.

Background

Musculoskeletal ultrasound has become increasingly prevalent in hospitals and clinics to aid in diagnosis and guide bedside procedures.[1-4] Advantages of musculoskeletal ultrasound as a diagnostic tool include immediate availability of high-resolution images, avoidance of ionizing radiation exposure, and minimization of patient discomfort.[5,6] Disadvantages include a relatively limited field of view compared to other imaging modalities, lack of visualization of deep structures due to shadowing from bones, and diagnostic accuracy that is dependent on operator skills.[7] The American Institute of Ultrasound in Medicine (AIUM), in collaboration with the American College of Radiology, has developed guidelines for the use of musculoskeletal ultrasound,[8,9] which include pathologies of joints, tendons, ligaments, soft tissues, and nerves. The American College of Rheumatology has published an evidence-based review of ultrasound to evaluate musculoskeletal conditions, such as arthrocentesis, intra-articular joint injections, aspiration of cysts or abscesses, and synovial biopsies.[10] This chapter reviews the normal ultrasound appearance of large joints, common

joint pathologies, and ultrasound-guided joint injection techniques.

Special Considerations

ANISOTROPY

Anisotropy is a common imaging artifact seen in musculoskeletal ultrasound and is defined as exhibition of properties with *different values* when measured in *different directions*.[11] Anisotropy is encountered when the ultrasound beam is not perpendicular to the plane of the structure being imaged, resulting in artifactual hypoechogenicity of the structure.[12] Reflective fibrous structures, primarily tendons and ligaments, exhibit more anisotropy than nerves or muscles. Thus, tendons are hyperechoic when imaged perpendicularly but may appear hypoechoic or even anechoic when imaged at an oblique angle, leading to potential misinterpretation of a tendon as a fluid collection. Experienced providers can use anisotropy to help differentiate normal tendons from other tissues by tilting the transducer and watching the tendon change from hyperechoic to hypoechoic compared to surrounding structures (Video 46.1).[13] Due to anisotropy and

427

other ultrasound artifacts, it is imperative to evaluate all potential abnormalities in both longitudinal and transverse planes (orthogonal planes) to reduce the risk of mistaking an artifact for pathology.

DOPPLER SETTINGS

The Doppler effect is defined as a shift in frequency of sound waves resulting from motion of the source, receiver, or reflector.[1,14] Doppler ultrasound is used in musculoskeletal ultrasound to identify increased tissue perfusion due to inflammation, in particular synovial inflammation.[15,16]

For the applications reviewed in this chapter, color or power Doppler modes are used exclusively (see Chapter 2 for a review of Doppler modes). Important color Doppler parameters include pulse repetition frequency (PRF), wall filter, and gain. The PRF represents the number of pulses emitted by the transducer per unit time. Lowering the PRF allows more time for the transducer to listen for returning echoes and increases the sensitivity for low flow states, such as perfusion of synovial tissue. The ideal PRF range for musculoskeletal ultrasound is between 0.5 and 1 kHz,[17] which is lower than the PRF for vascular Doppler exams. A wall filter is used to minimize effects of arterial pulsation on Doppler signal. The small synovial vessels have essentially no pulsatile wall motion, and therefore the wall filter should be minimized to optimize Doppler sensitivity. However, if the wall filter is set too low, "flash" artifact may be seen in the Doppler box from minimal transducer movements, obscuring the true Doppler signal.[14] In Doppler mode, gain regulates amplification of Doppler signals returning from tissues. When using color Doppler, adjust the gain by first increasing it until artifactual color Doppler signal is seen and then steadily decrease the gain until the artifactual Doppler signal disappears (Video 46.2).[17]

IMAGE ORIENTATION

In musculoskeletal ultrasound imaging, images have traditionally been oriented with the left side of the screen displaying medial or proximal structures and the right side displaying lateral or distal structures. In contrast, the left side of the screen in most point-of-care ultrasound imaging displays proximal structures or structures to the operator's left, regardless

of how the operator is facing the patient. Throughout this chapter, the traditional musculoskeletal ultrasound image orientation is followed with the left screen displaying medial/proximal structures and the right screen displaying lateral/distal structures.

Image Acquisition

The ultrasound machine should be positioned in front of the provider with the body part being scanned in between the provider and ultrasound screen to minimize head turning. Most musculoskeletal ultrasound exams are performed with a linear-array transducer, except for hip exams, which require the wider field of view and deeper penetration of a curvilinear transducer. In general, use the highest frequency that allows visualization of the bone surface. A frequency of 12 to 18 MHz is typically used for digits and wrists, 10 to 12 MHz for ankles, elbows, and knees, and 8 to 12 MHz for shoulders and hips.

SHOULDER

Nine standard views of the shoulder can identify the most common pathologies of the rotator cuff and biceps, acromioclavicular joint, and glenohumeral joint. The provider stands either in front of or behind the patient while the patient is in a seated position. Each view described next corresponds with Fig. 46.1.

1 Biceps Transverse View

Technique: Patient is sitting with the hand palm up on the thigh directly in front of shoulder. The transducer is horizontal with the greater tuberosity laterally and lesser tuberosity medially. Externally rotate the arm to evaluate for biceps subluxation (Video 46.3).

Findings: In a transverse plane, the biceps tendon is seen between the humeral tuberosities. The transducer angle should be adjusted to maximize echogenicity to identify any tendinopathy or tendon sheath effusion. Slide the transducer distally to the level of the pectoralis major insertion to avoid missing a biceps tendon tear.

1b Biceps Longitudinal View

Technique: Patient is sitting with the hand palm up on the thigh directly in front of the shoulder. Place the transducer vertically between the greater and lesser tuberosities. Press firmly with the distal transducer edge to position the transducer parallel to the tendon fibers to reduce anisotropy.

Findings: In a longitudinal plane, do not mistake the peribiceps tendon fat for the tendon itself—the fat does not have a fibrillar pattern like the tendon. Increased Doppler signal of the biceps sheath suggests inflammatory tenosynovitis. A recurrent branch of the anterior circumflex humeral artery runs lateral to the tendon sheath and should not be mistaken for hyperemia.

2 Subscapularis Longitudinal View

Technique: Patient is sitting, hand palm up, shoulder maximally externally rotated. Place the transducer horizontally over the lesser tuberosity.

Findings: Focus on the subscapularis tendon insertion site on the lesser tuberosity and that of the infraspinatus on the greater tuberosity. External rotation of the arm with slight translation of the transducer medially brings the subscapularis into view (see Video 46.3), whereas internal rotation of the arm with lateral translation of the transducer brings the infraspinatus into view.

2b Subscapularis Transverse View

Technique: Patient is sitting, hand palm up, shoulder maximally externally rotated. Place the transducer vertically over the lesser tuberosity.

Findings: Focus on the subscapularis tendon insertion site on the lesser tuberosity. The subscapularis tendon has a multipennate appearance—do not mistake this appearance for tendon injury.

3 Infraspinatus View

Technique: Patient is sitting with arm internally rotated across body. Transducer is placed horizontally over the lateral shoulder including the posterior edge of the greater tuberosity.

Findings: Focus on the infraspinatus tendon insertion site. The infraspinatus tendon can be followed posteriorly until the glenohumeral joint is reached with the transducer horizontal. Increase the depth setting and decrease the frequency until the bone contour is well visualized.

4 Glenohumeral View

Technique: Patient is sitting with the arm externally rotated. The glenohumeral joint is reached by following the infraspinatus tendon posteriorly with the transducer horizontal. The transducer is horizontal, posterior, parallel to the spine of the scapula, and centered over the humeral head, glenoid, and labrum.

Findings: The most sensitive region for showing shoulder joint effusion in a sitting patient is the caudal portion of the joint. Complete external rotation of the arm while viewing the posterior aspect of the glenohumeral joint

Anterior Left Shoulder

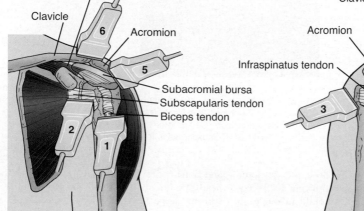

Posterior Left Shoulder

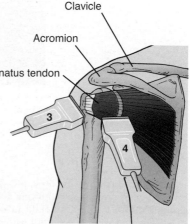

Supraspinatus tendon

Clavicle

6

Acromion

5

Subacromial bursa
Subscapularis tendon
Biceps tendon

2

1

Clavicle

Acromion

Infraspinatus tendon

3

4

Figure 46.1   Shoulder Ultrasound Examination.

Continued

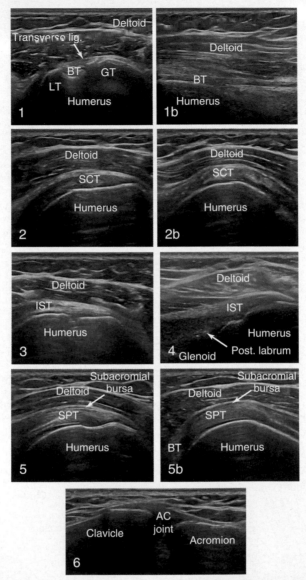

Figure 46.1, cont'd *1*, Biceps transverse view. *1b*, Biceps longitudinal view. *2*, Subscapularis longitudinal view. *2b*, Subscapularis transverse view. *3*, Infraspinatus view. *4*, Glenohumeral longitudinal view. *5*, Supraspinatus longitudinal view in Crass position. *5b*, Supraspinatus transverse view in modified Crass position. *6*, Acromioclavicular *(AC)* joint view. *BT*, Biceps tendon; *GT*, greater tubercle; *IST*, infraspinatus tendon; *lig.*, ligament; *LT*, lesser tubercle; *post.*, posterior; *SCT*, subscapularis tendon; *SPT*, supraspinatus tendon.

maximizes sensitivity for detection of joint effusion, with prior studies showing 100% sensitivity (30/30) for 8 mL of fluid in this position compared with 17% (5/30) with the arm in neutral position (Video 46.4, Video 46.5, Video 46.6).[18,19] The labrum, synovial capsule, and bone contours of the glenoid and humeral head should all be visualized. Normally, the labrum appears triangular shaped and is attached to the glenoid (Video 46.7). A torn labrum detaches from the glenoid with rotation of the arm (Video 46.8).

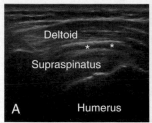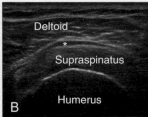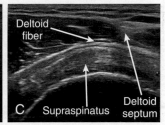

Figure 46.2   Subacromial Bursa. The supraspinatus tendon and distended subacromial bursa *(asterisks)* are demonstrated in longitudinal (A) and transverse (B) views. (C) Supraspinatus tendon in transverse view with some common imaging pitfalls: hypoechoic deltoid fiber can be mistaken for the subacromial bursa (the actual bursa is deep to it); deltoid septum casts a shadow on the supraspinatus, which could be mistaken for tendinosis or tear of the supraspinatus.

5 Supraspinatus Longitudinal View

Technique: Put the patient's arm in a "Crass" position (arm is maximally internally rotated with the dorsal surface of the hand on the mid-back), or "modified Crass" position (hand is in the back pocket with the elbow pointed posteriorly). The transducer is placed vertically over the tip of the greater tuberosity. To align the transducer parallel with the supraspinatus tendon, rotate the transducer to point the transducer orientation marker toward the acromion for the Crass position or toward the ear for the modified Crass position.

Findings: The supraspinatus tendon can be visualized in either the Crass or modified Crass position. Both of these positions help bring the supraspinatus out from under the acromion. The Crass or modified Crass position longitudinal views of the supraspinatus tendon should include visualization of the bone contour of the round, articular portion of the humeral head transitioning into the flat "footprint" portion of the greater tuberosity. As the supraspinatus fibers transition into infraspinatus fibers laterally, the bone transition becomes flat.[20] The supraspinatus fibers curve at their insertion onto the greater tuberosity creating anisotropy—the most common cause of a false-positive diagnosis of tendon tear.[21] Press in with the distal tip of the transducer to maximally brighten the distal tendon fibers (Fig. 46.2).

5b Supraspinatus Transverse View

Technique: Patient's arm is put in a Crass or modified Crass position (see above). The transducer is placed horizontally for a Crass

position or obliquely aligned with the xiphoid process for a modified Crass position.

Findings: The supraspinatus tendon should have similar thickness medially and laterally. If the tendon appears thin on one side of the screen, then the transducer is likely positioned oblique to the tendon. Visualization of the biceps tendon medial to the supraspinatus in a modified Crass transverse view ensures visualization of the most medial fibers of the supraspinatus, the fibers at greatest risk of injury. A potential pitfall is mistaking the shadow cast by the deltoid septum for a tear of the supraspinatus tendon in a transverse view, but orthogonal views should clarify this issue. In addition, the hypoechoic deep muscle fibers of the deltoid can be mistaken for the subacromial bursa (see Fig. 46.2; Video 46.9).[21]

6 Acromioclavicular Joint View

Technique: Position the patient sitting with the arm at the side. The transducer is horizontal and moved to the top of the shoulder across the clavicle and acromion to visualize the acromioclavicular joint.

Findings: Asymptomatic acromioclavicular joint capsule distention and osteophytes are common in older age groups.

ELBOW

Five standard views of the elbow are obtained to identify common flexor and extensor tendon origins, joint capsule, synovium, humerus, and ulna. The provider should sit in front of the patient. Arm extension is needed for anterior views, whereas 45 to 90 degrees of flexion is needed for other views. Each view described next corresponds with Fig. 46.3.

1 Antorior Longitudinal View

Technique: Patient is sitting with the elbow extended. Place the transducer anterior, vertically over the capitulum (distal lateral humerus), and sweep medially to a position over the trochlea (distal medial humerus). View the proximal joint capsule as well as the "seagull" over the joint cleft.

Findings: In a longitudinal view, the anterior elbow joint capsule will have a "seagull" appearance between the capitulum of the humerus and the radial head. The tissue in the joint cleft is the seagull's body, and the capsule spread over the bone to either side makes the wings. The "seagull" appearance disappears with a joint effusion because the capsule is pushed out of the joint cleft. The medial, humeroulnar portion of the joint is marked by the sharp, triangular coronoid process of the ulna, whereas the lateral, humeroradial portion of the joint has a square radial head.

1b Anterior Transverse View

Technique: With the elbow extended, place the transducer anterior, horizontally across the capitulum and trochlea of the distal humerus. Start over the hyaline cartilage–covered distal humerus, and sweep over the joint recess.

Findings: In a transverse plane, the hyaline coverage of the distal humerus has a "w" appearance. The transducer should be swept proximally from this point to the radial and coronoid fossae to avoid missing an effusion.

2 Lateral Longitudinal View

Technique: The elbow is flexed 90 degrees and internally rotated. The transducer is placed on the lateral epicondyle along the longitudinal plane of the common extensor tendons. Image the extensor tendon fibers rather than muscle.

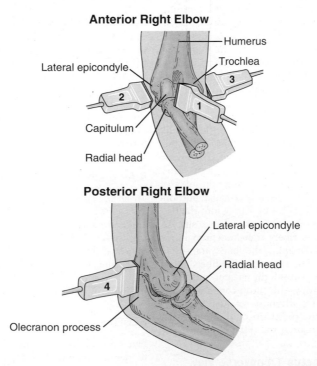

Figure 46.3 Elbow Ultrasound Examination. *1*, Anterior longitudinal view. *1b*, Anterior transverse view. *2*, Lateral longitudinal view. *3*, Medial longitudinal view. *4*, Posterior longitudinal view. *4b*, Posterior transverse view. *f*, Fossa; *lat*, lateral; *med*, medial; *p*, process; *ten*, tendon; *white arrows*, joint capsule; *yellow arrow*, joint cleft.

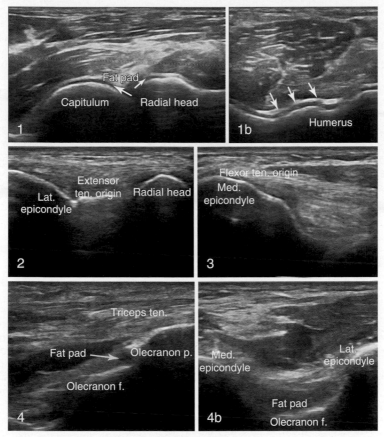

Figure 46.3, cont'd

Findings: The capsule of the joint appears just deep to the extensor tendon origin.

3 Medial Longitudinal View

Technique: The elbow is extended to 45 degrees and externally rotated to avoid awkward patient positioning. The transducer is placed longitudinally over the medial epicondyle.

Findings: The flexor tendon origin is seen with a relatively short tendon band. Medial collateral ligament tears can be visualized in this view.

4 Posterior Longitudinal View

Technique: Posterior views of the elbow are obtained with the elbow flexed at 90 degrees, internally rotated, and resting on the examining

table with the olecranon just off the edge of the table. The transducer is placed posterior, vertically from the olecranon across the olecranon fossa.

Findings: The posterior olecranon fossa is the most sensitive space to find an elbow joint effusion with ultrasound.[22] Erosions are commonly seen just proximal to the triceps insertion on the olecranon process. Keep in mind that the olecranon bursa is easily compressed by transducer pressure, and floating the transducer on a layer of gel will help avoid missing a small effusion.

4b Posterior Transverse View

Technique: The patient position is the same as the posterior longitudinal view. Place the

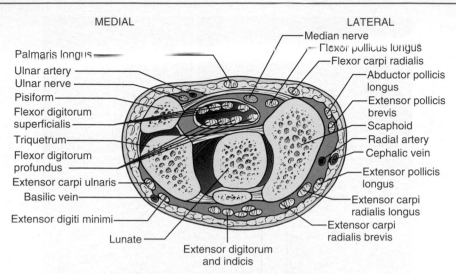

MEDIAL   LATERAL

Palmaris longus

Ulnar artery
Ulnar nerve
Pisiform
Flexor digitorum
superficialis
Triquetrum
Flexor digitorum
profundus
Extensor carpi ulnaris
Basilic vein
Extensor digiti minimi
Lunate

Median nerve
Flexor pollicus longus
Flexor carpi radialis
Abductor pollicis
longus
Extensor pollicis
brevis
Scaphoid
Radial artery
Cephalic vein
Extensor pollicis
longus
Extensor carpi
radialis longus
Extensor carpi
radialis brevis

Extensor digitorum
and indicis

Figure 46.4   Wrist Cross-Sectional Anatomy.

transducer posterior, horizontally over the olecranon fossa. Sweep the transducer through the olecranon fossa.

Findings: The posterior olecranon fossa is the most sensitive space to find an elbow joint effusion with ultrasound.[22]

WRIST

Eight standard views of the wrist exist to visualize the flexor and extensor tendons, joint compartments, and median nerve. The patient sits in front of the provider, with the palm pronated or supinated depending on the desired view. Excessive transducer pressure should not be applied to avoid missing fluid in the dorsal, medial, or lateral flexor tendon sheaths. A cross-sectional figure of the wrist is shown in Fig. 46.4, and each wrist view described below corresponds with Fig. 46.5.

1 Dorsal Transverse View

Technique: Position the hand palm down in a neutral position. Place the transducer horizontally across the wrist with one edge over Lister's tubercle and the other edge over the ulna. Slide from Lister's tubercle, through the scapholunate ligament, to the capitate. This view allows assessment of the dorsal tendons and can detect a disruption of the scapholunate ligament (Video 46.10).

Findings: When scanning the dorsal wrist, maintain a neutral position because extension

can lead to mistaking normal synovium for synovial hypertrophy. The normal extensor retinaculum of the dorsal wrist can be hypoechoic due to anisotropy and should not be mistaken for tenosynovitis.[23] Providers should remember that normal Doppler signal in the distal dorsal wrist from the carpal arch should not be mistaken for synovitis.

2 Dorsal Longitudinal View

Technique: The transducer is placed longitudinally over the center of the wrist (just ulnar to Lister's tubercle) and in line with the third metacarpal. Slide the transducer to both sides from this orientation.

Findings: Identify the radius, lunate, and capitate, and evaluate the joint capsule. The wrist should be in neutral position because synovial tissue will look more prominent if the wrist is extended. The lunate receives blood through a dorsal artery from the dorsal radiocarpal arch[24]; this vessel can be identified with color flow Doppler and should not be mistaken for an erosion. In addition, ulnar impaction syndrome can cause cystic changes to the ulnar aspect of the proximal lunate, which could be mistaken for an erosion.[25]

3 and 3b Radial Longitudinal and Transverse Views

Technique: Position the hand with the wrist rotated with the radial side up. Place the transducer longitudinally over the distal radius,

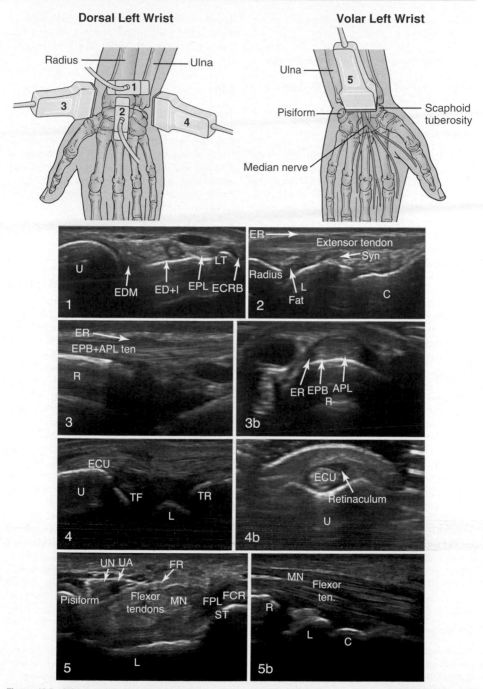

Figure 46.5 Wrist Ultrasound Examination. *1*, Dorsal transverse view. *2*, Dorsal longitudinal view. *3*, Radial longitudinal view. *3b*, Radial transverse view. *4*, Ulnar longitudinal view. *4b*, Ulnar transverse view. *5*, Volar transverse view. *5b*, Volar longitudinal view. *APL*, Abductor pollicis longus; *C*, capitate; *ECRB*, extensor carpi radialis brevis; *ECU*, extensor carpi ulnaris; *ED+I*, extensor digitorum and indicis; *EDM*, extensor digiti minimi; *EPB*, extensor pollicis brevis; *EPL*, extensor pollicis longus; *ER*, extensor retinaculum; *Fat*, normal joint fat/fibrous connective tissue; *FCR*, flexor carpi radialis; *FPL*, flexor pollicis longus; *FR*, flexor retinaculum; *L*, lunate; *LT*, Lister's tubercle; *MN*, median nerve; *R*, radius; *ST*, scaphoid tuberosity; *Syn*, normal synovial reflection; *TF*, triangular fibrocartilage; *TR*, triquetrum; *U*, ulna.; *UA*, ulnar artery; *UN*, ulnar nerve.

then rotate the transducer 90 degrees to obtain a transverse view.

Findings: Evaluate the first compartment tendons (extensor pollicis brevis and abductor pollicis longus). Radial views are most useful for evaluation of de Quervain's tendonitis (see "Pathologic Findings" below).

4 and 4b Ulnar Longitudinal and Transverse Views

Technique: Position the patient with the elbow flexed, and the hand and the wrist in a neutral position, slightly radially angled. Place the transducer longitudinally over the distal ulna, extensor carpi ulnaris (ECU), and triangular fibrocartilage. Rotate the transducer 90 degrees and place it over the ECU tendon in the ulnar sulcus to obtain transverse views.

Findings: Ulnar views are aimed at pathology of the ECU tendon, tenosynovium, and ulnar styloid, as well as the triangular fibrocartilage complex. In a longitudinal view, evaluate the triangular fibrocartilage complex for chondrocalcinosis. The ECU tendon can be evaluated for tenosynovitis, and ulnar erosions can be detected in transverse views.

5 Volar Transverse View

Technique: Position the hand with the palm up, slightly palmar flexed. Place the transducer horizontally from the scaphoid tuberosity to the pisiform. Tilt the transducer to view the median nerve.

Findings: Volar views are dedicated to evaluation of the median nerve, flexor tendons, and volar aspects of the wrist joint. The pisiform and scaphoid tuberosity are used as landmarks to identify the carpal tunnel. The median nerve is measured with the transducer perpendicular to the nerve axis, otherwise the cross-sectional nerve area may be falsely increased. The transducer should be angled to maximize brightness of the flexor tendons and epineurial lining of the median nerve to differentiate median nerve from flexor tendons.

5b Volar Longitudinal View

Technique: Position the hand with the palm up, slightly palmar flexed. Place the transducer longitudinally along the median nerve. Visualize the median nerve superficially and the radius, lunate, and capitate deep.

Findings: The flexor tendons and median nerve are seen superficially, and wrist bones are seen deeper. The wrist joint can be evaluated for volar synovitis. Sliding the transducer distally from the palm allows visualization of each flexor tendon and dynamic imaging can differentiate normal (Video 46.11) from abnormal flexor tendon sliding (Video 46.12).

HIP

Three standard views of the hip are obtained to visualize the hip joint capsule, iliopsoas tendons, gluteal tendons, and trochanteric bursa region. Deeper penetration is required to visualize the hip joint, and either a curvilinear transducer or virtual curvilinear setting on a linear transducer is used. Each view described next corresponds with Fig. 46.6.

1 and 1b Anterior Longitudinal and Transverse Views

Technique: Position the patient supine with the leg externally rotated by 15 degrees. The transducer is placed medial to the greater trochanter and below the inguinal ligament along a line between the anterior superior iliac spine and the superior patellar pole. Longitudinal views are obtained with the transducer vertical, and transverse views are obtained with the transducer horizontal. For an anterior longitudinal view, press in ("heel-toe") with the distal edge of the transducer to position it as parallel as possible to the portion of the joint capsule overlying the femoral head–neck junction.

Findings: Visualize the femoral head and neck, and joint recess and capsule. The joint capsule has to be clearly visualized to be able to detect a hip effusion deep to the capsule or an iliopsoas bursal effusion superficial to the capsule. Effusions in the hip joint should be suspected when the capsule is distended more than 7 mm, or 1 mm more than the asymptomatic side. This is the best hip view for joint aspiration. In addition, when the capsule is curved away from the concave femoral head–neck junction, an effusion or synovitis should be suspected.[26] Early avascular necrosis presents with hip pain and a noninflammatory hip effusion visible on ultrasound 65% of the time[27] but without visible changes to the bone contour. A herniation pit from femoroacetabular impingement could be mistaken for an erosion.[28] Iliopsoas bursitis appears as an anechoic fluid collection superficial to the joint capsule.

2 Lateral Longitudinal View

Technique: Lateral views are obtained with the patient in a lateral decubitus position with the

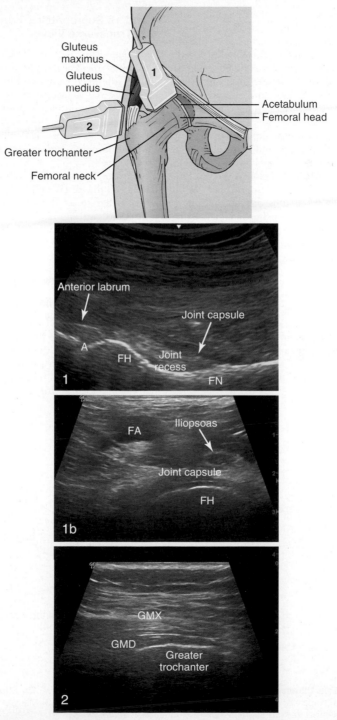

Figure 46.6 Hip Ultrasound Examination. *1,* Anterior longitudinal view. *1b,* Anterior transverse view. *2,* Lateral longitudinal view. *A,* Acetabulum; *FA,* femoral artery; *FH,* femoral head; *FN,* femoral neck; *GMD,* gluteus medius tendon; *GMX,* gluteus maximus muscle.

hip partially flexed. Place the transducer longitudinally over the greater trochanter, along the plane of the gluteus medius. The "peak" of the greater trochanter separates the gluteus minimus anteriorly from the gluteus medius posteriorly, which is best seen in a transverse plane. By positioning the transducer longitudinal to the fibers of the gluteus medius over the greater trochanter, providers can visualize the fascial plane between the gluteus medius and gluteus maximus tendons and muscles.

Findings: This is the best view to evaluate for trochanteric bursitis or gluteus medius tendonosis. The greater trochanteric bursa can be visualized only when it is distended. Sliding the transducer slightly proximally and visualizing the region between the gluteus medius and greater trochanter allows visualization of the subgluteal bursa when it is distended.

KNEE

Nine standard views exist to examine the knee and identify the knee joint capsule, femoral cartilage, quadriceps and infrapatellar tendons, medial and lateral menisci and collateral ligaments, and popliteal fossa. The patient should lie supine. Each view described below corresponds with Fig. 46.7.

1 and 1b Suprapatellar Longitudinal and Transverse Views

Technique: The patient should be supine. Flexion of the knee to 30 degrees or extension of the knee with quadriceps contraction maximizes the fluid seen in the suprapatellar recess.[29,30] The transducer is positioned midline, longitudinally over the quadriceps tendon to its insertion on the patella (Video 46.13). Turn the transducer 90 degrees to obtain transverse views.

Findings: Suprapatellar views permit evaluation of the distal quadriceps tendon and suprapatellar recess for an effusion. Maximal joint fluid can be viewed lateral of midline, where joint aspiration can be readily performed (Videos 46.14 and 46.15). Care must be taken to avoid excessive compression when evaluating for an effusion or prepatellar bursitis.

2 and 2b Infrapatellar Longitudinal and Transverse Views

Technique: Position the patient supine with the knee extended. Place the transducer vertically over the origin of the patellar ligament to its insertion on the tibial tuberosity for longitudinal views (Video 46.16). Place the transducer

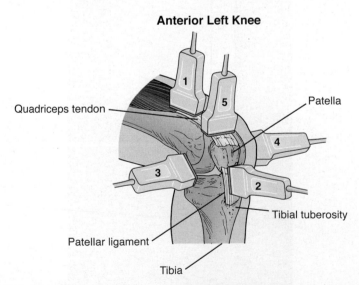

Anterior Left Knee

Figure 46.7 Knee Ultrasound Examination. *1*, Suprapatellar longitudinal view. *1b*, Suprapatellar transverse view. *2*, Infrapatellar longitudinal view. *2b*, Infrapatellar transverse view. *3*, Medial longitudinal view. *4*, Lateral longitudinal view. *5*, Suprapatellar maximum flexion transverse view. *6*, Posterior transverse view. *G*, Gastrocnemius (medial head); *LM*, lateral meniscus; *MCL*, medial collateral ligament; *MM*, medial meniscus; *PA*, popliteal artery; *asterisk*, where Baker's cyst would appear.

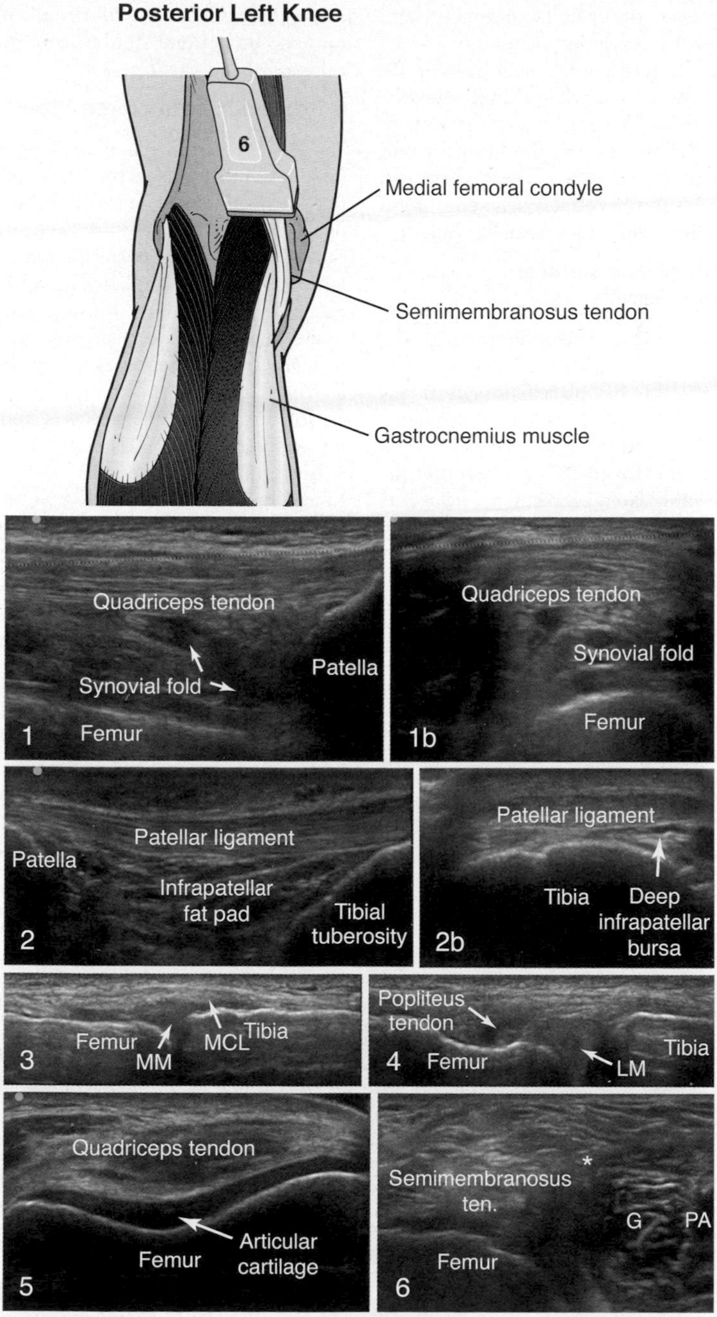

Figure 46.7, cont'd

horizontally over the patellar ligament and proximal tibia for transverse views.

Findings: The patellar ligament will be lax and partially anisotropic when viewed with the knee in extension. Thus, flexion of the knee to 30 degrees is helpful to pull the ligament taut and avoid anisotropic effect. These views can detect enthesitis of the patellar ligament (origin and insertion), as well as infrapatellar bursitis.

3 and 4 Medial and Lateral Longitudinal Views

Technique: Position the patient supine with the knee extended or flexed to 30 degrees. The transducer should be placed longitudinally over the medial and lateral collateral ligaments (Videos 46.17 and 46.18).

Findings: From the medial and lateral views, the medial and lateral collateral ligaments and outer edges of the menisci are seen. The menisci appear hypoechoic due to anisotropy and must be made maximally bright by transducer rocking to evaluate for a radial tear. Keep in mind that deep tears of the menisci that cause mechanical symptoms cannot be viewed with ultrasound.

5 Suprapatellar Maximum Flexion Transverse View

Technique: With the knee maximally flexed, place the transducer horizontally in a transverse plane over the distal femur and quadriceps tendon.

Findings: This view allows evaluation for a monosodium urate double contour, chondrocalcinosis, and cartilage loss.

6 Posterior Transverse View

Technique: Position the patient prone with the knee extended. Place the transducer horizontally to image the posterior knee in a transverse plane.

Findings: From a posterior view, identify the landmarks of the medial femoral condyle, the medial gastrocnemius muscle, and the semimembranosus tendon, because a Baker's cyst will emerge between these structures. Finding all three structures will prevent confusing an anisotropic semimembranosus tendon for a Baker's cyst. If a Baker's cyst is detected on a posterior transverse view, then a posterior longitudinal view is needed; a rounded cyst in a longitudinal view suggests it is intact, whereas a pointed distal end suggests that it has ruptured.[31]

ANKLE

Eleven standard views exist to examine the ankle to identify the joint capsule; the extensor, medial, lateral, and posterior tendons; the subtalar joint; and the retrocalcaneal bursa. The patient should be lying supine with the knee flexed and the foot flat against the examining table for the anterior views. All of the remaining views can be performed with the patient

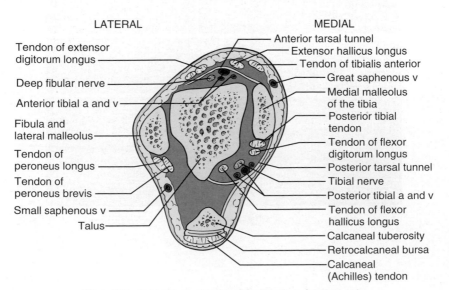

LATERAL

Tendon of extensor digitorum longus

Deep fibular nerve

Anterior tibial a and v

Fibula and lateral malleolus

Tendon of peroneus longus

Tendon of peroneus brevis

Small saphenous v

Talus

MEDIAL

Anterior tarsal tunnel

Extensor hallicus longus

Tendon of tibialis anterior

Great saphenous v

Medial malleolus of the tibia

Posterior tibial tendon

Tendon of flexor digitorum longus

Posterior tarsal tunnel

Tibial nerve

Posterior tibial a and v

Tendon of flexor hallicus longus

Calcaneal tuberosity

Retrocalcaneal bursa

Calcaneal (Achilles) tendon

Figure 46.8 Ankle Cross-Sectional Anatomy. *a*, Artery; *v*, vein.

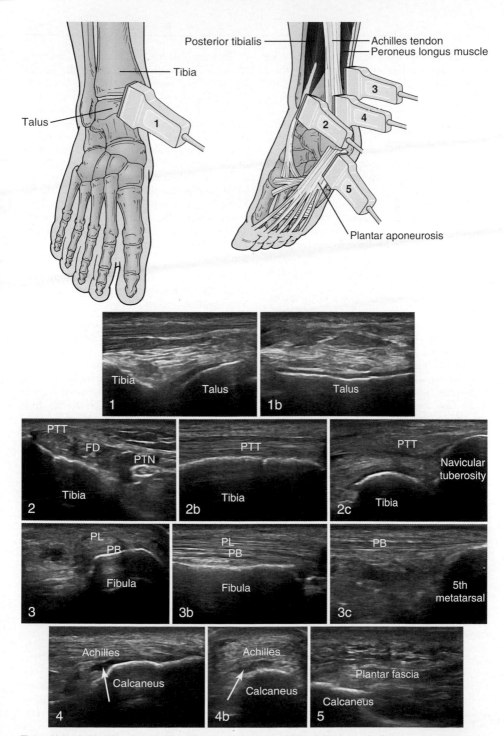

Figure 46.9 Ankle Ultrasound Examination. *1*, Anterior longitudinal view. *1b*, Anterior transverse view. *2*, Medial perimalleolar transverse view. *2b*, Medial perimalleolar longitudinal view. *2c*, Medial inframalleolar longitudinal view. *3*, Lateral perimalleolar transverse view. *3b*, Lateral perimalleolar longitudinal view. *3c*, Lateral inframalleolar longitudinal view. *4*, Posterior longitudinal view. *4b*, Posterior transverse view. *5*, Plantar longitudinal view. *FD*, Flexor digitorum; *PB*, peroneus brevis; *PL*, peroneus longus; *PTN*, posterior tibial nerve; *PTT*, posterior tibial tendon; *arrow*, retrocalcaneal bursa.

lying supine with the foot hanging off the edge of the examination table. A cross-sectional figure of the ankle is shown in Fig. 46.8. Each ankle view described below corresponds with Fig. 46.9.

1 and 1b Anterior Longitudinal and Transverse Views

Technique: Anterior views are obtained with the patient supine or sitting with plantar surface flat on the examining surface. Place the transducer anteromedially over the tibiotalar joint, vertically and then horizontally, for longitudinal and transverse views, respectively. The triangular anterior joint space is seen between the tibia, talus, and anterior tibial tendon. Start over the anterior distal tibia and sweep distally through the talus.

Findings: The anterior views focus on the capsular space between the tibia and talus, where the usual intracapsular fat can be displaced by an effusion (Video 46.19). The talar dome should be flat with an even anechoic cartilage lining. The extensor tendons (tibialis anterior, extensor hallucis longus, and extensor digitorum, from medial to lateral) do not normally have any surrounding effusion. Sliding the transducer laterally and slightly obliquely allows imaging of the sinus tarsi.

2, 2b, and 2c Medial Perimalleolar and Inframalleolar Longitudinal and Transverse Views

Technique: Position the patient supine or prone with the medial malleolus upwards. For perimalleolar medial views, place the transducer proximal and posterior to the medial malleolus to obtain transverse and longitudinal views. For an inframalleolar medial view, place the transducer from the navicular tuberosity to the tip of medial malleolus.

Findings: The medial ankle should be imaged with the transducer placed across the medial malleolus pointing straight back to the Achilles tendon; this position allows a pure transverse view of the medial tendons. For a longitudinal view, the transducer is placed along the axis of the posterior tibial tendon and then swept back until the flexor hallucis tendon is visualized. From the medial malleolus to the Achilles tendon, the medial tendons can be remembered with the mnemonic Tom (Tibialis posterior), Dick (flexor Digitorum), And Very Nervous (Artery, Vein, Nerve) Harry (flexor Hallucis). The medial inframalleolar view is

challenging due to the fan-shaped insertion of the posterior tibial tendon on the navicular and plantar surfaces of the first cuneiform. Tilting the transducer from bottom to top at the insertion on the navicular allows adequate visualization in most cases to detect enthesitis. Accessory ossicles, the os tibiale externum, are frequently found within the distal fibers of the posterior tibial tendon.[32] Normally, up to 4 mm of fluid can be seen in the posterior tibial tendon sheath just distal to the medial malleolus (Video 46.20).[33] The flexor hallucis longus tendon sheath communicates with the ankle or subtalar joint in half of all cases, so fluid within this sheath may be tracking from the joint.[34]

3, 3b, and 3c Lateral Perimalleolar and Inframalleolar Longitudinal and Transverse Views

Technique: Position the patient supine or prone with the lateral malleolus upwards. For perimalleolar lateral views, place the transducer proximal and posterior to the lateral malleolus to obtain transverse and longitudinal views. For an inframalleolar lateral view, place the transducer from the tuberosity of the fifth metatarsal to tip of the lateral malleolus.

Findings: Scanning of the lateral ankle is performed in the same manner as the medial side to visualize the lateral tendons. Both the lateral tendons and fibula can be seen in one view if the transducer is positioned posterior to anterior. The peroneus brevis is between the fibula and peroneus longus. The os perineum (small accessory bone) is found in the peroneus longus tendon as it dives under the lateral edge of the foot and should not be mistaken for pathology.[32] Normally, up to 3 mm of fluid can be seen in the peroneal tendon sheath just distal to the lateral malleolus.[33] The inframalleolar lateral view shows the enthesis of the peroneus brevis on the tuberosity of the fifth metatarsal bone.

4 and 4b Posterior Longitudinal and Transverse Views

Technique: Position the patient prone or kneeling with the foot extending over the edge of an examining surface. Place the transducer parallel to the Achilles tendon at its insertion on the proximal calcaneus for a longitudinal view, then rotate the transducer 90 degrees over the insertion of Achilles tendon on the calcaneus for a transverse view.

Findings: Do not mistake normal anisotropy of the distal insertion of the Achilles for a tendon tear. On gray scale imaging, you may need to apply subtle tension to the Achilles tendon to avoid anisotropy, but with Doppler scanning, tendon tension must be relaxed to avoid blanching of the small vessels.[35] A copious amount of gel needs to be used to adequately visualize the borders of the Achilles tendon in the posterior transverse view. The Achilles has a paratenon superficially but no synovial sheath. Thus, there cannot be tenosynovitis of the Achilles. The retrocalcaneal bursa usually has a few drops of fluid in it, but normally fluid does not extend past the edge of the calcaneus. Kager's fat pad should not be mistaken for a retrocalcaneal bursa effusion due to its hypoechogenicity.[32]

5 Plantar Longitudinal View

Technique: Position the patient prone or kneeling with the foot extending over the edge of an examining surface. Place the transducer vertically over the medial portion of calcaneus at the origin of the plantar fascia.

Findings: The plantar fascia can be visualized from the plantar aspect of the heel. At the origin of the aponeurosis, any erosive changes should be evaluated. Due to the thick keratin over the heel, the frequency setting may need to be lowered to allow for adequate tissue penetration to see the fascia and calcaneal border. The fascia should have an equal thickness at its origin and more distally. Thickening of the plantar fascia either at its origin or as fusiform swelling more distally is indicative of pathology.

Pathologic Findings

JOINT EFFUSION

One of the principal reasons for performing a musculoskeletal ultrasound evaluation is to detect fluid within a joint (Video 46.21), tendon sheath (Video 46.22), or bursa. One of the earliest uses of musculoskeletal ultrasound was to help diagnose a popliteal cyst.[36] On ultrasound imaging, fluid collections are anechoic, compressible, without Doppler flow, and create enhancement artifact (Video 46.23).[37,38] However, there are at least four exceptions to these characteristics. First, purulent or debris-filled collections can be isoechoic. This exception is particularly important to remember to avoid missing an abscess or septic arthritis.[39] Second, a fluid collection within a tightly confined ganglion cyst may not be compressible.[40] Third, fluid within a soft tissue collection may be actively circulating and mistaken for a blood vessel when using color Doppler. Last, some nonfluid structures with low impedance, such as neuromas, can also create enhancement artifact.[41]

An anisotropic tendon can be mistaken for a fluid collection. In the popliteal fossa, the semimembranosus tendon should be identified to help avoid this mistake (Fig. 46.10). Visualize any potential fluid collection in orthogonal planes to reduce the likelihood of mistaking a tendon for fluid due to anisotropy.

Due to its hypoechogenicity, muscle tissue can also mimic fluid. In the wrist and ankle, providers should be aware of muscle bellies

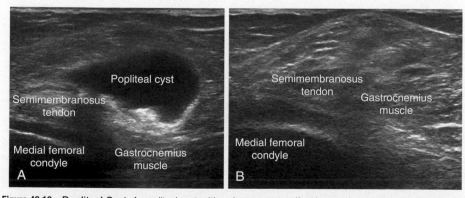

Figure 46.10   Popliteal Cyst. A popliteal cyst with enhancement artifact is seen in a transverse view through the popliteal fossa (A). The semimembranosus tendon can appear hypoechoic due to anisotropy and should not be mistaken for a fluid collection (B).

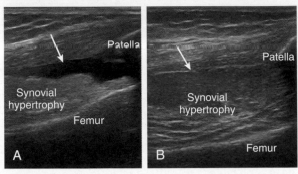

Figure 46.11   Synovial Hypertrophy. Suprapatellar longitudinal views of the knee showing the femur and patella. A knee effusion is seen *(arrow)* above an area of synovial hypertrophy (A), and absence of an effusion with substantial hypoechoic synovial hypertrophy is also seen (B, *arrow*).

that extend distally along with the tendons. Before diagnosing tenosynovial effusion, slide the transducer proximally to define the extent of the fluid collection and differentiate muscle striations from a fluid collection. Finally, sometimes it is difficult to distinguish fluid from hypoechoic synovium, especially in deep joints (Fig. 46.11). Increasing the gain and dynamic range settings can help differentiate between hypoechoic and anechoic material. Compressibility of fluid and lack of Doppler signal can also help make this distinction.

The significance of the presence and size of a joint effusion varies by the joint being examined. For example, a small effusion in a metatarsophalangeal joint will be of less clinical significance than a similar-sized effusion in a metacarpophalangeal joint.

SYNOVITIS

Synovial hypertrophy is defined as abnormal intra-articular tissue that is nondisplaceable, poorly compressible, usually hypoechoic, and may exhibit Doppler flow.[38] Synovitis usually refers to synovial hypertrophy in combination with inflammation and can be detected by a combination of two-dimensional and Doppler ultrasound images. Two-dimensional ultrasound can detect synovial hypertrophy and synovial effusion, whereas Doppler ultrasound can measure synovial hyperemia, a surrogate marker of inflammation (Videos 46.24 and 46.25). Studies have demonstrated a high sensitivity for the detection of inflammation using Doppler ultrasound.[42,43] The degree of Doppler signal correlates with the amount of vascular proliferation within the synovium on

histologic cross-sections[44,45] and the amount of contrast enhancement on magnetic resonance imaging.[42] However, not all synovial hyperemia exhibits Doppler flow,[45] and on the contrary, synovial Doppler signal can surround a noninflammatory effusion.[46]

Doppler ultrasound has been shown to detect small joint synovitis, and a methodology for semiquantitative measurement of Doppler signal has been validated in rheumatoid arthritis patients (Fig. 46.12).[47,48] Doppler signal in the biceps tendon sheath can help to differentiate inflammatory arthritis from degenerative causes of shoulder pain.[49] Furthermore, the presence of Doppler signal can be predictive of the future development of joint erosions in patients treated with disease-modifying antirheumatic drugs (DMARDs),[50-52] and loss of disease remission.[53,54] Studies have shown that Doppler signal scoring systems can identify patients in remission more accurately than patient-driven disease activity scores.[55,56]

EROSIONS

Outcome Measures in Rheumatology (OMERACT) has defined erosion as "an intraarticular discontinuity of the bone surface that is visible in two perpendicular planes."[38] When a cortical erosion is seen in one plane, a corresponding perpendicular view should be obtained for confirmation. Ultrasound is a more sensitive method to detect early erosions in inflammatory arthritis affecting the metacarpophalangeal joints compared with plain film radiography[57] and is highly sensitive for even small erosions seen on high-resolution computed tomography (CT) scans.[58] The

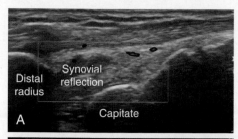

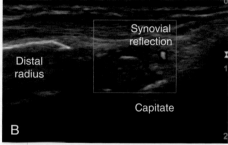

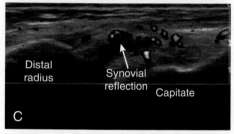

Figure 46.12 Synovitis. Synovial hyperemia is frequently graded on a 0–3 scale: Grade 0 = no Doppler signal in the synovium. The three dorsal longitudinal wrist images show varying grades of synovitis in the radiocarpal joint. (A) Grade 1+ = only one dot of red Doppler signal within the region of synovial hypertrophy. (B) Grade 2+ = >1 dot of Doppler signal, but less than half the volume of synovium is filled with Doppler signal. (C) Grade 3+ = more than half the synovial volume is filled with Doppler signal.

cortical bone has excellent reflective characteristics, which allows visualization of subtle cortical defects.[1] Ultrasound has greater sensitivity for erosions in joints with more acoustic windows, such as the second metacarpophalangeal joint compared with the fourth metacarpophalangeal joint.[59] Although erosions are usually associated with the presence of an inflammatory arthritis, small erosions of less than 2 mm can be detected in asymptomatic patients without a rheumatic disease.[60-62] Thus, the size and number of erosions detected is critical for disease specificity.[58,59] False-positive

erosive changes on ultrasound can result from detection of vascular channels on the volar aspect of metacarpophalangeal joints, and osteophyte changes that mimic erosions (Fig. 46.13).[63,64]

CRYSTAL DEPOSITION

Ultrasound can detect features of gout and calcium pyrophosphate arthropathy. A double contour sign, a hyperechoic line overlying a layer of hyaline cartilage, is an ultrasound finding in patients with gout. This finding should be distinguished from an "interface" sign, a thin hyperechoic line produced by a change in impedance as sound waves enter hyaline cartilage. A double contour sign is thicker, more irregular, and not limited to the area perpendicular to the incident sound waves.[65] In calcium pyrophosphate arthropathy, hyperechoic deposits can be seen *within* the hyaline cartilage layer versus *on the surface* of hyaline cartilage seen in gout (Fig. 46.14).[65] The double contour sign of gout was present in 60% of confirmed cases of gout that did not require urate-lowering therapy, and ultrasound detected tophi in 47% of these patients.[66] In a larger study of more than 800 subjects with crystal-proven diagnosis of acute monoarthritis, the sensitivity of double contour was 53% in patients without clinical tophi, compared with 72% in those with clinical tophi.[55] This study demonstrated that ultrasound features of both the double contour sign and tophus have an excellent specificity of greater than 90% for gout even in comparison to patients with calcium pyrophosphate arthropathy, although 16% of patients with calcium pyrophosphate deposition disease (CPPD) have at least one ultrasound feature typical for gout.

Gouty tophi appear as deposits with a heterogeneous echotexture, can be multilobular with a hypoechoic rim, and may have adjacent bone erosions.[65,67] Calcium pyrophosphate deposits are typically seen within fibrocartilage, such as the meniscus of the knee or triangular fibrocartilage complex of the wrist,[68] and ultrasound is substantially more sensitive than plain radiography to detect these lesions (Video 46.26).[69]

SOFT TISSUE NODULES

Ultrasound can be helpful in differentiating soft tissue nodules commonly encountered in

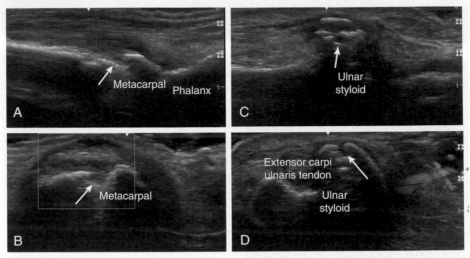

Figure 46.13 Erosions. Longitudinal (A) and transverse (B) views of a dorsal metacarpophalangeal joint. *Arrows* point to the region of bone erosion seen in both views. (B) The Doppler box demonstrates an absence of active hyperemia within the erosion and overlying synovial tissue. (C) and (D) Display longitudinal and transverse views of the dorsal ulnar styloid. *Arrows* point to erosions of the ulna (seen in 10% of rheumatoid arthritis patients within 6 months of disease onset).[64]

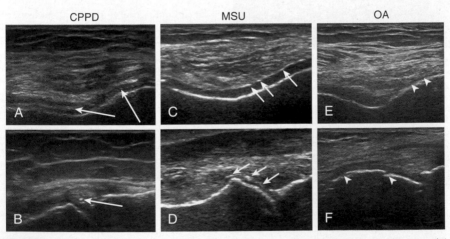

Figure 46.14 Crystal Arthritis. (A) Dorsal, flexed, transverse view of the femoral notch. *Arrows* point to calcium pyrophosphate deposits within the articular cartilage. (B) Medial knee joint line. *Arrow* points to calcium pyrophosphate deposits within the fibrocartilaginous medial meniscus. (C) Dorsal, flexed, transverse view of the femoral notch. *Arrows* point to monosodium urate *(MSU)* deposits over the superficial surface of the hyaline cartilage. (D) Longitudinal view of MSU deposits over the superficial surface of the hyaline cartilage at the first metacarpophalangeal joint *(arrows)*. Differentiation of MSU from calcium pyrophosphate is best made by assessing the location of crystal deposition in the cartilage, as well as by the specific combination of joint regions affected. (E) Dorsal, flexed, transverse view of the femoral notch with *arrowheads* pointing to asymmetric loss of cartilage on the right side compared with the left side of the femur, typical of osteoarthritis *(OA)*. (F) Longitudinal view of the dorsal medial femoral condyle, with *arrowheads* pointing to cortical irregularities deep to thinned cartilage seen in OA. *CPPD,* Calcium pyrophosphate deposition disease.

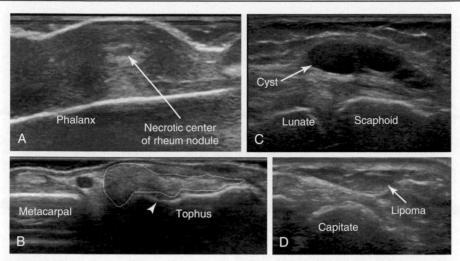

Figure 46.15   Soft Tissue Nodule. (A) A rheumatoid nodule is seen in a longitudinal view over a phalanx with regular shape, homogeneous echotexture, and an anechoic center. (B) A tophus *(outlined)* is seen in a transverse view over a metacarpal. Note the irregular shape, heterogeneous echotexture, and underlying erosion of the bone *(arrowhead)* in comparison with the normal metacarpal bone on the left. (C) A ganglion cyst is seen in a transverse view over the dorsal wrist. There is anechoic material within the cyst, it is noncompressible, and it is in the typical location of a ganglion cyst. (D) A lipoma is seen in a transverse view over the dorsal wrist. The location can create clinical confusion about whether this is a cyst, but its isoechoic contents with fibrous strands clearly distinguishes it from a cyst on ultrasound imaging.

patients with joint pain. Gouty tophaceous deposits on ultrasound are typically heterogeneous with small hyperechoic spots, and with a hypoechoic surrounding halo, when compared with surrounding fibrous tissue (Fig. 46.15). Tophi can have poorly defined borders and can have posterior acoustic shadowing.[70,71] Calcifications may or may not be present within the tophus and have not been shown to correlate with illness duration.[71] Hypervascularity may predict erosions and destruction of the adjacent bone (Videos 46.27 and 46.28).[72] A rheumatoid nodule, in comparison, is generally a homogeneous, poorly circumscribed collection of hypoechoic material with a central area of anechoic necrosis close to the bone surface.[73] Note, however, that there are rare exceptions where a tophus may appear less echoic than usual and thus may be mistaken for a rheumatoid nodule.[72] A multilobulated appearance is also more typical of a tophus than a rheumatoid nodule, which is typically single.[9]

Ultrasound also helps to differentiate between localized swelling that may be due to cysts, as opposed to synovitis. Cysts are characteristically noncompressible and maintain their shape on orthogonal views. Cysts will usually also have no Doppler signal and be anechoic if fluid-filled, although presence of some hyperechoic material within a cyst is possible.[74] An exception is a ruptured cyst, such as a ruptured popliteal cyst, that assumes a beak-shaped appearance on orthogonal view. Presence of Doppler signal may indicate that a vascular aneurysm is being visualized, rather than a cyst.

Tumors, although rare, will vary in appearance depending on the specific echogenic qualities of the comprising tissue. Lipomas are characteristically hyperechoic with no evidence of vascularity on color flow Doppler imaging. A subungual glomus tumor appears as a Doppler-positive, hypoechoic nodule on ultrasound. Synovial sarcomas appear as a hypoechoic lesion with absent flow on Doppler. Schwannomas on ultrasound are well-defined, oval, hypoechoic, hypovascular lesions that can be best distinguished by a nerve "tail" entering or exiting from the nodule.[75]

SOFT TISSUE CALCIFICATION

Calcium deposits have an echogenic appearance similar to bone and are easily identified on ultrasound. Characteristically, these deposits are hyperechoic, amorphous collections with or without posterior acoustic shadowing.

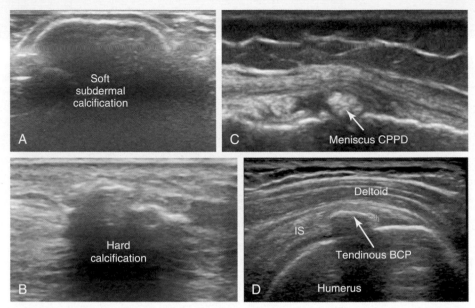

Figure 46.16 Soft Tissue Calcification. (A) "Soft" calcium deposits are just underneath the skin surface and observed as linear deposits with a smooth edge and posterior acoustic shadowing. (B) In distinction, "hard" calcium deposits are characterized by a jagged edge in the subcutaneous fat layer and posterior acoustic shadowing (this may or may not be present depending on the calcium thickness). (C) Calcium pyrophosphate deposition *(CPPD)* is seen within the medial meniscus of the knee. (D) Basic calcium phosphate *(BCP)* deposit is seen within the infraspinatus (IS) tendon of the shoulder.

It is important to note that presence of a calcium deposit does not always correlate with symptoms and should be used as a clue, rather than a confirmation of a clinical diagnosis. Doppler signal around the calcification is an indication of metabolic activity and increases the likelihood that the calcification is causing symptoms.[76]

Ultrasonography has long been used to identify and treat calcific tendonitis of the rotator cuff, with the supraspinatus tendon being the most frequently involved.[77] Studies suggest that involvement of supraspinatus, concurrent involvement of multiple additional tendons, size larger than 1.5 cm, fragmentation of the deposit, and positive Doppler all positively correlate with active symptoms.[84,78] Deposits have also been described as being "soft" or "hard" depending on their stage of formation and radiologic appearance. Soft deposits are localized, discrete, dense, and homogeneous with spontaneous healing tendency. Hard deposits are diffuse, fluffy, and heterogeneous with delayed and slow healing (Fig. 46.16).[79]

Presence of hyperechoic aggregates within fibrocartilage can be found in patients with CPPD in the knee menisci and the triangular fibrocartilage complex in the wrist. CPPD also manifests as hyperechoic aggregates within the hyaline cartilage. Presence of chondrocalcinosis has been shown to have high specificity and sensitivity for CPPD.[80]

Furthermore, calcium deposition within the muscle on ultrasound can be seen in inflammatory myopathies, along with other characteristic findings, such as increased Doppler signal. Discrete amorphous hyperechoic collections in the skin are characteristic of systemic sclerosis.[81]

Barbotage is a therapeutic modality for calcific rotator cuff tendonitis; it involves ultrasound-guided needling of the calcium deposit that softens it, making it more amenable to irrigation and aspiration (Video 46.29). It may also be followed by extracorporeal shock wave therapy of the involved area.[82,83]

TENOSYNOVITIS/RETINACULITIS

Tenosynovitis is inflammation of the fluid-filled sheath that surrounds tendons and can be seen with many mechanical and inflammatory conditions. Tenosynovitis has been defined by

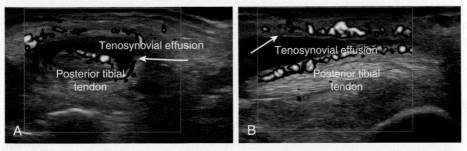

Figure 46.17 Tenosynovitis. Posterior tibial tendon in transverse (A) and longitudinal (B) views demonstrates tenosynovial effusion and tenosynovial thickening *(arrows)* with increased Doppler signal in both the tenosynovium and tendon.

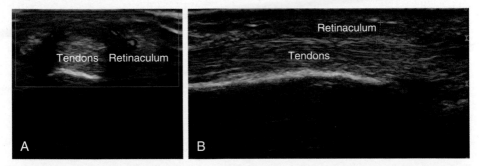

Figure 46.18 De Quervain's Tendonitis. Transverse (A) and longitudinal (B) views of the first compartment extensor tendons in a patient with de Quervain's tendonitis. The extensor pollicus brevis cannot be differentiated from the abductor pollicus longus in this image. The retinaculum, which is hypoechoic relative to the tendon, does not have the fibrillar tendon pattern in a longitudinal view and has some surrounding Doppler signal. The retinaculum surrounds the tendons from three sides, and the hyperechoic distal radius is directly deep to the tendons.

OMERACT as "hypoechoic or anechoic thickened tissue with or without fluid within the tendon sheath, which is seen in two perpendicular planes and which may exhibit Doppler signal."[38] Fluid sometimes appears as a "halo" around the tendon (Fig. 46.17; Videos 46.30 and 46.31) and is present in at least one wrist tendon in 49% of patients with rheumatoid arthritis.[84]

Pressure from the transducer can compress the fluid away from the region and collapse the sheath, resulting in false-negative exam. Hypoechoic, thickened tenosynovium can be confused with effusion but is not compressible, even though it may exhibit Doppler signal. Compression can help to distinguish tenosynovial effusion seen in inflammatory arthritis from thickened retinacular fibers seen in de Quervain's disease (Fig. 46.18) and trigger finger.[85]

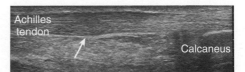

Figure 46.19 Achilles Tendonitis. Longitudinal view of the Achilles tendon. The *arrow* points to a region of fusiform swelling of the tendon. Notice the hypoechogenicity of the tendon fibers in the superficial part of the Achilles tendon and loss of some of the fibrillar pattern.

Inflamed regions of tendons, or tendonitis, appear hypoechoic with loss of fibrillar pattern and are thicker, suggesting tendon edema. A tendon tear can appear similar to tendonitis with a distinct break in fibrillar pattern.[86] Fusiform swelling of tendons is a typical finding in tendinosis (Fig. 46.19).[87,88] The posterior tibial tendon of the ankle is a common site affected by tenosynovitis or tendonitis in both mechanical and inflammatory conditions.[89]

Paratenonitis is the inflammation of the paratenon, nerve- and vessel-carrying tissue adherent to the tendon. It has classically been described in the Achilles tendon and often occurs in conjunction with Achilles tendinosis. Ultrasound can show edema lining the tendon acutely, and adhesions around the tendon with more chronic inflammation.[90]

ENTHESITIS

Enthesitis, or inflammation of the sites where tendons and ligaments insert onto bones, has a similar ultrasound appearance as tendonitis—hypoechogenicity, tendon thickening, and loss of fibrillar pattern at the attachment site. There may be features of bursitis, increased Doppler signal, cortical irregularities, or erosions of the bone proximal to the tendon attachment site (Fig. 46.20).[38] Enthesitis is a common feature in seronegative inflammatory arthritis, such as psoriatic arthritis.[91,92] Ultrasound is more sensitive than clinical exam for detecting enthesitis due to spondyloarthritis[92-94] and may be helpful for establishing a diagnosis of spondyloarthropathy.

BURSITIS

Bursas are paratendinous, fluid-filled sacs that aid in shock absorption and friction reduction.

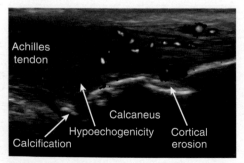

Achilles tendon

Calcaneus

Hypoechogenicity   Cortical erosion

Calcification

Figure 46.20 Enthesitis. Posterior longitudinal view of the ankle showing the calcaneus and Achilles tendon with extensive Doppler signal within the tendon at the enthesis, including the bone margin. Three additional features of inflammatory enthesitis are demonstrated: calcification with posterior shadowing in the region of the retrocalcaneal bursa, loss of normal tendon fibrillar pattern and hypoechogenicity, and cortical erosion.

Normally, a minimal amount of bursal fluid is present and is difficult to detect by ultrasound. Mechanical irritation, infection, and autoimmune diseases can increase bursal fluid. For example, the subdeltoid/subacromial bursa in the shoulder, which is barely visible normally, becomes distinctly hypoechoic between the supraspinatus and deltoid muscles and 2 mm thicker in disease states (see Fig. 46.2).[95,96] Sensitivity of ultrasound to detect subacromial bursitis is approximately 80%, with a specificity of 94% to 98%.[97] Finding bilateral subacromial bursitis can help establish a diagnosis of polymyalgia rheumatica[98] and differentiate between different causes of inflammatory shoulder pain.[99] When evaluating for subacromial bursitis, providers should avoid mistaking the deep hypoechoic muscle fibers of the deltoid for subacromial bursa. Deltoid muscle fibers extend from the acromion proximally to beyond the greater tuberosity distally, whereas the bursa is deep to the acromion proximally and extends to the tip of the greater tuberosity, or past the tip when it is distended with fluid.[21]

NERVE COMPRESSION

The first reports of using ultrasonography to assess peripheral nerves appeared in the 1990s with compression of the median nerve.[100,101] Ultrasonography has become an integral element in assessing patients with suspected peripheral neuropathies, including compression of the median, ulnar, posterior tibial, and posterior interosseous nerves, and complements the clinical examination and electromyography.[102] Furthermore, ultrasound is used to guide needle placement for perineural steroid injections.[103,104]

In a transverse cross section, a normal nerve is a well-demarcated, noncompressible round structure, which has small hypoechoic areas (nerve fascicles) within it that are separated by hyperechoic septae (interfascicular perineurium), giving it a "honeycomb-like" appearance (Video 46.32).[105] The longitudinal sections similarly reveal the fascicular architecture, leading to a "bundle of straws" appearance. Nerves are more echogenic than muscles but less echogenic than tendons. Normal nerves also show no signs of vascularization on color Doppler examination.[106]

The characteristic ultrasound finding of any peripheral nerve entrapment is hypoechoic enlargement of the nerve just proximal to the

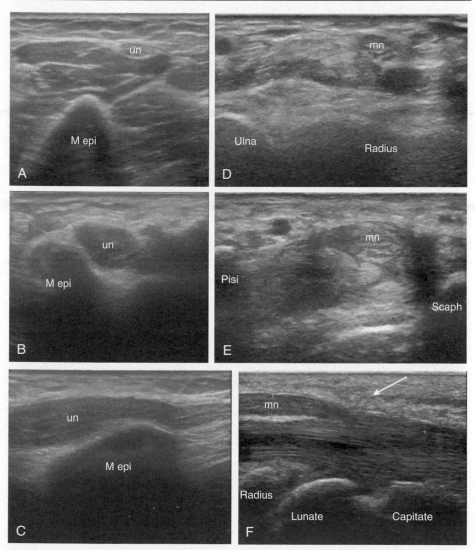

Figure 46.21 Compressive Neuropathies. (A) Ulnar nerve *(un)* (normal caliber) is seen in a transverse view, proximal to the cubital tunnel, and superficial to the medial epicondyle *(M epi)*. (B) Ulnar nerve is substantially swollen due to compression in the cubital tunnel. At this level it is in contact with the medial epicondyle. (C) Ulnar nerve in a longitudinal view demonstrating swelling proximal to the compression against the medial epicondyle. (D) Median nerve *(mn)* (normal caliber) is seen in a transverse view proximal to the carpal tunnel. (E) The median nerve is swollen at the entrance of the carpal tunnel, as defined by the pisiform and scaphoid tuberosity *(Scaph)*. (F) A change in the caliber of the median nerve is shown in a longitudinal view as it is compressed by the flexor retinaculum *(arrow)*. *pisi*, Pisiform bone.

entrapment site with distal tapering or transition to a normal size (Fig. 46.21; Videos 46.33 and 46.34).[107] This hourglass-like shape of the nerve trunk on longitudinal view helps to identify not just the location, but sometimes the etiology, of the compression.[105] Compression

results in increased intraneural vascular permeability resulting in intrafascicular edema that manifests as nerve swelling and increased cross-sectional area.

The widely accepted normal range for cross-sectional area of the median nerve is less than 0.08 to 0.12 cm². A median nerve cross-sectional area greater than 0.15 cm² or a difference in cross-sectional area measured at the level of the pisiform versus the forearm that is greater than 1.5 times is also considered a positive test.[100] Abnormal nerves may also show other characteristics on ultrasound that aid in diagnosis. These include altered "catching" movement, contour deformity, and positive Doppler. Pain or paresthesia may also be provoked by applying compression with a transducer to the altered nerve segment (sonographic Tinel's sign).[102]

Arthrocentesis

PRINCIPLES

Ultrasound can guide needle insertion into synovia and tendons to improve accuracy[108,109] and efficacy[110-113] over palpation of landmarks alone and can reduce procedural pain.[114,115] There are three techniques of ultrasound-guided needle insertion: indirect (static), direct (dynamic or real-time) out-of-plane transverse approach, and direct (dynamic or real-time) in-plane longitudinal approach. With indirect guidance, the target structure is identified with ultrasound in orthogonal planes, and the skin is marked over the needle insertion site. Depth of the target structure is noted, and a needle is inserted to this depth. In contrast, the direct insertion approach tracks the needle tip in real time as it is advanced toward the target tissue. Using a transverse out-of-plane approach, the transducer is held steady over the target, and the needle is inserted in the center of the long dimension of the transducer. The needle tip appears as a hyperechoic dot on the screen when the tip is within the plane of the ultrasound beam. If the needle trajectory is correct, then the needle tip is visualized advancing toward the target tissue. If not, then the needle must be withdrawn and reinserted on a different trajectory to reach the target tissue. Using a longitudinal in-plane approach, the transducer is held steady over the target, and the needle is inserted in the center of the short dimension of the transducer in the same plane as the ultrasound beam. The entire needle, not only the tip, is visualized advancing toward the target tissue. The advantage of the longitudinal in-plane approach is the ability to see the complete path of the needle and adjust the needle angle while advancing it to the target structure.

SHOULDER

Ultrasound guidance improves shoulder injection accuracy from 61% with the use of landmarks alone to 89% with the use of ultrasound.[116,117] This advantage is especially important when septic arthritis or bursitis is being considered. Studies have demonstrated better efficacy of ultrasound-guided glenohumeral joint injections[111,118] and subacromial bursal injections compared with landmark-guided techniques.[112,119,120] Ultrasound-guided shoulder injection is also significantly less painful compared with landmark-guided techniques.[121]

For subacromial bursa aspiration, the patient's arm should be put into a Crass or modified Crass position with the transducer positioned transverse to the supraspinatus tendon. The needle is usually inserted in a lateral to medial direction using a longitudinal in-plane approach. Compared with glenohumeral injections, the needle angle is shallow, and the needle should be well visualized on the ultrasound screen (Fig. 46.22A).

A long needle (3.5-inch spinal needle) is needed because of the shoulder joint's depth, and the tangential needle path used for in-plane ultrasound guidance, in contrast to the trajectory used when performing a landmark-guided shoulder arthrocentesis from a posterior approach. The needle is inserted inferolateral from the corner of the acromion and aimed anteromedially toward the coracoid process. The ultrasound transducer is parallel and just caudal to the spine of the scapula with the posterior glenoid and labrum in view (see Fig. 46.22B). Due to the relatively steep angle of the needle, the needle may be poorly visualized and needle visualization technology or beam steering may be helpful.

WRIST

Ultrasound can greatly aid in localizing fluid collections and improving success rate of diagnostic synovial fluid aspiration of small joints, like the wrist.[122] Furthermore, corticosteroid wrist injections performed with ultrasound guidance produce significantly better pain relief than those guided by landmarks.[123] For needle insertion in the wrist, the ultrasound transducer is placed transversely on the dorsal wrist. Radiocarpal joint effusions or synovium can be visualized just superficial to the scaphoid-lunate junction, whereas the

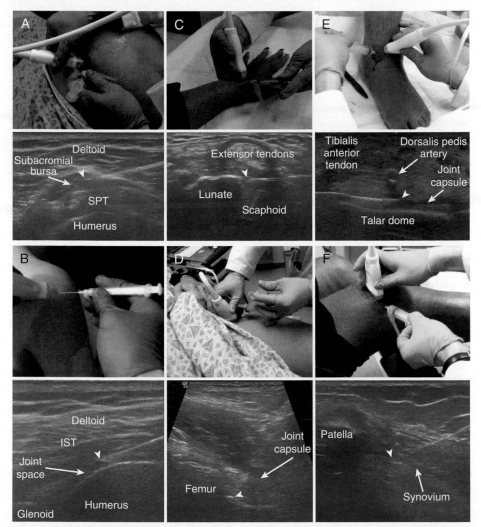

Figure 46.22 Ultrasound-Guided Needle Injection. Needle position is shown using a longitudinal in-plane approach. *Arrowheads* point to the needle tip in each image. Note that needle visibility is affected more by increasing needle angle than by increasing needle depth (compare images A, C, and E with B, D, and F). (A) Transverse view of the supraspinatus tendon in a modified Crass position. The humeral head, supraspinatus tendon, subacromial bursa, and deltoid are seen with the needle tip in the distended subacromial bursa. (B) Needle guidance into the glenohumeral joint. Using a longitudinal approach, the needle is inserted into the joint space deep to the deltoid and infraspinatus muscle, and superficial to the humeral head and glenoid. (C) Needle guidance into the radiocarpal joint. A needle is inserted using a longitudinal approach just superficial to the scaphoid and lunate and deep to the fourth compartment extensor tendons. (D) Needle guidance into the anterior hip joint. Using a longitudinal approach, the needle is inserted into the capsule and superficial to the femur. (E) Transverse approach to tibiotalar joint injection. The needle is inserted using a longitudinal approach in the joint capsule just superficial to the talar dome and deep to the dorsalis pedis artery. Note that the needle is inserted deep to the (anisotropic) tibialis anterior tendon. (F) Needle guidance into the synovial reflection of the knee. Using a longitudinal approach, the needle is inserted into the lateral parapatellar gutter near the patella. This approach can be useful for knees without effusions because the synovial fold can be difficult to see in the suprapatellar space. *Arrowheads*, Needle tip; *IST*, Infraspinatus tendon; *SPT*, supraspinatus tendon.

intercarpal synovial cavity can be found over the capitate. The needle can be inserted using a longitudinal in-plane approach to avoid overlying tendons and vessels while directing the needle to the synovial cavity (see Fig. 46.22C).

HIP

Two published studies showed 59 of 60 hip injections were performed successfully using ultrasound guidance.[124,125] There are no studies comparing ultrasound-guided versus landmark-guided needle insertion at the hip because hip joint injections are rarely done using landmarks.

In preparation for needle insertion, the hip joint should be visualized in an anterior longitudinal plane with emphasis on the capsule and joint recess overlying the femoral head–neck junction. A longitudinal in-plane approach with a 3.5 inch or longer needle is recommended. Avoid the medial circumflex femoral artery that may be found along the needle trajectory to the synovial capsule. Anesthetic should be injected along the needle path if there is any discomfort. Frequently, as long as intervening vessels are avoided, pain is experienced only when the needle traverses the joint capsule. Thus, anesthetic should be injected just superficial to the capsule before piercing it. Anesthetic flow within the capsule should be visualized before injecting corticosteroid or other medication into the joint (see Fig. 46.22D).

Needle visualization may be challenging because the needle path is steep relative to the transducer, especially in obese patients. Positioning the color flow Doppler box over the needle path may be helpful to identify the moving needle. Injection of anesthetic can also help to identify a poorly visualized needle. Finally, an alternative approach is positioning the transducer transversely over the femoral neck and joint recess and inserting the needle using a longitudinal in-plane approach with a shallower angle in a lateral to medial direction.

ANKLE

A sufficiently powered clinical study of ultrasound-guided versus landmark-guided needle placement in the ankle joint has not been performed, although studies suggest benefit of using ultrasound guidance. Cunnington found that 85% of ultrasound-guided ankle injections were accurate compared with 58% by palpation, but the numbers were too small for the difference to be statistically significant.[108] Cadaveric studies have found increased accuracy for ultrasound-guided needle placement into the sinus tarsi[126] and tarsometatarsal joints.[127]

When an ankle joint effusion is not clinically apparent, capsular distention can be visualized over the talar dome using ultrasound. The transducer should be placed transverse to the talar dome overlying the joint recess (see Fig. 46.22E). The needle can then be directed from medial to lateral into the joint capsule using a longitudinal in-plane approach. Placement of the transducer in a sagittal plane can also be used, but the needle trajectory is steeper with this approach.

An effusion of the subtalar joint into the sinus tarsi can be aspirated with the transducer obliquely placed from the lateral malleolus anterolaterally to the calcaneus, across the sinus tarsi. The needle can then be inserted with a transverse out-of-plane approach into the effusion.

KNEE

Although most knee effusions can be successfully aspirated without ultrasound guidance, patients with substantial adiposity around the knee, minimal effusion, or a history of poorly tolerated or unsuccessful needle placement may benefit from ultrasound guidance. A review of five studies evaluating knee arthrocentesis found ultrasound-guided needle placement into the knee to be 96% accurate versus 78% for those done by palpation ($P <$ .001).[116] Ultrasound-guided knee injection has also been shown to provide more than 50% pain reduction at 2 weeks to 90% of patients compared with 72% of patients injected with landmark-guided injection.[110] In addition, ultrasound-guided injection is substantially better tolerated by patients.[110,113,114]

Knee arthrocentesis can be performed using a lateral to medial approach with the ultrasound transducer transversely placed over the distal femur, just proximal to or lateral to the patella. The needle is directed in-plane to the synovial cavity in the suprapatellar recess or in the lateral gutter (see Fig. 46.22F; Video 46.35). Small effusions are easily compressible, and providers should avoid excessive transducer pressure that might displace the target fluid.

For a Baker's cyst aspiration, the patient should be placed prone and the transducer placed transversely on the medial femoral condyle at the origin of the cyst. The needle is directed using a longitudinal in-plane approach from medial to lateral into the cyst, avoiding the neurovascular bundle that is lateral to the cyst.

PEARLS AND PITFALLS

- Anisotropy is one of the most common imaging artifacts encountered in musculoskeletal ultrasound. Tilting the transducer normally changes tendon echogenicity compared with surrounding tissues and allows differentiation of normal from abnormal findings.
- Minimize transducer pressure to avoid unintended compression of superficial structures, especially fluid collections, which can lead to nonvisualization of musculoskeletal pathology.
- Power Doppler imaging with a low pulse repetition frequency (PRF) between 0.5 and 1 kHz is preferred to assess synovial hyperemia and assess for inflammation.
- A linear transducer is used to examine all joints with ultrasound, except the hip joint. A curvilinear transducer penetrates deeper to evaluate the hip joint.
- Complete external rotation of the arm while viewing the posterior aspect of the glenohumeral joint maximizes sensitivity for detection of joint effusion in the shoulder with a near 100% sensitivity.
- The anterior elbow joint capsule has a "seagull" appearance between the capitulum of the humerus and radial head; the "seagull" appearance disappears when a joint effusion is present because the capsule is pushed out of the joint cleft.
- Median nerve measurements on the volar aspect of the wrist should be performed with the transducer perpendicular to the nerve axis to avoid artificially increasing the cross-sectional nerve area.
- The anterior views of the hip joint are the best views to detect and aspirate a joint effusion, whereas the lateral longitudinal view of the hip is the best view to evaluate for trochanteric bursitis.
- Baker's cysts appear between the medial femoral condyle, medial gastrocnemius muscle, and semimembranosus tendon. Positively identifying all three structures avoids misinterpreting a tendon for a cyst, especially the semimembranosus tendon.
- A "double contour" sign is a hyperechoic line overlying a layer of hyaline cartilage that is an ultrasound finding of gout.
- Inflamed tendons, or tendonitis, appear hypoechoic with loss of fibrillar pattern and are thicker than normal.

CHAPTER 47

Pediatrics

Thomas W. Conlon ■ David O. Kessler ■ Erik Su

KEY POINTS

- Children are ideal candidates for ultrasound due both to their relatively high water content and small stature.
- Many similarities exist between children and adults in the use of ultrasound to guide diagnostic work-ups and bedside procedures.
- Pediatric point-of-care ultrasound use continues to expand as more providers receive training during graduate medical education or through continuing medical education courses.

Background

Point-of-care ultrasound is being used increasingly in the care of acutely ill pediatric patients. Some attributes of pediatric patients can facilitate or impede ultrasound imaging compared to adults. Compared to adults, children have relatively thinner chest walls, relatively higher body water content, and incomplete ossification of ribs that permit high-resolution visualization of the thorax using high-frequency transducers. Open fontanelles permit ultrasound assessment of the brain. However, some pediatric characteristics can make ultrasound imaging more challenging, including patient cooperation, narrow rib interspaces, ossified ribs in older children, and increased thermal loss of patients while exposed.[1]

Small transducers specifically designed for children are ideal to generate high-resolution

images through small windows. Large curvilinear transducers used in adults are often replaced by smaller footprint phased-array or microconvex transducers in children.

Current studies suggest that novice pediatric providers can learn to use ultrasound for procedural and diagnostic applications accurately and reliably.[2,3] Pediatric critical care fellowship programs report that 95% of academic pediatric intensive care units (ICUs) have access to a portable ultrasound machine, and 95% of emergency medicine fellowship programs report using ultrasound in their departments.[4,5] As point-of-care ultrasound is becoming a standard component of medical school curricula, more pediatric providers are entering practice knowledgeable and skilled in ultrasound. This chapter reviews the most common pediatric point-of-care ultrasound applications being used in clinical practice

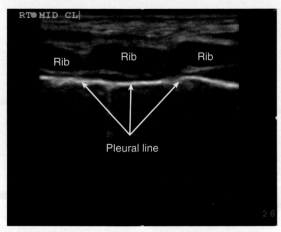

Figure 47.1 **Infant Ribs.** The pleural line can be visualized through the ribs of an infant due to incomplete rib ossification.

and highlights any important differences from adult imaging.

Lungs and Pleura

The normal and abnormal lung ultrasound findings described in Chapter 9 are similar in children (i.e., B-lines are seen with pulmonary edema, lung hepatization is seen with consolidation, etc.).[6] Pediatric providers often use a linear transducer to assess the lungs and pleura (Fig. 47.1). Orienting the transducer transversely, rather than longitudinally, in an intercostal space facilitates viewing the pleural line and parenchyma once the ribs are ossified after infancy.

PNEUMOTHORAX

A child with pneumothorax will have similar ultrasound findings as an adult, including absence of lung sliding, absence of B-lines, presence of a lung point, and presence of a barcode or stratosphere sign on M-mode imaging of the pleura.

Neonates have a high risk of pneumothorax, particularly premature infants, which is associated with high morbidity and mortality.[7] Ultrasound can reliably and rapidly detect pneumothorax in neonates. A study of sudden respiratory decompensation in 42 infants compared ultrasound versus clinical examination to diagnose pneumothorax with chest x-ray as the gold standard. This study found ultrasound was more sensitive (100% vs. 84%) and

specific (100% vs. 56%) than clinical examination. Further, performance of ultrasound was 15 minutes faster than chest x-ray with emergency drainage occurring prior to chest x-ray in 9 cases.[8] Findings supportive or contrary to a diagnosis of pneumothorax may be subtler with high-frequency oscillatory ventilation. Using M-mode, a barcode or stratosphere sign can be seen, similar to patients with pneumothorax during conventional ventilation, and use of M-mode over a lung point will yield a similarly patterned image (Fig. 47.2).

PLEURAL EFFUSIONS

Hemothorax, chylothorax, or simple effusions are common complications following congenital heart surgery.[9] High-frequency transducers assist in both identifying and differentiating simple versus complex pleural effusions (Fig. 47.3 and Video 47.1). The incidence of hemothorax in trauma is low in children versus adults due to increased thoracic compliance of children, though ultrasound can be used to rapidly diagnose hemothorax.[10]

LUNG AND AIRWAY DISEASE

Ultrasound detection of pneumonia in pediatric populations demonstrates a high specificity compared with chest radiography and strong correlation with clinical and laboratory data.[11,12] Bronchiolitis is a clinical entity unique to pediatrics that is common in children less than 2 years of age during winter. Lung ultrasound

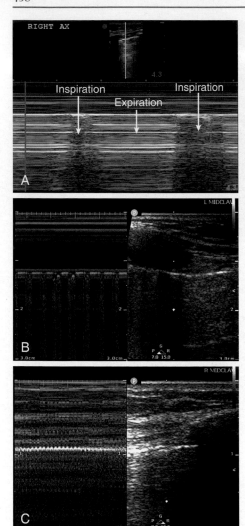

Figure 47.2 Pneumothorax With M-Mode Ultrasound. Alternating seashore and barcode signs due to a lung point are seen during conventional mechanical ventilation (A) and high-frequency oscillatory ventilation (B). Normal high-frequency oscillatory ventilation without pneumothorax is also shown (C).

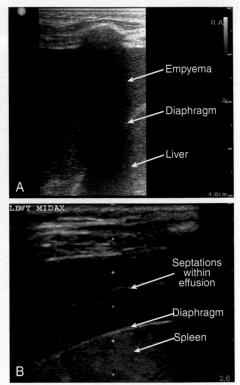

Figure 47.3 Complex Pleural Effusion. An empyema with increased echogenicity (A) and complex, septated effusion (B) are shown.

of bronchiolitis patients often shows a B-line pattern.[13,14] A lung ultrasound scoring system in infants with bronchiolitis admitted to a general pediatric ward found that ultrasound predicted supplemental oxygen dependence during admission with 99% sensitivity, 97% specificity, and 91% agreement between a pediatric provider and expert sonographer, suggesting a potential role for ultrasound severity scoring in bronchiolitis.[15] Use of ultrasound to distinguish bronchiolitis from bacterial pneumonia can spare children from unnecessary radiation exposure, prevent unnecessary antibiotic use, and reduce costs for families.

Lung ultrasound has also demonstrated benefit in grading newborn lung disease in the delivery bay. In a series of 54 newborns, a B-line dense parenchymal pattern at 2 hours of life was associated with non-invasive positive pressure ventilation failure and intubation by 24 hours of life with 89% sensitivity and 100% specificity.[16] Ultrasound has been used to characterize transient tachypnea of the newborn and identify acute pneumothorax as described previously, suggesting an important role for ultrasound in newborn resuscitation.[8,17]

DIAPHRAGM

Phrenic nerve injury from pediatric cardiothoracic surgery can lead to refractory respiratory failure and prolonged intubation, if not identified early in the postoperative period. Cardiac intensivists trained in ultrasound were able to identify evidence of phrenic nerve injury using ultrasound compared to fluoroscopy with 100% sensitivity and 100% specificity.[18] Diagnosing phrenic nerve injury at the bedside with ultrasound reduces the risk of complications from transporting and positioning the patient for a fluoroscopic exam, and reduces exposure to ionizing radiation. Diaphragm atrophy from prolonged intubation is associated with extubation failure in adults,[19] and ongoing studies may show similar benefits in children. Additionally, diaphragmatic excursion may be used to identify mainstem intubation in children (see "Procedural Applications" below).[20,21]

Heart

Focused cardiac ultrasound is used as an adjunct to other clinical data for management of a variety of hemodynamic conditions in children. The same views obtained from the subcostal, apical, and parasternal windows in adults are also obtained in children (see Chapter 14); however, one important difference is the apical and subcostal views are acquired by pediatric cardiologists with the screen orientation marker at the bottom of the screen (Fig. 47.4). Pediatric providers with advanced cardiac training may acquire additional views.[22]

Transducer selection is important as pediatric patients vary considerably in size. An adult phased-array transducer typically penetrates to a maximum depth of approximately 30 cm for use in older or obese children. Although a pediatric phased-array transducer may not penetrate as deep, it has a smaller face that is ideal for visualization of structures in between the ribs of children.

INTRAVASCULAR VOLUME STATUS

Multiple studies have investigated the use of point-of-care ultrasound for assessment of volume status in adults. Measurement of the inferior vena cava (IVC) size and collapsibility is one component of assessing volume status of adults. These techniques have been attempted to be applied to children; however, measuring respiratory variation of an infant's IVC is challenging because variation can equate to fractions of a millimeter over the respiratory cycle.

The IVC diameter changes with age, similar to other quantitative measurements.[23] Therefore, a ratio of the anterior-posterior diameter of the IVC and aorta is used as a relative index. A phased-array, curvilinear, or microconvex

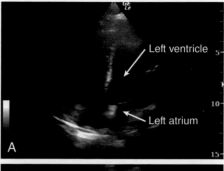

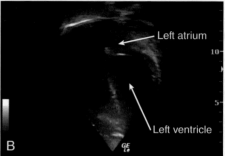

Figure 47.4   Apical 4-Chamber View. Most point-of-care users acquire cardiac images with the screen orientation marker in the top right side of the screen (A) compared to pediatric cardiologists, who position the screen orientation marker in the bottom right of the screen (B). Note the left-sided structures remain on the right side of the screen relative to the right-sided structures with either orientation.

transducer is placed in the midline immediately below the xiphoid process in a transverse orientation and the anterior-posterior aorta and IVC diameters are measured (Fig. 47.5). The point in the cardiac or respiratory cycle where measurements are obtained has not been standardized. This technique has been assessed in volume-depleted children in pediatric emergency departments (EDs), children receiving hemodialysis, and children in an austere medical mission setting.[24-27] From this aggregate data, a normal IVC to aorta ratio is likely between 0.8 and 1.2, with a ratio less than 0.8 suggesting intravascular hypovolemia, and a ratio greater than 1.2 suggesting fluid overload. Limitations include the ambiguity of when in the respiratory cycle measurements are obtained, and previous studies have attempted to use IVC measurements to assess volume depletion and not test for fluid responsiveness in shock.

Whether the patient is breathing spontaneously or receiving mechanical ventilation will affect the IVC ultrasound measurements

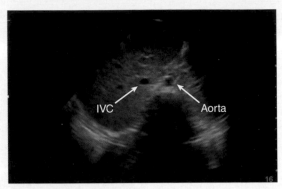

Figure 47.5   Inferior Vena Cava *(IVC)* and Aorta. A transverse view of the intrahepatic IVC and aorta is seen.

and their significance. Emerging evidence suggests that mechanical ventilation itself changes the IVC ultrasound characteristics such that pediatric volume status cannot be evaluated in the same manner during positive pressure ventilation as spontaneous breathing because increased intrathoracic pressure during positive pressure ventilation affects venous return and IVC compliance.[28] Therefore, use of quantitative IVC measurement to guide volume status assessment remains challenging and providers are encouraged to incorporate ultrasound findings with all other available data to guide decision-making.[29]

Using respiratory variation of the left ventricular outflow tract (LVOT) systolic blood flow velocity as an indicator of fluid responsiveness has been described in children.[30,31] Measurements are obtained from an apical 5-chamber view using pulsed-wave Doppler as described in adults (see Chapter 21). Variation of the LVOT velocity-time integral greater than 12% to 18% is suggestive of volume responsiveness, similar to variation of the oxygen saturation plethysmograph or arterial pressure tracings. This technique requires a narrower transducer face in small children because the pulsed-wave Doppler cursor must remain clear of the LVOT walls throughout the cardiac and respiratory cycles. Also, the sweep speed should be accelerated to separate each left ventricular (LV) contraction on the Doppler tracing.

CARDIAC FUNCTION

Regarding assessment of LV function, various studies have shown comparable accuracy of point-of-care ultrasound and comprehensive echocardiography in pediatric ED and ICU patients.[2,3,32-34] Cardiac function is evaluated qualitatively in children in a manner similar to that performed in adults. Providers should visualize the LV in multiple planes when assessing LV function. Qualitative assessment of LV function, or "eyeballing," is subject to user variability, but given that point-of-care ultrasound exams are usually performed in symptomatic patients, the pathologic findings may be more pronounced and easier to identify.

Though right ventricular (RV) physiology is important in several pediatric diseases, literature on pediatric point-of-care right heart assessment is sparse. Similar views as adults are used in children for a qualitative assessment. The RV free wall is relatively thicker in infants than adults due to the unique pulmonary vascular physiology of infants with increased RV afterload that is seen *in utero*.

STRUCTURAL PATHOLOGY

Anatomy of the great vessels and patent ductus arteriosus (PDA) has been an area of interest for neonatologists using point-of-care ultrasound. Though examination of PDA is common in some institutions, there is limited and conflicting evidence on the accuracy of ultrasound examinations performed by neonatologists.[22,35]

Concerns about abnormal cardiac structure are likely best assessed by providers with advanced echocardiographic training in structural heart disease. Point-of-care ultrasound may be beneficial as a screening modality in austere environments to identify patients needing more advanced imaging by expert echocardiographers.[36,37]

EXTRACORPOREAL MEMBRANOUS OXYGENATION AND CARDIAC ARREST

Point-of care ultrasonography can be used to assess patients receiving extracorporeal membranous oxygenation (ECMO). Guidelines on the use of echocardiography in ECMO have been published, and point-of-care ultrasound can assist in answering frequently encountered clinical questions.[38] Given the technical and personnel resources required for ECMO, providers are encouraged to corroborate point-of-care ultrasound findings with other data sources and collaborate with all involved specialties to guide management decisions.

Assessment of relative chamber sizes has utility in ECMO patients. Evaluation of the right heart and IVC can indicate relative chamber filling in the context of ECMO flow titration. LV size and function are relevant when weaning or titrating ECMO. Movement of the aortic valve can be monitored during recovery. Standard cardiac views are used in ECMO patients, but open chest incisions, postoperative dressings, and large lung volumes can limit acquisition of adequate cardiac views.

Cannula placement can be guided by point-of-care ultrasound. From a longitudinal IVC view, the base of the right atrium (RA) can be visualized during cannula placement. From a parasternal long-axis view, tilting the transducer and aiming the ultrasound beam toward the patient's right side acquires an RV inflow view. This view provides visualization of the RA and RV to guide placement of the access cannula from the superior vena cava (SVC) via internal jugular (IJ) vein or IVC via the femoral vein (see Chapter 17). The return cannula can be visualized in modified views of the aortic arch (see Chapter 14).

Use of point-of care ultrasound for assessment of cardiac arrest has been described in small pediatric series. Fourteen patients were described in one study where cardiac ultrasound was used for differentiation of potentially reversible causes of cardiac arrest.[39] Among those who had cardiac standstill, or an akinetic heart, return of spontaneous circulation (ROSC) was not achieved. However, one study described three patients with sonographic cardiac standstill who recovered cardiac function after receiving extracorporeal cardiopulmonary resuscitation (ECPR) and maybe cardiac standstill does not necessarily infer that ROSC

is impossible in children who have access to ECMO.[40] Though functional outcomes were dismal, the return of cardiac function suggests that cardiac standstill in isolation may not reliably predict ROSC failure in children.

Abdomen and Pelvis

Abdominal pain is a common presentation in children with a broad differential diagnosis that varies by age. Either a linear, curvilinear, or microconvex transducer can be used depending on the patient's size and the space being examined. Due to the small size of infants, a high-frequency transducer that generates high resolution images can be used to examine the abdomen.

MALROTATION

Bilious emesis, especially within the first week of life, raises immediate concern for malrotation with volvulus that must be promptly diagnosed. A linear transducer can be applied transversely over the mid-abdomen to visualize the aorta and IVC and locate the superior mesenteric artery (SMA) and superior mesenteric vein (SMV). Typically, the SMA is seen to the left of the SMV, similar to the aorta-IVC relationship. If the relationship is reversed, with the SMV seen on the patient's left relative to the SMA, concern should be raised for malrotation.

If the patient has bilious emesis, sonographic signs of obstruction due to volvulus would be expected. Several sonographic signs of small bowel inflammation, necrosis, or perforation have been described, including thickening of the bowel wall, intramural gas (the ultrasound equivalent of bowel *pneumatosis intestinalis*), and free fluid in the abdomen. Intramural air or pneumatosis appears as a strikingly bright pattern of thin, concentric, echogenic signal between the layers of bowel wall. Gas that escapes into the hepatic vasculature in severe bowel necrosis appears as a bright, echogenic signal in the hepatic portal veins. However, it is important to recall that gas signals in the hepatic venous vasculature can be due to inadvertent instillation of air through a lower extremity venous catheter. In volvulus, radiologists have described a whirlpool sign when using color flow Doppler over the inflamed bowel mass, indicating the SMV and mesentery are wrapped around the

SMA. Although fairly specific, this sign is not very sensitive and its absence can still miss the diagnosis.[41]

PYLORIC STENOSIS

Pyloric stenosis is the most common surgical cause of nonbilious emesis in the newborn period and typically presents between 4 and 12 weeks of age. Ultrasound is the primary modality used by radiologists to diagnose pyloric stenosis, and it can be performed by trained emergency medicine physicians.[42-44] The technique involves placing a linear transducer beneath the infant's sternum in a sagittal orientation, using the liver as an acoustic window, and following the antrum of the stomach medially until the pylorus is visible. The pylorus should be imaged in both short- and long-axis views, and may require the transducer to be held obliquely across the abdomen. Use warm gel and have the guardian cradle the patient in a semi-upright position to minimize discomfort.

To confirm that the structure is the stomach, trace it back to the area immediately below the left hemi-diaphragm. Allowing the infant to drink rehydration solution, water, or milk will fill the stomach, displace gas, and permit visualization of the stomach antrum and pylorus. The pylorus may be seen crossing immediately beneath the liver, or diving posteriorly particularly when the stomach is very distended (Fig. 47.6). Start with a depth of at least 6 cm,

and after identifying the pylorus, decrease the depth to focus on the area of interest.

Normally, the pylorus allows passage of gastric contents into the duodenum, and the fluid motion within the lumen is easily visualized by ultrasound. However, even a nonhypertrophied pylorus may demonstrate episodes of pylorospasm where the muscle sphincter closes and does not allow passage of contents, and therefore, one may need to observe for several minutes. An abnormally hypertrophied pylorus will not allow passage of any contents, except in rare circumstances where the stomach is so distended that pressure builds up and allows a very small volume of liquid to pass. In this scenario, pyloric stenosis can still be identified because the muscle wall will be very thickened (>3 mm) and the length of the pyloric channel wall will be elongated (>15 mm).[45-51] The muscle wall thickness is usually best appreciated and measured from a short-axis view where the concentric pylorus wall layers can be seen: (1) a thin bright serosal surface, (2) a thick, hypoechoic muscular layer, (3) a hyperechoic mucosal surface, and (4) the lumen, which is often completely obliterated due to hypertrophy. The thickness of the hypoechoic muscle layer should be measured in the top half of the cross-section closest to the transducer.

A thickened pylorus is often termed a "donut" sign from a short-axis view (Fig. 47.7). Thickness measured between 2 and 3 mm may indicate pylorospasm, early hypertrophy, or resolving hypertrophy and warrants further

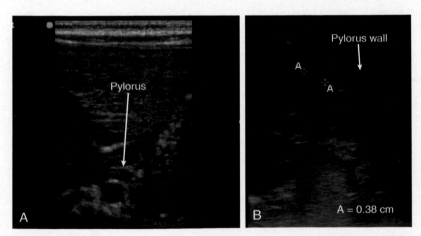

Figure 47.6 Pyloric Stenosis. A normal pylorus displaced downward by a distended stomach is seen (A) and an abnormal pylorus with a very thick wall (0.38 cm) are shown (B).

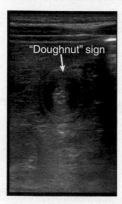

Figure 47.7 Pyloric Stenosis. A thickened pylorus (doughnut sign) is seen in pyloric stenosis.

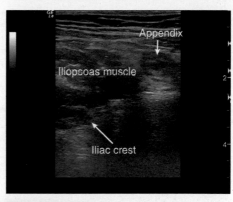

Figure 47.8 Appendix. The appendix is seen medial to the iliopsoas muscles and iliac crest in a short-axis view.

imaging by a radiologist and evaluation by a pediatric surgeon.

Other sonographic signs of pyloric stenosis include the "antral nipple" sign where part of the antrum buckles into the lumen of the enlarged fluid-filled stomach as pressure from peristalsis cannot propagate through the pylorus. This is best seen in a long-axis view of the stomach-pylorus interface. Sometimes the entire pylorus muscle may prolapse back into the stomach giving a rounded appearance to its edges (shoulder sign).

Narrow sections of the antrum can be misidentified as a normal pylorus, and these false negatives should be avoided by tracing the antrum in short-axis distally to make sure the smallest cross-section has been identified, and then sliding proximally to evaluate the confirmed section of pylorus. In difficult cases, repositioning the patient in a left or right lateral decubitus position may also help shift the pylorus into view.

APPENDICITIS

Appendicitis is one of the most common surgical emergencies associated with vomiting and abdominal pain in children. Due to the risks of radiation, ultrasound is the recommended initial modality to diagnose appendicitis in children.[52] When performed by skilled providers, ultrasound can closely approximate the sensitivity and specificity of computed tomography.[53,54] When used in a step-wise approach with other imaging modalities, ultrasound can improve the overall diagnostic accuracy of a

bedside examination while decreasing costs and exposure to ionizing radiation.[55-59]

A high-frequency linear transducer is preferred for this examination, but in obese children, a low-frequency transducer may be needed to visualize deep spaces where fluid or phlegmon may accumulate. Use copious amounts of gel to minimize inflicting pain, and start over the area of maximal tenderness. Gentle pressure with the transducer will push gas-filled loops of bowel aside and allow visualization of inflamed areas of bowel. Slowly tilt the transducer back and forth to thoroughly examine a section of the abdomen before moving to another location.

It is important to visualize all anatomic areas where the appendix can be located and where fluid can collect in the abdomen and pelvis. Abdominal or pelvic free fluid may offer a clue to pathology or even reveal an abscess or phlegmon from a perforated appendix (Video 47.2). One approach is to start in the most inferior portions of the abdomen both lateral and medial to the psoas muscle. On the lateral side, start by visualizing the iliopsoas muscle sitting within the right iliac bone in a short-axis view. Slowly slide the transducer rostrally until bowel is visualized, and continue until you have fully explored the area lateral to the psoas muscle up to the level of the umbilicus. This view is important with retrocecal appendices and atypical presentations. Certain conditions, such as pregnancy, predispose the appendix to being in an atypical location (Video 47.3). The medial side of the psoas muscle is where the appendix lies in the majority of patients (Fig. 47.8).

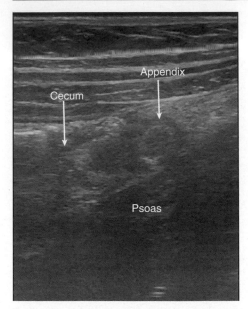

Figure 47.9 Appendix. The tubular appendix is seen adjacent to the gas-filled cecum in a short-axis view.

Once again, begin in the most inferior area with the bladder visualized medially and then slowly slide rostrally keeping the psoas muscle and iliac vessels in view laterally until passing the level of the umbilicus. If the appendix has not been identified, search for the cecum from a focused view of the psoas muscle and iliac vessels (Video 47.4). The cecum will appear as a gas- or fluid-filled structure with haustra appearing as irregular borders (Fig. 47.9; Video 47.5). Turn the transducer into a long-axis orientation over the psoas muscle while visualizing the cecum. In this orientation, search for the appendix by tilting the transducer laterally and medially.

The appendix typically comes off the most inferior portion of the cecum and ends in a blind loop. The blind loop should be seen in both short and long axes, avoiding oblique views (Fig. 47.10). Neither a normal nor abnormal appendix has peristalsis, which is one way to distinguish it from small bowel, although an inflamed or diseased small intestine may also lack peristalsis. The ileum joins the cecum approximately 2 cm from the distal end of the cecum. An abnormal appendix typically measures greater than 6 mm in diameter from outer wall to outer wall and does not compress with pressure from the transducer (Fig. 47.11).

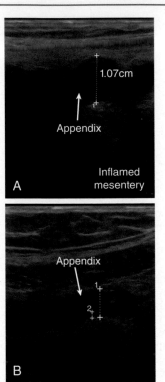

Figure 47.10 Distended Appendix. A distended appendix is seen in short-axis (A) and long-axis views (B).

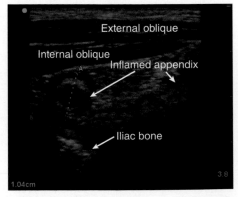

Figure 47.11 Inflamed Appendix. An inflamed, distended appendix is seen in a short-axis view and measures 1.04 cm in diameter.

Size alone is not truly enough to make a diagnosis of appendicitis in most cases. Secondary signs of appendicitis on ultrasound include surrounding mesenteric streaking (a smudged chalk appearance of tissues outlining the bowel

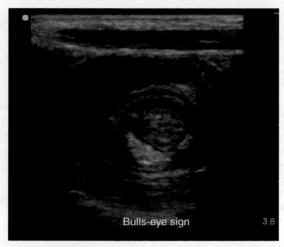

Figure 47.12 Intussusception. Multiple concentric layers of overlapping mesentery, fat, and bowel wall (bulls-eye sign) are seen in intussusception.

TABLE 47.1   Characteristics of a Normal and Inflamed Appendix, and Small Intestine

	Peristalsis	Compressible	Connects to Cecum	Blind End	Diameter
Appendix		✔	✔	✔	<6 mm
Appendicitis			✔	✔	>6 mm
Small intestine	✔	✔	✔		Variable

indicating echogenic fat), focal ileus (decreased or absent peristalsis of surrounding bowel), enlarged mesenteric lymph nodes, and abdominal free fluid (anechoic areas with sharp, irregular borders).[60] A fecalith may be visualized as a bright intraluminal object casting an acoustic shadow (Video 47.6). Of course, the area of concern should be tender when palpated with the transducer, otherwise the diagnosis should be questioned (Table 47.1).

INTUSSUSCEPTION

Intussusception can present with vomiting, abdominal pain, blood in the stool, and altered mental status. Intermittent symptoms should prompt evaluation for intussusception using point-of-care ultrasound. Novice providers have demonstrated rapid learning curves for diagnosing intussusception with ultrasound.[61,62]

Using a high-frequency linear transducer, start in the right lower quadrant over the ileocolic junction where more than 75% of intussusception occurs. Trace the large bowel in a square path around the abdomen by sliding superiorly on the right side (ascending colon), across to the left side (transverse colon), and then inferiorly on the left side (descending colon). When an intussusception is visualized in cross-section it appears as a large bullseye with multiple layers of mesentery, fat, and bowel wall forming concentric circles of varying echogenicity and measuring ≥2.5 cm in diameter (Fig. 47.12, Videos 47.7 and 47.8).

Small-bowel intussusception can mimic the appearance of ileocolic intussusception but will have a diameter less than 2.5 cm and may still demonstrate peristalsis. In a long-axis view, an intussusception may mimic the appearance of a kidney on ultrasound with a flattened "C" shape. Signs of advanced disease may include pockets of anechoic fluid trapped in between loops of bowel within the intussusception. Intramural air, appearing as echogenic foci within the bowel wall, is suggestive of ischemia and bowel wall injury and is associated with difficult or unsuccessful reduction.[63-67] Complete absence of blood flow on color Doppler imaging of the involved bowel is also a predictor of poor outcomes.[68,69]

PEDIATRIC BLUNT ABDOMINAL TRAUMA

In children, an extended focused assessment with sonography for trauma (e-FAST) can help identify injuries causing bleeding into the peritoneal, pericardial, or pleural spaces. Whereas no large randomized trials have demonstrated significant improvements in outcomes from an e-FAST as the initial diagnostic test, performance of an e-FAST has evolved to become standard practice in trauma centers, and findings can help in individual cases to decide on further imaging, disposition, or treatment.[70-77]

There are many similarities for conducting an e-FAST in pediatric and adult patients. An important difference is pediatric patients more frequently accumulate blood in the pelvis, as opposed to the right upper quadrant in adults.[70,78] The same technique is used in both adults and children (see Chapter 24).

Nervous System

Traditionally, pediatric diagnostic ultrasound imaging has included evaluation of the nervous system; however, literature on neurological ultrasound is limited. Although high-quality computerized tomography or functional testing, such as electroencephalogram (EEG), can provide definitive diagnoses in high-stakes neurological conditions, ultrasound is a potential screening tool to complement bedside evaluation and guide work-up of many neurological conditions.

NEUROSONOLOGY

The infant brain can be imaged through an open anterior or posterior fontanelle using a small 8 MHz curvilinear or microconvex transducer. The cerebral hemispheres are imaged in coronal and transverse planes by tilting or fanning the transducer in left to right and anterior to posterior directions, respectively (Fig. 47.13, Video 47.9). Neurosonology of the brain is the primary diagnostic modality for assessment of intraventricular hemorrhage in neonates. Neonatologists have been performing these examinations, although standards and protocols have not been well described.[79] Providers must be aware that bedside neurosonology is limited by provider expertise and in certain situations, including detection of extra-axial intracranial hemorrhages, small

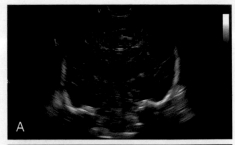
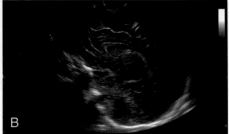

Figure 47.13 Neurosonology. Coronal (A) and sagittal (B) views of the infant brain are seen through the anterior fontanelle.

subdural hemorrhages lateral to the transducer's field of view, areas of ischemia without bleeding in acute stroke, and visualization of the posterior fossa and midbrain through the anterior fontanelle (see also Chapter 48).

TRANSCRANIAL DOPPLER

Transcranial Doppler (TCD) is an integral component of neurovascular assessment at the bedside in adults and children. It is a definitive modality for assessing flow acceleration in stenotic vessels and is routinely used for assessment of stroke risk, arteriospasm after subacute hemorrhage, and brain death.[80] Either dedicated TCD (one-dimensional ultrasound) or transcranial imaging (TCI) (two-dimensional Doppler ultrasound) can be used but are performed using different techniques. TCI is performed with a low-frequency ultrasound transducer, typically a phased-array transducer, that can penetrate bone, whereas a high-frequency microconvex transducer may be used in infants (Fig. 47.14, Video 47.10). Because the Doppler sample gate may be misaligned with the direction of flow when using TCI, some evidence suggests one-dimensional ultrasound may be more accurate.[81] Identifying flow changes in children on ECMO as a predictor of hemorrhage or other primary neurological event is a

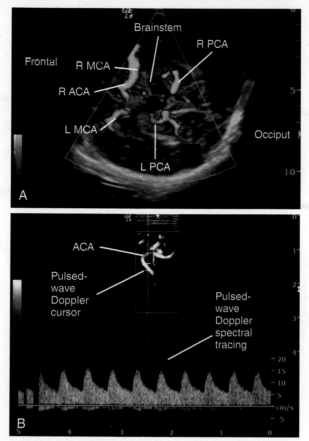

Figure 47.14 **Transcranial Doppler Ultrasound.** (A) Intracranial arteries are seen using color power Doppler ultrasound, and (B) pulsed-wave Doppler ultrasound is used to measure the flow of the anterior cerebral circulation through the temporal window. *ACA,* Anterior cerebral artery; *L,* left; *MCA,* middle cerebral artery; *PCA,* posterior cerebral artery; *R,* right.

potential application of TCD.[82] Several studies have examined the correlation of TCD values with intracranial pressure (ICP), but a meaningful association has not yet been established in pediatric patients.[83,84]

OPHTHALMIC—RETINA, GLOBE, AND IRIS

Ocular ultrasound is performed in a manner similar to that of adults (see Chapter 39). Because ultrasound gel can be irritating to the eye, ophthalmic lubricant can be used as the acoustic coupling media. Similar to adults, ocular ultrasound is useful for assessment of foreign body, trauma, pupillary reflex, and extraocular movements.[85,86] Within the

scope of a retinal assessment, retinoschisis as a sequela of abusive head trauma from shearing injury to the retina has been described in a cohort of abused children (Fig. 47.15).[87]

OPHTHALMIC—OPTIC NERVE SHEATH

The optic nerve sheath has been an area of interest as dilatation of the nerve sheath correlates with papilledema due to increased ICP.[88,89] A cohort of pediatric patients with increased ICP were found to have increased optic nerve sheath diameter (ONSD) measured 3 mm behind the retina.[90] However, generalization of this data raises questions about how the effects of growth and development alter

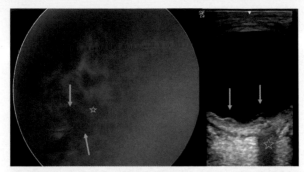

Figure 47.15   Retinoschisis. Areas of retinal detachment *(arrows)* are shown by ophthalmoscopy *(left)* and ultrasound *(right)*. *Star*, optic nerve.

this threshold across the age spectrum. Given that papilledema can persist despite resolution of increased ICP, as seen among craniosynostosis patients, one must consider the chronicity of intracranial hypertension. In patients with repeated episodes of hydrocephalus, studies demonstrate decreased concordance between ONSD measurements and intracranial hypertension.[91,92] Cadaveric data suggest that the dura of the optic nerve may not immediately return to normal size once ICP has been relieved.[93] Thus, changes in measurement of ONSD in patients with chronic intracranial hypertension are likely limited because preexisting increased ICP may affect its accuracy.[94-97]

Procedural Applications

Currently, most bedside procedures are performed with ultrasound guidance, and the most common procedural applications in pediatric acute care are described in the following section.

CENTRAL VENOUS ACCESS

Multiple national and international organizations support the use of ultrasound guidance for central venous catheter (CVC) insertion.[98-101] Most studies demonstrating benefits of ultrasound guidance in CVC placement were predominantly performed in adult patients. Patient anatomic variability and provider performance in trials of ultrasound-guided CVC placement in children has led to widespread use of ultrasound guidance.

Anatomic considerations include the smaller target vessel size and a higher likelihood for unintentional puncture of nearby structures in children compared to adults. Furthermore, pediatric patients have high rates of anatomic variation in common sites of central venous access, as well as higher rates of procedural complications, device failure, and infection compared to adults.[102-105]

Randomized trials have demonstrated that ultrasound-guided techniques are superior to landmark-based techniques in pediatric patients, predominantly in IJ CVC insertion.[106,107] Additionally, studies have demonstrated benefits of ultrasound-guided insertion of pediatric peripherally inserted central catheters (PICCs) and neonatal umbilical venous catheters.[108,109]

Due to the small size of pediatric necks and thoracic vessels, many experts advocate for use of ultrasound guidance to place CVCs in the brachiocephalic vein using a supraclavicular longitudinal approach. The transducer is placed parallel to and above the medial third of the clavicle, aiming the transducer face toward the center of the mediastinum. The transducer should be aligned over the brachiocephalic vein at the confluence of the IJ and subclavian veins. Literature supporting this approach has been published, but comparative trials among skilled providers are needed.[110,111] Additionally, placement of CVCs in the axillary vein at the level of the anterior axillary fold has been described in children.[112] For axillary vein cannulation, a linear-array transducer is placed transverse to the axillary vein with the vessel typically appearing relatively caudad to the pulsatile axillary artery (see Chapter 36, Fig. 36.12).

Although a common belief is that pediatric patients have a higher risk of infection with femoral CVCs due to soiling in the diaper, a

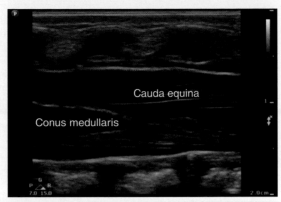

Figure 47.16 **Lumbar Spine.** A longitudinal view of an infant spine at the level of the conus medullaris with the cauda equina.

meta-analysis of CVC location and infection risk concluded that there was no difference in infection rate based solely on location.[113] Current pediatric literature supports the insertion of CVCs in the femoral vein as equivocal to other sites. (See also Chapter 36.)

PERIPHERAL VENOUS ACCESS

A meta-analysis demonstrated ultrasound guidance significantly improved the success rates of peripheral intravenous line (PIV) placement in adults.[114] Recent pediatric literature supports improved overall success rates (80% vs. 64%), reduced number of insertion attempts (1 vs. 3), and decreased number of needle redirections (2 vs. 10), in PIV placement performed by ED providers using ultrasound versus landmarks.[115] Although studies in adults suggest that long PIV catheters inserted with ultrasound guidance may have a lower failure rate than short catheters, an assessment of catheter length and duration has not been performed in children.[116,117] (See also Chapter 37.)

ARTERIAL ACCESS

The process of peripheral arterial cannulation is well described in Chapter 38. Cannulation of distal arteries (radial, ulnar, dorsalis pedis, or posterior tibial) is a common procedure, and studies have shown improved first-pass success rates and decreased complications when using ultrasound guidance versus landmarks (or Doppler methods) in pediatric patients.[118-121] A study of pediatric critical care trainees showed fewer attempts and faster radial artery

cannulation with the use of ultrasound guidance, regardless of the patient's body habitus or provider's level of training.[122]

LUMBAR PUNCTURE

Even though landmark-based lumbar puncture is commonly taught in pediatric training, most trainees demonstrate low first-pass success rates and failure to improve performance despite intensive training.[123] A randomized controlled study found a higher first-pass success rate (58% vs. 31%) and lower number of total attempts (1 vs. 2) with the use of ultrasound guidance in a pediatric ED.[124] In infants, visualization of the entire spinal cord, including the conus medullaris and cauda equina, is possible due to incomplete spinal ossification, which reveals obvious target sites for lumbar puncture (Fig. 47.16). (See also Chapter 43.)

INTUBATION

Though end-tidal CO_2 (ETCO$_2$) capnometry is considered a confirmatory test for verifying successful endotracheal intubation, false-negative ETCO$_2$ interpretations can arise in the setting of cardiac arrest or pulmonary embolism, and false-positive interpretations can arise in the setting of esophageal intubations following aggressive pre-intubation bag mask ventilation.[125] A prospective randomized trial using ultrasound to confirm endotracheal tube (ETT) position at the level of the cricothyroid membrane following intubation in the ED reported that ultrasound correctly identified the ETT location in all 50 patients. In two cases, proper

ETT position was confirmed despite negative $ETCO_2$ capnometry, as well as one case of esophageal intubation despite presence of $ETCO_2$.[126] In neonates and infants, studies have demonstrated the ability to directly visualize the endotracheal tube's tip position in greater than 80% of patients and strong correlation with radiographic position.[127,128] This technique relies on transmissibility of ultrasound through the neonatal mediastinal structures that have higher water content. In older infants and children, it is not possible to directly visualize the ETT through the sternum and ribs. However, diaphragmatic excursion is another method of assessing successful intubation. Finding unilateral diaphragm movement in a previously well child suggests mainstem intubation, and finding bilateral and equivalent diaphragm excursion suggests air is entering both lungs equally with the ETT in the trachea, though the exact tube position cannot be assessed with this technique.

PEARLS AND PITFALLS

- Because of incomplete ossification of bones and small size of children, a high-frequency linear transducer can often provide adequate penetration to image the thoracic and abdominal organs.
- Institutional standards should be established for acquiring pediatric heart images because pediatric cardiology traditionally has acquired images with the screen orientation marker in the lower right side of the screen.
- A normal range for inferior vena cava (IVC) diameter based on the size of a child has not been established, and therefore, a ratio of the IVC to aorta diameter is used that is normally 0.8 to 1.2.
- Assessment of cardiac chamber sizes and cannula position is a useful point-of-care ultrasound application in patients receiving extracorporeal membranous oxygenation.
- Ultrasound is the recommended initial modality to diagnose appendicitis in children, and when performed by skilled providers, ultrasound can closely approximate the sensitivity and specificity of computed tomography.
- When imaging through the anterior fontanelle in infants, high-quality images of the brain can be rapidly obtained with ultrasound.
- Although the presentation of various disease processes may be different in pediatric populations, the technique for evaluation and identification of pathophysiology is similar to adult techniques, and lessons learned from one population can complement the other.

CHAPTER 48

Neonatology

María V. Fraga ■ Thomas W. Conlon ■ Jae H. Kim ■ Erik Su

KEY POINTS

- Ultrasound guidance can reduce line manipulations and procedure time when inserting umbilical venous and arterial catheters, as well as peripherally inserted central catheters.
- The cartilaginous sternum and ribs of neonates facilitates thoracic ultrasound imaging of the heart, lungs, and mediastinal structures.
- Most neonatal providers are familiar with how to *interpret* brain ultrasound images acquired by radiology and can rapidly learn how to *perform* head ultrasound exams.

Background

Ultrasound has long been used in the management of critically ill neonates. It is an integral part of neurological monitoring for intraventricular hemorrhage, as well as for ongoing cardiac monitoring of congenital heart disease starting in the prenatal period. In recent years, ultrasound has become increasingly used by neonatologists, coupled with its central role in maternal-fetal medicine as a safe imaging modality that does not expose patients to ionizing radiation. More neonatologists are acquiring and interpreting basic ultrasound images in collaboration with primary imaging specialists to guide clinical decision-making,[1] and with increasing availability of ultrasound machines, basic point-of-care ultrasound skills will eventually become a standard skill set for most neonatologists.

Central Catheters

UMBILICAL VEIN AND ARTERY CATHETERS

Background

Central venous access is essential for newborns for adequate enteral nutrition and administration of intravenous medications. For neonates, umbilical catheters and peripherally inserted central catheters (PICCs) are most often inserted. The insertion of temporary central venous catheters in the subclavian, internal jugular, or femoral veins of neonates has increased in recent years due to availability of ultrasound guidance.

During umbilical venous catheter (UVC) insertion in newborns, point-of-care ultrasound has been used to verify accurate catheter tip position at the right atrium (RA)–inferior vena cava (IVC) junction. Use of ultrasound reduces line manipulations, procedure time, and number of radiographs.[2,3] Identification of the umbilical vein and arteries in neonates does not require ultrasound, and therefore, the primary function of ultrasound is guidance of catheter tip placement. A UVC is inserted in the umbilical vein, passed cephalad toward the left portal vein and ductus venosus, and positioned at the confluence of the RA and IVC. An umbilical arterial catheter (UAC) is passed caudad into the respective internal iliac artery, through one of the common iliac arteries, and positioned in the descending aorta (Fig. 48.1).

Technique

A phased-array transducer is generally preferred, but other transducer types capable of generating a sector-shaped image, such as a microconvex or linear transducer set to trapezoid mode,

471

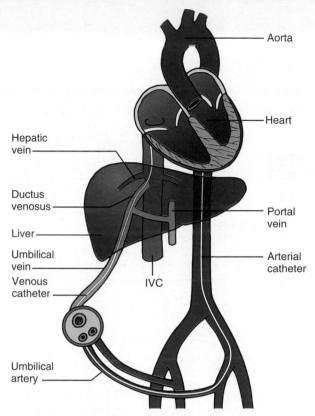

Figure 48.1 Anatomy of Neonatal Circulation. Location of umbilical venous and arterial catheters is shown. *IVC,* Inferior vena cava.

can be used for assessment of umbilical line tip location in neonates. A cardiac setting is most often used with the screen orientation indicator in the upper right corner.

For ultrasound-guided UVC insertion, two providers are ideally needed: one provider to advance the catheter and a second provider to perform the ultrasound imaging beneath the sterile drapes. A single operator can also perform this procedure with the abdomen sterilely prepped and draped from the umbilicus to the xiphoid process and with the probe covered in a sterile sheath. The transducer is placed on the upper abdomen with the orientation marker ("notch") pointed cephalad. The ultrasound beam is aligned parallel to the spine in order to visualize the intrahepatic IVC longitudinally. Before the UVC is seen in the IVC, only the UVC's dark shadow is seen in the ductus venosus, and the shadow is tracked as the catheter is advanced (Fig. 48.2 and Video 48.1). The shadow of the UVC is

the most obvious sign of the location of the catheter. Once the UVC enters the IVC, it is readily visible with ultrasound (Fig. 48.3 and Video 48.2). The catheter should be placed a bit further cephalad above the IVC-RA junction (about 0.5 cm) to keep it away from the liver where infusions may extravasate.

For ultrasound-guided UAC insertion, the transducer is optimally operated by a second provider. First, identify the descending abdominal aorta by placing the transducer in the midline superior to the umbilicus with the transducer orientation marker pointed cephalad. The muscular, pulsatile aorta is relatively easily identified with ultrasound. As the UAC is advanced, the tip becomes readily visualized as it approaches the liver. In general, UACs are easier to visualize than UVCs and are found left of midline and dorsal to UVCs (Fig. 48.4). The catheter tip should be placed slightly cephalad to the diaphragm which corresponds with T6 to T9. While targeting placement of

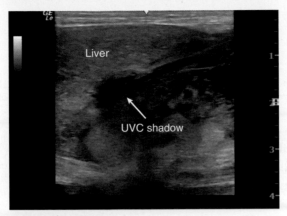

Figure 48.2   Umbilical Vein Catheter *(UVC)*. A UVC is seen within the ductus venosus from a longitudinal subcostal view. Note the prominent shadow cast by the UVC.

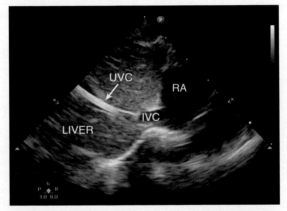

Figure 48.3   Right Atrial–Inferior Vena Cava *(IVC)* **Longitudinal View.** An umbilical vein catheter *(UVC)* is seen in the ductus venosus joining the IVC from a longitudinal subcostal view. *RA,* Right atrium.

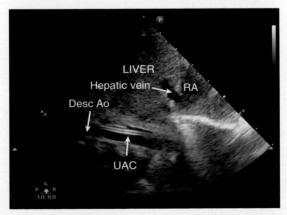

Figure 48.4   Umbilical Artery Catheter *(UAC)*. A UAC is seen in the descending aorta *(Desc Ao)* from a longitudinal subcostal view. *RA,* Right atrium.

the catheter tip slightly above the level of the diaphragm, the tip can be advanced under direct visualization until it appears in correct position. Placement of a UAC in a low position below the celiac trunk and renal arteries under ultrasound guidance may not be possible because of interference from bowel gas.

PERIPHERALLY INSERTED CENTRAL CATHETERS

Background

PICCs are used extensively for venous access in neonates. PICCs are inserted immediately after birth in neonates instead of UVCs when the ductus venosus is absent and after UVC removal, typically after 7 to 10 days of life.[4] Every baby with a birth weight <1500 g generally requires a PICC for delivery of fluids, nutrition, and medications. Data on catheter diameter and risk of thrombosis is limited; however, retrospective series suggest that limiting the catheter diameter to half of the vessel diameter may reduce the incidence of thrombosis.[5] PICCs are placed in both upper and lower extremity veins with the catheter tips in the superior vena cava (SVC) or IVC, respectively. For neonates, PICCs have been engineered to a miniscule 1 Fr size and come with a variety of insertion techniques. The small size of these catheters makes them difficult to see on plain radiographs and sometimes requires the injection of contrast agents to visualize the tip location. PICC catheters are visualized by ultrasound as hyperechoic structures.[6] For

PICC insertion, procedural time and manipulation are reduced when ultrasound guidance is used.[7]

Technique

The real-time needle visualization and insertion techniques used in newborns are the same as those used in children (see Chapters 36 and 47). Preferably, a second provider manipulates the transducer underneath the sterile drapes while the primary operator advances the catheter. The SVC can be visualized in neonates due to their cartilaginous chest walls. Place the transducer just to the left of the mid-sternum with the transducer orientation marker pointed cephalad to visualize the SVC. From this position, tilt the transducer toward the patient's right to bring the SVC into view deep to the prominent aorta. The PICC tip can be visualized as it is advanced into the SVC. The catheter can be seen in the SVC and should be placed just above or at the SVC–right atrial junction (Fig. 48.5). For lower extremity PICCs, the IVC is visualized from a subcostal longitudinal view, similar to UVC placement. The transducer should be centered longitudinally over the IVC for optimal visualization (Fig. 48.6).

For upper extremity PICCs, identify the tip with the arm flexed ~45 degrees at the elbow and armpit to ensure the deepest tip position is seen and ensure the catheter does not enter the RA. Similarly, for lower extremity PICCs, identify the tip with the knee and hip flexed at about 90 degrees to ensure the deepest tip position is seen.

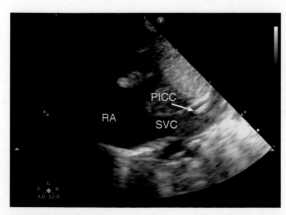

Figure 48.5 Superior Vena Cava (SVC) With Catheter. The tip of a peripherally inserted central catheter (PICC) is seen just above the SVC–right atrial (RA) junction.

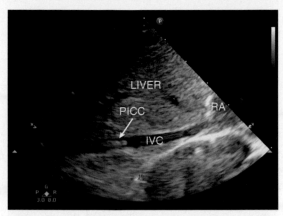

Figure 48.6 Inferior Vena Cava *(IVC)* With Catheter. The tip of a lower extremity peripherally inserted central catheter *(PICC)* is seen longitudinally in the IVC from a subcostal view. *RA*, Right atrium.

When difficulty is encountered in finding the catheter tip, the operator can flush a small amount of normal saline and the turbulent flow reveals the tip location. The tips of upper and lower extremity PICCs should be positioned at the superior and inferior cavoatrial junctions, respectively, to ensure adequate blood flow around the catheter to reduce the risk of thrombosis or cardiac arrhythmia. The catheter can become less visible or completely invisible if it is inserted beyond the SVC–RA junction because the turbulent flow of the RA will constantly move the catheter. If a lower extremity PICC is not visualized, the tip may be in the mid-abdomen and visualization can be obscured by bowel gas.

Endotracheal Tube Placement

BACKGROUND

Endotracheal tubes (ETTs) enter the nares or mouth and pass through the vocal cords to end midway between the thoracic inlet and carina. Localizing the ETT using ultrasound may present a technical challenge because air around the tube interferes with direct visualization of the tube. However, passage of the ETT into the trachea versus esophagus can be readily discerned using a small linear transducer placed transversely over the larynx in adults and pediatric patients.[8-11] In neonates, identification of the ETT is easier than adults or pediatric patients due to their cartilaginous sternum and ribs, and higher body water content. Confirmation of the ETT tip location from a

longitudinal view using a linear transducer has been shown in preterm and term infants.[12]

TECHNIQUE

Two important aspects of intubation can be assessed with ultrasound: confirmation and depth of ETT placement in the trachea. Confirmation of intubation success requires identification of the ETT within the trachea. During or immediately after the procedure, a linear transducer is placed in a transverse orientation above the suprasternal notch at the base of the neck. The ETT appears as a hyperechoic curved line in the trachea, and air within its lumen obscures visualization of other structures deep to the ETT (Fig. 48.7). If the ETT is misplaced in the esophagus, the trachea will be empty and the hyperechoic ETT will be seen in the adjacent esophagus to the left of the trachea. After confirming placement in the trachea, it is important to identify the depth of the ETT in the trachea. Rotate the infant's head to one side and place the transducer longitudinally over the middle to upper third of the sternum with the transducer marker pointing cephalad. In newborns, the sternum is cartilaginous and easily penetrated by ultrasound. The tracheal rings are seen as rectangular echogenic segments. Identify the tracheal markings diagonally across the screen and then look for the tip of the ETT as a hyperechoic line or spot in the trachea. To confirm the hyperechoic structure is the ETT, gently slide the ETT, no more than 0.5 cm in and out, and the tip should be seen moving on the screen

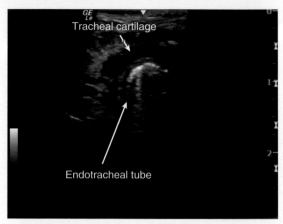

Figure 48.7 Endotracheal Tube (Transverse View). An endotracheal tube is seen within the trachea from a transverse view.

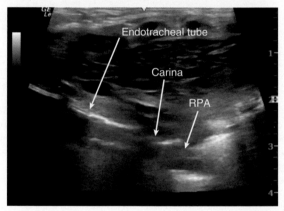

Figure 48.8 Endotracheal Tube (Longitudinal View). An endotracheal tube is seen within the trachea above the carina from a longitudinal view. *RPA,* Right pulmonary artery.

(Fig. 48.8 and Video 48.3). The carina is not readily seen by ultrasound but the right pulmonary artery (RPA) is a vascular landmark that can be used to identify the carina as the RPA is caudad to it.

Cardiac Ultrasound

BACKGROUND

Point-of-care cardiac ultrasound or echocardiography for hemodynamic evaluation of term and preterm infants is being increasingly performed by neonatologists. Ultrasound allows assessment of the complex and dynamic transitional circulation, variable responses of the immature myocardium in the early neonatal period, and the presence of intra- and extra-cardiac shunts

as a patent foramen ovale (PFO) or ductus arteriosus (PDA), respectively. The lack of reliable measurements to assess systemic blood flow has prompted neonatologists to use point-of-care cardiac ultrasound which offers new insights in the effects of the ductus arteriosus and pulmonary hemodynamics in patients with ongoing clinical instability. Point-of-care cardiac ultrasound permits rapid assessment of cardiac chamber size, function, and hemodynamics, allowing rapid diagnostic interpretation in a wide variety of settings, ranging from ambulatory clinics to intensive care units. Bedside ultrasound provides meaningful clinical data in real time to guide clinical decision-making[13,14] by providing a better understanding of the underlying physiological processes and monitoring responses to treatment. Some studies have demonstrated that routine use of point-of-care cardiac ultrasound in the neonatal period might lead to early identification of cardiovascular compromise that could expedite clinical management and potentially improve short-term outcomes.[15-18]

An important aspect of point-of-care cardiac ultrasound is the training of providers who use it. Accurate image acquisition and interpretation of cardiac images are essential skills in clinical practice to enable providers to augment their clinical assessment. Collaboration with pediatric cardiology is recommended for training, skill maintenance, and ongoing clinical support.

IMAGE ACQUISITION

Point-of-care cardiac ultrasound focuses primarily on the use of two-dimensional (2D) mode to evaluate the heart, and pulsed-wave Doppler (PWD), continuous-wave Doppler (CWD), color flow Doppler, and M-mode are used in specific cardiac applications. In term and preterm infants, a phased-array transducer with a frequency range of 8 to 12 MHz provides excellent resolution and adequate tissue penetration. Echocardiographic windows in newborns can be challenging due to their small size and lung hyperinflation, especially in preterm infants and neonates with bronchopulmonary dysplasia.

The principal cardiac views in neonatology are the same as those obtained in adult patients (see Chapter 14), with the addition of two unique views: the PDA and SVC views (Fig. 48.9, Videos 48.4–48.7).

- PDA view acquisition (Fig. 48.10 and Video 48.8): Place the transducer on the upper third of the sternum or in the suprasternal notch with the marker cephalad and aim the ultrasound beam slightly to the left of the midline to visualize the root of the left pulmonary artery (LPA) that will appear as a diverticulum at the distal end of the main pulmonary artery (MPA). The ductus arteriosus extends from the MPA just above the root of the LPA to the aortic arch.
- SVC view acquisition (Fig. 48.11 and Video 48.9): Place the transducer over the midsternum in a longitudinal plane, slightly to the left of the midline with the marker pointing cephalad. Tilt the transducer slightly to the right until the ascending aorta appears in view. Continue tilting to the right until the SVC appears in view connecting to the right atrium deep to the ascending aorta. This view is used primarily to measure the SVC maximum and minimum diameters. A subcostal SVC view is used to measure SVC blood flow velocities using PWD as described below.

IMAGE INTERPRETATION

Point-of-care cardiac ultrasound is usually focused on answering a specific clinical question. The following sections review some of the common clinical applications in a neonatal intensive care unit (NICU).

Cardiac Output

Systemic hypotension is a common problem in neonates, especially in preterm infants. Blood pressure is not a reliable surrogate marker of systemic organ perfusion because it cannot capture the complex cardiovascular hemodynamics during transitional circulation. Serial point-of-care cardiac ultrasound offers the advantage of revealing the physiologic nature of cardiovascular impairment: whether the underlying problem is preload, afterload, or myocardial contractility.

Evaluation of intravascular volume status and myocardial performance have been described previously (see Chapters 21 and 47). Similar techniques are used in pediatric and neonatal patients. Assessment of left ventricular stroke volume (SV) involves measuring the mean velocity of blood flow across the aortic valve from an apical 5-chamber view using PWD, and then determining the diameter of the aortic root from a parasternal long-axis view (Fig. 48.12; see also Figs. 21.4 and 21.5). The area under the waveform is used to calculate the velocity-time integral (VTI), which is a measure of the distance travelled by blood during each left ventricular contraction. Multiplying the VTI by the aortic cross-sectional area gives the SV, and multiplying the SV by the heart rate (HR) gives the left ventricular output (LVO). The LVO is divided by the patient's weight and expressed as mL/kg/min. In neonates, LVO must be used with caution. It might be falsely reassuring in the presence of a large PDA with significant systemic steal. Right ventricular output (RVO) is measured following the same approach but measuring blood flow across the pulmonic valve and using the pulmonary artery diameter. RVO reflects blood returning from the systemic circulation,

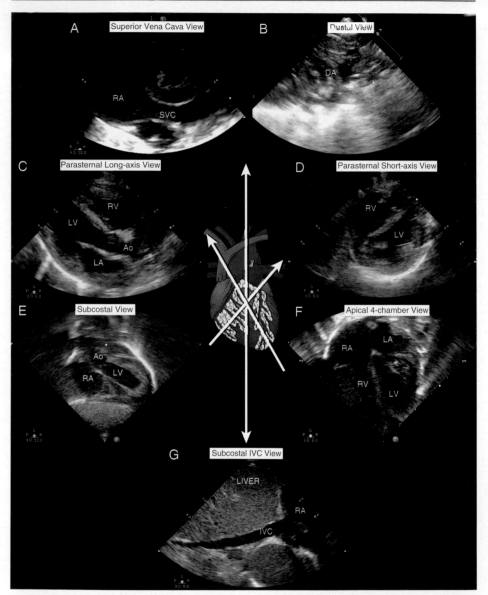

Figure 48.9   Basic Point-of-Care Cardiac Ultrasound Views in Neonates. The *arrows* depict the cardiac imaging planes to acquire the views shown. (A) Superior vena cava *(SVC)*, (B) Ductal, (C) Parasternal long axis, (D) Parasternal short axis, (E) Subcostal, (F) Apical 4-chamber, and (G) Subcostal inferior vena cava *(IVC)* views are shown. *Ao,* Aorta; *DA,* ductus arteriosus; *LA,* left atrium; *LV,* left ventricle; *RA,* right atrium; *RV,* right ventricle.

but similar to LVO, RVO can be confounded by the presence of an interatrial shunt.

SVC flow has been proposed as an alternative to measure venous return from the brain and upper body and is not confounded by any shunts.[19] SVC flow is calculated using the same concepts described above for LVO. A subcostal approach is used to measure SVC velocities using PWD because the ultrasound beam can be aligned with the direction of flow. The angle of insonation can be optimized by sliding the transducer inferiorly onto the abdomen to

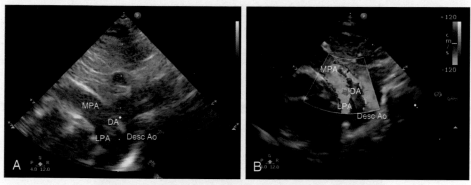

Figure 48.10 Patent Ductus Arteriosus View. (A) Two-dimensional view. (B) Color flow Doppler view. *DA,* Ductus arteriosus, *Desc Ao*; descending aorta; *LPA*, left pulmonary artery; *MPA*, main pulmonary artery.

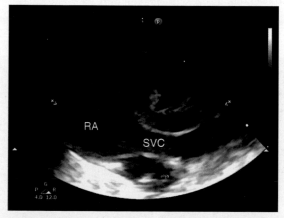

Figure 48.11 Superior Vena Cava View. *RA*, Right atrium; *SVC*, superior vena cava.

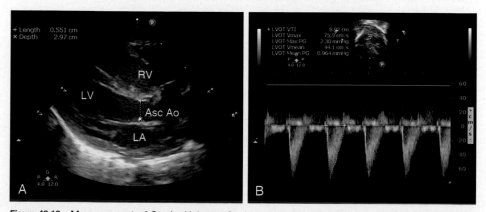

Figure 48.12 Measurement of Stroke Volume. Stroke volume is calculated by multiplying the cross-sectional area of the aorta from a parasternal long-axis view (A) by the aortic velocity time integral from an apical 5-chamber view using pulsed-wave Doppler (B). *Asc Ao*, Ascending aorta; *LA*, left atrium; *LV*, left ventricle; *RV*, right ventricle.

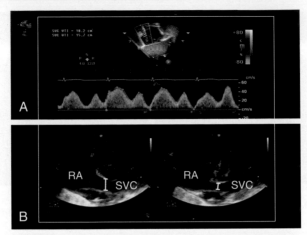

Figure 48.13 **Superior Vena Cava *(SVC)* Flow Measurement.** (A) The SVC flow is measured by placing the Doppler sample gate at the SVC–right atrial *(RA)* junction from a subcostal view. (B) The mean SVC diameter is calculated by averaging the SVC maximum diameter *(left)* and SVC minimum diameter by 2D *(right)*.

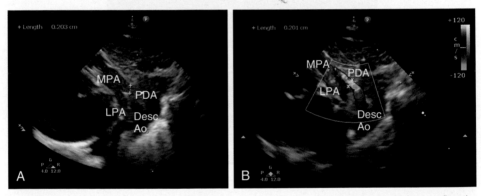

Figure 48.14 **Measurement of Ductus Arteriosus Diameter.** Color flow Doppler is used to confirm the location of the ductus arteriosus and calipers are used to measure the diameter. *Desc Ao*, Descending aorta; *LPA*, left pulmonary artery; *MPA*, main pulmonary artery; *PDA*, patent ductus arteriosus.

maximize visualization of flow within the SVC before its entry into the RA. A mid-sternal longitudinal view is used to measure the maximum and minimum SVC diameters to calculate the mean SVC diameter (Fig. 48.13). Normal SVC flow ranges from 40 to 120 mL/kg/min.

Patent Ductus Arteriosus

In preterm infants, the ductus arteriosus commonly fails to close in the early neonatal period, causing shunting of blood in a left to right direction, often with adverse hemodynamic consequences.[20-22] Prior to the advent of echocardiography, diagnosis of a PDA was based on clinical findings. However, the correlation between physical exam findings and presence of a PDA by echocardiography is poor

during the first week of life.[23,24] Echocardiography has become the standard diagnostic modality for PDA.

Characterization of a PDA includes measurement of the ductal diameter and assessment of the blood flow pattern. The internal diameter of the PDA is measured at its narrowest point using 2D and color flow Doppler from a ductal view (Fig. 48.14). Several studies have suggested that a ductal diameter greater than 2 mm defines a hemodynamically significant PDA that is unlikely to close spontaneously, but this assumption remains controversial. Although ductal size appears to be the most predictive of all markers, its value is questionable because a 2D estimate at a single point may not reflect the architecture of the ductus across its length.

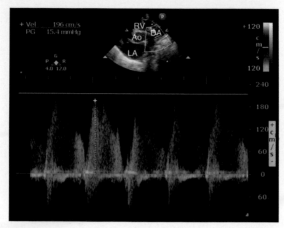

Figure 48.15 Measurement of Ductus Arteriosus Blood Flow Velocity. Pulsed-wave Doppler is used to measure ductal flow velocities showing a moderate-sized patent ductus arteriosus in this case. *Ao,* Aorta; *DA,* ductus arteriosus; *LA,* left atrium; *RV,* right ventricle.

Ductal size can also vary with oxygen saturation and surfactant administration.

The second assessment of a ductus arteriosus is measurement of transductal blood flow velocities (Fig. 48.15). Using PWD for velocities less than 2 m/s and CWD for velocities greater than 2 m/s, a ductal velocity of 1.5 to 2 m/s correlates with a moderate-sized PDA and velocities less than 1.5 m/s correlate with a large PDA.[25]

The increase in effective pulmonary blood flow may be estimated by the left atrium to aortic ratio (LA:Ao) and the LVO. However, neither measurement is reliable in the presence of an interatrial shunt.

The effect of ductal steal on systemic perfusion can also be quantified using SVC flow as a surrogate marker of systemic blood flow. High-volume transductal shunting is associated with low SVC flow, and low SVC flow has been correlated with an increased risk of intraventricular hemorrhage.[26,27] PWD can be used to evaluate blood flow in the descending aorta, celiac, and mesentery arteries, providing data on distal perfusion of the lower body.

However, despite many years of research, controversy still exists about the role of the ductus arteriosus in adverse outcomes and the best echocardiographic methods to predict these outcomes.

Pulmonary Hypertension

Persistent pulmonary hypertension (PPHN) is the leading cause of hypoxemic respiratory failure in newborns and it is diagnosed clinically and echocardiographically. A detailed anatomical examination to rule out structural congenital heart disease is mandatory before any functional assessment can be made. A quantitative assessment of pulmonary arterial pressure can be performed using the following techniques:

1. Measurement of right ventricular systolic pressure (RVSP): In the presence of tricuspid regurgitation, the RVSP can be calculated using the modified Bernoulli equation (Fig. 48.16):

$$RVSP = RA \text{ pressure} + [4 \times (\text{tricuspid regurgitation jet velocity})^2]$$

The RVSP is considered to be equivalent to the pulmonary artery systolic pressure because the pulmonic valve is open during right ventricular systole and the RV and pulmonary artery are in continuity.

2. Pulmonary pressure estimation in the presence of unrestrictive ductal flow: The peak velocity of transductal flow is used to calculate the pressure difference between the pulmonary and systemic circulation using the modified Bernoulli equation (Fig. 48.17). The direction of ductal flow can be used to estimate the severity of pulmonary hypertension.

3. Pulmonary artery acceleration time: Recent studies have shown that pulmonary artery acceleration time (PAAT) correlates with pulmonary artery pressures and pulmonary vascular resistance (PVR). In adults, the linear, inverse relationship between PAAT and mean pulmonary artery pressure (mPAP) was elucidated in the literature

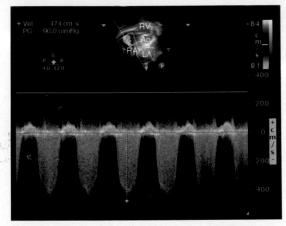

Figure 48.16 Right Ventricular Systolic Pressure. The maximum tricuspid regurgitation jet velocity is being measured using continuous-wave Doppler. Using the formula RVSP = RA pressure + [4 × (max tricuspid regurgitation jet velocity)^2], the pressure gradient across the tricuspid valve can be calculated to estimate the right ventricular systolic pressure. *Ao*, Aorta; *LA*, left atrium; *RA*, right atrium; *RV*, right ventricle.

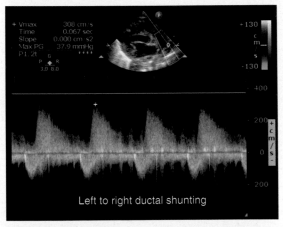

Figure 48.17 Pulmonary Pressure Gradient. The pressure gradient between the pulmonary and systemic circulation through ductus arteriosus is measured using continuous-wave Doppler.

in the 1980s. This relationship has only recently been explored in children. One study showed that PAAT can accurately predict pulmonary hypertension in children between the ages of 1.3 and 12.6 years.[28]

Pulmonary artery pressure can be estimated from the pulmonary artery Doppler waveforms using the ratio of PAAT to right ventricular ejection time (RVET) to correct for the HR. Acceleration time is measured as the time interval from the start of flow on the Doppler waveform's baseline to the peak velocity. RVET is the total time interval of right ventricular ejection (Fig. 48.18). PAAT/RVET ratios between

0.2 and 0.3 have been associated with moderately elevated pulmonary artery pressure and ratios less than 0.2 have been associated with severely elevated pulmonary artery pressure.[28] Several studies have shown that early detection of pulmonary hypertension by PAAT/RVET in preterm infants is a good predictor of late-onset chronic lung disease.[29]

In the absence of tricuspid regurgitation and a PDA, pulmonary artery pressure may be estimated using qualitative measures, including evaluation of the interventricular septal wall contour and motion. A qualitative assessment is performed from a parasternal short-axis

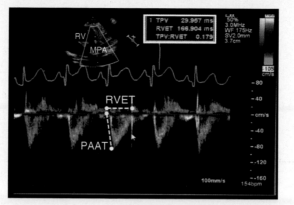

Figure 48.18 **Pulmonary Acceleration Time to Right Ventricular Ejection Time (PAAT:RVET) Ratio.** The PAAT and RVET are measured using pulsed-wave Doppler of the main pulmonary artery from a parasternal short-axis view. PAAT, pulmonary acceleration time is also called TPV, time to peak velocity. *MPA*, Main pulmonary artery; *RV*, right ventricle.

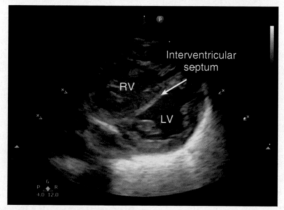

Figure 48.19 **Septal Flattening.** The interventricular septum appears flat, or "D" shaped, from a parasternal short-axis view due to elevated pulmonary artery pressure. *LV*, Left ventricle; *RV*, right ventricle.

view. The interventricular septum appears flat due to increased RV pressure (Fig. 48.19 and Video 48.10) or bowed toward the left ventricle in severe cases of elevated pulmonary artery pressures.

Lung and Pleural Ultrasound

BACKGROUND

The high extravascular water content and unossified thoracic rib cage of neonates allow for optimal ultrasound wave penetration for thoracic imaging. Transient tachypnea of the newborn (TTN), regardless of gestational age, is frequently encountered and is the most common cause of neonatal dyspnea. TTN results from pulmonary edema due to delayed absorption of fetal alveolar fluid. Its clinical diagnosis is frequently supported by chest radiography. TTN is typically a self-limited process requiring brief periods of respiratory support. It is important to differentiate TTN from other neonatal pulmonary processes including neonatal respiratory distress syndrome (RDS) or meconium aspiration syndrome (MAS). RDS is often, but not always, seen in more premature infants with immature lungs that lack surfactant. MAS is clinically suspected in neonates whose lungs and airways are exposed to meconium in utero and during delivery. Early identification of RDS and MAS allows timely and targeted treatment including administration of surfactant and empiric antibiotics. Although there are few studies describing use of lung ultrasound in neonates, the current data

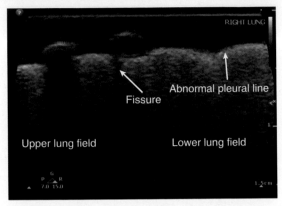

Figure 48.20   Double Lung Point Sign. Lung ultrasound in transient tachypnea of the newborn shows dense B-lines in the lower lobes and normal findings (A-lines) in the upper lobes. Fluid is seen in the fissure separating the lobes.

suggest ultrasound may be used to characterize and differentiate these pathologic processes. Furthermore, ultrasound allows for rapid identification of pneumothorax, another common and life-threatening cause of tachypnea in neonates. See Chapters 9, 10, and 47 for further discussion of lung ultrasound.

IMAGE ACQUISITION

It is important to use a systematic approach for a lung ultrasound examination comparing both right and left lungs for normal and pathologic processes (see Chapter 8). High-frequency linear, microconvex, or phased-array transducers are commonly used for lung ultrasound imaging. The transducer orientation marker is pointed cephalad, and in general, lungs are imaged in a longitudinal plane to maximize visualization of pleural sliding. Transverse lung images may be obtained for additional views when focusing on a specific pathologic finding.

IMAGE INTERPRETATION

By lung ultrasound, TTN has been characterized with high specificity by the "double lung point" sign: compact coalescent B-lines in the lower lung fields and normal A-lines in the upper lung fields.[30] Demarcation of upper and lower lung fields due to edema within the fissures can also be seen. A double lung point sign had a high sensitivity and specificity for TTN and was not observed in healthy infants, infants with RDS, atelectasis, pneumothorax, pneumonia, or pulmonary hemorrhage (Fig. 48.20).[31] Notably, lung consolidation is

not frequently encountered in patients with TTN and identification of this finding should suggest an alternative diagnosis.

RDS is the most common cause of neonatal respiratory failure and mortality. By ultrasound, RDS uniformly demonstrates consolidative processes with air bronchograms along with confluent B-lines. Such findings differentiate RDS from TTN with high sensitivity and specificity.[32,33] Ultrasound characterization of MAS demonstrates heterogenous abnormalities including B-line prevalence, consolidation, and air bronchograms.[34,35]

Neurological Ultrasound

BACKGROUND

Ultrasound evaluation of the neonatal brain is possible via the open soft tissue windows of the anterior and posterior fontanelles, and the open sutures between the cranial bones. Most neonatologists are familiar with viewing brain ultrasound images captured by diagnostic radiology specialists.[36] Point-of-care ultrasound can provide excellent views of the general brain architecture, especially the two lateral ventricles in the evaluation of hemorrhage or calcification, and the parenchyma in the early evaluation of ischemia. Point-of-care ultrasound imaging of the brain is particularly useful when intraventricular hemorrhage may be responsible for acute deterioration or hemodynamic instability, especially when diagnostic sonography services are not readily available. Detection of increased intracranial pressure, extra-axial bleeding (i.e., subdural hemorrhage),

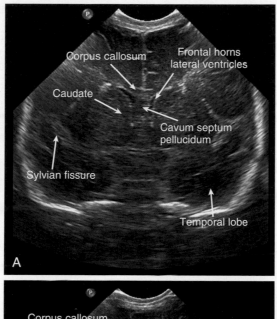

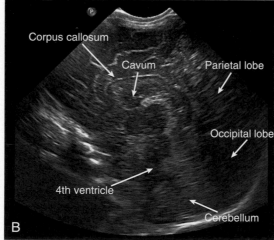

Figure 48.21 Brain Ultrasound Views. (A) Coronal frontal view, and (B) sagittal midline view.

cerebral edema, and arterial or venous stroke have not been well studied with point-of-care ultrasound and other imaging modalities, such as computed tomography or magnetic resonance imaging, are recommended.

Image Acquisition

The standard brain ultrasound views are (1) coronal views from the frontal lobe to the occiput and (2) sagittal views from left parietal cortex to the right parietal cortex (Fig. 48.21).

For coronal views, place the transducer in a transverse position over the center of the anterior fontanelle with the transducer marker pointed toward the patient's right side. Center the brain image on the screen. To obtain a sequence of coronal views, start with the transducer tilted anteriorly to capture frontal views of the brain and then tilt the transducer posteriorly toward the patient's occiput. Capture a minimum of six still images as you gradually tilt or sweep the transducer posteriorly toward the occiput. Next, to acquire sagittal views, rotate the transducer 90 degrees into a sagittal plane with the transducer marker pointing anteriorly toward the front of the head. Keep the transducer centered on the fontanelle. The radiology convention is for

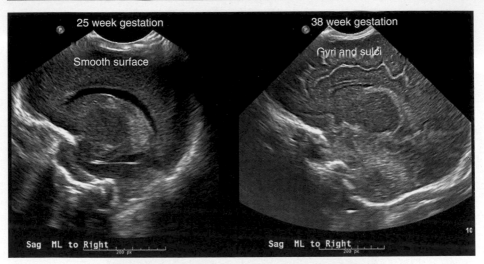

Figure 48.22 Preterm Versus Term Infant Brain. A smooth brain surface with absent gyri and sulci of a preterm infant versus a term infant is seen from a sagittal view.

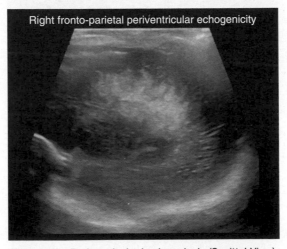

Figure 48.23 Periventricular Leukomalacia (Sagittal View).

the posterior brain to be viewed on the right side of the screen. From the midline, tilt the transducer toward the left and right sides to view both hemispheres of the brain, and take at least four still images on each side. Additional views can be obtained through the posterior fontanelle to image the occipital cortex using the same steps described above.

Image Interpretation

Neonatologists must be aware of the normal variants of the brain architecture depending on gestational age. Whereas the brain surface appears smooth in premature infants, gyri and sulci must be evident in the brains of term infants (Fig. 48.22).

Interpretation of brain ultrasound images is a common skill for neonatologists because reviewing images is generally a routine part of most providers' workflow for early and late neurological injury. Most neonatologists have ample experience in interpreting brain ultrasound images for common pathologies, such as periventricular leukomalacia (Fig. 48.23),

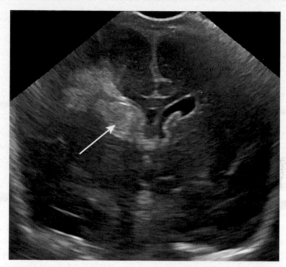

Figure 48.24   Intraventricular Hemorrhage. A grade IV intraventricular hemorrhage *(arrow)* is seen from a coronal frontal view.

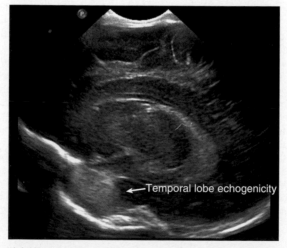

←Temporal lobe echogenicity

Figure 48.25   Intracranial Hemorrhage. Increased temporal lobe echogenicity which corresponds with temporal lobe hemorrhage is seen from a sagittal view.

intraventricular hemorrhage (Fig. 48.24), and intracranial hemorrhage (Fig. 48.25). Due to the small size of the fontanelles, it is best to provide sweeping images of the brain by tilting the transducer in both directions to obtain sectional views. It is important to remember that visualization is limited by the wedge-shaped footprint of the transducer, and lesions can be missed in the parietal regions lateral to the imaging window.

PEARLS AND PITFALLS

- Umbilical catheters
  - Identifying the umbilical vein catheter tip: Once a portion of the catheter shadow is seen, rotate the transducer slightly to create the longest shadow along the imaging plane to ensure the catheter is maximally seen.
  Look for the actual catheter tip as

it approaches the right atrium from the inferior vena cava. Moving the catheter a few millimeters in and out can provide reassurance the tip has been identified.

- Positioning the transducer for a umbilical arterial catheter (UAC) tip: Place a UAC catheter tip posterior to the right atrium, which represents approximately T8.
- Peripherally inserted central catheters (PICCs)
  - The tip can be difficult to localize, and if you are uncertain about the tip location, then pull the catheter back until the tip is identified with certainty.
  - Detecting a low-lying PICC may be difficult due to bowel gas; rotating the infant slightly to the left or right may permit a better view.
- Endotracheal tubes (ETTs)
  - Rotate the head to one side to access the upper chest and neck, but avoid too much rotation, flexion, or extension of the neck as these movements can shift the ETT position.
  - If you are having difficulty finding the midline structures, look for the aortic trunk which is the most visible and prominent vascular landmark in the midline. To locate the carina, look for a cross-sectional view of the right pulmonary artery on the lesser curvature of the aorta.
  - The tip of the ETT may be difficult to visualize initially and gently moving the ETT in and out less than 5 mm can make the tip easier to identify.

- Cardiac ultrasound
  - Measure the maximum and minimum superior vena cava (SVC) diameters during the cardiac cycle and use the mean to calculate the SVC flow. Low SVC flow is associated with an increased incidence of intraventricular hemorrhage.
  - Tricuspid regurgitation jet velocity may underestimate right ventricular systolic pressure in the absence of a complete Doppler envelope.
- Pulmonary ultrasound
  - In neonates with impending respiratory failure, transient tachypnea of the newborn should not be suspected if lung ultrasound shows consolidation.
  - Pleural effusions can be seen in patients with transient tachypnea of the newborn (TTN), respiratory distress syndrome (RDS), and meconium aspiration syndrome (MAS) and cannot be used to distinguish between these disease entities.
- Neurological Ultrasound
  - To obtain the highest-quality images, stay centered on the anterior fontanelle as much as possible. Tilting the transducer, rather than sliding it, is the key to acquiring the highest-quality images.
  - Multiple coronal images of both cerebral hemispheres and sagittal images of the posterior fossa structures should be obtained to avoid missing important findings.

Ultrasound Program Management

CHAPTER 49

Competence, Credentialing, and Certification

Paru Patrawalla ■ Uché Blackstock

KEY POINTS

- An increasing number of point-of-care ultrasound applications are now required components of training in certain specialties, and training standards for attaining competency are being developed for medical students, postgraduate trainees, and physicians in practice.

- Although several professional societies have stated explicit curricular goals for training in point-of-care ultrasound, there are few studies examining evaluation methods for achieving and maintaining competency.

- National certification or board examination in point-of-care ultrasound does not exist; however, various training pathways offer certificates of training that can assist physicians in obtaining institutional privileges to use point-of-care ultrasound.

Background

The American Medical Association (AMA) has long recognized that ultrasound has diverse applications and is used by a wide range of physicians and disciplines. In 1999, the AMA stated "that ultrasound imaging is within the scope of practice of appropriately trained physicians."[1] Point-of-care ultrasound includes a subset of organ-specific ultrasound applications utilized by different medical specialties varying in breadth and depth. Frontline medical specialties, such as critical care medicine, typically perform a breadth of ultrasound examinations, whereas system-specific specialties, such as

rheumatology, typically perform more in-depth examinations of specific organs or structures.[2-6]

Specialty-specific guidelines for point-of-care ultrasound applications, training standards, and competency assessments are undergoing rigorous evaluation and primarily focus on the expectations for practicing physicians. The American College of Emergency Physicians (ACEP) published a compendium establishing emergency ultrasound imaging standards and practice guidelines to better define training, proficiency, and credentialing of providers using emergency ultrasound.[7-9] The American College of Chest Physicians (ACCP) and the Société de Réanimation de Langue Française

(SRLF) defined the specific components of competency in general critical care ultrasound, basic critical care echocardiography, and advanced critical care echocardiography in 2009.[2] Critical care medicine societies, including the Society of Critical Care Medicine (SCCM), have individually or collaboratively further defined training standards for critical care ultrasound.[10-14] In addition, combined professional society guidelines have emerged that mention training and competency, such as the American Society of Echocardiography (ASE) and ACEP consensus statement on focused cardiac ultrasound in emergent settings. As a result, many providers, particularly those trained prior to the inclusion of ultrasonography in graduate medical education (GME), have sought local and national training courses organized by professional societies and private education companies.

In recognition of its utility and widespread use, point-of-care ultrasound has become a required component of training in several specialties' residency and fellowship programs, as defined by the Accreditation Council for Graduate Medical Education (ACGME) in the United States.[15-17] GME programs have taken a prominent stance to include ultrasound education in numerous specialties, and undergraduate medical education (UME) followed suit by integrating ultrasound into the preclinical and clinical curricula.[18-23]

Although these statements give explicit goals for training in ultrasound particularly at the level of practicing physicians or postgraduate trainees, specific training methods or standards to achieve these goals are often broadly defined. Our understanding of learning curves for various applications of point-of-care ultrasound, and minimal requirements for achieving and maintaining competency and expertise is currently limited.

Definitions

The processes of both attaining and demonstrating the requisite knowledge and skills to use ultrasound safely and effectively require an understanding of four important terms.

Competence is the inherent state of possessing the cognitive and technical skills necessary to perform a specific task or range of tasks. The criteria that constitute competence are often difficult to define. Criteria for professional competence of physicians have typically been set by ACGME, American Board of Medical Specialties, and professional societies. Some professional societies have broadly described training pathways to achieve competence that may include specific criteria to define competence in the use of point-of-care ultrasound and other specialty-specific procedures.[2,8,10,11,13]

Competency-based education (CBE) is a framework for training that has not been well defined until recently. Frank et al. defined CBE as "an approach to preparing physicians for practice that is fundamentally oriented to graduate outcome abilities and organized around competencies derived from an analysis of societal and patient needs. It deemphasizes time-based training and promises greater accountability, flexibility, and learner-centeredness."[24] For point-of-care ultrasound, CBE assumes outcomes-based assessments to ensure that providers have a basic set of knowledge and skills that they can integrate into clinical practice as independent users of ultrasound.

Certification is the method by which an internal or external body formally attests to the competence of a provider. In the United States, certification indicates that the provider has met the knowledge and skills required to be competent to practice a specialty. Currently, there is no formal external certificate of competency, or "board," in point-of-care ultrasound that is offered by the American Board of Medical Specialties in the United States. Some institutions have developed internal certification pathways for the use of point-of-care ultrasound. The ACCP and Society of Hospital Medicine (SHM) offer certificates of completion for training in critical care or point-of-care ultrasound, but these certificates are not certificates of competency.

Credentialing and privileging are governed by the rules and regulations of an individual provider's hospital and department, where that entity grants an individual permission to practice a certain set of skills, duties, and procedures. Credentialing is the process by which a department or hospital verifies a provider's qualifications, such as board certification and medical licenses. Privileging is the process by which an institution grants a provider permission to perform patient care activities based on their scope of practice and competence. Currently, the following pathways are being used to grant providers privileges to use point-of-care ultrasound: documentation of a provider's completion of an ACGME-accredited postgraduate training program that included ultrasound training, completion of an internal certification pathway, fulfillment of specialty-specific competency requirements, completion of a professional society's certificate of training, or attestations from providers or peers.

The following sections describe in detail current training standards for point-of-care ultrasound using competency-based assessments, including UME, GME, and continuing medical education (CME) pathways for providers in practice.

Training Standards and Competency-Based Education

Point-of-care ultrasound includes many different organ- and disease-specific applications, and the relevance of each application differs for each provider's practice. Use of ultrasound independently by a provider requires competence in several areas, including basic ultrasound knowledge (physics, machine controls, normal and abnormal anatomy), image acquisition, image interpretation, and clinical integration.

TRAINING PATHWAYS

Ultrasound training is a continuum for an individual learner as they progress from medical school through residency and fellowship and into clinical practice. However, training recommendations are developing at different rates for each stage of medical education—UME, GME, and CME—differ in the breadth and depth of competency requirements. The pathways to achieve competency in ultrasonography are best described at the GME and CME levels, although there are emerging recommendations at the UME level.

- UME-based pathway: There are emerging recommendations for curricular milestones in ultrasound that should be included in medical schools[19]; however, currently there are no national requirements to include ultrasound training in UME.
- GME-based pathway: Aside from the specialty of radiology, the ACGME has delineated minimal education requirements for general ultrasound training in certain specialties with a broad scope of practice, including emergency medicine and critical care medicine, and for specific ultrasound

applications in certain specialties with a narrower scope of practice, including anesthesiology, sports medicine, obstetrics/gynecology, pulmonary disease, gastroenterology, cardiology, endocrinology, rheumatology, physical medicine and rehabilitation, urology, colorectal surgery, thoracic surgery, vascular surgery, and ophthalmology.[25] Specific and detailed training requirements have been well established only for emergency medicine.[8]

- CME-based pathway: Recommendations have been made by ACEP[8,9] for minimal education requirements and competency assessment for physicians who completed Emergency Medicine residency training without ultrasound training. Competence in critical care ultrasound has been defined in statements by ACCP/SRLF[2] and SCCM,[11] and training standards are further delineated in consensus statements on critical care ultrasound.[10,14]

COMPETENCY-BASED EDUCATION IN ULTRASOUND

CBE is a framework for training that focuses on the expected learning outcome (developing competency in point-of-care ultrasound). For ultrasound, a competency-based program includes the following components:
1. Introductory course with didactics, image interpretation practice, and hands-on image acquisition practice based on specialty-specific guidelines
2. Deliberate, supervised practice with targeted feedback at the bedside with patients
3. Competency assessment or a mastery standard that must be met
4. Skill maintenance and quality assurance

Training Duration

The amount of time needed to attain minimal competency standards for core applications is unknown. However, multiple studies have shown that focused training sessions for several hours ("boot camps") or multiple, focused sessions over several days, with or without a requirement for proctored exams, can effectively train providers in several core applications, including lung/pleural,[26] vascular diagnostic,[27,28] and cardiac ultrasound.[29-35] Despite the success of such focused training approaches, competency cannot always be determined using absolute cutoffs for number of examinations performed.[36,37] Based on international expert consensus in critical care medicine, at least 10 hours of training for general critical care ultrasound and 10 additional hours for basic echocardiography are recommended for introductory training.[14] Further study is needed on learning curves and the minimal amount of training required for achievement of competency.

Introductory Course

- UME-based pathway: Current literature describes several methods for introductory training, including workshops incorporating ultrasound into preclinical courses on anatomy and physiology,[38,39] integrating ultrasound with rotations during the clinical years,[40,41] and vertical curricula spanning all years of training.[20,42]
- GME-based pathway: An introductory course may be offered by the training program as a series of lectures and hands-on practice sessions, or trainees can attend a regional or national training course in their specialty.
- CME-based pathway: Practicing physicians can attend regional or national courses developed by professional societies, which have been shown to be effective for introductory training.[43] Alternatively, some introductory didactic knowledge and image interpretation can be obtained via prerecorded didactics available online or by DVD, but hands-on experience and practice are mandatory.

Achieving Mastery Through Deliberate Practice

Supervised deliberate practice to achieve mastery has been shown to be a successful method of obtaining competence in several procedures, including ultrasound-guided vascular access and thoracentesis.[44-47] Deliberate practice, or repetition with focused feedback,[48] is an important adjunct to review and advance techniques in image acquisition, image interpretation, and clinical integration.

- UME-based pathway: There are no specific guidelines on how to incorporate deliberate practice at the UME level. However, published experiences from medical schools who have developed competency-based curricula can serve as a guide to medical schools looking to initiate an ultrasound training program.[20,42]

- GME-based pathway: Having ultrasound-trained faculty guide deliberate practice of trainees with direct bedside supervision and feedback, and review of saved ultrasound examinations, is the recommended approach. ACEP has defined specific requirements for the number and type of ultrasound examinations for emergency medicine residents.[8] Current consensus guidelines in critical care medicine do not specify the number of examinations that need to be completed to achieve mastery for critical care medicine fellows.[14]
- CME-based pathway: Ideally, practicing physicians should pursue deliberate practice with an experienced physician or sonographer. However, in settings where a more experienced provider is not available, remote review of ultrasound examinations, either in real-time or recorded images, can be provided by some professional societies. Another approach is to compare point-of-care ultrasound exam findings to the confirmatory exam from the requisite subspecialty as a means of self-evaluation to improve one's image acquisition and interpretation skills.

Competency Assessment and Skill Maintenance

Competency in each core ultrasound application should be assessed diligently. Current methods to assess competency include written exams to assess knowledge, and objective structured clinical exams, simulation-based testing, video review, and bedside observation of skills, to assess image acquisition and interpretation skills. Numerous studies have reported methods for competency assessment and validation of evaluation tools that can be referenced when developing a new program.[49-52] It is important to build in a process for quality assurance with periodic evaluation for skill maintenance.

- UME-based pathway: Competency assessments in medical schools are nascent; however, there are several comprehensive competency-based training programs that have described their evaluation methods.[42]
- GME-based pathway: This may be determined at a national level. For example, the ACGME requirement for obstetrics/gynecology residency training is a minimum performance of 50 obstetric and 50 transvaginal ultrasound exams. ACEP recommends at least 25 documented and reviewed cases

for each core application and a minimum of 150 total emergency ultrasound examinations for Emergency Medicine.[8] Specific requirements do not yet exist for most other specialties, and may be determined and documented by an individual program director.

- CME-based pathway: A similar standard for competency assessment exists for providers learning ultrasound after completing GME. ACEP recommendations for emergency medicine are similar to those required during residency.[8] Minimal requirements will depend on individual institutions for physicians in other fields. The Certificates of Completion in ultrasound training offered by ACCP and SHM were not designed to serve as certificates of competency. Rather, these certificates serve as evidence for completing a standardized training pathway that has been endorsed by large national professional societies that represent a specialty.

Certification

Certification is an attestation of a provider's competence in point-of-care ultrasound. Certification can be external through a national certifying body, typically a specialty board or professional society, or internal through a provider's local institution. At present, there is no national board certification in point-of-care ultrasound that grants external certification for competency in point-of-care ultrasound. However, certain specialty boards, such as emergency medicine, include competency in point-of-care ultrasound based on completing residency training and receiving national board certification in emergency medicine.

The National Board of Echocardiography (NBE) has the most established program for certification in disciplines related to echocardiography. Certification requirements include passing the examination of special competence for one of several levels of echocardiography, completion of formal training, and achieving minimum numbers of interpreted and performed studies. Physicians without formal cardiovascular medicine training cannot be certified by the NBE; however, many physicians without formal cardiovascular medicine training have received "testamur" status for taking the written echocardiography board examination. Starting in 2019, the NBE is going to

offer a new board certification in Advanced Critical Care Echocardiography.[53]

ACEP first published specialty-specific ultrasound guidelines in 2001, and the most recent update to the guidelines was published in 2017.[8] Although they have not developed a specialty-specific examination, the tenets of CBE underlie ACEP's recommendations.

ACCP has developed comprehensive programs for providers seeking rigorous training in critical care ultrasound using a framework of CBE.[43] The Certificates of Completion offered by ACCP and SHM require didactic and hands-on training, formative assessment of cognitive and technical skills, development of an online portfolio, and a final summative written and hands-on assessment.

Initial Credentialing and Privileging

Clinical privileges are governed by the rules and regulations of an individual institution. A hospital's credentialing and privileging body should reference specialty-specific guidelines, as well as a provider's prior experience and competency assessments. Ideally, a responsible party, most often the ultrasound director or a member of a multi-specialty ultrasound committee, will assess a provider's point-of-care ultrasound skills prior to granting privileges to use ultrasound in clinical practice. Hospital credentialing and privileging bodies in collaboration with different departments will need to decide if point-of-care ultrasound applications are core privileges or separate privileges. Certain well-established applications of ultrasound, such as ultrasound-guided central venous catheterization, may be designated core privileges, whereas other less common point-of-care ultrasound applications may be designated separate privileges. The policy on privileging for ultrasound imaging from the AMA is shown in Table 49.1.[1]

Maintenance of Competency

Competency should be maintained by performing a minimal number of each core application annually. The exact minimum required to maintain competency is unknown and will differ for each core application. CME to learn new point-of-care ultrasound applications and provide deliberate practice is important

TABLE 49.1   American Medical Association (AMA) Policy H-230.960 on Privileging for Ultrasound Imaging

1. AMA affirms that ultrasound imaging is within the scope of practice of appropriately trained physicians.
2. AMA policy on ultrasound acknowledges that broad and diverse use and application of ultrasound imaging technologies exist in medical practice.
3. AMA policy on ultrasound imaging affirms that privileging of the physician to perform ultrasound imaging procedures in a hospital setting should be a function of hospital medical staffs and should be specifically delineated on the department's Delineation of Privileges Form.
4. AMA policy on ultrasound imaging states that each hospital medical staff should review and approve criteria for granting ultrasound privileges based upon background and training for the use of ultrasound technology and strongly recommends that these criteria are in accordance with recommended training and education standards developed by each physician's respective specialty. (Res. 802, I-99; Reaffirmed: Sub. Res. 108, A-00; Reaffirmed: CMS Rep. 6, A-10.)

for skill maintenance and progression of expertise.[48]

Periodic assessments of image acquisition and interpretation skills through quality assurance measures should be conducted with timely feedback given to providers. Ordering confirmatory studies to assess and improve a provider's image acquisition and interpretation skills may be incorporated into maintenance of competency. Provider-specific data on outcomes of ultrasound-guided procedures, such as central venous access, arterial line placement, thoracentesis, and chest tube placement, should be monitored at regular intervals.

Reprivileging

Hospitals require renewal of privileges at least every 2 years. When applying for reappointment to a medical staff with clinical privileges, the reappointment process should include measures of current competence in point-of-care ultrasound. The number of ultrasound-guided procedures performed, CME activities attended, and quality assurance reviews performed, should be used to assess a provider's appropriateness for re-privileging.

Conclusions

Point-of-care ultrasound is a field that is rapidly expanding in nearly all specialties. Although development and adoption of a universally-accepted external certification pathway in point-of-care ultrasound does not currently exist, the specific components that define competency have been described. Training

standards for attaining competency are being developed at the UME, GME, and CME levels. Providers seeking point-of-care ultrasound privileges will need to comply with local requirements defined by their institution.

PEARLS AND PITFALLS

- When providers desiring to use point-of-care ultrasound are meeting resistance from other specialists, it is important to recall AMA Policy H-230.960 on Privileging for Ultrasound Imaging which states, "that ultrasound imaging is within the scope of practice of appropriately trained physicians."
- In addition to emergency medicine, several other specialties require point-of-care ultrasound training during graduate medical education: critical care medicine, obstetrics/gynecology, pulmonary disease, ophthalmology, urology, colorectal surgery, vascular surgery, and rheumatology.
- Certification is an attestation of a provider's competence in point-of-care ultrasound and can be external through a specialty board or professional society, or internal through a local institution. Currently, there is no board certification in point-of-care ultrasound.
- The Certificates of Completion offered by ACCP and SHM are certificates for completing the training program

and are not considered certificates of competency.

- When an experienced physician or sonographer is not available to supervise deliberate practice, comparing point-of-care ultrasound exam findings to the confirmatory exam is a method to improve one's diagnostic accuracy.
- Starting in 2019, the National Board of Echocardiography (NBE) will be offering a new board certification in Advanced Critical Care Echocardiography.

CHAPTER 50

Equipment, Workflow, and Billing

Laura K. Gonzalez ■ Shideh Shafie ■ Eitan Dickman

KEY POINTS

- When purchasing an ultrasound machine, providers should consider the scope of examinations and clinical setting when selecting the make and model, transducers, and software packages.
- A structured quality assurance process is an important component of a clinical point-of-care ultrasound program.
- Appropriately acquired and interpreted point-of-care ultrasound exams are eligible for billing when the required supporting documentation is included.

Background

The use of point-of-care ultrasound has expanded rapidly over the past 20 years. In 2013, the United States ultrasound sales market hit a record high of 1.44 billion dollars with projected growth to 1.88 billion dollars by 2018.[1] Although approximately half of these sales represented expenditures in traditional imaging specialties such as radiology, 47% of the total sales were due to increased demand for compact hand-carried ultrasound machines designed specifically for point-of-care applications.[2] With the increasing demand, manufacturers have responded by creating unique devices with a broad range of options and features. This chapter reviews important considerations when selecting an ultrasound machine, establishing a workflow, instituting billing, and understanding medicolegal risk.

Ultrasound Equipment

SIZE

When choosing a point-of-care ultrasound machine, size is an important consideration. In general, smaller ultrasound machines have less functionality (e.g., spectral Doppler may not be an available feature), but smaller machines are more portable and less expensive. Thus one must balance portability, functionality, and cost (Table 50.1).

For rapid response and code teams, it is important to buy a compact machine, such as a handheld device, that can be rapidly moved to the bedside of critically ill patients. In an intensive care unit, emergency department, or hospital ward, a portable ultrasound machine on a cart that multiple providers can use may be preferred. With most portable ultrasound machines attached to a cart, the footprint of the cart is as important a consideration as the size of the machine itself. For other clinical settings, such as outpatient clinics, the machine may be stationed in one examination room; thus, a larger ultrasound machine with increased functionality may be a better choice.

POWER SOURCE

Battery power determines how long an ultrasound machine can be used without requiring charging, which affects portability. Battery life should allow several hours of scanning, giving providers the freedom to perform several ultrasound examinations without being tethered by an electrical cord. Through USB ports, the ultrasound machine may also serve as a power source for other devices, such as a printer,

TABLE 50.1 **Comparison of Point-of-Care Ultrasound Machines**

	Large Devices	Laptop-Style Devices	Tablet Devices	Pocket Devices	Probes (connected to tablet)
	Images courtesy of Philips Ultrasound (Bothell, WA)	Image courtesy © FUJIFILM SonoSite, Inc. All rights reserved. Reproduced with permission.	Image courtesy © FUJIFILM SonoSite, Inc. All rights reserved. Reproduced with permission.	Courtesy of GE Healthcare.	Images courtesy of Samsung (Tablet), Philips Ultrasound (Bothell, WA)
Imaging modes	2-Dimensional Color Doppler Tissue Doppler Spectral Doppler M-Mode 3-Dimensional[a]	2-Dimensional Color Doppler Tissue Doppler Spectral Doppler M-Mode	2-Dimensional Color Doppler M-Mode	2-Dimensional Color Doppler M-Mode[a]	2-Dimensional Color Doppler M-Mode[a]
Transducers	L, C, P, EC, TEE	L, C, P, EC, TEE	L, C, P	P, (P/L)[b]	L, C, P
Size	100+ lbs (with cart)	10–15 lbs (without cart)	1–4 lbs (without cart)	1 lb	<1 lb
Battery life	2–3 hr	2 hr	1 hr	1.5 hr	Varies by tablet
Screen size	16+ inches	12 inches	8 inches	3.5 inches	Varies by tablet
Cost	$60–$100,000[c]	$30–$50,000[c]	$15–$30,000[c]	$5–$10,000	$2–$8000[d]

[a]Feature offered in some models.
[b]One manufacturer offers a probe with both phased- and linear-array function.
[c]Approximate cost of standard ultrasound unit with two transducers.
[d]Cost per probe without a tablet.
C, Curvilinear transducer; EC, endocavitary transducer; L, linear-array transducer; P, phased-array transducer; TEE, transesophageal transducer.

video recorder, gel warmer, bar-code scanner, wireless bridge, or other institution-specific devices. The start-up time of an ultrasound machine is an important consideration, especially when caring for acutely ill patients with potentially life-threatening conditions. A long start-up time is a barrier to use, particularly when patient care decisions must be made emergently.

TRANSDUCER SELECTION

The clinical applications that are most likely to be performed determine the types of transducers needed. Phased-array, linear-array, curvilinear, and endocavitary probes are the most common types of transducers, and at a minimum, a linear- and phased-array transducer are needed. Transducers can be easily damaged because they have fragile internal construction and damaged transducers often cannot be repaired. The cost of replacing a typical transducer ranges from $6000 to $12,000. Selection of transducers that are sufficiently durable for high-acuity, ambulatory settings with multiple users is crucial. Many manufacturers offer service contracts to repair or replace damaged transducers, and it is important to ensure that the machine vendor is able to ship replacement transducers in a timely manner in order to minimize disruption of using the ultrasound machine.

FEATURES AND FUNCTIONS

The buttons for selecting the mode and exam type, and adjusting the depth and gain must be easily identified. Many machines have a button that resets the gain to the default setting for a particular exam type. In addition to a freeze button to capture still images, most machines have a cine-loop function. The cine-loop function records video clips ranging from 2 to 60 seconds. Providers can scroll through a cine-loop and select the highest quality still images for storage. Other features, such as Doppler ultrasound, tissue harmonics, elastography, and spatial compounding, may be important depending on the practice setting. A practical consideration is selecting an ultrasound machine with an ergonomic control panel. Trackballs can be more precise and easier to use with a gloved hand compared to trackpads, but they are also more susceptible to being damaged or clogged by ultrasound

gel. Calculation packages can be included to perform certain ultrasound exams, such as fetal ultrasonography. The capability of transferring images in Digital Imaging and Communications in Medicine (DICOM) format is needed for most image archiving systems.

MAINTENANCE

Transducers may serve as vectors of bacterial transmission and should be disinfected before and after each patient contact.[3] Ultrasound transducers should never be autoclaved or subjected to high heat, electricity, or pressure because the piezoelectric elements are very sensitive and easily damaged. Transducers that do not make contact with mucous membranes must be cleaned with nonabrasive soap, or low- or intermediate-level disinfectant wipes after each use. Transducers that make contact with mucous membranes, including endocavitary probes, require a disposable cover and should be cleaned with nonabrasive soap and water followed by high-level disinfection after each use. Other transducers such as transesophageal probes can be used without a disposable cover but must undergo high-level disinfection after use. When imaging a grossly infected or bloody surface, a disposable transducer cover should be used followed by high-level disinfection. Transducers exposed to patients with *Clostridium difficile* infection must be cleaned with a hypochlorite-based or hydrogen-peroxide solution to kill the bacterial spores. Consult institutional policies for local transducer disinfection requirements. Specific recommendations can also be found in the Centers for Disease Control's (CDC) *Guideline for Disinfection and Sterilization in Healthcare Facilities*[4] or in the American Institute of Ultrasound Medicine's (AIUM) *Guidelines for Cleaning and Preparing External and Internal Use Probes Between Patients.*[5] Information about appropriate disinfectants should be obtained from the ultrasound manufacturer, the CDC, or the United States Food and Drug Administration (FDA) website.[6] Adherence to these guidelines will ensure transducer longevity and compliance with infection control practices.

Many manufacturers include a service warranty, whereas the purchase of an ultrasound machine while others offer purchase of a separate contract which often costs 10% to 15% of the total purchase price per year. At a minimum, we recommend purchasing a comprehensive service warranty, especially when multiple healthcare providers will be using the same machine. Additionally, ultrasound machines require periodic software updates which can be coordinated with the machine vendor or the institutional biomedical engineering department.

Workflow

Administrative policies, including proper use and maintenance of ultrasound equipment, as well as protocols outlining integration of ultrasound findings into clinical decision pathways, should be established. Documentation requirements for billing and quality assurance of ultrasound exams must be developed and made familiar to all providers. Most modern ultrasound machines have operating systems that allow for customization based on the clinical environment, which can further increase workflow efficiency. A standardized approach for ultrasound use in emergent situations, especially cardiac arrest, should be outlined. In emergent situations, demographic patient data is rarely entered, and a workflow that allows providers to review and attach patient identifiers to images retrospectively is advantageous in this situation.

"Back end" workflow includes extracting, reviewing, and archiving images from an ultrasound machine. Various options for data transfer are available. Images may be stored on the hard drive of the machine itself, but this method is not ideal for long-term storage due to limited capacity and access. Another option is to print still images and store them with the patient's medical record, but printed images degrade with time and scanned images often have low resolution. Currently, transmitting images wirelessly or via a data or USB port to an image bank is becoming the most common method of storing ultrasound images. Wireless transmission of data is advantageous for several reasons, including allowing providers to share ultrasound images without delay, and should be considered once a point-of-care ultrasound program has been established. Images must be transmitted in an acceptable format, DICOM being the most common format, to be part of an image bank or electronic medical record. Image archiving is essential for education, quality assurance, and billing, and should not be overlooked when developing a point-of-care ultrasound program.

QUALITY ASSURANCE

Reviewing images to assess individual providers' technical and interpretive skills is a key component of quality assurance (QA). Images should be linked to a report that contains the following information: patient demographics, indications for the ultrasound exam, views obtained, findings, and interpretation of images. A more comprehensive report, such as that suggested by American College of Emergency Physicians' (ACEP) 'Emergency Ultrasound Standard Reporting Guidelines,' may be desired.[7] Providing specific feedback and tracking provider metrics are components of a quality assurance process. Noncredentialed providers should have their ultrasound images reviewed for quality assurance purposes, and should refrain from making clinical decisions based on self-obtained images until credentialed.

Currently, there is no national certifying body for point-of-care ultrasonography. Some institutions have developed pathways to grant privileges to providers—some grant specific privileges for each point-of-care ultrasound application, whereas others grant general privileges which encompass all common applications of point-of-care ultrasonography per specialty. Many hospital policies on point-of-care ultrasound are modeled after guidelines published by professional societies, such as ACEP and American College of Chest Physicians.[8,9] Different models to privilege providers have been described but generally include a provisional period of acquiring and interpreting images that are reviewed by an ultrasound director. Once proficiency has been consistently demonstrated, the provider is given privileges to apply and integrate point-of-care ultrasound into patient care. Ultrasound directors continue to periodically review providers' ultrasound exams to ensure performance standards are met, and five or more hours of annual continuing medical education in ultrasound is recommended for providers.[8]

IMAGE STORAGE

Recording and archiving images is a necessary component of ultrasound program workflow. Retrievable images are needed for continuity of patient care and for fulfilling billing requirements. Stored images can be reviewed to verify and monitor changes of normal and pathologic findings, guide clinical decision-making, and assess provider skills for credentialing and privileging.

Ease of use for both clinicians performing the ultrasound exams and ultrasound directors reviewing the images is important when selecting an image archiving system. The Picture Archiving and Communications System (PACS) used by most hospital radiology departments may be used for archiving point-of-care ultrasound images, but some radiology departments prefer to archive point-of-care ultrasound images separately. Alternatively, third party image archiving platforms designed specifically for point-of-care ultrasound images are commercially available. These platforms typically store images on a dedicated local server or a cloud-based virtual server.

When choosing between a shared PACS versus a separate point-of-care ultrasound image archiving system, there are pros and cons to consider. With PACS, images are immediately available for other providers and can be compared to other imaging that has been performed. Additionally, maintenance and backup of a PACS is usually provided by the hospital. If a hospital-wide PACS is used, policies should be drafted to distinguish point-of-care ultrasound images from radiology department images, and the responsibilities of each department for interpretation, quality assurance, and billing of images stored in the hospital's PACS should be delineated. Teaching institutions must decide the workflow for educational images obtained by trainees. If the images are archived in PACS, it is recommended to store trainee or new provider images separately to avoid other providers making clinical decisions based on educational images.

Selecting a third party image archiving system, rather than PACS, may be advantageous to avoid possible overlap with radiology images because point-of-care ultrasound has a distinct workflow, especially at teaching institutions. Some commercially available image archiving systems have specific features to address the unique educational, billing, and quality assurance considerations of point-of-care ultrasound.

Prior to purchasing a point-of-care ultrasound image archiving system, it is important to review the technical specifications for compatibility with the ultrasound machines to connect and upload images into the system. Other important considerations include the ability to query the database of stored images for billing, credentialing, and research purposes; initial purchase and recurring maintenance costs; customer service; and compliance with institutional information security policies.

Billing

Billing for use of point-of-care ultrasound for diagnostic purposes or procedural guidance has specific requirements. Reimbursement patterns and rules vary by region or country, though many concepts discussed here are generalizable. In the United States, there are two components of billing: a professional fee and a technical fee. The professional fee is reimbursement for the provider's interpretation of images, and the technical fee accounts for costs associated with acquiring images, including the ultrasound machine, staff, and supplies. In a private clinic setting where the provider owns and maintains an ultrasound machine, the technical and professional fee are usually billed together. In a hospital setting in which the ultrasound machine is owned by the hospital, providers can bill for the professional component, and the hospital can bill for the technical component. It is essential to be knowledgeable with the most recent billing requirements and work in collaboration with local billing experts to ensure regulatory compliance.

A distinct report and archived image(s) are both required in order to bill for a diagnostic ultrasound exam. An indication for the study should be documented and supported by the history and physical examination. The documentation used for billing should be identifiable and retrievable in the medical record. The report should include the following information: operator, type of exam (limited or complete), organs imaged, indication, findings, impression, and provider's signature. To encourage compliance, a report template is recommended. Some ultrasound machines generate reports at the bedside using templates included with the purchase of the ultrasound machine.

When billing for point-of-care ultrasound exams in the United States, the Current Procedural Terminology (CPT) system is used. The CPT codes, maintained by the American Medical Association (AMA), are a series of codes that indicate services rendered by physicians. There are specific CPT codes for both complete and limited ultrasound exams. To bill for a complete exam, there must be an attempt at diagnostic scrutiny of all organs and vascular structures within the anatomical area described. However, most point-of-care ultrasound exams focus on specific anatomic structures to answer a single diagnostic question and are billed as limited ultrasound exams.

In addition to the standard CPT codes, modifiers may be used that provide additional information. For example, the −26 modifier indicates that the bill is only for the professional component of the examination; the −76 modifier indicates a repeat ultrasound exam performed by the same physician or physician group. There are multiple other modifiers that may be relevant to specific clinical scenarios.

CPT codes for billing ultrasound-guided bedside procedures either combine the procedure and use of ultrasound into one code, or have a separate code for use of ultrasound guidance. For example, thoracentesis is billed with imaging guidance (32555) or without imaging guidance (32554). Paracentesis is also billed with imaging guidance (49083) and without imaging guidance (49082). In contrast, insertion of a central venous catheter is billed separately (36555) from use of real-time ultrasound visualization to guide insertion (76937). When utilizing point-of-care ultrasound for procedural guidance, it is important to note that one can bill for both the diagnostic ultrasound exam, such as a limited abdominal ultrasound exam, as well as the procedure itself.

A review of current CPT guidelines with local billing and compliance experts should be performed prior to starting to bill for use of point-of-care ultrasound.[10] More information regarding billing issues can be found in society-specific documents such as the American College of Emergency Physician's *Emergency Ultrasound Coding and Reimbursement Document.*[10]

Medicolegal Issues

Point-of-care ultrasonography is a relatively young field and uptake by different specialties continues to expand. Similar to other aspects of medical care, this field is subject to litigation, and it is important to utilize point-of-care ultrasound within established standards of care as defined by local and national guidelines. Two legal reviews of emergency physician-performed ultrasonography over a 20-year span identified no cases in which a lawsuit was based on

performance or interpretation of a point-of-care ultrasound exam; however, there were five lawsuits due to failure to perform a point-of-care ultrasound exam.[11,12] A similar study of neonatologist and pediatric subspecialty-performed point-of-care ultrasound exams over a 25-year period revealed a similar absence of lawsuits based on point-of-care ultrasound use.[13]

Point-of-care ultrasound may instead be regarded as a medicolegally protective modality, expediting the recognition and management of life-threatening conditions and decreasing procedural complications.[14,15] The AMA is supportive of physicians utilizing point-of-care ultrasound, guided by training standards developed by individual specialties. The importance of a rigorous quality assurance and credentialing program is emphasized by the AMA.[16] The performance and interpretation of point-of-care ultrasound exams is more focused than complete exams performed by radiology, and this is an important distinction to communicate to patients. Generalized statements such as, "everything looks fine," should be avoided. Instead, an accurate reflection of the scope of the limited ultrasound exam should be conveyed, which not only provides explicit information to the patient but may also be helpful in preventing litigation related to use of this technology. For example, if a focused ultrasound exam is performed of the abdominal aorta, the patient should be informed about the presence or absence of an abdominal aortic aneurysm, rather than implying that the entire abdomen is normal. Clinician-performed sonography can be an immensely helpful tool in the hands of well-trained providers. However, compliance with the policies and protocols regarding the incorporation of this technology into clinical practice is essential.

PEARLS AND PITFALLS

- Provider and departmental needs should be considered when purchasing an ultrasound machine. Important considerations include the portability, transducer types, imaging modes, software packages, and manufacturer's warranty or service plan.
- For infection control, it is important to identify an approved brand of low- to intermediate-level disinfectant wipes that is recommended by the institution

and manufacturer for cleaning the transducers. Making the disinfectant wipes readily available, such as attaching them to the stand of the ultrasound machine, can improve compliance with cleaning the machine and transducers.

- Workflows and protocols for incorporating point-of-care ultrasound into clinical practice need to be developed with input from key stakeholders prior to launching widespread use.
- Requirements to receive institutional privileges to use point-of-care ultrasound are generally negotiated between specialties using point-of-care ultrasound, imaging specialties, primarily radiology and cardiology, and hospital administration. Several professional organizations have published specialty-specific recommendations for privileging.
- Billing for diagnostic point-of-care ultrasound examinations requires documentation of the findings and archiving of ultrasound images. It is essential to work with local billing and compliance experts to stay updated with the latest billing requirements.
- Although no lawsuits based on performance or interpretation of a point-of-care ultrasound exam have been documented, providers should be aware of the legal liability when using point-of-care ultrasonography. When properly documented and communicated to patients, use of point-of-care ultrasound can actually be protective from medicolegal liability.

Page numbers followed by "*f*" indicate figures, "*t*" indicate tables, "*b*" indicate boxes, and "*e*" indicate online content.